Physiology, Pathophysiology and Clinical Management in Maternal-Fetal Medicine

Physiology, Pathophysiology and Clinical Management in Maternal-Fetal Medicine

Editor: Ella Gilbert

AMERICAN
MEDICAL PUBLISHERS
www.americanmedicalpublishers.com

AMERICAN
MEDICAL PUBLISHERS
www.americanmedicalpublishers.com

Cataloging-in-Publication Data

Physiology, pathophysiology and clinical management in maternal-fetal medicine / edited by Ella Gilbert.
p. cm.
Includes bibliographical references and index.
ISBN 979-8-88740-379-3
1. Obstetrics. 2. Obstetrics--Pathophysiology. 3. Obstetrics--Treatment. 4. Perinatology.
5. Fetus--Diseases. 6. Pregnancy--Complications. 7. Prenatal diagnosis. I. Gilbert, Ella.
RG526 .P49 2023
618.2--dc23

American Medical Publishers,
41 Flatbush Avenue,
1st Floor, New York,
NY 11217, USA

ISBN 979-8-88740-379-3 (Hardback)

Contents

Preface

The purpose of the book is to provide a glimpse into the dynamics and to present opinions and studies of some of the scientists engaged in the development of new ideas in the field from very different standpoints. This book will prove useful to students and researchers owing to its high content quality.

Maternal-fetal medicine refers to a subdivision of medicine that aims to manage the health concerns of the fetus and mother before, during and after the delivery of the baby. It is concerned with taking care of pregnant women who are suffering from chronic conditions like diabetes, hypertension, and kidney and heart disease. It also focuses on the clinical management of pregnancy-related complications, such as twin or triplet pregnancies, pre-eclampsia and preterm labor, along with women whose fetus is at risk. Congenital abnormalities, genetic diseases, maternal infections and diseases can pose a risk to the fetus. The occurrence of infections is common when a woman is pregnant, as the immune system is suppressed naturally. Maintenance of human pregnancy needs strictly regulated tolerance mechanisms and immune interactions, which comprise molecular, microvesicular and cellular transport of biological signaling and information between fetus and mother. Maternal-fetal medicine manages all the conditions related with pregnancy and helps in achieving better patient outcomes. This book unravels the recent studies in maternal-fetal medicine. It is appropriate for students and professionals seeking detailed information on the physiology, pathophysiology and clinical management in this area of medicine.

At the end, I would like to appreciate all the efforts made by the authors in completing their chapters professionally. I express my deepest gratitude to all of them for contributing to this book by sharing their valuable works. A special thanks to my family and friends for their constant support in this journey.

Editor

1

Placental Morphologic Similarities Between ZIKV-Positive and HIV-Positive Pregnant Women

Daiane Cristine Martins Ronchi[1], Mineia Alessandra Scaranello Malaquias[1], Patrícia Zadorosnei Rebutini[1], Letícia Arianne Panini do Carmo[1], Plínio Cézar Neto[1], Emily Scaranello Marini[1], Amanda Prokopenko[1], Seigo Nagashima[1], Camila Zanluca[2], Claudia Nunes Duarte dos Santos[2] and Lúcia de Noronha[1]*

[1] Laboratory of Experimental Pathology, Postgraduate Program of Health Sciences, School of Medicine, Pontifícia Universidade Católica do Paraná, Curitiba, Brazil, [2] Molecular Virology Laboratory, Instituto Carlos Chagas, Fundação Oswaldo Cruz, Curitiba, Brazil

***Correspondence:**
Lúcia de Noronha
lnno.noronha@gmail.com

Zika virus (ZIKV) caused global concern due to Brazil's unexpected epidemic, and it was associated with congenital microcephaly and other gestational intercurrences. The study aimed to analyze the placenta morphometric changes of ZIKV-infected pregnant women (ZIKV group; n = 23) compared to placentas of HIV-infected (HIV group; n = 24) and healthy pregnant women (N-control group; n = 22). It also analyzed the relationship between the morphometric results and pathological alterations on conventional microscopy, gestational trimester of infection, and presence of the congenital Zika syndrome (CZS). There was a significant increase in area ($p = 0.0172$), as well as a higher number of knots ($p = 0.0027$), sprouts ($p < 0.0001$), and CD163 +Hofbauer cells (HCs) ($p < 0.0001$) in the ZIKV group compared to the N-control group, suggesting that villous dysmaturity and HCs hyperplasia could be associated with ZIKV infections. The HIV group had a higher area ($p < 0.0001$), perimeter ($p = 0.0001$), sprouts ($p < 0.0001$), and CD163 + HCs ($p < 0.0001$) compared to the N-control group, demonstrating that the morphometric abnormalities found in the ZIKV and HIV group are probably similar. However, when ZIKV and HIV groups are compared, it was observed a higher number of sprouts ($p = 0.0066$) and CD163+ HCs ($p < 0.0001$) in the first one, suggesting that placental ZIKV congenital changes could be more pronounced.

Keywords: Zika virus, HIV, vertical transmission, placenta, morphometric analysis

INTRODUCTION

During pregnancy, Zika virus (ZIKV) infection has been associated with fetal malformations, such as microcephaly, lissencephaly, cerebellar hypoplasia, hydrocephalus, polymicrogyria, abnormal development of the corpus callosum, and changes in neuronal migration and subcortical calcifications that configure the Congenital Zika Syndrome (1–9).

Recently, ZIKV caused global concern due to the unexpected epidemic of infection in Brazil, associated with congenital microcephaly and abortions, both of which have been more common when ZIKV infection occurred during the first trimester of gestation. Besides, severe cerebral malformations have not been described when the infection occurred in the third trimester, suggesting that the brain's abnormal development associated with ZIKV could become the organogenesis period (10, 11).

CZS has been associated with placental alterations like an increase in the number of syncytial knots and sprouts, stromal disorders, villous immaturity, Hofbauer cells (HCs) hyperplasia, and vascular abnormalities (12, 13). The direct infection and replication of ZIKV in placenta tissues can be triggered by the infection of HCs (placental macrophage) in the chorionic villi (10). HCs appear to be the most frequently observed ZIKV-positive cells in the naturally infected human placentas and also may remain persistently infected until delivery. Even in the placenta samples with a short interval between the acute phase of infection and delivery time, ZIKV appears to be detected exclusively in HCs. Furthermore, villous immaturity may be related to congenital disorders caused by ZIKV infection, and it is also associated with an increase in HCs. The persistence of ZIKV-positive HCs in full-term placentas may indicate that these cells could provide a viral source for continued fetal infection and may be responsible for the transplacental transmission mediated by its migratory ability to reach the fetal vessels (12).

Human immunodeficiency virus (HIV) has also been associated with abortion, stillborn, preterm delivery, and other gestational intercurrences, but not with the congenital syndrome. However, the effects of HIV on the placentas remain poorly understood. The main target of HIV is CD4 T lymphocytes, but other cells expressing CD4 are also infected, like monocytes, macrophages, and dendritic cells, where HCs are included. Some of the alterations described include chorioamnionitis and deciduitis, and villitis, an increase in the number of syncytial knots and sprouts, stromal disorders like fibrin deposition and fibrosis, abnormalities of the villous maturation and infarction. Other authors have described placentas of HIV-infected pregnant with no pathological alterations on the conventional microscopy. On the other hand, morphometric techniques have usually shown alterations in villus diameter and perimeter, suggesting changes in villous maturation (14–18).

Given that, despite having different vertical transmission routes and outcomes, both HIV and ZIKV may produce similar morphological changes in placental tissues, such as villous immaturity and hyperplasia of HCs. Severe villitis, for example, does not appear to be a common form of placental injury in both cases. In addition, these two viruses can break through the placental barrier causing only subtle morphological alterations, resulting in placentas of the usual histological aspect under conventional microscopy (14–18).

Because of this, the present study aimed to analyze the placental morphometric changes in ZIKV-infected pregnant women and compare these changes with that found in HIV-infected pregnant women, considering gestational trimester of infection, presence of CZS, and pathological alterations on conventional microscopy as variables. In addition, this study also compares both groups (ZIKV and HIV) to the placentas of healthy (non-infected) pregnant women.

MATERIALS AND METHODS

Ethical Approvals

The Brazilian National Ethics Committee approved the presented study under the number CAAE: 42481115.7.0000.5248. The authors confirm that all methods were carried out following relevant guidelines and regulations. Furthermore, the sample collection followed all relevant ethics and safety protocols. The data that support the findings of this study are available from the corresponding author upon reasonable request.

Samples

The ZIKV-infected placenta group (ZIKV group) comprises 23 placentas that were formalin-fixed paraffin-embedded (FFPE) (12). The 23 patients gave birth to 15 term healthy and eight malformed babies, between 34 and 40 gestational weeks (average = 38; median = 38; SD = 2.17). All the 15 term healthy babies (37–40 gestational weeks) are alive. Of the eight malformed babies, five were preterm (34–36 gestational weeks). Still, regarding this group of malformed babies, four of them are alive, two had perinatal death and two were stillborn. The 23 mothers have at least two positive tests for ZIKV infection: anti-ZIKV IgM positive in the maternal blood and/or colostrum, positive RT-PCR in the maternal blood and/or urine, positive RT-PCR in the frozen placenta samples, positive RT-PCR and/or immunohistochemical test in the FFPE placenta samples. The newborn/stillborn additional samples were also positive: brain tissue RT-PCR and anti-ZIKV IgM in the blood (12).

The HIV-infected placenta group (HIV group) consisted of 24 FFPE placenta samples of HIV-positive pregnant women with no comorbidities. Pregnant women gave birth to healthy newborns between 33 and 40 weeks (average = 38.08; median = 38; SD = 1.99) of gestation in 2004 to 2005, when ZIKV was not circulating in Brazil. The placentas showed no pathological changes on the conventional microscopy. We did not observe villous maturation changes, and weights of the newborns were normal for gestational age (average = 2789.29 g; median = 2730 g; SD = 497.19 g; min-max = 1780–3890 g). Maternal age of this group ranged from 17 to 42 years (average = 26; median = 26; SD = 6.53). The placentas were from pregnant women who had been diagnosed with HIV before or during their pregnancy. The newborns were followed up until their HIV infection condition was defined as negative. All the babies are alive e HIV-seronegative. The viral loads and CD4/CD8 ratio were measured three to six times for most patients. The viral loads ranged from 13047.5 to 5760 (copies), and the CD4/CD8 ratio ranged from 0.65 to 0.35 during the 9 months of pregnancy. Antiretroviral therapy was administered at least 1 month before the birth in all patients (16).

The non-infected placenta group (N-control group) comprises 22 pregnant women that had prenatal without comorbidities. They gave birth to healthy newborns, between 34 and 40 gestational weeks (average = 38.19; median = 38; SD = 1.65), from 2004 to 2005, when ZIKV was not circulating in Brazil. The placentas did not present anatomopathological alterations. We did not observe villous maturation changes, and weights of the newborns were normal for gestational age (average = 2957.27 g; median = 2887.5 g; SD = 762.63 g; min–max = 1770–4410 g). Maternal age of this group ranged from 15 to 40 years (average = 26.06; median = 24; SD = 7.14). The pregnant woman and the newborn were followed up until discharge from the hospital (16).

The samples of three groups were matched by gestational age, which varied from 33 to 38 weeks. All the pregnant women were submitted to laboratory tests for congenital intrauterine infections (*TORCH = toxoplasmosis, rubella, cytomegalovirus, syphilis, and herpes*) with negative results. Analysis of gestational age showed no significant differences between the groups.

Morphometric Analysis

Histological sections of all placentas were stained with hematoxylin & eosin (H&E) to evaluate the perimeter, diameter, and area of villi, the number of sprouts, syncytial knots, and villi numbers per medium power field (MPF). H&E sections were photographed at a magnification of 200× (MPF) using the Scanner Axion Scan.Z1, generating an average of 5,000 images. Unfocused, with artifacts, non-villous tissue representative (membranes, cord, decidua) images were excluded. The remaining images selected (about 1,000) had 100% of the field occupied with placental villi and were randomized to obtain about 100 images for each case of the three groups.

For all placentas, the perimeter, diameter, area of the villi, and basal membrane thickness were measured using Image-Pro Plus® 4 software, based on freehand drawing on 100 consecutive villi. After freehand villus' contour, the program provided perimeter, diameters (major), area, and basal membrane thickness in micrometers or square micrometers ($\mu m/\mu m^2$) (16).

To evaluate the syncytial knots and sprouts per villi, the same 100 MPF/H&E images were used and submitted to simple counting of these microscopic structures (12).

Immunohistochemical Analysis

Histological sections of the placentas were fixed on electrically charged glass slides and subsequently dewaxed with heated xylol (37°C), dehydrated with successive baths of absolute ethyl alcohol, and rehydrated with water. Methyl alcohol and hydrogen peroxide were used to block endogenous peroxidase and distilled water and hydrogen peroxide for the second block. They were incubated with anti-CD163 primary antibody (type: polyclonal/rabbit; clone/code: 14215; dilution: 1:1000; source: Thermo Fisher) for 1 h and with secondary antibody associated with the dextran polymer (Spring Bioscience, Pleasanton, USA) for 30 min. DAB/substrate complex (DAB, DakoCytomation) was added onto the slides, followed by counterstaining with Mayer's hematoxylin, dehydration with ethyl alcohol baths, clarification with xylol, and blending with Canada balsam (12).

The 30 HPF (high power field = 400×) were analyzed by counting the number of villi and CD163+ HCs per villi in all three study groups.

The images were obtained from random sample regions without the interference of an observer. The morphometric measurements and the score of CD163 positive cells were performed blindly.

Statistical Analyses

The results were described by means, standard deviations, medians, minimum, and maximum values. The comparison of the groups concerning quantitative variables was performed using the non-parametric Kruskal-Wallis test or t-test. The Shapiro-Wilk test evaluated the normality condition. Values of $p < 0.05$ indicated statistical significance. The data were analyzed using the IBM SPSS Statistics v.20.0 software. Armonk, NY, USA: IBM Corp.

RESULTS

Morphometric Alterations of the HIV and ZIKV Groups

The analysis of the area ($p = 0.0172$) and the number of knots ($p = 0.0027$), sprouts ($p < 0.0001$), and CD163+ HCs ($p < 0.0001$) in the ZIKV group demonstrated larger immature chorionic villi with a higher number of knots and sprouts and HCs hyperplasia when compared with the N-control group (**Figure 1** and **Supplementary Figure 1**).

HIV group placentas with no pathological alterations on conventional microscopy also showed changes in villous maturation and HC hyperplasia by morphometry analysis compared to the N-control group. The area ($p < 0.0001$), perimeter ($p = 0.0001$), number sprouts ($p < 0.0001$), and CD163+ HCs ($p < 0.0001$) of HIV group were higher than the N-control group (**Figure 1** and **Supplementary Figure 1**).

The ZIKV group placentas showed higher values of the number of sprouts ($p < 0.0066$) and CD163+ HCs ($p < 0.0001$) compared to the HIV group (**Figure 1** and **Supplementary Figure 1**).

Trimester of ZIKV Infection

Morphometric analyses were performed in placental samples from mothers who were infected with ZIKV during the first (n = 4), second (n = 8), and third trimesters of pregnancy (n = 6). In five placenta samples, the trimester of infection was unknown. The perimeter ($p = 0.0292$), number of knots ($p = 0.0062$), sprouts ($p < 0.0001$), and CD163+ HCs ($p < 0.0001$) showed significant differences by the trimester of infection. The most relevant differences were observed between the second trimester and third trimester of infection versus the N-control group, revealing second-/third-trimester ZIKV placentas with villous dysmaturity and HCs hyperplasia compared to the control placentas (**Table 1**).

Pathological Alterations

ZIKV group placentas with and without pathological alterations by conventional microscopy were compared. It was observed that placentas with pathological changes presented higher diameter ($p = 0.0226$), perimeter ($p = 0.0212$), number of knots ($p = 0.0101$), number of sprouts ($p < 0.0001$), and CD163+ HCs ($p < 0.0001$) compared to placentas without pathological alterations (**Table 1**). However, placentas considered within normal standards also presented morphometric changes characterized by higher area, perimeter, number of knots, sprouts, and CD163+ HCs compared to the N-control group ($p < 0.05$).

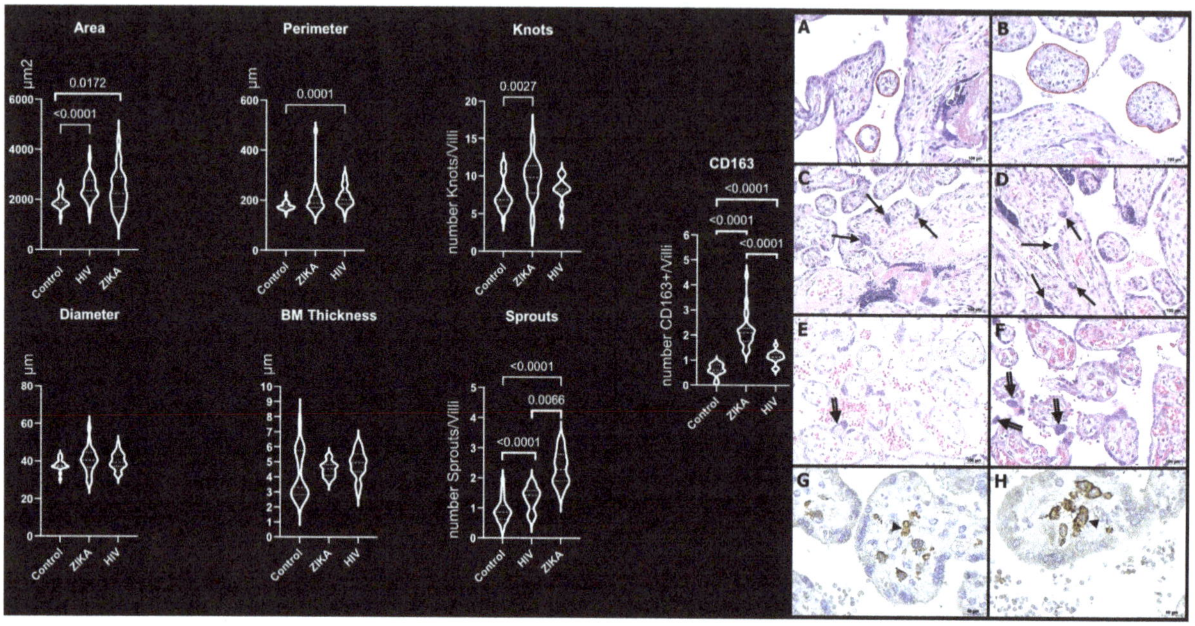

FIGURE 1 | Morphometric analysis of placental specimens from women infected with ZIKV during the pregnancy compared to the HIV and N-control groups. Perimeter, diameter, and basal membrane (BM) thickness in μm; area in μm^2; number of knots, sprouts, and CD163+ HCs per villi (CD163/villi). Photomicrography of a placental sample stained with H&E showing the perimeter of villi (red freehand drawing) in N-control group **(A)** and ZIKV group **(B)**; the number of syncytial knots/villi (arrows) in N-control group **(C)** and ZIKV-group **(D)**; the number of sprouts/villi (double arrows) in N-control group **(E)** and ZIKV group **(F)**. Original magnification: 200×. Scale bars: 100 μm. Photomicrography of immunostaining with CD163 highlighting Hofbauer cell (arrowhead) in the N-control group **(G)** and ZIKV group **(H)**. Original magnification: 400×. Scale bars: 50 μm.

Congenital Zika Syndrome

The status of the newborns (with or without CZS) was also analyzed. The diameter ($p = 0.0109$), area ($p = 0.0102$), perimeter ($p = 0.0035$), number of knot ($p = 0.0054$), number of sprouts ($p < 0.0001$), and CD163+ HCs ($p < 0.0001$) were higher in placentas of newborns with CZS compared with placentas of newborns without this condition (**Table 1**).

DISCUSSION

Morphometric Alterations of HIV and ZIKV Groups

The findings showed significant enlargement of the area of the ZIKV group when compared with the N-control group. A higher number of knots, sprouts, and CD163+ HCs were also noticed.

Syncytial knots are syncytiotrophoblasts' specializations, and their severe increase in late gestation indicates early maturation (12). Syncytial sprouts are markers of trophoblast proliferation; they are seen frequently during early pregnancy and are increased in the villous dysmaturity (19, 20).

HCs, the most frequently ZIKV-positive cells, are placental villous macrophages of fetal origin, and alterations in their numbers (hyperplasia) and biological features are associated with complications in pregnancy. HCs play a role in diverse functions, such as placental vasculogenesis, immune regulation, and the secretion of enzymes and cytokines across the maternal-fetal barrier. In addition, there is some evidence suggesting the involvement of HCs in the development of placental villi (12).

This study's findings corroborate with studies that showed a delay in villous maturation and signs of the HCs hyperplasia in ZIKV-infected placentas. These alterations could damage the chorionic villi, such as calcification, necrosis, Wharton jelly sclerosis, fibrin deposition, and a significant villi size increase (11, 21–23). We could conclude that all of the anatomopathological parameters could be confirmed by the morphometric data and may be used to describe ZIKV-infected placentas.

Other findings showed that the HIV group had a larger area, perimeter, number of sprouts, and CD163+ HCs compared to the N-control group. Studies also revealed that placentas exposed to HIV infection exhibited the following microscopic features: edema, villous immaturity, focal necrosis of trophoblasts, numerous HCs, intervillous fibrin deposition, and chorangiosis (17, 18, 24). However, when those patterns are subtle or minimal, pathologists cannot make the diagnosis. Given that, morphometric techniques may be helpful to identify subtle abnormalities.

Rabelo et al. (22) showed ZIKV NS1 protein in the decidual and endothelial cells of the maternal decidua and CTB, STB, and HCs in the third trimester placental tissues associated with an HIV-exposed, but uninfected, infant with severe congenital Zika syndrome. Nonetheless, the maternal HIV infection could have contributed to the permissiveness of other placental cell types to ZIKV infection.

Finally, when both groups (ZIKV and HIV) were compared, no statistically significant results were found, except for the number of

TABLE 1 | Median (max-min) and *p*-value of morphometric data in the gestational trimester of infection, presence of placenta pathological alterations, and CZS.

Variables	N-CONTROL	Gestational Trimester of Infection[†] First (n = 4)	Second (n = 8)	Third (n = 6)	*p*	Pathological Alterations of Placenta on Conventional Microscopy§ No (n = 15)	Yes (n = 8)	*p*	Congenital Zika Syndrome* No (n = 15)	Yes (n = 8)	*p*
Diameter (µm)	37.6 (43.4–30.4)	38.3 (46.3–29.1)	40.2 (45.3–32.1)	39.8 (44.6–29.1)	NS	40.1 (50.6–29.1)	44.9 (57.7–36.6)	**0.0226**	40.0 (45.3–29.1)	45.5 (57.7–36.6)	**0.0109**
Area (µm²)	1867 (2496–1314)	1812.9 (3536.9–1228.8)	2119.4 (2927.2–1377.9)	2241.8 (2917.7–1527.3)	NS	2165.1 (3671.2–1228.8)	2907.4 (4354.4–1673.3)	NS	2119.4 (2927.2–1228.8)	2897.1 (4354.4–1673.3)	**0.0102**
Perimeter (µm)	174 (219–148)	174.2 (237.2–142.2)	182.1 (477.7–163.2)	186.2 (203.8–154.3)	**0.0292[a]**	181.2 (477.7–142.2)	208.9 (257.6–163.2)	**0.0212**	180.3 (477.7–142.2)	214.0 (257.6–176.9)	**0.0035**
Number of knots/villi	6.9 (11.7–4.2)	9.9 (11.6–7.9)	11.1 (14.3–9.3)	8.6 (15.5–4.7)	**0.0062[a]**	9.8 (15.5–4.7)	10.2 (11.6–3.5)	**0.0101**	10.1 (15.5–4.7)	9.8 (11.6–3.5)	**0.0054**
Number of sprouts/villi	0.9 (1.9–0.3)	1.9 (3.2–1.6)	2.4 (3.1–1.4)	2.1 (2.6–1.8)	**<0.0001[b]**	2.4 (3.2–1.6)	2.0 (3.3–1.4)	**<0.0001**	2.2 (3.2–1.4)	2.8 (3.3–1.7)	**<0.0001**
Number of cells CD163+/villi	0.6 (1.0–0.1)	2.7 (3.3–2.0)	2.2 (2.3–1.7)	1.9 (2.3–1.7)	**<0.0001[c]**	2.0 (2.4–1.3)	2.5 (4.4–1.7)	**<0.0001**	2.0 (2.4–1.3)	2.8 (4.4–1.4)	**<0.0001**

Analysis only for the ZIKV group.
[†]Five cases of unknown gestational trimester.
[§]Main pathological findings: umbilical artery agenesis (1), mild acute funisitis (1), and villous immaturity (6).
**Major central nervous malformations: microcephaly (3), spina bifida (1), hydrocephalus (2), and encephalocele (1).*
[a]p value refers to the second trimester vs. N-control.
[b]p-value refers to the e third trimester vs. N-control and first vs. the third trimester.
[c]p-value refers to the third trimester vs. N-control; first vs. the second and third trimester. Kruskal-Wallis test and t-test; values of $p < 0.05$ indicated statistical significance.
NS, not significant p-value.
Bold values = Statistically significant values.

sprouts and CD163+ HCs higher in the ZIKV group. Thus, it seems that HCs hyperplasia and sprouting/dysmaturity villi may be more pronounced and characteristic in the ZIKV-infected placentas (12, 17). Even though placental changes, such as dysmaturity and hyperplasia of HCs, can be seen in other maternal-fetal diseases, such as congenital infections (TORCH) and diabetes, in the absence of these comorbidities, this aspect may help the pediatric pathologists to suspect the diagnosis of ZIKV vertical transmission. This study also demonstrates that the morphometrical abnormalities finding in ZIKV and HIV groups are very similar, despite having different vertical transmission routes and outcomes since ZIKV is a teratogenic virus and HIV is not. In addition, vertical HIV transmission is much rarer than that of ZIKV, but it can increase perinatal and intrauterine deaths (**Supplementary Figure 1**) (14, 17, 18).

Trimester of ZIKV Infection

When the gestational trimester of infection was analyzed, it was observed that most of the differences between the ZIKV and N-control groups appear to be when infection occurred in the second or third trimester. Since all newborns of this study were in the third trimester (term or preterm), the shorter time that elapsed between the moment of ZIKV infection and the birth may be an explanation for more pronounced changes in these placentas.

The number of HCs also showed differences between groups, suggesting that these cells may have early hyperplasia, and this hyperplasia seems to be maintained throughout the gestational period, although it decreases in intensity over the months. This fact appears to agree with the hypothesis that these cells can work as a reservoir of ZIKV (12, 25).

Regardless of the trimester in which the infection occurred, as ZIKV is detected in placental cells until the end of pregnancy, it is plausible to speculate that the infection of the fetus could happen as a secondary event. In some cases, those abnormalities are only detected months after the delivery (20, 26–29).

Pathological Alterations

Fifteen of 23 ZIKV group placentas were diagnosed without pathological alterations for the pediatric pathologist. However, eight of them had pathological alterations on conventional microscopy, mainly villous immaturity. When placentas with and without pathological alterations were compared, placentas diagnosed with villous immaturity had a higher diameter, perimeter, number of knots, and CD163+ cells. This means that pathologists probably identified those alterations on conventional microscopy and, altogether, termed villous immaturity, so they did not need morphometry techniques to make these diagnoses.

On the other hand, ZIKV-group placentas with no pathological alterations also showed higher diameter, perimeter, and number of knots, sprouts, and CD163+ cells to the N-control group. Therefore, conventional microscopy cannot identify subtle alterations that morphometry could find.

Congenital Zika Syndrome

This study showed significant enlargement of the villi's diameter, area, and perimeter and the number of sprouts and CD163+ HCs in the group that had CZS. In addition, eight infants had fetal malformations related to ZIKV infection during pregnancy. However, 15 women had the onset of ZIKV symptoms during pregnancy and gave birth to infants without CZS.

This study observed that ZIKV causes essential alterations in the placenta's villous, leading to congenital disorders, stillborn, and neonatal death. We could also conclude that morphometric parameters may be biomarkers for CZS since they are more pronounced in malformed newborns. These data could help in the clinical follow-up of newborns with subclinical congenital disorders or even unapparent at birth.

In conclusion, there are placental dysmaturity alterations after ZIKV infection during pregnancy. Very similar placental alterations could be demonstrated on the HIV-infected pregnant women, but sprouting and HCs hyperplasia may be less pronounced in this group. Also, the morphometric analysis revealed villous dysmaturity even in placentas diagnosed within the usual standards by the routine exams. The second and third gestational trimester infections generated more villous dysmaturity and HCs hyperplasia than those pregnant women who became infected in the first trimester. In addition, placentas whose babies had CZS showed more pronounced changes than those without CZS. These alterations may help understand the aspect of ZIKV infection related to placental damage and congenital disabilities and possible deficiencies that might appear after birth.

ETHICS STATEMENT

The studies involving human participants were reviewed and approved by the ethics committee of the Oswaldo Cruz Foundation (Fiocruz) Brazilian National Ethics Committee of Human Experimentation. The patients/participants provided their written informed consent to participate in this study.

AUTHOR CONTRIBUTIONS

LN, CZ, and CNDS contributed to the study design. CZ performed the experiments. SN prepared the materials for analyses. DCMR, PZR, LAPC, PCN, and AP performed the morphometric analyses. PZR participated in the patient follow-up. MASM and ESM participated in sample identification/distribution. DCMR, MASM, PZR, and LN analyzed the results and wrote the manuscript. All authors contributed to the article and approved the submitted version.

FUNDING

This research was funded by Fiocruz, CNPq (439968/2016-0), CAPES Zika Fast Track 481-2016 (88887.116626/2016-01), and Fundação Araucária (CP04/2016). CNDS and LN have a CNPq fellowship.

SUPPLEMENTARY MATERIAL

Supplementary Figure 1 | Illustrative figure shows the morphometric differences between N-control and ZIKV group and between N-control and HIV group, respectively. However, it also represents similar morphometrics results when the ZIKV group was compared with the HIV group. The N-control group's syncytial membranes are more efficient in exchanges because the vessels are closer to the cytotrophoblast. In ZIKV- and HIV-infected placentas, villus increases in size, moving the vessel away from the trophoblast layer, distancing the syncytiotrophoblast membranes cause intrauterine death, premature, low birth weight babies, and/or other malformations. Created with www.biorender.com.

REFERENCES

1. Neu N, Duchon J, Zachariah P. TORCH Infections. *Clin Perinatol* (2015) 42 (1):77–103(viii). doi: 10.1016/j.clp.2014.11.001
2. Noronha Ld, Zanluca C, Azevedo ML, Luz KG, Santos CN. Zika Virus Damages the Human Placental Barrier and Presents Marked Fetal Neurotropism. *Mem Inst Oswaldo Cruz* (2016) 111(5):287–93. doi: 10.1590/0074-02760160085
3. Ayres CFJ. Identification of Zika Virus Vectors and Implications for Control. *Lancet Infect Dis* (2016) 16(3):278–9. doi: 10.1016/S1473-3099
4. Solomon IH, Milner DA, Folkerth RD. Neuropathology of Zika Virus Infection. *J Neuroinfect Dis* (2016) 7(2):220. doi: 10.4172/2314-7326.1000220
5. Hughes BW, Addanki KC, Sriskanda AN, McLean E, Bagasra O. Infectivity of Immature Neurons to Zika Vírus: A Link to Congenital Zika Syndrome. *EBioMedicine* (2016) 10):65–70. doi: 10.1016/j.ebiom.2016.06.026
6. Oehler E, Watrin L, Larre P, Leparc-Goffart I, Lastère S, Valour F, et al. ZIKV Infection Complicated by Guillain-Barré Syndrome: Case Report, French Polinesia, December 2013. *Euro Surveill* (2014) 19(9):1–3. doi: 10.2807/1560-7917.es2014.19.9.20720
7. Brasil P, Pereira JP, Moreira ME, Nogueira RMR, Damasceno L, Wakimoto M, et al. Zika Virus Infection in Pregnant Women in Rio De Janeiro. *N Engl J Med* (2016) 375:2321–34. doi: 10.1056/NEJMoa1602412
8. Melo AS, Aguiar RS, Amorim MMR, Arruda MB, Melo FO, Ribeiro STC, et al. Congenital Zika Virus Infection: Beyond Neonatal Microcephaly. *JAMA Neurol* (2016) 73:1407–16. doi: 10.1001/jamaneurol.2016.3720
9. Schuler-Faccini L, Ribeiro EM, Feitosa IM, Horovitz DDG, Cavalcanti DP, Pessoa A, et al. Brazilian Medical Genetics Society–Zika Embryopathy Task Forceet. Possible Association Between Zika Virus Infection and Microcephaly–Brazil, 2015. Morb. *Mortal Wkly Rep* (2016) 65:59–62. doi: 10.15585/mmwr.mm6503e2
10. Petersen LR, Jamieson DJ, Powers AM, Honein MA. Zika Virus. Baden LR, Editor. *N Engl J Med* (2016) 374(16):1552–63. doi: 10.1056/NEJMra1602113
11. Bhatnagar J, Rabeneck DB, Martines RB, Reagan-Steiner S, Ermias Y, Estetter LBC, et al. Zika Vírus RNA Replication and Persistence in Brain and Placental Tissue. *Emerging Infect Dis* (2017) 23(3):405–14. doi: 10.3201/eid2303.161499
12. Noronha L, Zanluca C, Burger M, Suzukawa AA, Azevedo M, Rebutini PZ, et al. Zika Virus Infection At Different Pregnancy Stages: Anatomopathological Findings, Target Cells and Viral Persistence in Placental Tissues. *Front Microbiol* (2018) 9:2266. doi: 10.3389/fmicb.2018.02266
13. Souza AS, Dias CM, Braga FDCB, Terzian ACB, Estofolete CF, Oliani AH, et al. Fetal Infection by Zika Virus in the Third Trimester: Report of 2 Cases. *Clin Infect Dis* (2016) 63:1622–5. doi: 10.1093/cid/ciw613
14. Maartens G, Celum C, Lewin SR. HIV Infection: Epidemiology, Pathogenesis, Treatment, and Prevention. *Lancet* (2014) 384(9939):258–71. doi: 10.1016/S0140-6736(14)60164-1
15. Yang SW, Cho EH, Choi SY, Lee YK, Park JH, Kim MK, et al. Dc-SIGN Expression in Hofbauer Cells may Play an Important Role in Immune Tolerance in Fetal Chorionic Villi During the Development of Preeclampsia. *J Reprod Immunol* (2017) 124:30–7. doi: 10.1016/j.jri.2017.09.012
16. Baurakiades E, Martins APC, Moreschi V, Souza CDA, Abujamra K, Saito AO, et al. Histomorphometric and Immunohistochemical Analysis of Infectious Agents, T-cell Subpopulations and Inflammatory Adhesion Molecules in Placentas From HIV-seropositive Pregnant Women. *Diagn Pathol* (2011) 6:101. doi: 10.1186/1746-1596-6-101
17. López CL, Pires ARC, Fonseca EC, Rodrigues FR, Braga Neto AR, Herdy GVH, et al. Anatomopathological Characterization of Placentas From HIV+ Patients Associated With p24 Expression. *J Bras Patol Med Lab* (2013) 49 (6):437–45. doi: 10.1590/S1676-24442013000600010
18. Obimbo MM, Zhou Y, McMaster MT, Cohen CR, Qureshi Z, Ong'ech J, et al. Placental Structure in Preterm Birth Among HIV-positive Versus HIV-negative Women in Kenya. *J Acquir Immune Defic Syndr* (2019) 80(1):94–102. doi: 10.1097/QAI.0000000000001877
19. Loukeris K, Sela R, Baergen RN. Syncytial Knots as a Reflection of Placental Maturity: Reference Values for 20 to 40 Weeks Gestational Age. *Pediatr Dev Pathol* (2010) 13:305–9. doi: 10.2350/09-08-0692-OA.1
20. Aagaard KM, Lahon A, Suter MA, Arya RP, Seferovic MD, Vogt MB, et al. Primary Human Placental Trophoblasts are Permissive for Zika Virus (ZIKV) Replication. *Sci Rep* (2017) 7:41389. doi: 10.1038/srep41389
21. Tabata T, Petitt M, Puerta-Guardo H, Michlmayr D, Wang C, Fang-Hoover J, et al. Zika Virus Targets Different Primary Human Placental Cells, Suggesting Two Routes for Vertical Transmission. *Cell Host Microbe* (2016) 20(2):155–66. doi: 10.1016/j.chom.2016.07.002
22. Rabelo K, Fernandes RCSC, Souza LJ, Souza TL, Santos FB, Nunes PCG, et al. Placental Histopathology and Clinical Presentation of Severe Congenital Zika Syndrome in a Human Immunodeficiency Virus-Exposed Uninfected Infant. *Front Immunol* (2017) 8:1704. doi: 10.3389/fimmu.2017.01704
23. Zare Mehrjardi M, Shobeirian F. The Role of the Placenta in Prenatally Acquired Zika Virus Infection. *Virus Dis* (2017) 28(3):247–9. doi: 10.1007/s13337-017-0399-z
24. Anderson VM. The Placental Barrier to Maternal HIV Infection. *Obstet Gynecol Clin North Am* (1997) 24(4):797–820. doi: 10.1016/s0889-8545(05)70345-4
25. Zanluca C, De Melo VCA, Mosimann ALP, dos Santos GIV, dos Santos CND, Luz K. First Report of Autochthonous Transmission of Zika Virus in Brazil. *Mem Inst Oswaldo Cruz* (2015) 110(4):569–72. doi: 10.1590/0074-02760150192
26. Aragão M, Holanda A, Brainer-Lima A, Petribu NCL, Castillo M, van der Linden V, et al. Nonmicrocephalic Infants With Congenital Zika Syndrome Suspected Only After Neuroimaging Evaluation Compared With Those With Microcephaly At Birth and Postnatally: How Large is the Zika Virus "Iceberg"? *AJNR Am J Neuroradiol* (2017) 38:1427–34. doi: 10.3174/ajnr.A5216
27. Ventura L, Ventura C, Lawrence L, van der Linden V, van der Linden A, Gois AL, et al. Visual Impairment in Children With Congenital Zika Syndrome. *J AAPOS* (2017) 21:295–9. doi: 10.1016/j.jaapos.2017.04.003
28. Luo H, Winkelmann ER, Fernandez-Salas I, Li L, Mayer SV, Danis-Lozano R, et al. Zika, Dengue and Yellow Fever Viruses Induce Differential Anti-Viral Immune Responses in Human Monocytic and First Trimester Trophoblast Cells. *Antiviral Res* (2018) 151:55–62. doi: 10.1016/j.antiviral.2018.01.003
29. Sheridan MA, Yunusov D, Balaraman V, Alexenko AP, Yabe S, Verjovski-Almeida S, et al. Vulnerability of Primitive Human Placental Trophoblast to Zika Virus. *Proc Natl Acad Sci* (2017) 114(9):E1587–96. doi: 10.1073/pnas.1616097114

2

IgG Fc Glycosylation Patterns of Preterm Infants Differ with Gestational Age

Nele Twisselmann[1*†], *Yannic C. Bartsch*[2†], *Julia Pagel*[1,3], *Christian Wieg*[4], *Annika Hartz*[1], *Marc Ehlers*[2,5] *and Christoph Härtel*[1]

[1] *Department of Pediatrics, University of Lübeck and University Medical Center Schleswig-Holstein, Lübeck, Germany,* [2] *Laboratories of Immunology and Antibody Glycan Analysis, Institute for Nutrition Medicine, University of Lübeck and University Medical Center Schleswig-Holstein, Lübeck, Germany,* [3] *Department of Infectious Diseases and Microbiology, University of Lübeck and University Medical Center Schleswig-Holstein, Lübeck, Germany,* [4] *Department of Neonatology, Hospital Aschaffenburg-Alzenau, Aschaffenburg, Germany,* [5] *Airway Research Center North (ARCN), German Center for Lung Research (DZL), University of Lübeck, Lübeck, Germany*

Correspondence:
Nele Twisselmann
nele.twisselmann@uksh.de

Preterm infants acquire reduced amounts of Immunoglobulin G (IgG) via trans-placental transfer as compared to term infants which might explain their high susceptibility for infections. The reduced amount of IgG antibodies also results in a lower amount of anti-inflammatory Fc N-galactosylated and -sialylated IgG antibodies. This reduction or, even more, a qualitative shift in the type of IgG Fc glycosylation might contribute to the increased risk for sustained inflammatory diseases in preterm infants. It was the aim of our explorative study to investigate the IgG Fc glycosylation patterns in preterm infants of different gestational ages compared to term infants and mothers of preterm infants. In plasma samples of preterm infants (n = 38), we investigated IgG concentrations by use of ELISA. Furthermore, we analyzed IgG Fc glycosylation patterns in plasma of preterm infants (n = 86, 23–34 weeks of gestation), term infants (n = 15) and mothers from preterm infants (n = 41) using high performance liquid chromatography. Extremely low gestational age infants (born <28 weeks of gestation during second trimester) had reduced IgG concentrations and decreased proportions of galactosylated (84.5 vs. 88.4%), sialylated (14.5 vs. 17.9%) and bisecting N-acetylglucosamine-containing (8.4 vs. 10.8%) IgG Fc N-linked glycans as compared to preterm infants born ≥28 weeks of gestation (during third trimester) and term infants. Increased non-galactosylated (agalactosylated, 16.9 vs. 10.6%) IgG Fc N-linked glycans were associated with the development of chronic inflammatory bronchopulmonary dysplasia (BPD). However, mothers of preterm infants born during second or third trimester of pregnancy did not show significant differences in IgG Fc glycosylation patterns. Thus, the IgG Fc glycosylation patterns of preterm infants depend on their gestational age. Although lack of bisecting N-acetylglucosamine has been associated with less inflammatory effector functions, the decreased IgG Fc galactosylation and sialylation with lower gestational age suggest a rather pro-inflammatory pattern. The difference in IgG Fc glycosylation patterns between preterm infants and mothers of preterm infants suggests a selective enrichment of IgG glyco forms in preterm infants, which might contribute to or result of the development of sustained inflammatory diseases like BPD.

Keywords: newborn, trans-placental transfer, IgG antibodies, IgG Fc glycosylation, mothers, galactosylation, sialylation, preterm infants

INTRODUCTION

The adaptation of women during pregnancy leads to a feto-maternal immune tolerance, which is disrupted in the settings of preterm birth. Reasons for preterm birth are often associated with rather pro-inflammatory conditions at the feto-maternal interface (e.g., infection, age, stress) (1). With a compromised and immaturely developed immune system, preterm infants are exposed to the extrauterine environment leading to a high susceptibility for infections and sustained lung inflammation, such as bronchopulmonary dysplasia (BPD) of particular very early preterm infants (2–4).

The endogenous Immunoglobulin G (IgG) production in infants starts within 1–3 months after term birth (5). Therefore, specific immune protection of infants against pathogens is provided by the active transport of IgG through the placenta probably exclusively via the neonatal Fc receptor (FcRn) (6–10). However, IgG concentrations of the fetus are largely diminished in the second trimester of pregnancy. Specifically, during week 17–22 of gestation only 5–10% of maternal IgG concentrations are transported via the placenta, which rises to 50% during week 28–32 of gestation (11). Hence, reduced IgG concentrations in preterm infants might contribute to their predisposition for infection (9).

In addition, a resulting reduced total amount of anti-inflammatory galactosylated and sialylated IgG antibodies (12) or, even more, qualitative changes in the type of IgG Fc glycosylation might have an impact on the specific risk profile of preterm infants including inflammation-mediated diseases. IgG Fc glycosylation patterns are characterized as follows: IgG molecules bare an N-glycosylation site on the conserved asparagine at position 297 (N297) of each heavy chain CH2 domain. The glycan is composed of a biantennary core heptasaccharide comprised of four N-acetylglucosamines (GlcNAc) and three mannoses (**Figure 1A**). The core structure can be further modified by addition of fucose, bisecting GlcNAc (bisection), galactose (G), or sialic acid (S) (13, 14).

IgG Fc glycosylation patterns are clinically relevant, as a shift toward more non-galactosylated (agalactosylated; G0) glycans has been linked to inflammation-mediated immune diseases (15–19). Animal models have verified that the absence or presence of galactose and sialic acid themselves can influence the inflammatory properties of IgG, i.e., pro-inflammatory [high proportion of agalactosylated glycan structures; (19, 20)] or anti-inflammatory [high proportion of galactosylated and sialylated glycan structures; (19, 21–27)]. IgG Fc glycosylation patterns without bisecting GlcNAc have been associated with reduced affinity to classical Fcγ receptors and instead less inflammatory conditions (28). The IgG Fc glycosylation pattern thereby influences not only the effector function of antigen-specific IgG in form of immune complexes, but also the immune modulatory effect of total IgG (12, 19, 21–26).

In humans, IgG Fc glycosylation patterns are variable and influenced by several factors, such as genetics, gender, age, and disease state (29–31). During pregnancy, the degree of galactosylation and sialylation of IgG antibodies increases whereas the degree of bisecting GlcNAc slightly decreases (32–36), which may contribute to the tolerance at the feto-maternal interface. Recent data from cord blood samples have confirmed that the proportion of galactosylated and sialylated IgG is higher in infants at term birth compared to older children as expected from the IgG Fc glycosylation pattern of pregnant women (37).

However, the IgG Fc glycosylation patterns of preterm infants, which are highly susceptible to infection and sustained inflammation, have not been studied yet. It was the primary objective of our explorative study to investigate the Fc glycosylation patterns in the context of preterm birth. We hypothesized that IgG Fc glycosylation patterns of preterm infants are comparable to their mother's type of IgG Fc glycosylation (feto-maternal tolerance) or are polarized toward more inflammatory properties, which might contribute to or result of the development of sepsis and sustained lung inflammation.

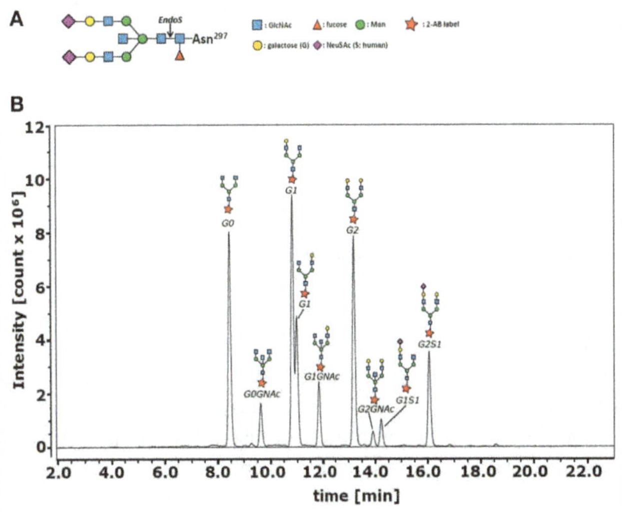

FIGURE 1 | IgG Fc N-glycan structure and representative chromatogram of IgG Fc N-glycans. **(A)** The glycan structure is composed of a biantennary core heptasaccharide comprised of N-acetylglucosamines (GlcNAc or GNAc, blue) and mannoses (Man, green). The core structure can be further modified by addition of fucose (Fuc), bisecting GlcNAc (GNAc, blue), galactose (G, yellow), or sialic acid (Neu5Ac, purple). **(B)** The different Fc N-glycan modifications G0, G0GNAc, G1, G1GNAc, G2, G2GNAc, G1S1, G2S1 and G2S2 (not marked in this sample analysis) were detected using hydrophilic interaction liquid chromatography (representative chromatogram), where glycans with higher hydrophobicity (e.g., more sugar units) were retained longer by the column. Glycan composition of collected fractions containing individual peaks was previously identified by MALDI-TOF analysis (38).

MATERIALS AND METHODS

Study Cohort

We performed an explorative study in two tertiary care centers for neonates as part of our Immunoregulation of the Newborn (IRoN) study. Samples and clinical data were obtained from infants born between January 1st, 2012 and May 1st, 2015 (center 1; analyzed plasma IgG concentration of infants at mean ± SD 23 ± 2 days of life) and October 1st, 2014 and August

1st, 2017 (center 2; analyzed IgG Fc glycosylation at mean ± SD 32 ± 5 days of life). The inclusion criteria were preterm infants with gestational age ≥23.0 and ≤35.0 weeks without lethal abnormalities, and written informed consent provided by parents or a legal representative. At center 2 (IgG Fc glycosylation), term infants served as controls (blood withdrawal with routine newborn screening at 48–72 h of life). Form mothers of preterm infants born in center 2, we were able to obtain maternal blood from a routine sampling immediately after birth.

Ethics

Written informed consent was obtained from parents on behalf of the infants enrolled into our studies. The study parts were approved by the local committee on research in human subjects at the University of Lübeck (center 2) and by the local committee on research in human subjects at Ärztekammer Bayern (center 1), respectively. All blood samples were obtained within a medically required blood withdrawal procedure. The additional blood volume obtained for research purposes (<1% of whole body blood volume per blood sampling) was in line with current guidelines of the European Medical Agency on the investigation of medicinal products in term and preterm infants; Committee for Medicinal Products for Human Use and Pediatric Committee (39).

Definitions

Gestational age was calculated from the best obstetric estimate based on early prenatal ultrasound and obstetric examination.

Early-onset sepsis (EOS) was defined as sepsis, clinical or culture-proven, occurring within the first 72 h of life.

Late-onset sepsis (LOS) was defined as sepsis, clinical or culture-proven, occurring after the first 72 h of life.

Clinical sepsis was defined as condition when neonatologists decided to treat the infant with antibiotics and continued for at least 5 days due to the following reasons: ≥2 clinical signs of systemic inflammatory response: temperature >38°C or <36.5°C, tachycardia >200/min, new onset or increased frequency of bradycardias or apneas, hyperglycemia >140 mg/dl, base excess <-10 mval/l, changed skin color, increased oxygen need; and at least one laboratory sign: C-reactive protein >10 mg/L, platelet count <100/nl, immature/total neutrophil ratio >0.2, white blood cell count <5/nl (NeoKISS).

Blood culture-confirmed sepsis was defined as clinical sepsis with proof of causative agent in the blood culture.

Necrotizing enterocolitis (NEC) and focal intestinal perforation (FIP) were defined as surgery due to spontaneous intestinal perforation or necrotizing enterocolitis (Bell stage ≥2).

Intraventricular hemorrhage (IVH) was defined according to Papile ultrasound criteria.

Bronchopulmonary dysplasia (BPD) was defined as need for oxygen supplement and/or respiratory support at corrected age of 36 weeks.

Cause of preterm delivery was determined at the discretion of the attending obstetrician, specifically: (1) preterm labor (labor refractory to tocolytic agents) or **amniotic infection syndrome** [AIS; labor ± rupture of membranes, maternal fever (≥39.0°C), and/or one of the following signs: increased maternal inflammatory markers without any other cause (CRP > 10 mg/l or elevation of white blood cell count >15.000/μl), fetal tachycardia, painful uterus and foul-smelling cervical discharge]; (2) pre-eclampsia (pregnancy-induced maternal hypertension, oedema, proteinuria), pathological Doppler (e.g., Arteria umbilicalis Doppler, Ductus venosus flow, Arteria cerebri media Doppler), intrauterine growth restriction as diagnosed by the attending specialist for antenatal ultrasound,

TABLE 1 | Summary of patient demographics from center 1 (IgG quantification).

	<28 weeks	≥28 weeks	Total
n	19	19	38
Gestational age [weeks]	26.4 ± 1.0	30.9 ± 1.9	28.7 ± 2.7
Birth weight [g]	853 ± 160	1261 ± 255	1057 ± 295
Male Gender	11 (58)	8 (42)	19 (50)
Multiple	5 (26)	6 (32)	11 (29)
EOS	0 (0)	0 (0)	0 (0)
LOS	4 (21)	4 (21)	8 (21)
NEC	0 (0)	0 (0)	0 (0)
FIP	1 (5)	0 (0)	1 (3)
IVH	4 (21)	2 (11)	6 (16)
BPD	11 (58)	3 (16)	14 (37)
Cause of delivery			
Preterm labor or AIS	8 (42)	5 (26)	13 (34)
Pathological doppler, placental abruption, pre-eclampsia	8 (42)	8 (42)	16 (42)
Others	3 (16)	6 (32)	9 (24)

EOS, early-onset sepsis; LOS, late-onset sepsis; NEC, necrotizing enterocolitis; FIP, focal intestinal perforation; IVH, intraventricular hemorrhage; BPD, bronchopulmonary dysplasia; AIS, amnion infection syndrome. Data are described as mean ± standard deviation or n (%).

or placental abruption; and (3) others, including cholestasis, etc.

Sample Collection

Peripheral blood (EDTA) samples were stored at room temperature and processed within 24 h after withdrawal. Samples were spun down for 6 min at 1,500 rpm. The clear plasma fraction was transferred and immediately stored at −80°C until further use.

IgG ELISA

A 96 well plate was coated with anti-human IgG-Fc primary antibody (Bethyl, Laboratories, Montgomer, TX). After blocking residual binding sites, plasma dilutions were added. Intravenous immunoglobulin (IVIG, Biotech, Dreieich, Germany) was used as standard. Plasma IgG concentration was detected with horse radish peroxidase-conjugated anti-human-IgG-Fc antibody (Bethyl, Laboratories, Montgomer, TX) and assay developed with TMB substrate (BD Biosciences).

IgG Purification and IgG-Fc Glycan Analysis

Total IgG was purified from human plasma samples using Protein G coupled agarose beads (Genetex, San Antonio, TX) in a 96 well filter plate (Merck, Darmstadt, Germany). In brief, 50 µl settled beads were constituted by washing 3 times with 200 µl

TABLE 2 | Summary of patient demographics from center 2 (IgG Fc glycosylation; infants and mothers of preterm infants).

	<28 weeks	≥28 weeks	Term infants	Total
INFANTS				
n	43	43	15	101
Gestational age [weeks]	26.1 ± 1.2	29.8 ± 1.6	39.6 ± 1.2	29.7 ± 4.7
Birth weight [g]	809 ± 232	1260 ± 229	3220 ± 656	1359 ± 871
Male Gender	26 (60)	18 (42)	8 (53)	52 (51)
Multiple	11 (26)	14 (33)	2 (13)	27 (27)
EOS	13 (30)	6 (14)	1 (7)	20 (20)
LOS	22 (51)	6 (14)	0 (0)	28 (28)
NEC	2 (9)	0 (0)	0 (0)	2 (2)
FIP	4 (9)	0 (0)	0 (0)	4 (4)
IVH	12 (28)	2 (5)	0 (0)	14 (14)
BPD	14 (33)	7 (16)	0 (0)	21 (21)
Cause of delivery				
Preterm labor or AIS	31 (72)	27 (63)	1 (7)	59 (58)
Pathological doppler, placental abruption, pre-eclampsia	6 (14)	13 (30)	1 (7)	20 (20)
Others	6 (14)	3 (7)	13 (87)	22 (22)
MOTHERS				
n	16	25		41
Age of mother at birth [years]	33 ± 6	32 ± 4		32 ± 5
Gestational age [weeks]	25.8 ± 1.6	31.2 ± 2.1		29.1 ± 3.3
Birth weight [g]	756 ± 279	1484 ± 511		1200 ± 562
Male Gender	11 (69)	11 (44)		22 (54)
Multiple	2 (13)	4 (16)		6 (15)
EOS	7 (44)	2 (8)		9 (22)
LOS	9 (56)	1 (4)		10 (24)
NEC	2 (13)	0 (0)		2 (5)
FIP	2 (13)	0 (0)		2 (5)
IVH	4 (25)	0 (0)		4 (10)
BPD	6 (38)	0 (0)		6 (15)
Cause of delivery				
Preterm labor or AIS	9 (56)	14 (56)		23 (56)
Pathological doppler, placental abruption, pre-eclampsia	3 (19)	8 (32)		11 (27)
Others	4 (25)	3 (12)		7 (17)
MOTHER-INFANT-PAIRS				
n	12	8	0	20

EOS, early-onset sepsis; LOS, late-onset sepsis; AIS, amnion infection syndrome; NEC, necrotizing enterocolitis; FIP, focal intestinal perforation; IVH, intraventricular hemorrhage; BPD, bronchopulmonary dysplasia. Data are described as mean ± standard deviation or n (%).

of PBS and applying negative pressure on a vacuum manifold. Protein G was than incubated with 200 μl of a 1:4 plasma dilution (50 μl plasma volume) for 2 h at room temperature with agitation. Unspecific plasma proteins were washed away 5 times with 200 μl of PBS. IgG was eluted three times with 100 μl of 100 mM formic acid (pH 2.5). Elution was neutralized by adding 10 μl of 1 M ammonium bicarbonate into each elution fraction. IVIG (Biotech, Dreieich, Germany) was used as standard.

From the purified IgG, Fc N-glycan composition was analyzed as previously described (38). Briefly, Fc N-linked glycans were enzymatically released with recombinant endoglycosidase S (EndoS) from *Streptococcus pyogenes*. EndoS hydrolyses specifically the IgG Fc N-glycan of IgG after the first GlcNAc (**Figure 1A**). The N-glycans were purified using self-made graphitized carbon columns (Fisher Scientific, Hampton, NH) and labeled with anthranilamide (Sigma-Aldrich). The labeled glycans were analyzed by hydrophilic interaction liquid chromatography–high performance liquid chromatography (HPLC) on a Dionex Ultimate 3000 (Thermo Fischer Scientific, Waltham, Mass) by using an Xbridge XP BEH Glycan column (1.7 μm, 100 × 2.1 mm i.d.; Waters, Milford, Mass). As previously described (38), glycan composition was identified by MALDI-TOF analysis of collected fractions containing individual peaks. N-glycans with higher hydrophobicity (e.g., more sugar units) were retained longer in the column (**Figure 1B**).

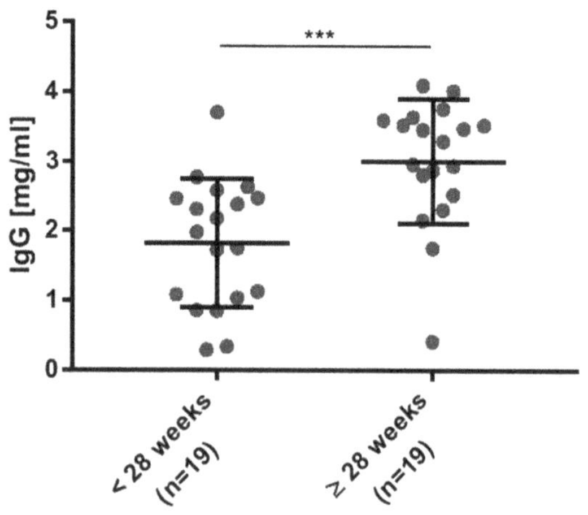

FIGURE 2 | Plasma IgG concentrations were significantly decreased in preterm infants born at lower gestational ages. ELISA data for detection of human IgG-Fc parts. Intravenous immunoglobulin (IVIG) was used as a standard to estimate the plasma IgG concentration (mean ± SD, Mann-Whitney test). ***$p < 0.001$.

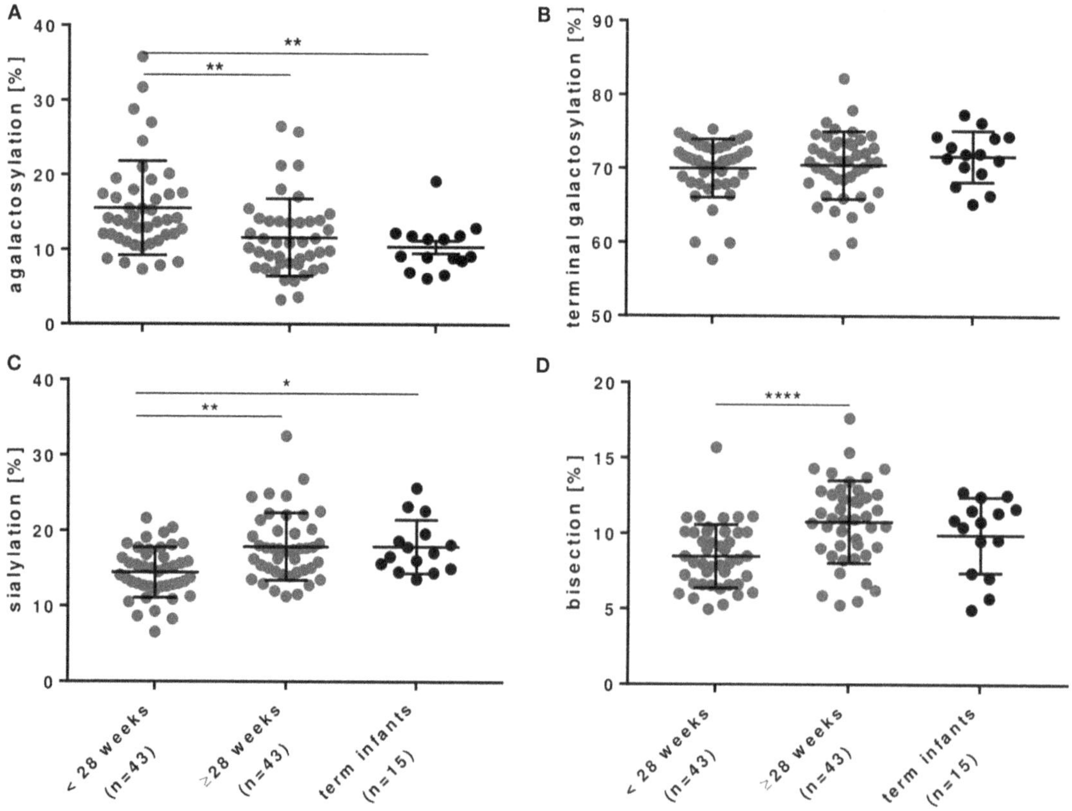

FIGURE 3 | IgG Fc glycosylation in preterm infants is dependent on gestational age. **(A)** IgG with agalactosylated Fc glycans were significantly increased, whereas **(B)** IgG with terminally galactosylated Fc glycans were unchanged and IgG with **(C)** sialylated and **(D)** bisecting Fc glycans were significantly decreased in preterm infants born <28 weeks of gestational age. Term infants served as controls (mean ± SD, Kruskal-Wallis test). *$p < 0.05$, **$p < 0.01$, ***$p < 0.0001$.

The area under the curve (AUC) of the following nine glycan peaks were identified: G0, G0GlcNAc, G1, G1GlcNAc, G2, G2GlcNAc, G1S1, G2S1, and G2S2. Sialylated glycans with bisecting GlcNAc were not detected. The relative proportion of the individual peaks of a sample was calculated by dividing AUC of the individual curve by the AUC of the sum of all nine identified peaks and this multiplied by 100 (for raw data see **Supplementary Tables 1, 2**). For presentation, the four following groups were defined and percentages of the groups calculated as the sum of the percentages of the individual glycan proportions: (1) agalactosylation: G0 ± bisecting GlcNAc; (2) terminal galactosylation: G1 ± bisecting GlcNAc, G2 ± bisecting GlcNAc; (3) sialylation: G1S1, G2S1, G2S2; (4) bisection: G0 + bisecting GlcNAc, G1 + bisecting GlcNAc, G2 + bisecting GlcNAc.

Statistical Analysis

All data were analyzed using GraphPad Prism®version 7. After testing for normal distribution, Kruskal-Wallis test followed by Dunn's multiple comparisons test or the Mann-Whitney test was used for not normally distributed data. Correlations were evaluated using Spearman correlation. Two-way ANOVA followed by Bonferroni's multiple comparison test was done for correlation with clinical parameter. The threshold for

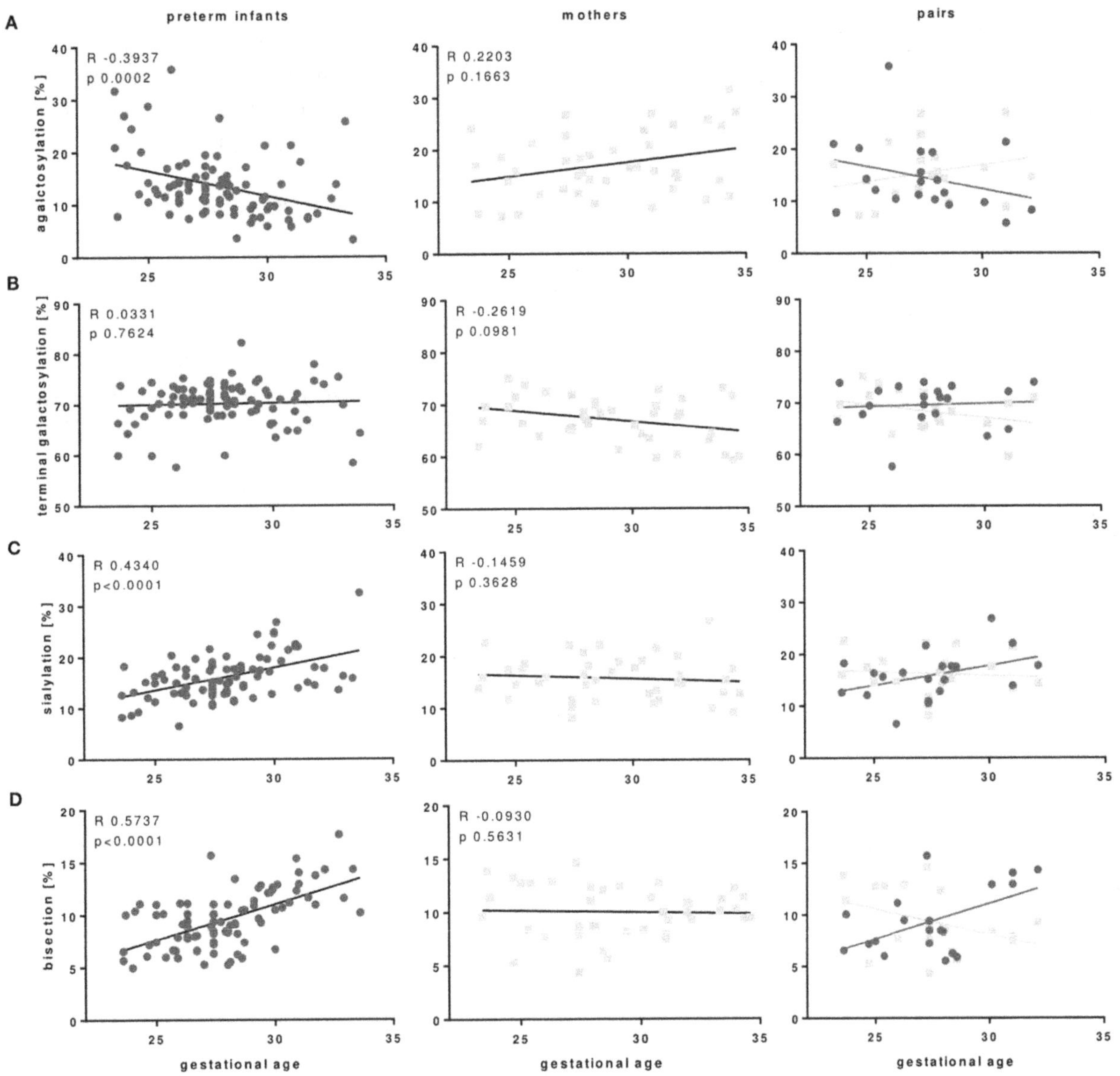

FIGURE 4 | IgG Fc glycosylation patterns of preterm infants but not IgG Fc glycosylation of mothers of preterm infants correlate with gestational age of infants. **(A)** IgG with agalactosylated Fc glycans of preterm infants correlated negatively with gestational age, while Fc agalactosylation of mothers of preterm infants does not correlate with gestational age of their infants. **(C)** Sialylated and **(D)** bisecting Fc glycans correlated positively with gestational age of preterm infants which is not seen in Fc glycosylation of mothers from preterm infants. Terminal galactosylation **(B)** showed no correlation with gestational age in both preterm infants and mothers (Preterm infants: $n = 86$, mothers: $n = 41$, mother-infant-pairs: $n = 20$, Spearman correlation).

significance was a p-value < 0.05 depicted as *, < 0.01 as **, < 0.001 as ***, and <0.0001 as ****.

RESULTS

Clinical Characteristics

We recruited a cohort of preterm infants in two centers and collected plasma from peripheral blood samples and key clinical outcome parameters. In samples of center 1 we analyzed plasma IgG concentrations and in samples of center 2 we investigated IgG Fc glycosylation. To analyze whether plasma IgG concentrations and Fc glycosylation patterns differ with gestational age, we divided the cohort in 2 gestational age groups (center 1/center 2: ≥23(+0 days) and ≤27(+6) weeks, $n = 19/n = 43$; ≥28(+0) and ≤34(+6) weeks, $n = 19/n = 43$; **Tables 1, 2**).

The cohort of center 1 (plasma IgG concentration) was also selected for a matched pair analysis of BPD diagnosis vs. no BPD. For this matched pair analysis early onset sepsis cases were excluded, and late onset sepsis cases were equal in both groups. In center 2, we also analyzed IgG Fc glycosylation patterns of term infants ($n = 15$) and mothers of preterm infants ($n = 41$) (**Table 2**). For a subgroup of preterm infants and mothers from center 2, we were able to analyze mother-infant-pairs ($n = 20$).

TABLE 3 | IgG Fc glycosylation patterns in infants of different gestational age groups depicted in **Figure 3** (mean ± SD).

	<28 weeks	≥28 weeks	Term infants
Agalactosylation (%)	15.5 ± 6.3	11.6 ± 5.2	10.4 ± 3.3
Galactosylation (%)	84.5 ± 6.3	88.4 ± 5.2	89.6 ± 3.3
Terminal galactosylation (%)	70.0 ± 3.9	70.5 ± 4.6	71.7 ± 3.5
Sialylation (%)	14.5 ± 3.4	17.9 ± 4.5	17.9 ± 3.6
Bisection (%)	8.4 ± 2.1	10.8 ± 2.7	9.9 ± 2.5

Plasma IgG Concentrations Were Decreased in Preterm Infants Born at Lower Gestational Ages

As outlined in **Figure 2**, IgG was detectable in infants born <28 weeks of gestational age and increased significantly with

TABLE 4 | IgG Fc glycosylation patterns of preterm infants associated with (i) gender and clinical parameters defining (ii) cause of birth, (iii) bronchopulmonary dysplasia (BPD) or (iv) sepsis (early and late onset sepsis cases included) (mean ± SD, two-way ANOVA, multiple comparison within group to adjust for gestational age).

	<28 weeks		≥28 weeks	
(i)	**Male ($n = 26$)**	**Female ($n = 17$)**	**Male ($n = 18$)**	**Female ($n = 25$)**
Agalactosylation (%)	15.0 ± 6.5	16.3 ± 6.1	12.4 ± 6.3	11.1 ± 4.2
Galactosylation (%)	85.0 ± 6.5	83.7 ± 6.1	87.6 ± 6.3	88.9 ± 4.2
Terminal galactosylation (%)	70.3 ± 3.7	69.6 ± 4.3	70.9 ± 5.5	70.1 ± 3.8
Sialylation (%)	14.7 ± 3.5	14.1 ± 3.2	16.7 ± 4.0	18.8 ± 4.7
Bisection (%)	8.8 ± 2.3	8.0 ± 1.8	11.1 ± 3.4	10.6 ± 2.2
(ii)	**Preterm labor or AIS ($n = 31$)**	**All other causes ($n = 12$)**	**Preterm labor or AIS ($n = 27$)**	**All other causes ($n = 16$)**
Agalactosylation (%)	15.2 ± 5.6	16.4 ± 8.0	11.3 ± 4.0	12.2 ± 6.9
Galactosylation (%)	84.8 ± 5.6	83.6 ± 8.0	88.7 ± 4.0	87.8 ± 6.9
Terminal galactosylation (%)	70.0 ± 3.4	70.0 ± 5.3	71.2 ± 3.7	69.3 ± 5.8
Sialylation (%)	14.8 ± 3.0	13.6 ± 4.0	17.5 ± 4.1	18.6 ± 5.1
Bisection (%)	8.3 ± 1.8	9.0 ± 2.8	9.8 ± 2.3 ***	12.5 ± 2.7
(iii)	**BPD ($n = 14$)**	**No BPD ($n = 29$)**	**BPD ($n = 7$)**	**No BPD ($n = 36$)**
Agalactosylation (%)	17.0 ± 6.4	14.8 ± 6.2	16.9 ± 8.1*	10.6 ± 3.8
Galactosylation (%)	83.0 ± 6.4	85.2 ± 6.2	83.1 ± 8.1*	89.4 ± 3.8
Terminal galactosylation (%)	69.5 ± 4.2	70.3 ± 3.8	66.6 ± 5.4	71.2 ± 4.1
Sialylation (%)	13.5 ± 2.9	14.9 ± 3.5	16.5 ± 4.6	18.2 ± 4.5
Bisection (%)	8.4 ± 2.2	8.5 ± 2.1	10.9 ± 2.5	10.8 ± 2.8
(iv)	**Sepsis ($n = 27$)**	**No sepsis ($n = 16$)**	**Sepsis ($n = 11$)**	**No sepsis ($n = 32$)**
Agalactosylation (%)	16.6 ± 7.2	13.8 ± 3.9	14.8 ± 7.3	10.5 ± 3.8
Galactosylation (%)	83.4 ± 7.2	86.2 ± 3.9	85.2 ± 7.3	89.5 ± 3.8
Terminal galactosylation (%)	69.5 ± 4.6	70.8 ± 2.4	68.8 ± 5.5	71.1 ± 4.2
Sialylation (%)	13.9 ± 3.5	15.4 ± 3.0	16.4 ± 3.7	18.4 ± 4.7
Bisection (%)	8.7 ± 2.4	8.2 ± 1.6	12.1 ± 2.1	10.4 ± 2.8

*IgG Fc agalactosylation is additionally depicted in **Figure 5**. *p < 0.05, ***p < 0.001.*

gestational age. Plasma IgG concentrations were not different in a matched pair analysis of preterm infants developing BPD vs. no BPD diagnosis (data not shown).

IgG Fc Glycosylation Patterns Depend on Gestational Age of Preterm Infants

As outlined in **Figures 3, 4** and **Table 3**, preterm infants had a higher proportion of agalactosylated (accordingly lower proportion of galactosylated) IgG Fc N-glycans with decreasing gestational age ($R = -0.3937$, $p = 0.0002$). No difference in agalactosylated IgG Fc glycans was observed between infants born ≥28 weeks of gestation and term controls. Further, no correlation between terminal galactosylation of IgG and gestational age in preterm infants was found ($R = 0.0331$, $p = 0.76$). However, also IgG Fc sialylation was significantly lower in preterm infants born <28 weeks as compared to infants born ≥28 weeks of gestation and term infants (correlation with gestational age; $R = 0.4340$, $p < 0.0001$). The proportion of IgG glycans with bisecting GlcNAc also correlated with gestational age ($R = 0.5737$, $p < 0.0001$).

IgG Fc Glycosylation Shows Differences Between Preterm Infants and Mothers of Preterm Infants

In the comparison of maternal with neonatal IgG Fc glycosylation patterns we did not find the same correlation between IgG Fc glycosylation patterns in mothers of preterm infants with the gestational age of their infants which we observed between the IgG Fc glycosylation patterns of preterm infants with their gestational age (**Figure 4**).

Clinical Correlation of IgG Fc Glycosylation in Preterm Infants

For the cause of preterm delivery bisecting IgG Fc glycosylation was significantly decreased in preterm infants born ≥28 weeks of gestation with preterm labor or amnion infection syndrome (AIS) as compared to other preterm delivery reasons (**Table 4**).

For the development of BPD, preterm infants born < or ≥28 weeks of gestation had respectively, a tending or significant increased proportion of agalactosylated IgG as compared to preterm infants without BPD (**Figure 5** and **Table 4**). A similar

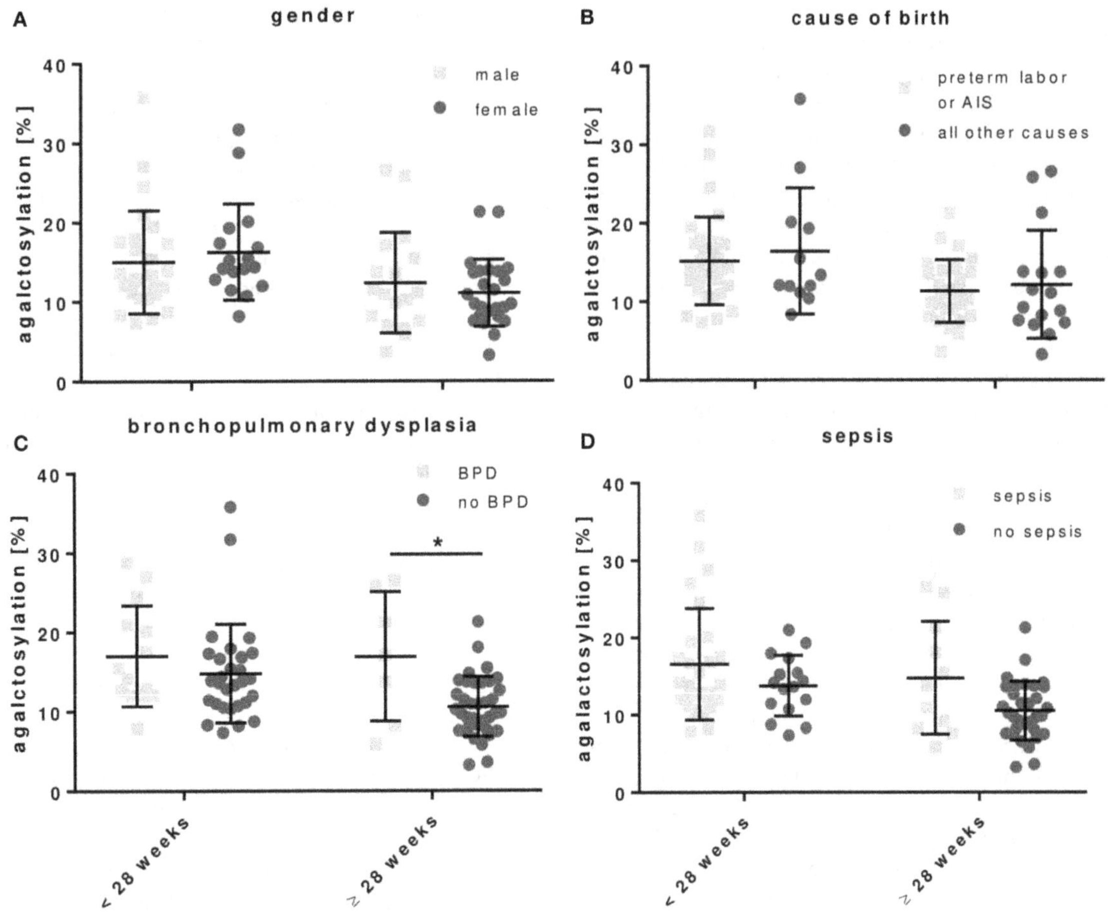

FIGURE 5 | Agalactosylated IgG Fc N-glycans show a tendency to increase in preterm infants developing bronchopulmonary dysplasia (BPD). The correlation was done with (i) gender and clinical parameters defining, (ii) cause of birth, (iii) BPD, and (iv) sepsis (early and late onset sepsis cases included) for all preterm infant groups (mean ± SD, two-way ANOVA, multiple comparison within groups to adjust for gestational age). *$p < 0.05$.

tendency, which was however not significant, was observed in preterm infants with sepsis (**Figure 5** and **Table 4**). No differences in IgG Fc glycosylation were found for the gender (**Figure 5** and **Table 4**).

DISCUSSION

To our knowledge, this is the first explorative study investigating IgG Fc glycosylation patterns in peripheral blood of preterm infants. We noted that IgG Fc glycosylation patterns of preterm infants differ with gestational age whereas the patterns of mothers, as described in the literature (32, 33), did not differ with gestational age of their offspring. Preterm infants born <28 weeks of gestation displayed an IgG Fc glycosylation pattern characterized by a higher proportion of agalactosylated IgG (reduced proportion of galactosylated IgG) and a reduced proportion of sialylated and bisecting IgG. The pattern of Fc glycosylation from mothers, however, did not differ between the second and third trimester of pregnancy suggesting an enrichment of IgG glyco forms in extremely low gestational age infants. This novel finding needs further prospective in-depth-analysis, how these IgG Fc glyco forms are enriched in the smallest, most vulnerable infants, whether they contribute to or are a result of dysregulated immune responses and sustained inflammation like BPD, and how they function.

We were able to confirm that IgG antibodies are transported through the placenta during second trimester of pregnancy, but in a much less amount in infants born <28 weeks of gestation as compared to infants born ≥28 weeks of gestation. In our setting, IgG concentration of preterm infants ≥28 weeks of gestation were still below the levels of term born infants (clinical reference values for infants between 1 and 3 months of age are 2.5–7.5 mg/ml IgG, Immunology laboratory of the medical clinic in Freiburg, Germany, 2007).

Our current understanding of IgG Fc glycosylation patterns and its functional role for the immune system is that different Fc N-linked glycan structures can influence the inflammatory properties of IgG antibodies. Galactosylation and sialylation of total serum IgG but also of antigen-specific IgG in form of immune complexes were shown to mediate more anti-inflammatory effector functions (12, 19, 21–27) whereas a shift toward more agalactosylated and bisecting glycan structures has been associated with pro-inflammatory effects (19, 20, 28). IgG glycosylation of pregnant women in the Fc part was shown to be similar during second and third trimester of pregnancy and directed toward an anti-inflammatory pattern as compared to non-pregnant woman (32, 33). This pattern was also previously found in cord blood samples of term infants (35, 37) and was suggested to contribute to the condition of feto-maternal tolerance and permissive microbiota establishment after birth. In the context of preterm birth, however, the IgG Fc glycosylation patterns are different between infants born during second and third trimester and it is yet unknown whether immune dysregulation derives from a pro-inflammatory setting, i.e., reduced galactosylation and sialylation, or from an anti-inflammatory effect due to reduced bisection leading to lower affinities to activating Fcγ receptors. For this reason, functional studies are needed determining which IgG Fc glycosylation pattern is dominant. We showed that reduced bisection was associated with birth pathology, especially preterm labor and amnion infection syndrome (AIS) suggesting a role of Fc glycosylation patterns for preterm birth. Additionally, we showed a trend of increased IgG Fc agalactosylation in inflammatory-mediated diseases of preterm infants (i.e., chronic lung disease) supporting the hypothesis of a pro-inflammatory effect.

Since IgG of infants in the first month of life are mainly of maternal origin (5), several studies investigated the role of trans-placental transfer through FcRn to be selective for certain Fc glycosylation. *In vitro*, FcRn has a higher affinity to galactosylated IgG (40). A few studies showed a transfer of more galactosylated IgG to infants born at term by comparing IgG glycosylation in healthy pregnant women and umbilical cord blood of term infants (35, 41, 42). In another study, a similar IgG Fc glycosylation pattern between maternal sample and cord blood was reported (43). In our setting, IgG Fc glycosylation patterns in peripheral blood revealed a difference between preterm infants born during second and third trimester compared to IgG Fc glycosylation of mothers from preterm infants which is not changing over the second and third trimester. The reduced galactosylation, sialylation and bisection in extremely preterm infants might reflect the enrichment of certain IgG glyco forms at lower gestation. Since endogenous IgG production slowly starts at 1–3 months (5), we assumed that detected IgG in preterm infants is still of maternal origin. Several mechanisms for the enrichment of the described IgG glyco forms in preterm infants born <28 weeks of gestation might be possible. First, a selective IgG transport via the placenta might play a role in early stages of pregnancy. Second, trimming (44) or extracellular modification (45) of the sugars from IgG Fc glycans in the circulation of early preterm infants might result in a dominance of the detected IgG Fc glycosylation pattern. Third, IgG in breast milk might modify the IgG Fc glycosylation pattern also it only contains about 0.01–0.06 mg/ml in women from western countries (46).

Taken together, our findings suggest an enrichment of certain IgG glyco forms in extremely low gestational age infants and that a high proportion of "pro-inflammatory" agalactosylated IgG Fc N-glycans in those infants might contribute to or result from inflammation-mediated diseases. However, IgG Fc agalactosylation was not significantly associated with the diagnosis of BPD or sepsis in extremely preterm infants, only with the diagnosis of BPD in preterm infants born ≥28 weeks of gestation. Future studies need to evaluate larger cohorts using multivariable linear regression accounting for possible confounding factors. Furthermore, functional *in vitro* and *in vivo* studies are needed to reveal consequences for effector functions of IgG glycosylation pattern in term and preterm infants.

The use of peripheral blood from infants in contrast to umbilical cord blood has the advantage not to be contaminated with maternal blood in the context of clinical sampling. Despite the limited sample volumes, we obtained peripheral blood samples of highly vulnerable infants. Our data are hypothesis-generating and add another component to the discussion of intravenous substitution of pooled immunoglobulins

(IVIg) to preterm infants. Large trials have shown no benefit (INIS trial) with regard to sepsis risk or neurodevelopmental outcome (47), but to e.g., reduction of the inflammatory cytokine IL-6 (48). However, the role of IgG Fc glycosylation has never been reflected in the context of IVIg treatment in preterm infants and also not in the context of BPD. The effect might be beneficial in sustained inflammation of preterm infants, if the intravenous immunoglobulins would be immunomodulatory with higher proportions of galactosylation and sialylation, since this would simulate more closely the measured IgG glycosylation patterns in term infants and might mediate anti-inflammatory effects in preterm infants.

In summary, our data suggest that IgG Fc glycosylation patterns differ in preterm infants and their mothers suggesting an enrichment of certain IgG glyco forms in early stages of gestation. Further investigations with a larger cohort are needed to determine the enrichment and functional role of the observed IgG Fc glycosylation pattern in early preterm infants and to verify its correlation with sustained inflammation of preterm infants.

AUTHOR CONTRIBUTIONS

NT, YB, JP, AH, ME, and CH contributed conception and design of the study. CH and CW provided clinical samples. YB performed experiments and HPLC analysis. NT correlated HPLC analysis with clinical data and performed statistical analysis. NT and YB wrote first draft of the manuscript. All authors contributed to manuscript revision, read and approved the submitted version.

FUNDING

NT was supported by a grant of the Friedrich-Ebert-Stiftung (financed by the German Ministry of Education and Research, BMBF). JP was supported by a grant of the German Centre of Infection Research (DZIF; financed by the German Ministry of Education and Research, BMBF). AH was supported by grants from the IRTG 1911 (financed by the German Society of Research, DFG). CH was funded by the BMBF (PRIMAL clinical study, No. 01GL1746A), the University of Lübeck and Lübeck-Hilfe für krebskranke Kinder e.V.

ACKNOWLEDGMENTS

We are indebted to the patients and their families for their participation and the physicians of the local NICU for their generous collaboration in this study. We thank Matthias Collin for the EndoS. The experimental work of ME's laboratories was supported by the Else-Kröner-Fresenius Foundation (2014_A91) and the German Research Foundation (DFG; EH 221/8-1, /9-1, /10-1, /11-1, Research Training Group (GRK) 1727, Clinical Research Unit (CRU) 303, SFB/TR 654 and Excellence cluster 306 Inflammation at Interfaces).

REFERENCES

1. Arck PC, Hecher K. Fetomaternal immune cross-talk and its consequences for maternal and offspring's health. *Nat Med Rev.* (2013) 19:548–56. doi: 10.1038/nm.3160
2. Stoll BJ, Hansen NI, Bell EF, Walsh MC, Carlo WA, Shankaran S, et al. Trends in care practices, morbidity, and mortality of extremely preterm neonates, 1993-2012. *JAMA J Am Med Assoc.* (2015) 314:1039–51. doi: 10.1001/jama.2015.10244
3. Niedermaier S, Hilgendorff A. Bronchopulmonary dysplasia–an overview about pathophysiologic concepts. *Mol Cell Pediatrics* (2015) 2:2. doi: 10.1186/s40348-015-0013-7
4. Kan B, Razzaghian HR, Lavoie PM. An immunological perspective on neonatal sepsis. *Trends Mol Med.* (2016) 22:290–302. doi: 10.1016/j.molmed.2016.02.001
5. Morell A, Skvaril F, Hitzig WH, Barandun S. IgG subclasses: development of the serum concentrations in 'normal' infants and children. *J Pediatr.* (1972) 80:960–4.
6. Jauniaux E, Jurkovic D, Gulbis B, Liesnard C, Lees C, Campbell S. Materno-fetal immunoglobulin transfer and passive immunity during the first trimester of human pregnancy. *Hum Reprod.* (1995) 10:3297–300. doi: 10.1093/oxfordjournals.humrep.a135906
7. Gonçalves G, Cutts FT, Hills M, Rebelo-Andrade H, Trigo FA, Barros H. Transplacental transfer of measles and total IgG. *Epidemiol Infect.* (1999) 122:273–9. doi: 10.1017/S0950268899002046
8. Firan M, Bawdon R, Radu C, Ober RJ, Eaken D, Antohe F, et al. The MHC class I-related receptor, FcRn, plays an essential role in the maternofetal transfer of γ-globulin in humans. *Int Immunol.* (2001) 13:993–1002. doi: 10.1093/intimm/13.8.993
9. Silveira Lessa AL, Krebs VL, Brasil TB, Pontes GN, Carneiro-Sampaio M, Palmeira P. Preterm and term neonates transplacentally acquire IgG antibodies specific to LPS from *Klebsiella pneumoniae*, *Escherichia coli* and *Pseudomonas aeruginosa*. *FEMS Immunol Med Microbiol.* (2011) 62:236–43. doi: 10.1111/j.1574-695X.2011.00807.x
10. Fouda GG, Martinez DR, Swamy GK, Permar SR. The impact of IgG transplacental transfer on early life immunity. *ImmunoHorizons* (2018) 2:14–25. doi: 10.4049/immunohorizons.1700057
11. Malek A, Sager R, Kuhn P, Nicolaides KH, Schneider H. Evolution of maternofetal transport of immunoglobulins during human pregnancy. *Am J Reprod Immunol.* (1996) 36:248–55. doi: 10.1111/j.1600-0897.1996.tb00172.x
12. Maddur MS, Kaveri SV, Bayry J. Circulating normal IgG as stimulator of regulatory T cells: lessons from intravenous immunoglobulin. *Trends Immunol.* (2017) 38:789–92. doi: 10.1016/j.it.2017.08.008
13. Arnold JN, Wormald MR, Sim RB, Rudd PM, Dwek RA. The impact of glycosylation on the biological function and structure of human immunoglobulins. *Annu Rev Immunol.* (2007) 25:21–50. doi: 10.1146/annurev.immunol.25.022106.141702
14. Jefferis R. Glycosylation as a strategy to improve antibody-based therapeutics. *Nat Rev Drug Discov.* (2009) 8:226–34. doi: 10.1038/nrd2804
15. Ercan A, Cui J, Chatterton DE, Deane KD, Hazen MM, Brintnell W, et al. Aberrant IgG galactosylation precedes disease onset, correlates with disease activity, and is prevalent in autoantibodies in rheumatoid arthritis. *Arthritis Rheum.* (2010) 62:2239–48. doi: 10.1002/art.27533
16. Wuhrer M, Selman MH, McDonnell LA, Kümpfel T, Derfuss T, Khademi M, et al. Pro-inflammatory pattern of IgG1 Fc glycosylation in multiple sclerosis cerebrospinal fluid. *J Neuroinflammation.* (2015) 12:235. doi: 10.1186/s12974-015-0450-1

17. Vučković F, Krištić J, Gudelj I, Teruel M, Keser T, Pezer M, et al. Association of systemic lupus erythematosus with decreased immunosuppressive potential of the IgG glycome. *Arthritis Rheumatol.* (2015) 67:2978–89. doi: 10.1002/art.39273
18. Trbojević Akmačić I, Ventham NT, Theodoratou E, Vučković F, Kennedy NA, Krištić J, et al. Inflammatory bowel *disease* associates with proinflammatory potential of the immunoglobulin G glycome. *Inflammatory Bowel Dis.* (2015) :1237–47. doi: 10.1097/MIB.0000000000000372
19. Bartsch YC, Rahmöller J, Mertes MMM, Eiglmeier S, Lorenz FKM, Stoehr AD, et al. Sialylated autoantigen-reactive IgG antibodies attenuate disease development in autoimmune mouse models of lupus nephritis and rheumatoid arthritis. *Front Immunol.* (2018) 9:1183. doi: 10.3389/fimmu.2018.01183
20. Van Beneden K, Coppieters K, Laroy W, De Keyser F, Hoffman IE, Van den Bosch F, et al. Reversible changes in serum immunoglobulin galactosylation during the immune response and treatment of inflammatory autoimmune arthritis. *Ann Rheum Dis.* (2009) 68:1360–5. doi: 10.1136/ard.2008.089292
21. Kaneko Y, Nimmerjahn F, Ravetch JV. Anti-inflammatory activity of immunoglobulin G resulting from Sc sialylation. *Science* (2006) 313:670–3. doi: 10.1126/science.1129594
22. Karsten CM, Pandey MK, Figge J, Kilchenstein R, Taylor PR, Rosas M, et al. Anti-inflammatory activity of IgG1 mediated by Fc galactosylation and association of FcγRIIB and dectin-1. *Nat Med.* (2012) 18:1401–6. doi: 10.1038/nm.2862
23. Oefner CM, Winkler A, Hess C, Lorenz AK, Holecska V, Huxdorf M, et al. Tolerance induction with T cell-dependent protein antigens induces regulatory sialylated IgGs. *J Allergy Clin Immunol.* (2012) 129:1647–55.e13. doi: 10.1016/j.jaci.2012.02.037
24. Anthony RM, Wermeling F, Ravetch JV. Novel roles for the IgG Fc glycan. *Ann N Y Acad Sci.* (2012) 1253:170–180. doi: 10.1111/j.1749-6632.2011.06305.x
25. Hess C, Winkler A, Lorenz AK, Holecska V, Blanchard V, Eiglmeier S, et al. T cell-independent B cell activation induces immunosuppressive sialylated IgG antibodies. *J Clin Invest.* (2013) 123:3788–96. doi: 10.1172/JCI65938
26. Collin M, Ehlers M. The carbohydrate switch between pathogenic and immunosuppressive antigen-specific antibodies. *Exp Dermatol.* (2013) 22:511–4. doi: 10.1111/exd.12171
27. Lilienthal GM, Rahmöller J, Petry J, Bartsch YC, Leliavski A, Ehlers M. Potential of murine IgG1 and human IgG4 to inhibit the classical complement and Fcγ receptor activation pathways. *Front Immunol.* (2018) 9:958. doi: 10.3389/fimmu.2018.00958
28. Davies J, Jiang L, Pan LZ, LaBarre MJ, Anderson D, Reff M. Expression of GnTIII in a recombinant anti-CD20 CHO production cell line: expression of antibodies with altered glycoforms leads to an increase in ADCC through higher affinity for FC gamma RIII. *Biotechnol Bioeng.* (2001) 74:288–94. doi: 10.1002/bit.1119
29. Ruhaak LR, Uh HW, Beekman M, Koeleman CA, Hokke CH, Westendorp RG, et al. Decreased levels of bisecting GLcNAc glycoforms of IgG are associated with human longevity. *PLoS ONE* (2010) 5:e12566 doi: 10.1371/journal.pone.0012566
30. Pučić M, KneŽević A, Vidič J, Adamczyk B, Novokmet M, Polašek O, et al. High throughput isolation and glycosylation analysis of IgG–variability and heritability of the IgG glycome in three isolated human populations. *Mol Cell Proteomics* (2011) 10:M111.010090. doi: 10.1074/mcp.M111.010090
31. Dekkers G, Rispens T, Vidarsson G. Novel concepts of altered immunoglobulin G galactosylation in autoimmune diseases. *Front Immunol.* (2018) 9:553. doi: 10.3389/fimmu.2018.00553
32. van de Geijn FE, Wuhrer M, Selman MH, Willemsen SP, de Man YA, Deelder AM, et al. Immunoglobulin G galactosylation and sialylation are associated with pregnancy-induced improvement of rheumatoid arthritis and the postpartum flare: results from a large prospective cohort study. *Arthritis Res Ther.* (2009) 11:R193. doi: 10.1186/ar2892
33. Bondt A, Rombouts Y, Selman MHJ, Hensbergen PJ, Reiding KR, Hazes JMW, et al. Immunoglobulin G (IgG) fab glycosylation analysis using a new mass spectrometric high-throughput profiling method reveals pregnancy-associated changes. *Mol Cell Proteomics* (2014) 13.11:3029–39. doi: 10.1074/mcp.M114.039537
34. Jansen BC, Bondt A, Reiding KR, Lonardi E, de Jong CJ, Falck D, et al. and Wuhrer M. Pregnancy-associated serum N-glycome changes studied by high-throughput MALDI-TOF-MS. *Sci Rep.* (2016) 6:23296. doi: 10.1038/srep23296
35. Jansen BC, Bondt A, Reiding KR, Scherjon SA, Vidarsson G, Wuhrer M. MALDI-TOF-MS reveals differential N-linked plasma-and IgG-glycosylation profiles between mothers and their newborns. *Sci Rep.* (2016) 6:34001. doi: 10.1038/srep34001
36. Bondt A, Hafkenscheid L, Falck D, Kuijper TM, Rombouts Y, Hazes JMW, et al. ACPA IgG galactosylation associates with disease activity in pregnant patients with rheumatoid arthritis. *Ann Rheum Dis.* (2018) 77:1–7. doi: 10.1136/annrheumdis-2018-212946
37. De Haan N, Reiding KR, Driessen G, Van Der Burg M, Wuhrer M. Changes in healthy human IgG Fc-glycosylation after birth and during early childhood. *J Proteome Res.* (2016) 15:1853–61. doi: 10.1021/acs.jproteome.6b00038
38. Epp A, Hobusch J, Bartsch YC, Petry J, Lilienthal GM, Koeleman CAM, et al. Sialylation of IgG antibodies inhibits IgG-mediated allergic reactions. *J Allergy Clin Immunol.* (2018) 141:399–402.e8. doi: 10.1016/j.jaci.2017.06.021
39. Pediatric Committee of the European Union (PDCO) (2006). Available online at: https://www.ema.europa.eu/en/human-regulatory/overview/paediatric-medicines/paediatric-regulation
40. Dashivets T, Thomann M, Rueger P, Knaupp A, Buchner J, Schlothauer T. Multi-angle effector function analysis of human monoclonal IgG glycovariants. *PLoS ONE* (2015) 10:e0143520. doi: 10.1371/journal.pone.0143520
41. Williams PJ, Arkwright PD, Rudd P, Scragg IG, Edge CJ, Wormald MR, et al. Selective placental transport of maternal IgG to the fetus. *Placenta* (1995) 16:749–56. doi: 10.1016/0143-4004(95)90018-7
42. Kibe T, Fujimoto S, Ishida C, Togari H, Wada Y, Okada S, et al. Glycosylation and placental transport of immunoglobulin G. *J Clin Biochem Nutr.* (1996) 21:57–63. doi: 10.3164/jcbn.21.57
43. Einarsdottir HK, Selman MHJ, Kapur R, Scherjon S, Koeleman CAM, Deelder AM, et al. Comparison of the Fc glycosylation of fetal and maternal immunoglobulin G. *Glycoconj J.* (2013) 30:147–57. doi: 10.1007/s10719-012-9381-6
44. Yang WH, Aziz PV, Heithoff DM, Mahan MJ, Smith JW, Marth JD. An intrinsic mechanism of secreted protein aging and turnover. *Proc Natl Acad Sci USA.* (2015) 112:13657–62. doi: 10.1073/pnas.1515464112
45. Jones MB, Oswald DM, Joshi S, Whiteheart SW, Orlando R, Cobb BA. B-cell-independent sialylation of IgG. *Proc Natl Acad Sci USA.* (2016) 113:7207–12. doi: 10.1073/pnas.1523968113
46. Ruiz L, Espinosa-Martos I, García-Carral C, Manzano S, McGuire MK, Meehan CL, et al. What's normal? immune profiling of human milk from healthy women living in different geographical and socioeconomic settings. *Front. Immunol.* (2017) 8:696. doi: 10.3389/fimmu.2017.00696
47. Ohlsson A, Lacy JB. Intravenous immunoglobulin for suspected or proven infection in neonates. *Cochrane Database Syst Rev.* (2015) CD001239. doi: 10.1002/14651858.CD001239.pub5
48. Liu P, Li L, Fan P, Zheng J, Zhao D. High-dose of intravenous immunoglobulin modulates immune tolerance in premature infants. *BMC Pediatr.* (2018) 18:74. doi: 10.1186/s12887-018-1055-5

3

Inhibition of Tryptophan Catabolism is Associated with Neuroprotection During Zika Virus Infection

Fernanda Martins Marim[1,2,3], *Danielle Cunha Teixeira*[2,3], *Celso Martins Queiroz-Junior*[2,3,4], *Bruno Vinicius Santos Valiate*[1,3], *Jose Carlos Alves-Filho*[5], *Thiago Mattar Cunha*[5], *Robert Dantzer*[6], *Mauro Martins Teixeira*[1,2,3], *Antonio Lucio Teixeira*[7*] and *Vivian Vasconcelos Costa*[2,3,4*]

[1] Department of Biochemistry and Immunology, Institute of Biological Sciences, Universidade Federal de Minas Gerais, Belo Horizonte, Brazil, [2] Research Group in Arboviral Diseases, Institute of Biological Sciences, Universidade Federal de Minas Gerais, Belo Horizonte, Brazil, [3] Center for Drug Research and Development of Pharmaceuticals, Institute of Biological Sciences, Universidade Federal de Minas Gerais, Belo Horizonte, Brazil, [4] Departament of Morphology, Institute of Biological Sciences, Universidade Federal de Minas Gerais, Belo Horizonte, Brazil, [5] Center for Research in Inflammatory Diseases (CRID), Department of Pharmacology, Ribeirao Preto Medical School, Universidade de São Paulo, Ribeirão Preto, Brazil, [6] Department of Symptom Research, The University of Texas MD Anderson Cancer Center, Houston, TX, United States, [7] Department of Psychiatry and Behavioral Sciences, McGovern Medical Houston, The University of Texas Health Science Center at Houston, Houston, TX, United States

***Correspondence:**
Vivian Vasconcelos Costa
vivianvcosta@gmail.com;
vivianvcosta@ufmg.br
Antonio Lucio Teixeira
altexr@gmail.com

Zika virus (ZIKV) is an arbovirus belonging to *Flaviviridae* family that emerged as a global health threat due to its association with microcephaly and other severe neurological complications, including Guillain-Barré Syndrome (GBS) and Congenital Zika Syndrome (CZS). ZIKV disease has been linked to neuroinflammation and neuronal cell death. Neurodegenerative processes may be exacerbated by metabolites produced by the kynurenine pathway, an important pathway for the degradation of tryptophan, which induces neuronal dysfunction due to enhanced excitotoxicity. Here, we exploited the hypothesis that ZIKV-induced neurodegeneration can be rescued by blocking a target enzyme of the kynurenine pathway, the Indoleamine 2,3-dioxygenase (IDO-1). RT-PCR analysis showed increased levels of IDO-1 RNA expression in undifferentiated primary neurons isolated from wild type (WT) mice infected by ZIKV *ex vivo*, as well as in the brain of ZIKV-infected A129 mice. Pharmacological inhibition of IDO-1 enzyme with 1-methyl-D-tryptophan (1-MT), in both *in vitro* and *in vivo* systems, led to significant reduction of ZIKV-induced neuronal death without interfering with the ability of ZIKV to replicate in those cells. Furthermore, *in vivo* analyses using both genetically modified mice ($IDO^{-/-}$ mice) and A129 mice treated with 1-MT resulted in reduced microgliosis, astrogliosis and Caspase-3 positive cells in the brain of ZIKV-infected A129 mice. Interestingly, increased levels of CCL5 and CXCL-1 chemokines were found in the brain of 1-MT treated-mice. Together, our data indicate that IDO-1 blockade provides a neuroprotective effect against ZIKV-induced neurodegeneration, and this is amenable to inhibition by pharmacological treatment.

Keywords: ***Zika virus*, IDO-1, neuroinflammation, neuronal death, microgliosis**

INTRODUCTION

ZIKV is an arbovirus belonging to the family *Flaviviridae*, genus *Flavivirus*, composed of positive sense, single-stranded RNA. ZIKV was first isolated from a rhesus monkey in 1947 in the Zika forest (Uganda) and humans' infection was reported in Nigeria in 1954 (1). Epidemiological studies suggest that *Zika virus* had a wide geographical distribution, being introduced in Brazil between 2013 and 2015, causing a major epidemic (2) when there was an increase in cases of microcephaly and the incidence of Guillain-Barré syndrome (GBS) (3). ZIKV transmission occurs mainly by culicids of the genus *Aedes* (4), however, other transmission routes such as blood transfusion, sexual transmission and maternal-fetal transmission have already been demonstrated (5).

In humans, the disease caused by ZIKV manifests in about 20% of cases and is characterized by mild clinical symptoms such as fever, headache, myalgia, rash, conjunctivitis and joint pain (6). However, fetal brain samples from infected mothers have shown that ZIKV is able to break through biological placental barriers to infect developing neural cells inducing neuroinflammation, neuronal death, and neurodegeneration, therefore, leading to microcephaly and congenital Zika syndrome, both of which eventually manifest as fetal brain abnormalities (7–11).

The mechanism by which ZIKV exerts these neurological effects has been related to induction of neuronal excitotoxicity, a pathological process mediated by excessive glutamatergic activity (12), infection, activation, and apoptosis of neural progenitor cells, mature neurons, and glial cells with concomitant inflammation (13). Cell death and neurodegenerative processes can be exacerbated by metabolites produced by the kynurenine pathway (KP), an important pathway of degradation of tryptophan, at least in part due to excitotoxicity. Kynurenine pathway is induced by the activation of Indoleamine-2,3-dioxygenase (IDO-1) enzyme in the presence of proinflammatory cytokines, generating several neuroprotective and neurotoxic metabolites (14, 15).

IDO-1 is found in macrophages, monocytes, microglia, astrocytes, and neurons (16, 17) and is considered the major enzyme involved in tryptophan degradation (18). Imbalances in levels of KP metabolites have been associated with neurodegenerative disorders including Huntington's, Alzheimer's, and Parkinson's diseases and other brain disorders as well as several cancers (19). IDO-1 has been linked to neurodegenerative diseases, and have been studied as a possible therapeutic target (19–23).

1-methyl-D-tryptophan (1-MT) is a methylated tryptophan, acting as a competitive IDO-1 inhibitor (24). Recent studies have shown its ability to improve responses to many anticancer therapies and to boost immunity in infectious diseases (24).

In this study we explored the hypothesis that ZIKV-induced neurodegeneration can be rescued by blocking the enzyme IDO-1 that catalyzes the rate-limiting step in KP.

MATERIAL AND METHODS

Animals and Ethics

This study was carried out in accordance with the recommendations of the Brazilian Government (law 11794/2008a) and approved by the Committee on Animal Ethics of Universidade Federal de Minas Gerais (UFMG) (protocol no.106/2020 CEUA/UFMG). All mice were 5 to 8 weeks old and were kept under specific-pathogen-free conditions at 23°C on a 12-h light/12-h dark cycle with food and water provided *ad libitum*. Experiments were conducted using wild-type C57BL/6 mice, type I interferon receptor deficient mice (A129) on SV129/Ev background, and deficient mice in the enzyme indoleamine 2,3-dioxygenase (IDO-$1^{-/-}$) on C57BL/6 background at the Immunopharmacology Laboratory at ICB-UFMG. C57BL/6 mice were purchased from Biotério Central of UFMG, A129 mice were originally purchased from B&K Universal Limited (United Kingdom) and IDO-$1^{-/-}$ were kindly provided by Universidade de São Paulo (USP).

Mouse Experiments

Mice were inoculated with ZIKV by intravenous (I.V) route (tail vein) with $4x10^3$ PFU of ZIKV in a volume of 200 µl PBS or by intracranial (i.c) route with 1x 10^6 PFU of ZIKV in a volume of 20 µl PBS. In some experiments, mice were treated orally with 10 mg/animal of the Indoleamine 2,3-dioxygenase enzyme inhibitor (1-MT), 1 hour after infection and every 24 hours. Clinical symptoms were monitored daily and severely ill mice with a ≥ 20% weight decrease were euthanized. On day 5 after infection (the peak of ZIKV infection), the animals were euthanized to obtain spleen, brain, optic nerve and eye. For primary culture experiments (neurons), brains from mouse embryos on the fifteenth day of the embryonic period (E15) were collected to obtain neuronal cultures.

Virus

A low-passage-number clinical isolate of ZIKV (HS-2015-BA-01), isolated from a viremic patient with symptomatic infection in Bahia State, Brazil, in 2015, was used. The complete genome of the virus is available at GenBank under the accession no. KX520666. Virus stocks were propagated in C6/36 *Aedes albopictus* cells and were titrated in CCL-81 Vero cells as described previously (25).

Intraocular Pressure Measurement (IOP)

The IOP was measured on days 0, 3 and 5 after ZIKV infection using an applanation tonometer (Tono-Pen Vet - Reichert Technologies, NY, USA), as previously described (26–28).

Virus Titration

The viral load on mouse tissues (brain, eye, optic nerve and spleen) and in the supernatant of cell culture samples was determined by plaque assay in CCL-81 Vero cells, as previously described (25). Plaque counts were computed as p.f.u. per gram of tissue mass or milliliter of supernatant.

Evaluation of Inflammatory Markers

The brain tissue was homogenized in a buffer containing protease inhibitors (100 mg of tissue per 1 mL of extraction solution; 0.4 mol/L NaCl, 0.05% Tween 20, 0.5% BSA, 0.1 mmol/L phenylmethyl sulfonil fluoride, 0.1 mmol/L benzethonium chloride, 10 mmol/L EDTA, and 20 KI aprotinin). The brain homogenate was centrifuged at 3000 × *g* for 10 min at 4°C, and the supernatant was collected to determine the concentration of cytokines by ELISA. The cytokines (TNF and IL-1β) and chemokines (CCL5 and CXCL1) levels in the brain of mice were measured using DuoSet ELISA kits antibodies (R&D Systems) in accordance with the manufacturer's instructions. Neutrophil accumulation in mouse brains was also indirectly measured by determining the level of myeloperoxidase activity, according to a previous study (29).

Brains Sections and Staining

For histopathological scoring, brain samples were stained with hematoxylin and eosin (H&E) and the analyses was performed in cerebral cortex and hippocampus sections in a blinded manner according to previous studies (29, 30). Briefly, each brain region was graded on a four-point scale: 0, no tissue damage; 1, minimal tissue damage and/or mild inflammation; 2, mild tissue damage and/or moderate inflammation; 3, severe tissue damage and high inflammation; 4, necrosis with loss of tissue elements and presence of cellular debris. Meningeal inflammation was also graded on a four-point scale: 0, no inflammation; and points between 1 and 4 were assigned when there were one to four layers of cellular inflammation, respectively. The final score was calculated as a sum of cerebral cortex added to the score obtained from the meningeal inflammation analysis, totalizing a maximum of 8 points. For immunostaining analyses, brain samples were processed and sections from hippocampus, striatum, and prefrontal and motor cortex of mice were stained for microglia (IBA1 Polyclonal Antibody – Invitrogen), astrocytes (S100-β polyclonal antibody – Abcam) and apoptosis (Caspase-3 Monoclonal Antibody – Invitrogen) according to manufacturer's instructions (Vector Elite kit - Vector Laboratories) as described in as previously described (31). Image acquisition and analysis were performed using an Olympus BX 41 microscope (Olympus). The images presented in the article are representative of one of those experiments.

Primary Neurons Cell Cultures

Neuronal cultures were prepared from the cortex and striatal regions of E15 of C57BL/6 wild-type mouse embryo brains. After dissection, the brain tissue was submitted to trypsin digestion followed by cell dissociation using a fire-polished Pasteur pipette. Neuronal cells were plated onto poly-L-ornithine-coated dishes in neurobasal medium supplemented with N2 and B27 supplements (Gibco), 2 mM GlutaMAX (Gibco) and 50 g/ml penicillin/streptomycin (Sigma), incubated at 37°C and 5% CO_2 for 5 days. Infection was performed with ZIKV (MOI of 0.1), followed by an adsorption period of 1 h. Wells were washed with incomplete medium and each well was replaced by a final volume of complete neurobasal medium. In some experiments, neuronal cultures were treated with 3, 10, 30 or 100 μM of the Indoleamine 2,3-dioxygenase enzyme inhibitor every 24h. Beside the kinetic experiments, all experiments evaluating the effects of 1-MT on primary neurons were performed after 48 h of ZIKV infection. At the time point, the supernatant was collected for quantification of viral load while the cells adhered to the plate were used in the cell death assay.

Neuronal Cell Viability

Neuronal cell death was assessed by LIVE/DEAD Cell Viability Assays after 48 hours of ZIKV infection, as previously described (27). Briefly, the neuronal cell culture was stained with 2 μM calcein acetoxymethyl ester (AM) and 2 μM ethidium homodimer -1. After 10 minutes, the neuronal culture was immediately visualized by a FLoid Cell Imaging Station fluorescence microscope (Thermo Fisher Scientific). Images were captured and the fractions of live (green, calcein AM) and dead (red, ethidium homodimer -1) cells in the same field of view were evaluated. Cell viability was analyzed, and the quantification was performed using the ImageJ software. Data are reported as the percentage of dead cells out of the total number of cells.

Real-Time RT-PCR

RNA was isolated using TRIzol™ reagent in accordance with the manufacturer's instructions (Invitrogen). RNA was resuspended in 30 μL of nuclease-free water, and its concentration was analyzed by Nanodrop spectrophotometer. cDNAs were prepared from 2 μg of total RNA extracted in a 10 μL final reverse transcription reaction. RT-qPCR was performed from 10x diluted cDNA using SYBR Green PCR Master Mix (Applied Biosystems). Real-time was performed in a 7500 Fast Real-Time PCR System (Applied Biosystems). The appropriate primers were used to amplify a specific fragment corresponding to specific gene targets as follows: GAPDH F: 5'-ACG GCC GCA TCT TCT TGT GCA- 3'; GAPDH R: 5' -CGC CCA AAT CCG TTC ACA CCG A- 3; IDO-1 F: 5'-TCA AAG CAA TCC CCA CTG TAT CC- 3'; IDO-1 R: 5' -TCC ACA AAG TCA CGC ATC CTC- 3'. All data are presented as relative expression units after normalization to GAPDH gene, and measurements were conducted in duplicate.

Statistical Analysis

Results were expressed as Mean ± SEM for the number of independent experiments. GraphPad Prism (GraphPad Software, Inc) was used to analyze data using different-tests as appropriate and $P < 0.05$, $P < 0.01$, $P < 0.001$ and $P < 0.0001$

indicate the levels of statistical significance. Additional information is indicated in *Figure Legends*.

RESULTS

IDO-1 Expression Is Enhanced Upon ZIKV Infection *In Vitro* and *In Vivo*

The KP is segregated into two distinct branches triggering neurotoxic and neuroprotective metabolites. The first step of KP converts the essential amino acid L-tryptophan to N-formylkynurenine and is regulated by rate-limiting enzymes, being the Indoleamine 2,3-dioxygenase 1 (IDO-1) the main enzyme contributing to the production of kynurenines during inflammatory conditions (32). Therefore, differential mRNA expression of IDO-1 was investigated in non-infected and ZIKV-infected primary neuron cultures from cortex and striatal regions obtained from wild type (WT) C57BL/6 mice embryo brains. After 48 hours of ZIKV infection, there was an increase in the levels of IDO-1 when compared to Mock control in primary neuron cultures (**Figure 1A**). Additionally, increased levels of IDO-1 expression were also seen in the brain of A129 mice infected with ZIKV, 5 days upon infection, peak of disease manifestation in these mice, when compared to Mock littermates (**Figure 1B**). These results clearly demonstrate that ZIKV infection induced increased expression of IDO-1 enzyme *in vitro* and *in vivo*.

1-MT Inhibitor Reduces Neuronal Death in ZIKV Primary Neurons

Subsequently, we evaluated the effect of blockade of IDO-1 enzyme *in vitro*. Previous studies by our group have shown that undifferentiated neuronal cultures are highly susceptible to ZIKV infection, inducing neuronal death (27, 33). Then, we tested whether the IDO-I inhibitor, 1-methyl-D-tryptophan (1-MT) would reduce ZIKV-induced neuronal cell death. For that, primary neuronal cultures obtained from the corticostriatal region of C57BL/6 embryo brains were infected with ZIKV (MOI 0.1) and treated with 1-MT at concentrations of 3; 10; 30 and 100 μM. After 48 hours following infection, the supernatant was collected to evaluate viral load by plaque assay and cells were subjected to cell viability assays. ZIKV neuronal infection resulted in 10^9 PFU/mL in the culture supernatants, and *in vitro* IDO-1 inhibition with 1-MT did not interfere with ability of the virus to replicate in these cells. The highest 1-MT concentration triggered some reduction of the viral load (**Figure 2A**). Nevertheless, 1-MT treatment induced a significant reduction of neuronal cell death, in all evaluated concentrations (**Figures 2B, C**). At the concentration of 100 μM 1-MT, cytotoxicity was detected in infected cells, but without reaching statistical difference.

IDO-1 Inhibition Did Not Prevent ZIKV-Induced Clinical Manifestations as Well as Virus Replication in A129 Mice

Further, we investigated the effects of IDO-1 inhibition during ZIKV infection *in vivo*. For that, A129 mice were inoculated (i.v) with 4 x 10^3 PFU of ZIKV and, after 1 hour, they were treated with 1-MT and every 24 hours until euthanasia (**Figure 3A**). Five days after infection, peak of disease manifestation in this model, spleen, brain, optic nerve and eye of the animals were collected. In accordance with previous studies from our group (27), there was significant body weight loss in the ZIKV group when compared to Mock control. Similarly, infected mice treated

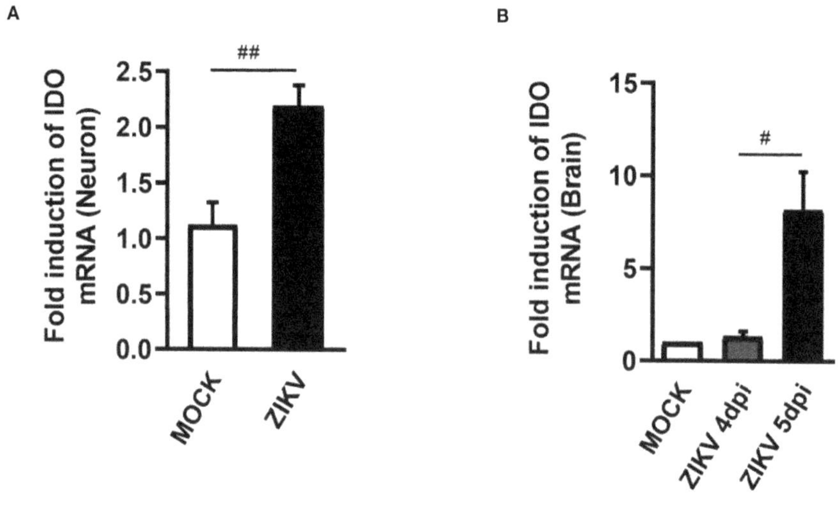

FIGURE 1 | IDO-1 expression induced by ZIKV infection. **(A)** Primary culture of cortical-striatal neurons from C57BL/6 mice on D5 were infected with ZIKV (MOI 0.1) and after 48 hours the cells were harvested. **(B)** Type I interferon receptor deficient mice (A129) were inoculated (i.v) with 4x10^3 PFU/200 μL of ZIKV. At day 4 and 5 of infection, the brain was harvested. RNA extraction and subsequent Real time PCR analysis of IDO-1 expression in the brain and neuronal primary culture was done. Results are expressed as mean ± SEM and are representative of two independent experiments. Statistically significant differences were assessed by Mann Whitney test. (#) for *P < 0.05* and (##) for *P < 0.01*.

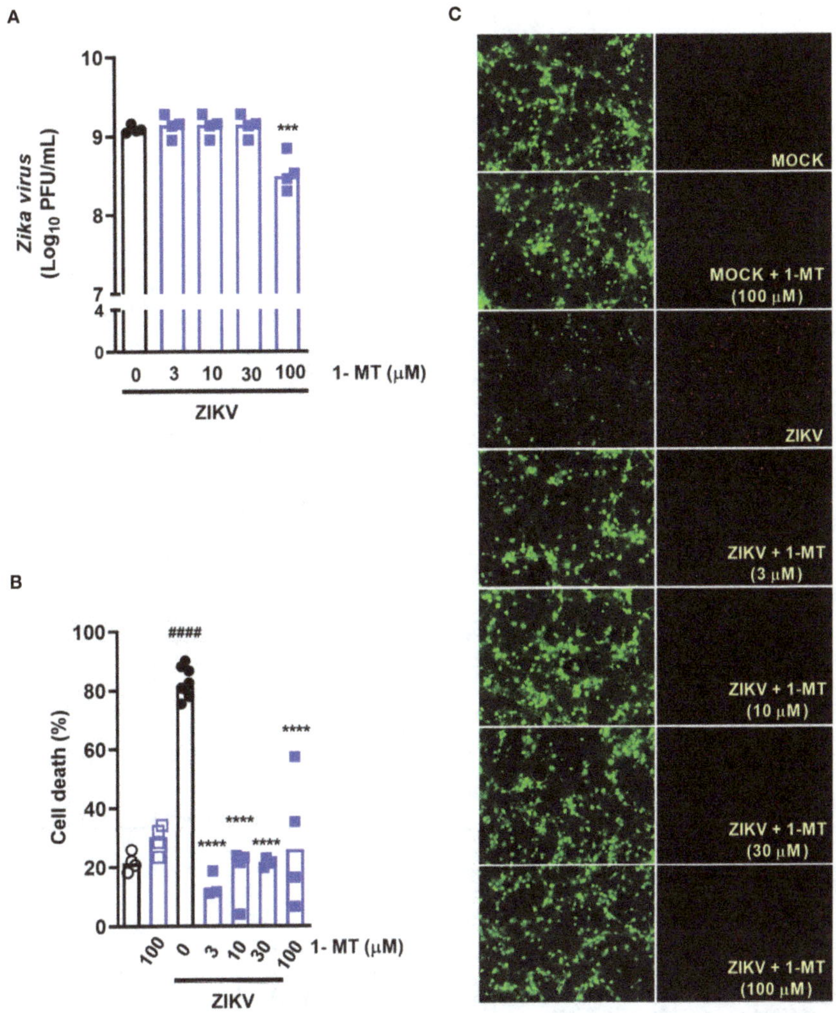

FIGURE 2 | IDO-1 inhibition in primary undifferentiated neurons infected by ZIKV. Primary culture of cortical-striatal neurons on D5. Neuronal culture from C57BL/6 mice were infected with ZIKV (MOI 0.1) and treated with 1-MT inhibitor at concentrations of 3; 10; 30 and 100 μM. After 48 hours, **(A)** the supernatant was collected to assess viral load, **(B)** cell death was assessed using the LIVE/DEAD Cell Viability Assay. **(C)** Representative images of infected and uninfected neurons stained with calcein AM (green indicates live cells) and ethidium homodimer (red indicates dead cells). All results are expressed as median and are representative of at least two independent experiments. Statistically significant differences were assessed by One-way ANOVA plus Holm-Sidak's or Tukey's comparisons test. (####) for $P < 0,0001$ compared to the MOCK group; (***) for $P < 0,001$ and (****) for $P < 0,0001$ compared to the ZIKV group.

with 1-MT lost as much weight as the ZIKV group (**Figure 3B**). Ophthalmic alterations induced by ZIKV infection were also evaluated through the measurement of intraocular pressure (IOP), but no significant differences were detected between infected groups, treated or not with 1-MT (**Figure 3C**). Moreover, 1-MT treatment of ZIKV-infected mice did not interfere with viral loads detected in the brain (**Figure 3D**), optic nerve (**Figure 3E**), eye (**Figure S1A**) or spleen (**Figure S1B**). No significant differences were detected in neutrophils recruitment to the brain (**Figure 3F**). Although 1-MT did not prevent viral replication, it induced larger production of the chemokines CCL5 (**Figure 3G**) and CXCL1 (**Figure 3H**) in the brain of infected mice when compared to non-treated ZIKV group, but there was no difference in TNF (**Figure 3I**) and IL -1β (**Figure 3J**) levels. Overall, the results show that IDO-1 inhibition was not able to reduce clinical manifestations induced by ZIKV-infection, as well as virus replication in A129 mice.

IDO-1 Inhibition Prevents Microgliosis, Astroglioses and Caspase-3 Expression of Cells in the Brain of ZIKV Infected Mice

Infection of A129 mice with ZIKV triggered histopathological signs of brain inflammation and tissue damage. Histopathological analysis of the brain revealed mild gliosis and meningitis 5 days after ZIKV infection. Such changes were similar in non-treated and 1-MT-treated ZIKV-infected mice (**Figures 4A, B**). Despite such evidence, 1-MT treatment prompted a significant reduction in the number of IBA-1

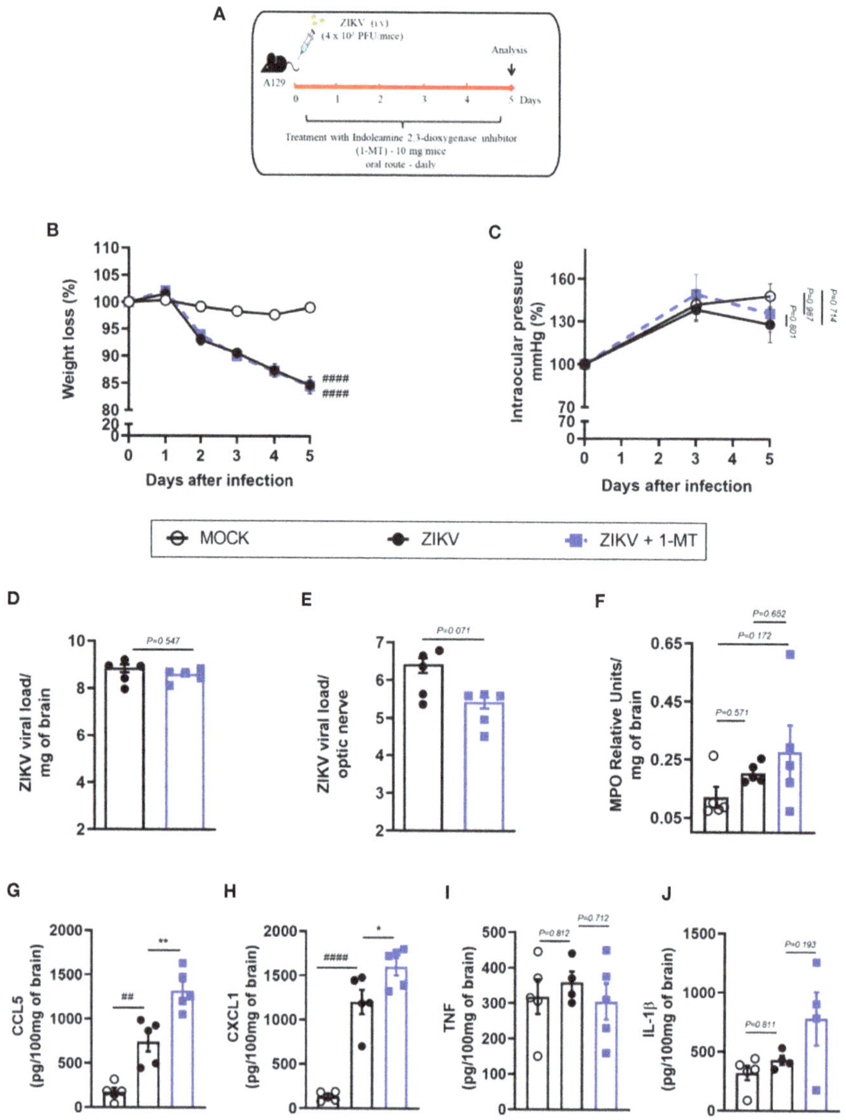

FIGURE 3 | Clinical signs and inflammatory parameters in A129 mice infected by ZIKV treated or not with 1-MT inhibitor. **(A)** Experimental schematic representation of experimental strategy. A129 were inoculated (i.v) with $4x10^3$ PFU/200µL of ZIKV and treated daily with 1-MT. **(B)** The body weight was evaluated daily and **(C)** the intraocular pressure was analyzed on days 0, 3 and 5. At day 5 of infection, **(D)** the brain and **(E)** optical nerve was harvested for plaque assay analysis. **(F)** Measurement of myeloperoxidase activity (neutrophil accumulation) and **(G–J)** chemokine/cytokine production was assessed in mouse brain of animals. All results are expressed as mean and error bar indicate the standard error (SEM) and are representative of at least two independent experiments. Statistically significant differences were assessed by Two-way ANOVA plus Tukey's comparisons test **(A, B)**, Mann Whitney test **(D, E)** and One-way ANOVA **(F–J)** plus Tukey's comparisons test. (##) for $P < 0{,}01$ and (####) for $P < 0{,}0001$ when compared to the MOCK group. (*) for $P < 0{,}05$ and (**) for $P < 0{,}001$ compared to the ZIKV group.

positive cells (IBA-1$^+$ cells) in the cerebral cortex of infected mice (**Figures 4C, D**). In addition, there was significant reduction in the number of astrocytes (S100β$^+$ cells) in 1-MT-treated group when compared to non-treated ZIKV infected group (**Figures 4E, F**). Another important feature of ZIKV infection is neurodegeneration, including cell death. In this regard, treatment of infected mice with 1- MT decreased the number of brain Caspase-3-positive cells (Caspase-3$^+$ cells), which is suggestive of reduced apoptosis (**Figures 4G, H**).

Effects of ZIKV Infection in Indoleamine 2,3-Dioxigenase 1 (IDO-1$^{-/-}$) Deficient Mice

In view of the effects observed after 1-MT treatment and the potential contribution of this pathway in preventing neurodegeneration, we also evaluated ZIKV infection in genetically modified Indoleamine 2,3-dioxigenase 1 deficient (IDO-1$^{-/-}$) mice. Since C57BL/6 mice are resistant to ZIKV infection (27, 34, 35), ZIKV infection was performed by intracerebral route by inoculation of with 1 x 10^6 PFU of

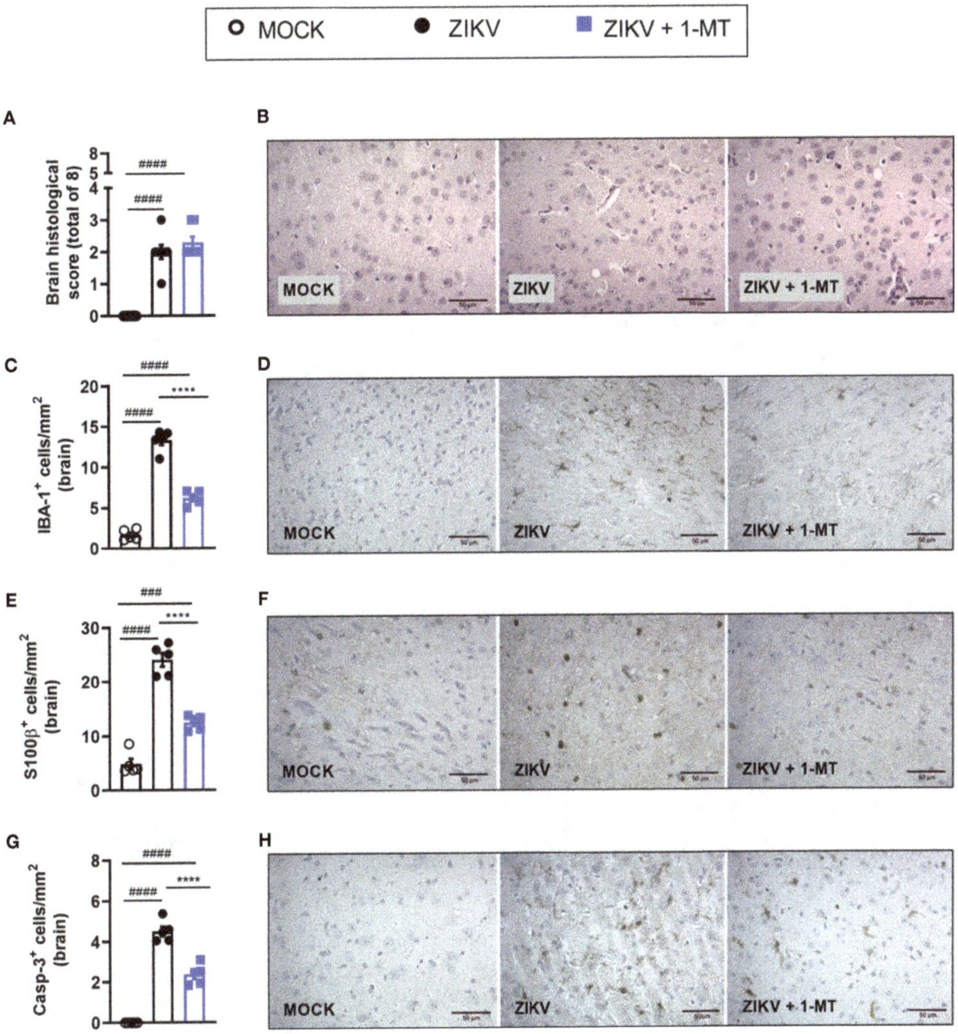

FIGURE 4 | Morphometric analysis of the brain of A129 mice infected by ZIKV, treated or not with 1-MT inhibitor. A129 were inoculated (i.v) with 4x10^3 PFU/200μL of ZIKV and treated daily with 1-MT. **(A)** Semiquantitative analysis (histopathological score) after H&E staining of brain sections of ZIKV-infected mice 5 days after infection. **(C, E, G)** Immunostaining of **(C)** IBA-1$^+$, **(E)** S100-β$^+$ and **(G)** Caspase-3 was performed in the brains of mice. **(B, D, F, H)** Representative images from brain sections. All results are expressed as mean and error bar indicate the standard error (SEM) and are representative of at least two independent experiments. Statistically significant differences were assessed by One-way ANOVA plus Tukey's comparisons test. (###) for *P < 0,001* and (####) for *P < 0,0001* when compared to the MOCK group. (****) for *P < 0,0001* compared to the ZIKV group.

ZIKV (i.c) in both WT C57BL/6 and IDO-1$^{-/-}$ mice (**Figure 5A**). Body weight loss was significantly higher in C57BL/6 and IDO-1$^{-/-}$ mice infected with ZIKV than in their respective controls (**Figure 5B**). Furthermore, there was no significant change in the IOP levels between WT and IDO-1$^{-/-}$ ZIKV-infected groups (**Figure 5C**). Regarding viral replication, no viable virus (assessed by plaque assay) or ZIKV genome (RT-PCR) was detected in the brain of ZIKV-infected WT or IDO-1$^{-/-}$ mice. Accordingly, no difference in MPO levels was detected into mice's brains (**Figure 5D**). Finally, as demonstrated during 1-MT treatment, intracranial ZIKV infection also led to increased production of inflammatory mediators, such as CCL5 (**Figure 5E**) and CXCL1 (**Figure 5F**) in both WT and IDO-1$^{-/-}$ ZIKV mice. Production of TNF and IL-1β in WT and IDO-1$^{-/-}$ was analogous to Mock (**Figures 5G, H**). Additionally, in a pattern similar to that observed in A129 mice treated with 1-MT, brain histopathological analysis of C57BL/6 and IDO-1$^{-/-}$ infected mice revealed mild gliosis and meningitis in both infected experimental groups (**Figures 6A, B**). Accordingly, reduced microgliosis, astrogliosis and apoptosis were found in infected IDO-1$^{-/-}$ mice in comparison to ZIKV infected WT littermates as demonstrated by reduction of the number of IBA-1 (**Figures 6C, D**), S100β (**Figures 6E, F**) and Caspase-3 (**Figures 6G, H**) positive cells of mice's brain sections. Furthermore, the morphology of the Caspase-3-stained cells, especially the nucleus morphology, comprised both neurons and glial cells.

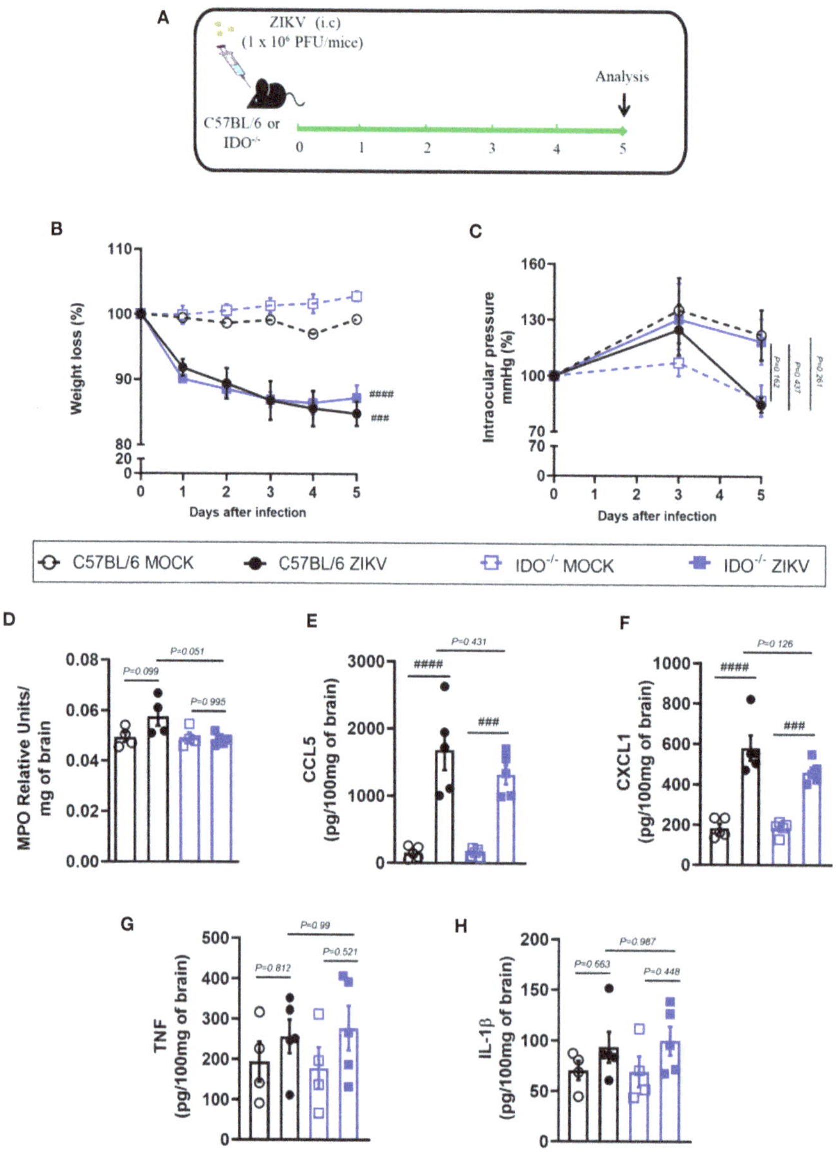

FIGURE 5 | Clinical signs and inflammatory parameters after ZIKV infection of WT and IDO$^{-/-}$ mice infected by ZIKV. **(A)** Experimental schematic representation of experimental strategy. C57BL/6 and IDO-1$^{-/-}$ were inoculated (intracranial) with 1x10^{6} PFU/20µL of ZIKV. **(B)** The body weight was evaluated daily and **(C)** the intraocular pressure was analyzed on days 0, 3 and 5. At day 5 of infection, **(D)** the brain was harvested and myeloperoxidase absorbance analysis and **(E–H)** chemokine/cytokine production was assessed. All results are expressed as mean and error bar indicate the standard error (SEM) and are representative of at least two independent experiments. Statistically significant differences were assessed by Two-way ANOVA plus Tukey's comparisons test **(B, C)** and One-way ANOVA plus Tukey's comparisons test (D-H). (###) for *P < 0,001* and (####) for *P < 0,0001* compared to the MOCK group.

DISCUSSION

Several studies have reported the tropism of the ZIKV to different cellular types, tissues and body fluids. Meanwhile, ZIKV-tropism to the CNS is the most harmful feature to the host and may cause neurodegeneration and other neuronal dysfunctions. Despite its association with neurological diseases, such as microcephaly, GBS and CZS, there are no current approved therapies for the treatment of this important pathogen (36). In order to develop effective therapies, a better understanding of the pathogenicity resulting from the virus-host interaction is required. Global analysis of gene expression shows that ZIKV infection prompts significant dysregulation of several host factors associated with neural development, immune response, cell death, among others (37, 38). In the present study, we evaluated the potential neuroprotective effect of the blockade of IDO-1 enzyme by using a genetically approach (IDO-1$^{-/-}$ mice) or a pharmacological strategy (1-MT inhibitor), *in vitro* and *in vivo*. The main results

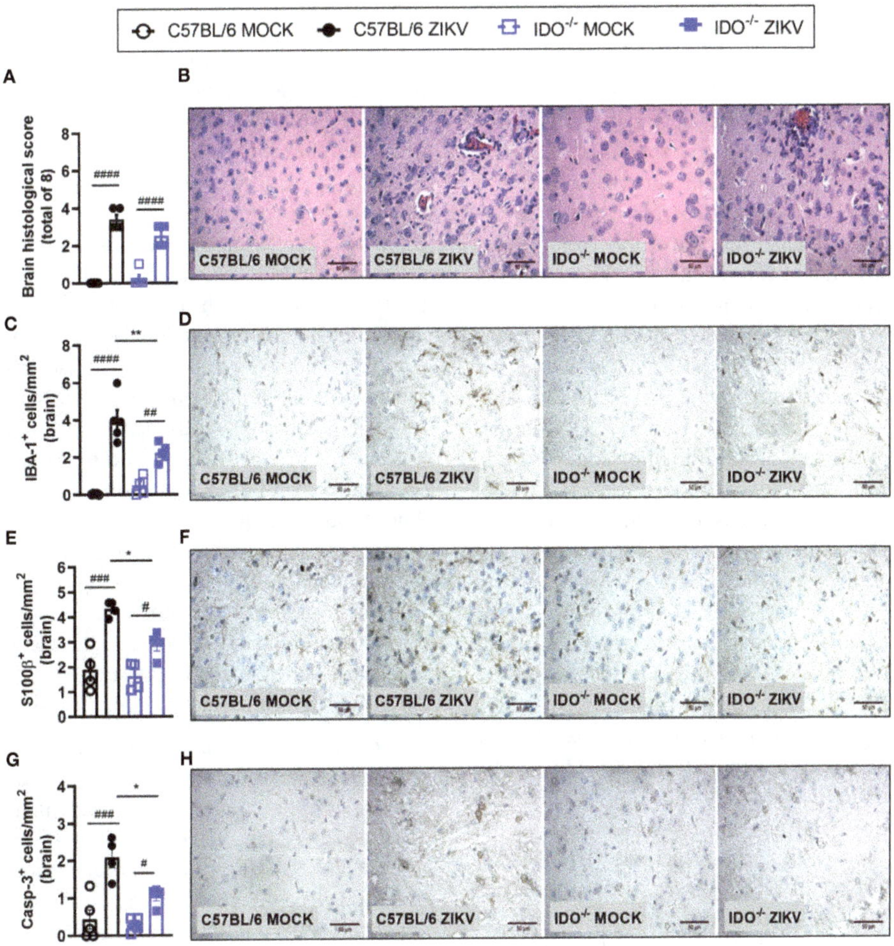

FIGURE 6 | Morphometric analysis of the brain of WT and IDO$^{-/-}$ mice infected by ZIKV. C57BL/6 and IDO-1$^{-/-}$ were inoculated (intracranial) with 1x10^6 PFU/20µL of ZIKV. **(A)** Semiquantitative analysis (histopathological score) after H&E staining of brain sections of ZIKV-infected mice 5 days after infection. **(C, E, G)** Immunostaining of **(C)** IBA-1$^+$, **(E)** S100-β$^+$ and **(G)** Caspase-3 was performed in the brains of mice. **(B, D, F, H)** Representative images from brain sections. Results are expressed as mean and error bar indicate the standard error (SEM) and are representative of at least two independent experiments. Statistically significant differences were assessed by One-way ANOVA plus Tukey's comparisons test (#) for $P < 0,05$, (##) for $P < 0,01$ and (###) for $P < 0,001$ and (####) for $P < 0,0001$ when compared to the MOCK group. (*) for $P < 0,05$ and (**) for $P < 0,01$ compared to the ZIKV group.

were: (I) increased levels of IDO-1 expression after ZIKV infection; (II) reduction of neuronal death upon 1-MT treatment; (III); massive reduction of ZIKV-induced microgliosis, astrogliosis and apoptosis in IDO$^{-/-}$ mice and after 1-MT administration in A129 mice. Overall, these data indicate a neuroprotective effect induced by IDO-1 inhibition after ZIKV infection *in vivo* and *in vitro*.

IDO-1 is the first rate-limiting of the KP responsible for converting tryptophan into several downstream kynurenine metabolites. This enzyme is expressed by many cell types, including macrophages, microglia, dendritic cells, astrocytes, fibroblasts, and epithelial cells (32) and is commonly induced by proinflammatory cytokines. In the current study, we showed that ZIKV infection increased levels of IDO-1 expression in mice's brain and also in primary neuron culture obtained from embryonic brains of mice. These results demonstrate that Indoleamine-2,3-dioxygenase, or IDO-1, is activated by the inflammatory response induced by ZIKV. In this context, we next, evaluated the effects of the inhibition of IDO-1 on ZIKV infection *in vitro* and *in vivo* systems. We found that a pharmacological inhibition in primary neurons infected by ZIKV did not prevent viral replication but induced less cell death. Likewise, human monocyte-derived macrophages induce IDO-1 expression upon West Nile virus (WNV), *via* TNF and NF-KB signaling, but IDO was not essential for the control of WNV infection (39). Similarly, 1-MT treatment of ZIKV-infected mice did not interfere with the ability of ZIKV to replicate in the brain, optic nerve, eye or spleen tissues. Additionally, no significant difference in neutrophil recruitment was observed between treated and non-treated ZIKV-infected mice. At the same time, chemokines relevant for the migration of monocytes, lymphocytes, as well as for neutrophil traffic, such as CCL5 and CXCL1, respectively, had increased levels in 1-MT treated ZIKV mice. We also evaluated ZIKV infection in IDO-1$^{-/-}$ mice and WT mouse model. Corroborating the pharmacological data, the absence of IDO did not interfere with clinical signs, viral replication or inflammatory parameters, although microgliosis, astrogliosis and caspase-3 expression reduced after infection. Chemokine signaling plays an important homeostatic role and modulates neuroprotective processes on different stimuli, orchestrating the action of neurons-microglia-astrocytes to preserve brain damage (40). In pathological processes, pro-inflammatory cytokines and chemokines are robustly induced and can lead IDO-1 activity and tryptophan associated metabolites (39, 41, 42). IDO-1 inhibition in Influenza virus infection does not affect leukocyte infiltration or viral clearance, thus, blockade of IDO-1 could play a beneficial role in host protection (43–45). These data show that pharmacological inhibition or genetic ablation of IDO-1 did not completely prevent brain inflammation, but reduced brain damage and cell death.

ZIKV can infect almost all CNS cells, including neurons, glial cells, endothelial cells and pericytes. Activated CNS-resident cells could be the source of proinflammatory cytokines and chemokines such as CCL5 and CXCL1, found in ZIKV-infected brain tissue. ZIKV infection and replication are associated with brain damage and, as consequence, severe neurological symptoms (8, 27). The mechanisms by which ZIKV exert these effects involve neuronal excitotoxicity and apoptosis of microglia, astrocytes and other cells. Our group has shown that neuronal cell death induced by ZIKV is associated with excitotoxicity mediated by the release of glutamate and other neurotoxic factors such as TNF and IL-1β, inducing the activation of NMDA (N-methyl-d-aspartate receptor) receptors (27, 33). Accordingly, treatment with Memantine (an FDA-approved allosteric NMDA receptor antagonist) *in vivo* and *in vitro* was effective to prevent ZIKV-induced cell death and neurodegeneration but did not interfere with the ability of the virus to replicate. Furthermore, administration of Ifenprodil (a selective inhibitor of the NMDA receptor, specifically for the GluN1 and GluN2B subunits) in a primary neuron culture rescues ZIKV-induced neurotoxicity (27, 33). IDO expression in Huntington's disease is chronically elevated, inducing neurotoxicity, and IDO inhibition reduces neurotoxicity sensitivity and neuroprotective role (46).

Cell death and neurodegenerative processes can be exacerbated by metabolites produced by KP. Kynurenine metabolism is directly associated with several neurodegenerative and neurological diseases, such as Alzheimer's disease, multiple sclerosis, and stroke (23, 47). In accordance with recent studies from our group (27, 33, 48), infection of A129 mice induced brain inflammation and tissue damage, and we found mild gliosis and meningitis in all infected mice groups. However, pharmacological inhibition or deletion of IDO-1 (IDO$^{-/-}$) prompted a significant reduction of IBA-1 positive cells in the brain's mice, suggesting less microglia activation. It appears that microglia activation is dependent on IDO-1 (49, 50). In a similar pattern, we found a reduction in the number of astrocytes (S100β positive cells). Microglia and activated astrocytes produce several inflammatory mediators, including IL-1β, TNF, glutamate, nitric oxide (NO) among others, which can trigger neuronal death after ZIKV infection (33). In addition, ZIKV-induced neurodegeneration can be caused by loss of structure or function of neurons. Recent studies demonstrated that ZIKV is able to induce apoptosis of neuronal cells *in vitro* (33) and *in vivo* (28). In this regard, we have shown that treatment of infected mice with 1-MT decreased the number of brain Caspase-3-positive cells, which is suggestive of reduced apoptosis. According to cell morphology, especially the nucleus, these cells comprised both neurons and glial cells, however, co-localization assays were not performed (Caspase-3/IBA-1 or Caspase-3/S100β or NeuN/Caspase-3). Although ZIKV-induces neuronal damage, it is unclear whether neuronal death is due to direct neurotoxicity or secondary to the activation of microglia and astrocytes. Apoptosis can be a result from inflammatory mediators released by the activated microglia or induced in a non-cell autonomous manner, triggering cell death of uninfected neurons by releasing cytotoxic factors (33). These data suggest the pharmacological or genetic inhibition of IDO-1 prevents microglial activation, astrogliosis and apoptosis in the brain of ZIKV infected, without preventing clinical outcomes.

Development of efficient therapies against viral infections, such as ZIKV, is important for the control and reduction of clinical symptoms, viral load, neuroinflammation, and mainly, neurodegeneration. A combination of compounds that could prevent ZIKV-induced neurodegeneration with viral replication (antiviral drugs) represents the ideal treatment. Meanwhile, no approved antiviral drugs are available. Recently, our group showed that a therapeutic administration of an antiviral peptide (AH-D) significantly reduced viral loads in serum, spleen, brain and optical nerve throughout the course of ZIKV infection (30). Additionally, we also demonstrated the efficacy of the 7-Deaza-7-fluoro-2'-C-methyl adenosine (DFMA), a nucleoside analogue, which showed significant antiviral effects against ZIKV *in vitro* and *in vivo* systems, especially when administered prophylactically and at early times after ZIKV infection (48). These compounds open a new perspective to evaluate the synergic effect of a neuroprotective drug such as 1-MT along with an antiviral drug against ZIKV-induced disease in an early future.

In conclusion, our data indicate that IDO-1 inhibition exerts a neuroprotective role in CNS reducing the microglial activation, astrogliosis and apoptosis without antiviral effect. Further studies are required to elucidate the mechanisms of neuroprotection obtained by ablation of IDO-1 and it will be important to evaluate whether the combination of neuroprotective drugs, such 1-MT, and antiviral like AH-D or DFMA could be the treatment for ZIKV infection.

ETHICS STATEMENT

The animal study was reviewed and approved by Committee on Animal Ethics of Universidade Federal de Minas Gerais (UFMG) (protocol no.106/2020 CEUA/UFMG).

AUTHOR CONTRIBUTIONS

FM, JA-F, TC, MT, AT, and VC designed the study. FM, DT, CQ-J, and BV conducted the experiments and analysis of the data. FM, AT, and VC interpreted the results. FM, CQ-J, AT, and VC wrote the first draft of the paper. RD, MT, AT, and VC obtained funding. All authors contributed to the article and approved the submitted version.

FUNDING

This work was supported by the Grants from National Institute of Science and Technology in Dengue and Host-microorganism Interaction (INCT dengue), which is a programme sponsored by the Brazilian National Science Council (CNPq, Brazil) and the Minas Gerais Foundation for Science (FAPEMIG, Brazil). This work also received support from Coordenação de Aperfeiçoamento de Pessoal de Nível Superior - CAPES/Brazil (grant no CAPES: 88881.130741), ZIKALLIANCE consortium - 734548, Financiadora de Estudos e Pesquisa (FINEP 01.16.0050.00, Brazil), Conselho Nacional de Desenvolvimento Cientifico e Tecnológico (CNPq) under grants: 425359/2018 and 440423/2016-13, Fundação de Amparo à Pesquisa do Estado de Minas Gerais (FAPEMIG, Brazil) - APQ-02281- 18) and by L'Oréal-Unesco-ABC For Women in Science Program). Also, this work was funded by NIH (R01 CA193522 and R01 NS073939) and an MD Anderson Cancer Support Grant (P30 CA016672).

ACKNOWLEDGMENTS

We thank Ilma Marçal and Tania Colina for technical support during the study.

SUPPLEMENTARY MATERIAL

Supplementary Figure 1 | Viral load in the eye and spleen of A129 mice infected by ZIKV, treated or not with 1-MT inhibitor. A129 were inoculated (i.v) with 4x10^3 PFU/200µL of ZIKV and treated daily with 1-MT. **(A)** Eye and **(B)** spleen was harvested for plaque assay analysis. All results are expressed as mean and error bar indicate the standard error (SEM) and are representative of at least two independent experiments. Statistically significant differences were assessed by One-way ANOVA plus Tukey's comparisons test.

REFERENCES

1. Macnamara FN. Zika Virus: A Report on Three Cases of Human Infection During an Epidemic of Jaundice in Nigeria. *Trans R Soc Trop Med Hyg* (1954) 48(2):139–45. doi: 10.1016/0035-9203(54)90006-1
2. Baud D, Gubler DJ, Schaub B, Lanteri MC, Musso D. An Update on Zika Virus Infection. *Lancet* (2017) 390(10107):2099–109. doi: 10.1016/S0140-6736(17)31450-2
3. Campos GS, Bandeira AC, Sardi SI. Zika Virus Outbreak, Bahia, Brazil. *Emerg Infect Dis* (2015) 21(10):1885–6. doi: 10.3201/eid2110.150847
4. Cunha MS, Esposito DL, Rocco IM, Maeda AY, Vasami FG, Nogueira JS, et al. First Complete Genome Sequence of Zika Virus (Flaviviridae, Flavivirus) From an Autochthonous Transmission in Brazil. *Genome Announc* (2016) 4 (2):e00032-16. doi: 10.1128/genomeA.00032-16
5. Kurscheidt FA, Mesquita CSS, Damke G, Damke E, Carvalho A, Suehiro TT, et al. Persistence and Clinical Relevance of Zika Virus in the Male Genital Tract. *Nat Rev Urol* (2019) 16(4):211–30. doi: 10.1038/s41585-019-0149-7
6. Duffy MR, Chen TH, Hancock WT, Powers AM, Kool JL, Lanciotti RS, et al. Zika Virus Outbreak on Yap Island, Federated States of Micronesia. *N Engl J Med* (2009) 360(24):2536–43. doi: 10.1056/NEJMoa0805715
7. Cugola FR, Fernandes IR, Russo FB, Freitas BC, Dias JL, Guimaraes KP, et al. The Brazilian Zika Virus Strain Causes Birth Defects in Experimental Models. *Nature* (2016) 534(7606):267–71. doi: 10.1038/nature18296
8. Garcez PP, Loiola EC, Madeiro da Costa R, Higa LM, Trindade P, Delvecchio R, et al. Zika Virus Impairs Growth in Human Neurospheres and Brain Organoids. *Science* (2016) 352(6287):816–8. doi: 10.1126/science.aaf6116
9. Noronha L, Zanluca C, Azevedo ML, Luz KG, Santos CN. Zika Virus Damages the Human Placental Barrier and Presents Marked Fetal Neurotropism. *Mem Inst Oswaldo Cruz* (2016) 111(5):287–93. doi: 10.1590/0074-02760160085
10. Dallmeier K, Neyts J. Zika and Other Emerging Viruses: Aiming at the Right Target. *Cell Host Microbe* (2016) 20(4):420–2. doi: 10.1016/j.chom.2016.09.011
11. Saiz JC, Martin-Acebes MA. The Race To Find Antivirals for Zika Virus. *Antimicrob Agents Chemother* (2017) 61(6):e00411-17. doi: 10.1128/AAC.00411-17
12. Dong XX, Wang Y, Qin ZH. Molecular Mechanisms of Excitotoxicity and Their Relevance to Pathogenesis of Neurodegenerative Diseases. *Acta Pharmacol Sin* (2009) 30(4):379–87. doi: 10.1038/aps.2009.24
13. Marim FM, Camargos VN, Queiroz-Junior CM, Costa VV. Zika Virus Infection and Potential Mechanisms Implicated in Neuropsychiatric Complications. In: AL Teixeira, D Macedo, BT Baune, editors. *Perinatal Inflammation and Adult Psychopathology: From Preclinical Models to Humans*. Springer (2020). p. 207–22.
14. O'Connor JC, Andre C, Wang Y, Lawson MA, Szegedi SS, Lestage J, et al. Interferon-Gamma and Tumor Necrosis Factor-Alpha Mediate the Upregulation of Indoleamine 2,3-Dioxygenase and the Induction of Depressive-Like Behavior in Mice in Response to Bacillus Calmette-Guerin. *J Neurosci* (2009) 29(13):4200–9. doi: 10.1523/JNEUROSCI.5032-08.2009
15. Campbell BM, Charych E, Lee AW, Moller T. Kynurenines in CNS Disease: Regulation by Inflammatory Cytokines. *Front Neurosci* (2014) 8:12. doi: 10.3389/fnins.2014.00012
16. Guillemin GJ, Cullen KM, Lim CK, Smythe GA, Garner B, Kapoor V, et al. Characterization of the Kynurenine Pathway in Human Neurons. *J Neurosci* (2007) 27(47):12884–92. doi: 10.1523/JNEUROSCI.4101-07.2007
17. Jones SP, Guillemin GJ, Brew BJ. The Kynurenine Pathway in Stem Cell Biology. *Int J Tryptophan Res* (2013) 6:57–66. doi: 10.4137/IJTR.S12626
18. Lob S, Konigsrainer A, Zieker D, Brucher BL, Rammensee HG, Opelz G, et al. IDO1 and IDO2 Are Expressed in Human Tumors: Levo- But Not Dextro-1-Methyl Tryptophan Inhibits Tryptophan Catabolism. *Cancer Immunol Immunother* (2009) 58(1):153–7. doi: 10.1007/s00262-008-0513-6
19. Maddison DC, Giorgini F. The Kynurenine Pathway and Neurodegenerative Disease. *Semin Cell Dev Biol* (2015) 40:134–41. doi: 10.1016/j.semcdb.2015.03.002
20. Zadori D, Klivenyi P, Szalardy L, Fulop F, Toldi J, Vecsei L. Mitochondrial Disturbances, Excitotoxicity, Neuroinflammation and Kynurenines: Novel Therapeutic Strategies for Neurodegenerative Disorders. *J Neurol Sci* (2012) 322(1-2):187–91. doi: 10.1016/j.jns.2012.06.004

21. Giil LM, Midttun O, Refsum H, Ulvik A, Advani R, Smith AD, et al. Kynurenine Pathway Metabolites in Alzheimer's Disease. *J Alzheimers Dis* (2017) 60(2):495–504. doi: 10.3233/JAD-170485
22. Hestad KA, Engedal K, Whist JE, Farup PG. The Relationships Among Tryptophan, Kynurenine, Indoleamine 2,3-Dioxygenase, Depression, and Neuropsychological Performance. *Front Psychol* (2017) 8:1561. doi: 10.3389/fpsyg.2017.01561
23. Colpo GD, Venna VR, McCullough LD, Teixeira AL. Systematic Review on the Involvement of the Kynurenine Pathway in Stroke: Pre-Clinical and Clinical Evidence. *Front Neurol* (2019) 10:778. doi: 10.3389/fneur.2019.00778
24. Fox E, Oliver T, Rowe M, Thomas S, Zakharia Y, Gilman PB, et al. Indoximod: An Immunometabolic Adjuvant That Empowers T Cell Activity in Cancer. *Front Oncol* (2018) 8:370. doi: 10.3389/fonc.2018.00370
25. Costa VV, Fagundes CT, Valadao DF, Avila TV, Cisalpino D, Rocha RF, et al. Subversion of Early Innate Antiviral Responses During Antibody-Dependent Enhancement of Dengue Virus Infection Induces Severe Disease in Immunocompetent Mice. *Med Microbiol Immunol* (2014) 203(4):231–50. doi: 10.1007/s00430-014-0334-5
26. Foureaux G, Franca JR, Nogueira JC, Fulgencio Gde O, Ribeiro TG, Castilho RO, et al. Ocular Inserts for Sustained Release of the Angiotensin-Converting Enzyme 2 Activator, Diminazene Aceturate, to Treat Glaucoma in Rats. *PloS One* (2015) 10(7):e0133149. doi: 10.1371/journal.pone.0133149
27. Costa VV, Del Sarto JL, Rocha RF, Silva FR, Doria JG, Olmo IG, et al. N-Methyl-D-Aspartate (NMDA) Receptor Blockade Prevents Neuronal Death Induced by Zika Virus Infection. *mBio* (2017) 8(2):e00350–17. doi: 10.1128/mBio.00350-17
28. Camargos VN, Foureaux G, Medeiros DC, da Silveira VT, Queiroz-Junior CM, Matosinhos ALB, et al. In-Depth Characterization of Congenital Zika Syndrome in Immunocompetent Mice: Antibody-Dependent Enhancement and an Antiviral Peptide Therapy. *EBioMedicine* (2019) 44:516–29. doi: 10.1016/j.ebiom.2019.05.014
29. Amaral DC, Rachid MA, Vilela MC, Campos RD, Ferreira GP, Rodrigues DH, et al. Intracerebral Infection With Dengue-3 Virus Induces Meningoencephalitis and Behavioral Changes That Precede Lethality in Mice. *J Neuroinflamm* (2011) 8:23. doi: 10.1186/1742-2094-8-23
30. Jackman JA, Costa VV, Park S, Real A, Park JH, Cardozo PL, et al. Therapeutic Treatment of Zika Virus Infection Using a Brain-Penetrating Antiviral Peptide. *Nat Mater* (2018) 17(11):971–7. doi: 10.1038/s41563-018-0194-2
31. Doria JG, de Souza JM, Silva FR, Olmo IG, Carvalho TG, Alves-Silva J, et al. The mGluR5 Positive Allosteric Modulator VU0409551 Improves Synaptic Plasticity and Memory of a Mouse Model of Huntington's Disease. *J Neurochem* (2018) 147(2):222–39. doi: 10.1111/jnc.14555
32. Fujigaki H, Yamamoto Y, Saito K. L-Tryptophan-Kynurenine Pathway Enzymes are Therapeutic Target for Neuropsychiatric Diseases: Focus on Cell Type Differences. *Neuropharmacology* (2017) 112(Pt B):264–74. doi: 10.1016/j.neuropharm.2016.01.011
33. Olmo IG, Carvalho TG, Costa VV, Alves-Silva J, Ferrari CZ, Izidoro-Toledo TC, et al. Zika Virus Promotes Neuronal Cell Death in a Non-Cell Autonomous Manner by Triggering the Release of Neurotoxic Factors. *Front Immunol* (2017) 8:1016. doi: 10.3389/fimmu.2017.01016
34. Rossi SL, Tesh RB, Azar SR, Muruato AE, Hanley KA, Auguste AJ, et al. Characterization of a Novel Murine Model to Study Zika Virus. *Am J Trop Med Hyg* (2016) 94(6):1362–9. doi: 10.4269/ajtmh.16-0111
35. Dowall SD, Graham VA, Rayner E, Atkinson B, Hall G, Watson RJ, et al. A Susceptible Mouse Model for Zika Virus Infection. *PloS Negl Trop Dis* (2016) 10(5):e0004658. doi: 10.1371/journal.pntd.0004658
36. Boldescu V, Behnam MAM, Vasilakis N, Klein CD. Broad-Spectrum Agents for Flaviviral Infections: Dengue, Zika and Beyond. *Nat Rev Drug Discov* (2017) 16(8):565–86. doi: 10.1038/nrd.2017.33
37. Sun X, Hua S, Chen HR, Ouyang Z, Einkauf K, Tse S, et al. Transcriptional Changes During Naturally Acquired Zika Virus Infection Render Dendritic Cells Highly Conducive to Viral Replication. *Cell Rep* (2017) 21(12):3471–82. doi: 10.1016/j.celrep.2017.11.087
38. Chang Y, Jiang Y, Li C, Wang Q, Zhang F, Qin CF, et al. Different Gene Networks are Disturbed by Zika Virus Infection in a Mouse Microcephaly Model. *Genomics Proteomics Bioinf* (2021). doi: 10.1016/j.gpb.2019.06.004
39. Yeung AW, Wu W, Freewan M, Stocker R, King NJ, Thomas SR. Flavivirus Infection Induces Indoleamine 2,3-Dioxygenase in Human Monocyte-Derived Macrophages *Via* Tumor Necrosis Factor and NF-kappaB. *J Leukoc Biol* (2012) 91(4):657–66. doi: 10.1189/jlb.1011532
40. Trettel F, Di Castro MA, Limatola C. Chemokines: Key Molecules That Orchestrate Communication Among Neurons, Microglia and Astrocytes to Preserve Brain Function. *Neuroscience* (2020) 439:230–40. doi: 10.1016/j.neuroscience.2019.07.035
41. Ito H, Ando T, Ogiso H, Arioka Y, Saito K, Seishima M. Inhibition of Indoleamine 2,3-Dioxygenase Activity Accelerates Skin Wound Healing. *Biomaterials* (2015) 53:221–8. doi: 10.1016/j.biomaterials.2015.02.098
42. Hoshi M, Osawa Y, Ito H, Ohtaki H, Ando T, Takamatsu M, et al. Blockade of Indoleamine 2,3-Dioxygenase Reduces Mortality From Peritonitis and Sepsis in Mice by Regulating Functions of CD11b+ Peritoneal Cells. *Infect Immun* (2014) 82(11):4487–95. doi: 10.1128/IAI.02113-14
43. Fox JM, Sage LK, Huang L, Barber J, Klonowski KD, Mellor AL, et al. Inhibition of Indoleamine 2,3-Dioxygenase Enhances the T-Cell Response to Influenza Virus Infection. *J Gen Virol* (2013) 94(Pt 7):1451–61. doi: 10.1099/vir.0.053124-0
44. Lin YT, Lin CF, Yeh TH. Influenza A Virus Infection Induces Indoleamine 2,3-Dioxygenase (IDO) Expression and Modulates Subsequent Inflammatory Mediators in Nasal Epithelial Cells. *Acta Otolaryngol* (2020) 140(2):149–56. doi: 10.1080/00016489.2019.1700304
45. Kim SB, Choi JY, Uyangaa E, Patil AM, Hossain FM, Hur J, et al. Blockage of Indoleamine 2,3-Dioxygenase Regulates Japanese Encephalitis *Via* Enhancement of Type I/II IFN Innate and Adaptive T-Cell Responses. *J Neuroinflamm* (2016) 13(1):79. doi: 10.1186/s12974-016-0551-5
46. Mazarei G, Budac DP, Lu G, Lee H, Moller T, Leavitt BR. The Absence of Indoleamine 2,3-Dioxygenase Expression Protects Against NMDA Receptor-Mediated Excitotoxicity in Mouse Brain. *Exp Neurol* (2013) 249:144–8. doi: 10.1016/j.expneurol.2013.08.007
47. Huang YS, Ogbechi J, Clanchy FI, Williams RO, Stone TW. IDO and Kynurenine Metabolites in Peripheral and CNS Disorders. *Front Immunol* (2020) 11:388. doi: 10.3389/fimmu.2020.00388
48. Del Sarto JL, Rocha RPF, Bassit L, Olmo IG, Valiate B, Queiroz-Junior CM, et al. 7-Deaza-7-Fluoro-2'-C-Methyladenosine Inhibits Zika Virus Infection and Viral-Induced Neuroinflammation. *Antiviral Res* (2020) 180:104855. doi: 10.1016/j.antiviral.2020.104855
49. Herrera-Rios D, Mughal SS, Teuber-Hanselmann S, Pierscianek D, Sucker A, Jansen P, et al. Macrophages/Microglia Represent the Major Source of Indolamine 2,3-Dioxygenase Expression in Melanoma Metastases of the Brain. *Front Immunol* (2020) 11:120. doi: 10.3389/fimmu.2020.00120
50. Zhang S, Zong Y, Ren Z, Hu J, Wu X, Xiao H, et al. Regulation of Indoleamine 2, 3-Dioxygenase in Hippocampal Microglia by NLRP3 Inflammasome in Lipopolysaccharide-Induced Depressive-Like Behaviors. *Eur J Neurosci* (2020) 52(11):4586–601. doi: 10.1111/ejn.15016

4

Elevated Soluble PD-L1 in Pregnant Women's Serum Suppresses the Immune Reaction

*Mai Okuyama [1,2], Hidetoshi Mezawa [2], Toshinao Kawai [3] and Mitsuyoshi Urashima [1,2]**

[1] Division of Molecular Epidemiology, The Jikei University School of Medicine, Tokyo, Japan, [2] Department of Pediatrics, The Jikei University School of Medicine, Tokyo, Japan, [3] Division of Immunology, National Center for Child Health and Development, Tokyo, Japan

***Correspondence:**
Mitsuyoshi Urashima
urashima@jikei.ac.jp

Background: Programmed death-ligand 1 (PD-L1) is expressed not only on some cancer cells, but also on the outer surface of placental syncytiotrophoblasts, which is assumed to induce maternal immune tolerance to fetal tissue via programmed death-1 (PD-1) receptors on T cells. Recently, levels of soluble forms of PD-L1 (sPD-L1) were reported to be higher in the serum of pregnant women (PW) than in non-pregnant women (non-PW). However, there have been no reports of the functional significance of PW's serum containing high sPD-L1 levels. Therefore, the aim of the present study was to clarify the role of sPD-L1 in the sera of PW as an immunosuppressive molecule by *in vitro* assays.

Methods: As a *post-hoc* analysis of our previous cohort study, 330 pairs of serum from PW during the third trimester and cord blood (CB) from paired offspring without major complications were examined. Serum levels of sPD-L1 and sPD-1 were measured by ELISA. On mixed lymphocyte culture (MLC), ^{3}H-thymidine uptakes in the presence of PW's, offspring's, or non-PW's serum were compared. Peripheral blood mononuclear cells (PBMCs) were cultured in the presence of PW's serum stimulated with PHA, and then cytokine levels were measured in supernatants by multiple cytokine analysis with or without anti-PD-L1blocking antibody.

Results: The median sPD-L1 level was 8.3- and 6.9-fold higher in PW than in offspring and non-PW, respectively, whereas sPD-1 levels were lower in PW and offspring than in non-PW. On MLC, ^{3}H-thymidine uptake in the presence of autoantigen was strongly reduced by co-culture with serum of both PW and offspring, compared with serum of non-PW. In contrast, uptake in the presence of alloantigen was moderately inhibited by PW's serum, whereas it was less suppressed by offspring's serum, compared with non-PW's serum. In the culture of PBMCs, tumor necrosis factor-α, interferon gamma, interleukin (IL)-2, and IL-4 levels were significantly higher in the presence of anti-PD-L1 blocking antibody than in culture not treated with antibody (all $P < 0.05$) or culture treated with isotype control antibody (all $P < 0.05$).

Conclusion: The levels of sPD-L1 are elevated in PW's serum, which may, at least in part, suppress maternal immunity.

Keywords: PD-1, PD-L1, cord blood, pregnant woman, serum, MLC, IFN-γ

INTRODUCTION

Programmed death-ligand 1 (PD-L1) is expressed on some cancer cells to suppress anti-tumor immunity by interacting with the programmed death-1 (PD-1) receptor expressed on T cells (1). Indeed, blocking this interaction by administering monoclonal antibodies targeting either the PD-1 or PD-L1 molecule improves the prognosis of cancer patients (2, 3). By immunohistochemical staining with anti-PD-L1 antibody, PD-L1 was proven to be highly expressed on the outer surface of syncytiotrophoblasts on chorionic villi in placenta facing the maternal blood stream in the uterus, but not on the inner aspect of the syncytiotrophoblasts facing chorionic villous stroma, as well as not on cytotrophoblasts facing fetal blood vessels (4–6). It has long been the immunological paradox of pregnancy that, even though tissues of the fetus including the placenta express allogeneic paternal antigen in addition to autogenic maternal antigen, they are not rejected by maternal immune systems. Thus, this paradox may be explained at least in part by PD-L1 being highly expressed on placenta; like cancer cells, PD-L1 on the placenta suppresses T cells attached to the placenta and induces immune tolerance to fetal tissues via PD-1 receptors on T cells. In fact, blockade of the PD-1 pathway by anti-PD-L1 monoclonal antibody during pregnancy increased abortions in mice (7).

Both PD-L1 and PD-1 exist in membrane-bound form and induce local or peripheral immune tolerance by maintaining the quiescence of autoreactive T cells. Recently, soluble forms of PD-L1 and PD-1 (sPD-L1 and sPD-1), which are considered to be generated by proteolytic cleavage of the membrane-bound forms, have been detected in the serum of cancer patients (8, 9). ELISA has confirmed that sPD-L1 binds to PD-1 (10). In addition, a recent meta-analysis showed that a higher level of sPD-L1 is associated with worse overall survival of cancer patients (11), indicating that sPD-L1 may work as a systemic suppressor of anti-tumor immunity, in addition to local suppression of anti-tumor immunity by membrane-bound PD-L1 on cancer cells. In 2018, sPD-L1 levels were reported to be higher in the serum of pregnant women (PW) than in non-pregnant women (non-PW), and postpartum women (12). In contrast to sPD-L1, sPD-1 may block the interaction between PD-L1 and PD-1 on T cells by competitive inhibition (13), resulting in enhanced activity of autoreactive T cells and contributing to anti-cancer effects. These experimental results were further supported by both an animal model in which sPD-1-producing virotherapy successfully improved the prognosis of tumor-bearing mice (14) and clinical evidence in which non-small cell lung cancer patients with increased serum levels of sPD-1 showed prolonged survival (15). However, there have been no reports regarding serum sPD-1 levels in PW or the functional significance of elevated sPD-L1 levels in PW's serum. Therefore, the aim of the present study was to clarify the role of sPD-L1 in sera of PW as an immunosuppressive molecule by *in vitro* assays.

METHODS

Study Design

As a *post-hoc* analysis, 330 pairs of PW and their offspring were randomly selected from our previous cohort study (16) conducted at Shiomidai Hospital, a general hospital in Kanagawa Prefecture, Japan. The inclusion criteria were: PW $\geq$ 20 years old at enrollment; lack of major complications, such as gestational diabetes mellitus, pregnancy-induced hypertension, pre-eclampsia, preterm labor, or the need for emergent cesarean section; and lack of high-risk fetal conditions, such as twins, intrauterine growth retardation, and congenital malformations. PW were enrolled from June 2011 to September 2012. Because sPD-L1 levels vary with age, 20 commercial serum samples from non-pregnant healthy women in their twenties and thirties were initially purchased for use as age-matched controls. To compare serum sPD-L1 levels among non-PW with known smoking status, 21 commercial serum samples from non-pregnant healthy women were also purchased: non-smokers, $n = 7$; past smokers, $n = 7$; and current smokers, $n = 7$.

Ethics

The study protocol was approved by the ethics committee at the Jikei University School of Medicine, the clinical study committee at Jikei Hospital, and the institutional review board at Shiomidai Hospital. Clinical data and samples were anonymized immediately after their collection at birth in a non-linkable fashion. Data monitoring was performed in the Division of Epidemiology, the Jikei University School of Medicine, with all data monitored and fixed by HM, who did not participate in ELISA measurements or statistical analyses. All women provided their written, informed consent. The serum samples used for controls were purchased from Tokyo Future Style, Inc. (Tsukuba, Ibaraki, Japan).

Measurement of sPD-L1 and sPD-1 Levels

Serum samples were collected from PW at 34 weeks of gestation. The offspring's serum (5–10 mL) was sampled from the placental side after placental delivery at birth. The serum samples were stored at $-80°C$ prior to use. Serum levels of sPD-L1 and sPD-1 were measured by MO, using ELISA kits from Abcam (Cambridge, MA, USA) and RayBiotech (Norcross, GA, USA), respectively, according to the manufacturers' protocols. Each sample was tested in triplicate for sPD-L1 and in duplicate for sPD-1, with the medians used for analysis. The lower detection limits for ELISA were 3.9 pg/mL for sPD-L1 and 20 pg/mL for sPD-1. The upper detection limits for ELISA were 1,300 pg/mL for sPD-L1 and 6,000 pg/mL for sPD-1.

Mixed Lymphocyte Culture

Reactions of lymphocytes in the presence of either autoantigen or alloantigen were measured by ^{3}H-thymidine uptake using a mixed lymphocyte culture (MLC) assay system at SRL Inc (Hachioji, Tokyo, Japan). Briefly, peripheral blood mononuclear cells (PBMCs) were obtained from three healthy male volunteers, named A, B, and C. For the MLC assay with autoantigen, fresh PBMCs were co-cultured with 13-Gy-irradiated PBMCs from the same donor in three patterns, i.e., fresh A—irradiated A, fresh B—irradiated B, and fresh C—irradiated C. For the MLC assay with alloantigen, fresh PBMCs were co-cultured with 13-Gy-irradiated PBMCs from different donors in four patterns, i.e., fresh A—irradiated B, fresh A—irradiated C, fresh B—irradiated A, and fresh C—irradiated A. These cells were cultured for 5 days with RPMI1640 and 20% of either a mixture of serum samples from PW, offspring, or non-PW, randomly selected from the cohort of this study. Each kind of serum was a mixture of at least 10 samples. Cells were pulsed with ^{3}H-thymidine during the last 17.5 h of incubation and counted in a liquid scintillation counter (Microplate Scintillation and Luminescence Counter; Perkin Elmer, Inc, Waltham, MA, USA). This MLC experiment was repeated for three sets using the same serum samples.

Cytokine Assay

PBMCs were obtained from a healthy female volunteer. Then, 2.0×10^4 PBMCs per well in 96-well U-bottom plates were co-cultured with RPMI1640 and a mixture of serum samples derived from at least 10 PW randomly selected from the cohort of this study. The serum concentration was brought to 5%, and treated with 5 μg/ml of phytohemagglutinin (PHA) (J-CHEMICAL, Inc., Chuo-ku, Tokyo, Japan) for stimulation. Samples treated with anti-PD-L1 blocking antibody (5 μg/ml) (Monoclonal Antibody MIH1, Functional Grade, eBioscience, San Diego, CA, USA), isotype control (5 μg/ml) (mouse IgG1 kappa Isotype Control, Functional Grade, eBioscience), and samples without antibody were cultured according to the method of Andorsky et al. (17). After 72 h of culture, supernatants were harvested from culture, and tumor necrosis factor-α (TNF-α), interleukin 6 (IL-6), interferon gamma (IFN-γ), IL-2, and IL-4, as markers of broad immune responses, were measured by quantitative multiplex detection using the Human Magnetic Luminex Screening Assay (R&D System, Minneapolis, MN, USA), since these cytokines were reported to be secreted from PBMCs stimulated by PHA (18).

Statistical Analyses

Because the skewness test showed that sPD-L1 levels and sPD-1 levels were not normally distributed, their levels were compared among control non-PW, PW, and CB using the Kruskal-Wallis rank test (KW test). If the result of the KW test was significant, then the Mann-Whitney test was used to compare between two groups. Spearman's rank correlation, represented as rho, with linear regression was used to quantify the strengths of associations between two continuous variables: rho $\geq$0.4, strong; 0.4> rho $\geq$0.2, moderate; and rho <0.2, weak. The test for trends across ordered groups developed by Cuzick (19) was used to examine the relationships between anthropometric measurements at birth and quartiles of sPD-L1. Multivariate analysis with linear regression was performed to adjust for potential confounders of the associations between anthropometric data and sPD-L1 quartiles, gestational weeks, and sex of offspring. For ^{3}H-thymidine uptake on MLC, as well as production levels in cytokine assays, the KW test and the Mann-Whitney test were used to compare among three groups and between two groups, respectively. Stata version 14.0 software (StataCorp, College Station, TX, USA) was used for all analyses. Values of $P < 0.05$ were considered significant. These analyses were not corrected for multiple comparisons.

RESULTS

Participants' Characteristics

In a *post-hoc* manner, 330 pairs of PW and offspring were analyzed in this study; the demographic and clinical data are shown in **Table 1**. Moreover, 20 serum samples from non-PW were used as controls.

Serum Levels of sPD-L1 and sPD-1 Among PW, Offspring, and Non-PW

Serum levels of sPD-L1 were first compared among PW, offspring, and non-PW to find significant differences (KW test: $P = 0.0001$) (**Figure 1A**). The median level of sPD-L1 was 8.3-fold higher in the serum of PW than in offspring ($P < 0.0001$) and 6.9-fold higher in PW than in non-PW ($P < 0.0001$). The median level of sPD-L1 was lower in offspring than in non-PW ($P = 0.003$). Then, serum sPD-1 levels were compared among the three groups to find significant differences (KW test: $P = 0.0006$) (**Figure 1B**). In the serum of non-PW, the median level of sPD-1 was 4.8-fold higher than in serum of PW ($P = 0.0003$), and 4.6-fold higher than in serum of offspring ($P = 0.0001$). However, the sPD-1 level was not significantly different between PW and offspring ($P = 0.72$). The median sPD-1/sPD-L1 ratio of non-PW was 41.6-fold higher than in PW ($P < 0.0001$) and 4.6-fold higher than in offspring ($P = 0.001$), and the ratio of offspring was 9.1-fold higher than in PW ($P < 0.0001$) (**Figure 1C**).

Collinearity of sPD-L1 and sPD-1 Serum Levels Between PW and Paired Offspring

The sPD-L1 levels in PW had a strong positive association with those in offspring (Spearman's rho = 0.40; $P < 0.0001$) (**Figure 2A**). The sPD-1 levels in PW also had a strong positive association with those in offspring (Spearman's rho = 0.54; $P < 0.0001$) (**Figure 2B**). In contrast, there were no associations

TABLE 1 | Participants' characteristics.

	Pregnant women *n* = 330	Offspring *n* = 330	Non-pregnant women *n* = 20
Age (y) mean (*SD*)	32 (5)	–	29 (7)
Female ratio (%)	100%	48%	100%
Body height (cm) mean (*SD*)	158.6 (5.2)	48.7 (1.9)	
Body weight (kg) mean (*SD*)	52.9 (8.1)	3.057 (0.410)	
Weight change (kg) mean (*SD*)	8.6 (3.6)		
Gestational weeks mean (*SD*)	38.7 (1.3)		
Apgar score, median (25–75%)			
1 min		9 (8–9)	
5 min		9 (9–10)	

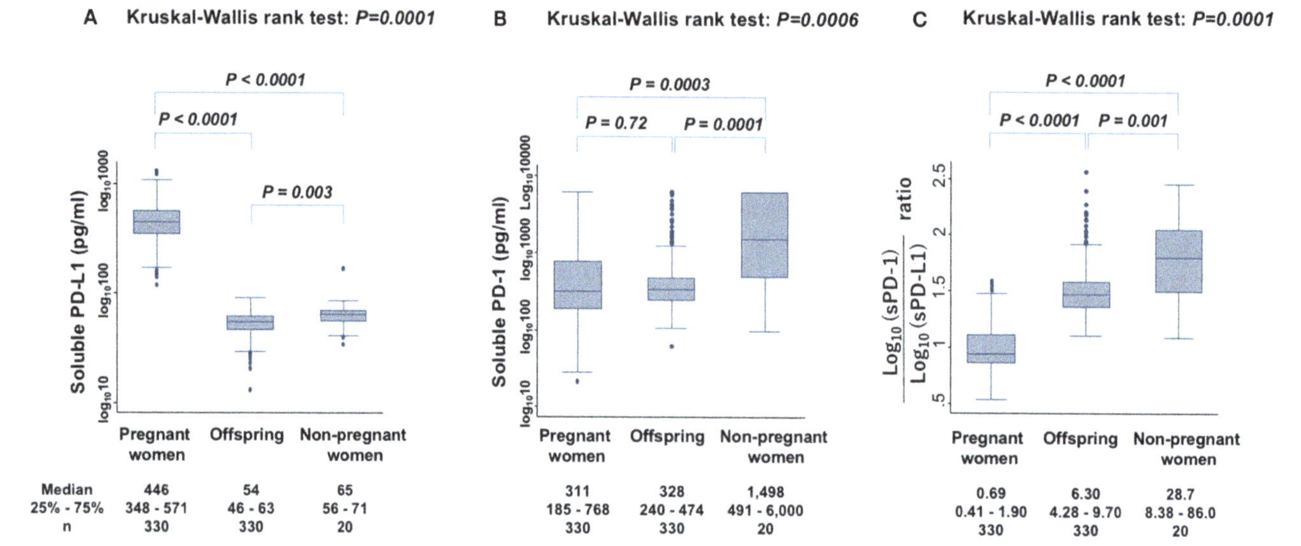

FIGURE 1 | Levels of sPD-L1 **(A)**, sPD-1 **(B)**, and the ratio of sPD-1 to sPD-L1 **(C)** in serum from PW, offspring, and non-PW controls. The Kruskal-Wallis rank test (KW test) was used for comparisons among three groups. The Mann-Whitney test was used to compare two groups. Values were transformed by the common logarithm ($\log_{10}$) prior to analysis and are shown in the graph, although the median and 25–75th percentiles are presented as absolute values.

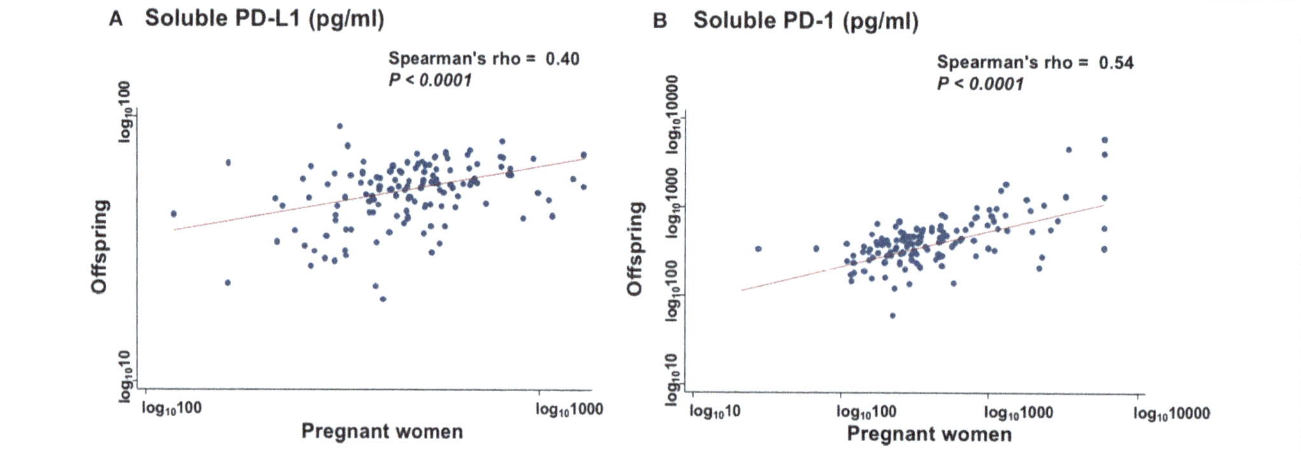

FIGURE 2 | Collinearity levels of sPD-L1 **(A)** and sPD-1 **(B)** in serum between PW and matched offspring. Spearman's rank correlation with linear regression was used to quantify the strength of association; sPD-L1 values were transformed by common logarithm ($\log_{10}$) prior to analysis.

between sPD-L1 and sPD-1 levels in serum of PW and of offspring.

Mixed Lymphocyte Culture

Level of ^{3}H-thymidine uptake in the presence of autoantigen (**Figure 3A**) and alloantigen (**Figure 3B**) were compared among three groups: PW, offspring, and non-PW. In the presence of autoantigen, median ^{3}H-thymidine uptake was strongly reduced by co-culture with serum from both PW (57% reduction; $P = 0.047$) and offspring (78% reduction; $P = 0.02$), compared with that of non-PW. On the other hand, there was no difference in the uptake between sera from PW and offspring. In the presence of alloantigen, ^{3}H-thymidine uptake was moderately reduced by co-culture with serum from PW (23% reduction; $P = 0.005$), and not significantly reduced by co-culture with offspring's sera ($P = 0.33$), compared with that of non-PW.

Cytokine Assay

In the presence of PW's sera, anti-PD-L1 blocking antibody increased the secretion of TNF-α (**Figure 4A**), IFN-γ (**Figure 4B**), IL-2 (**Figure 4C**), and IL-4 (**Figure 4D**), significantly more than samples without antibody or those treated with isotype antibody (all $P < 0.05$). On the other hand, the levels of these cytokines did not show significant difference between samples without antibody and those treated with isotype antibody. There was a similar tendency for IL-6, but it was not significant (data not shown).

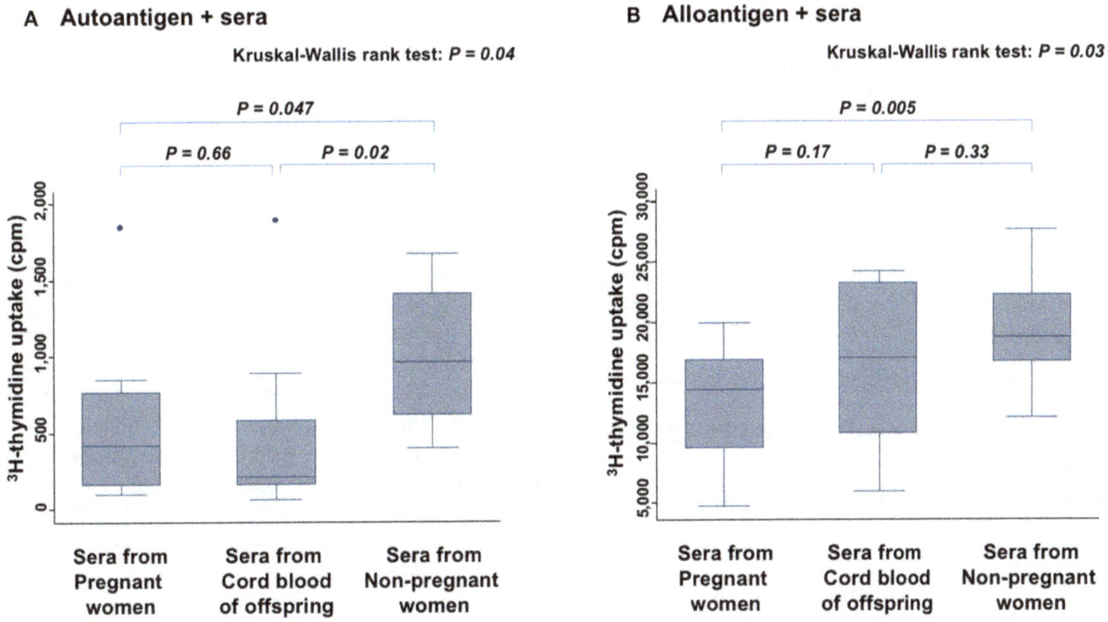

FIGURE 3 | Mixed lymphocyte culture assays in the presence of autoantigen **(A)** and alloantigen **(B)**. Levels of ^{3}H-thymidine uptake of peripheral blood mononuclear cells (PBMCs) are compared among sera from PW, offspring, and non-PW. The Kruskal-Wallis rank test (KW test) was used for comparisons among three groups. The Mann-Whitney test was used to compare two groups.

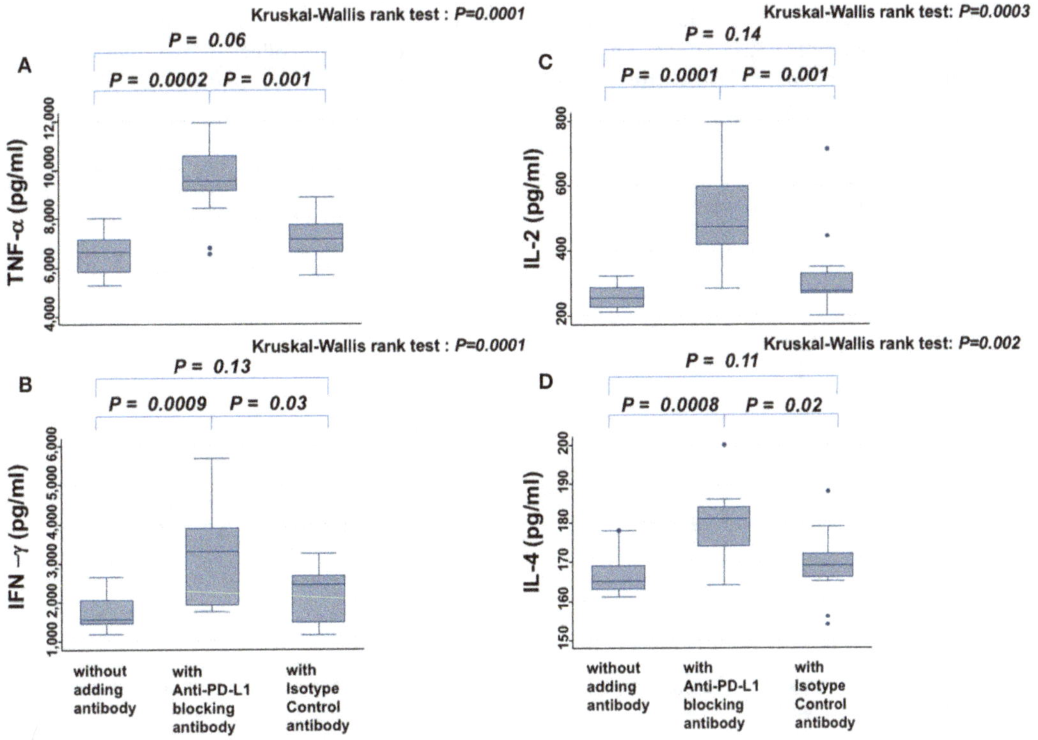

FIGURE 4 | Cytokine assay. Levels of TNF-α **(A)**, IFN-γ **(B)**, IL-2 **(C)**, and IL-4 **(D)** secreted from PBMCs in the presence of PHA and PW's serum are compared among samples without antibody, those treated with anti-PD-L1 blocking antibody, and those treated with isotype control antibody. The Kruskal-Wallis rank test (KW test) was used for comparisons among the three groups. If there was a significant difference, the Mann-Whitney test was used to compare two groups.

Levels of sPD-L1 and Smoking Status in PW and Non-PW

The levels of sPD-L1 were compared among non-smokers, past smokers, and current smokers among PW to find significant differences (KW test: $P = 0.0006$) (**Figure 5A**). The sPD-L1 levels were 13 and 31% lower in past and in current smokers, respectively, than in non-smokers. Serum levels of sPD-L1 were also measured among non-PW (KW test: $P = 0.03$) (**Figure 5B**). In particular, the sPD-L1 levels were 27% lower in current smokers than in non-smokers plus past smokers (Mann-Whitney test: $P = 0.03$), whereas there was no significant difference in sPD-L1 levels between non-smokers and past smokers.

Offspring Anthropometric Measurements and sPD-L1 Levels in PW

Offspring anthropometric measurements at birth were compared with serum sPD-L1 levels in PW as both quartiles and continuous variables.

The median body weight at birth in the highest sPD-L1 quartile (Q4) was 270 g heavier than in the lowest quartile (Q1). Thus, there was a significant trend for increased body weight with higher levels of sPD-L1 (trend test, $P < 0.0001$) and a moderate Spearman's rho (0.24, $P < 0.0001$) (**Supplementary Figure 1**). On multivariate adjustment with gestational weeks and offspring's sex, body weight remained a significant factor.

The median body height of the highest quartile (Q4) of sPD-L1 was 0.6 cm taller than that of the lowest quartile (Q1). There was thus a significant trend for increased body height with higher levels of sPD-L1 (trend test, $P < 0.0001$) and a weak Spearman's rho (0.13, $P = 0.02$) (**Supplementary Figure 2**). On multivariate adjustment with gestational weeks and offspring sex, body height remained a significant factor.

The median head circumference of the highest quartile (Q4) of sPD-L1 was 0.4 cm longer than that of the lowest quartile (Q1). There was thus a significant trend for increased head circumference with higher levels of sPD-L1 (trend test, $P = 0.009$) and a weak Spearman's rho (0.15, $P = 0.007$) (**Supplementary Figure 3**). On multivariate adjustment with gestational weeks and offspring sex, head circumference remained a significant factor.

The median chest circumference of the highest quartile (Q4) of sPD-L1 was 0.5 cm longer than that of the lowest quartile (Q1). There was thus a significant trend for increased chest circumference with higher levels of sPD-L1 (trend test, $P < 0.0001$) and a moderate Spearman's rho (0.21, $P = 0.0001$) (**Supplementary Figure 4**). On multivariate adjustment with gestational weeks and offspring sex, chest circumference remained a significant factor.

DISCUSSION

In the present study, the median serum sPD-L1 level in PW during the third trimester was high, 8.3-fold higher than in offspring and 6.9-fold higher than in healthy age-matched non-PW controls. Although serum levels of sPD-L1 were reported to increase throughout gestation (12) when blood samples from 30 PW were collected, this increase of sPD-L1 in PW was reconfirmed by expanding the sample size to 330 PW, and their offspring's CB was found to have lower levels of

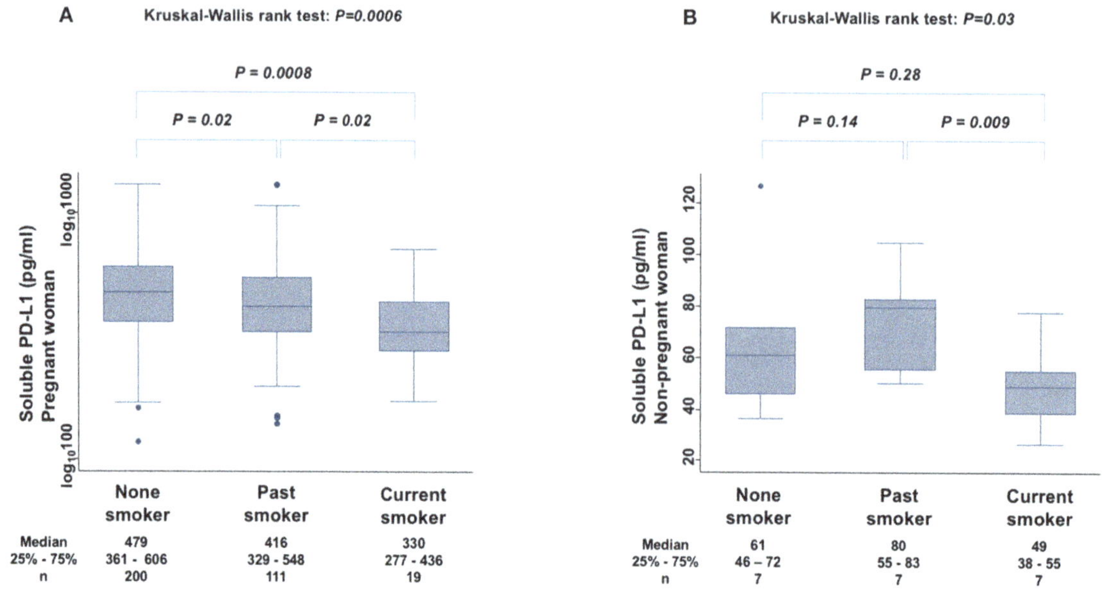

FIGURE 5 | Relationship between sPD-L1 levels and smoking status in PW **(A)** and in non-PW **(B)**. The Kruskal-Wallis rank test (KW test) was used for comparisons among three groups: non-smoker, past smoker, and current smoker. The Mann-Whitney test was used to compare two groups; sPD-L1 values were transformed by the common logarithm ($\log_{10}$) prior to analysis and are shown in the graph **(A)**, although the median and 25–75th percentiles are presented as absolute values.

sPD-L1 than the serum of non-PW. In contrast to sPD-L1, sPD-1 levels were lower in PW and offspring than in non-PW. Opposite to sPD-L1, sPD-1 was reported to competitively inhibit the interaction between PD-L1 and PD-1 on T cells (13). Therefore, it was assumed that when both increased sPD-L1 and decreased sPD-1 are present in the serum of PW, the immune reaction may be more suppressed than in offspring with decreased sPD-L1 and decreased sPD-1 in the serum. Thus, in serum from PW, the sPD-1/sPD-L1 ratio was very low and could inhibit lymphocyte proliferation in response to both autoantigen and alloantigen. In serum from offspring's CB, the sPD-1/sPD-L1 ratio was moderately low and could inhibit lymphocyte proliferation in response to autoantigen, but not significantly to alloantigen. To clarify whether the elevated sPD-L1 protein in PW's serum contributes to immune suppression, *in vitro* experiments of cytokine production assays with PHA stimulation, where an attempt was made to block specific functions of sPD-L1 in PW's serum with anti-PD-L1 antibody, were added. These experiments showed that various cytokines were increased in the presence of anti-sPD-L1 blocking antibody, suggesting that the elevated sPD-L1 protein in PW's serum may be functional, able to suppress broad immune reactions, and may thus be considered to protect the placenta and fetus from maternal immunosurveillance, at least in part.

With respect to clinical data, levels of sPD-L1 in PW showed a negative association with smoking. It has been well reported that maternal smoking impairs placental structure and function (20, 21). In addition, expression of PD-L1 mRNA in trophoblasts was reported to be increased with rising oxygen concentrations and decreased rapidly by a low oxygen concentration (5). On the other hand, administration of PD-L1 protein was demonstrated to protect against pre-eclampsia in the rat (22). Judging from these lines of evidence, it was then assumed that smoking may decrease oxygen supply to the placenta and secretion of sPD-L1 to the maternal blood stream, and the decreased sPD-L1 may further impair placental function and reduce sPD-L1 secretion to form a vicious circle. Of interest, even among non-PW, serum levels of sPD-L1 were suppressed in current smokers. PD-L1 is usually expressed on the macrophage lineage (23). Smoking impairs alveolar macrophage activation (24), which can be normalized by smoking cessation (25). In this case, smoking may be assumed to suppress sPD-L1 levels through impaired macrophage function.

There are several limitations of the present study. First, PW with major complications, such as gestational diabetes mellitus, pregnancy-induced hypertension, pre-eclampsia, preterm labor, or the need for emergent cesarean section, and who lacked high-risk fetal conditions, such as twins, intrauterine growth retardation, and congenital malformation, were excluded. Thus, associations between sPD-L1 levels of PW and these complications could not be examined. Instead, associations with smoking status and with fetal growth were examined to show that serum sPD-L1 levels can be a biomarker of placental function. Second, functional assays were added to support the hypothesis that sPD-L1 in addition to PD-L1 expressed on the surface of the placenta suppresses the maternal immune reaction to reject the placenta and fetus. It was demonstrated that the serum of PW showed stronger suppressive effects on autogenic and allogeneic immune reactions than serum of non-PW. Moreover, this suppressive effect of PW's sera was blocked using anti-PD-L1 antibody, as demonstrated by cytokine production assays. Third, MLC, which is used to evaluate the possibility of graft vs. host or host vs. graft disease in the field of bone marrow transplantation or organ transplantation, was used to examine immune reactions in the presence of PW's serum, considering the immunological paradox of pregnancy. However, there are many other types of functional assays. Fourth, since placental tissue was not collected in this cohort, for example, direct interactions between syncytiotrophoblasts and T cells could not be examined. Instead, the focus was not on membrane-bound PD-L1 molecules expressed on syncytiotrophoblasts, but on the soluble form of PD-L1 in the serum of PW. Fifth, sPD-L1 was measured at only one point in the third trimester during pregnancy. Sixth, placental PD-L1 protein expression was not measured by immunohistochemistry.

In conclusion, this is the first study to measure both sPD-L1 and sPD-1 levels in the serum of PW, as well as paired offspring, and it showed that: (1) sPD-L1 levels were very high in the serum of PW in the third trimester, but low in paired offspring; (2) sPD-1 levels were lower in both PW and offspring than in non-PW; (3) there was a strong correlation of sPD-1 levels, as well as sPD-L1 levels, between PW and offspring; (4) on MLC, ^{3}H-thymidine uptake in the presence of autoantigen was strongly reduced by co-culture with sera from both PW and offspring, compared with non-PW's serum, while uptake in the presence of alloantigen was moderately inhibited by sera from PW, but it was not significantly suppressed by offspring's serum, compared with non-PW's serum; (5) adding the anti-PD-L1 blocking antibody to sera from PW raised cytokine secretion (6); and, finally, sPD-L1 levels in PW and in non-PW were suppressed by smoking.

The novel finding of this study was that PW's serum may suppress both autogenic and allogeneic immune reactions, whereas offspring's serum may suppress mainly the autogenic immune reaction and only partly allogeneic immune reactions. It was further shown that anti-PD-L1 antibody impairs the immunosuppressive effects of PW's serum, and it was suggested that elevated sPD-L1 levels in PW's sera may be functional and play, at least in part, a role in suppressing the maternal immune reaction to alloantigen, i.e., placenta and fetus. Further research is needed to confirm this.

AUTHOR CONTRIBUTIONS

MO and MU conceptualized and designed the study, drafted the initial manuscript, and reviewed and revised the manuscript. TK and HM collected and fixed clinical data and reviewed and revised the manuscript. MU performed experiments and analyzed data statistically. All authors approved the final manuscript.

FUNDING

This work was supported by JSPS KAKENHI Grant Number JP16K09074 and by The Jikei University School of Medicine.

ACKNOWLEDGMENTS

We would like to thank the pregnant women who agreed to provide blood samples and demographic data for this research project, and the doctors and nurses at Shiomidai Hospital for their time in obtaining informed consent and for data collection at birth. The authors are also grateful to Prof. Hiroyuki Ida for assistance in organizing the study team.

REFERENCES

1. Boussiotis VA. Molecular and biochemical aspects of the PD-1 checkpoint pathway. *N Engl J Med.* (2016) 375:767–78. doi: 10.1056/NEJMra1514296
2. Topalian SL, Hodi FS, Brahmer JR, Gettinger SN, Smith DC, McDermott DF, et al. Safety, activity, and immune correlates of anti-PD-1 antibody in cancer. *N Engl J Med.* (2012) 366:2443–54. doi: 10.1056/NEJMoa1200690
3. Brahmer JR, Tykodi SS, Chow LQ, Hwu WJ, Topalian SL, Hwu P, et al. Safety and activity of anti-PD-L1 antibody in patients with advanced cancer. *N Engl J Med.* (2012) 366:2455–65. doi: 10.1056/NEJMoa1200694
4. Veras E, Kurman RJ, Wang TL, Shih IM. PD-L1 expression in human placentas and gestational trophoblastic diseases. *Int J Gynecol Pathol.* (2017) 36:146–53. doi: 10.1097/PGP.0000000000000305
5. Holets LM, Hunt JS, Petroff MG. Trophoblast CD274 (B7-H1) is differentially expressed across gestation: influence of oxygen concentration. *Biol Reprod.* (2006) 74:352–8. doi: 10.1095/biolreprod.105.046581
6. Petroff MG, Chen L, Phillips TA, Azzola D, Sedlmayr P, Hunt JS. B7 family molecules are favorably positioned at the human maternal-fetal interface. *Biol Reprod.* (2003) 68:1496–504. doi: 10.1095/biolreprod.102.010058
7. Guleria I, Khosroshahi A, Ansari MJ, Habicht A, Azuma M, Yagita H, et al. A critical role for the programmed death ligand 1 in fetomaternal tolerance. *J Exp Med.* (2005) 202:231–7. doi: 10.1084/jem.20050019
8. Zhu X, Lang J. Soluble PD-1 and PD-L1: predictive and prognostic significance in cancer. *Oncotarget* (2017) 8:97671–82. doi: 10.18632/oncotarget.18311
9. Frigola X, Inman BA, Lohse CM, Krco CJ, Cheville JC, Thompson RH, et al. Identification of a soluble form of B7-H1 that retains immunosuppressive activity and is associated with aggressive renal cell carcinoma. *Clin Cancer Res.* (2011) 17:1915–23. doi: 10.1158/1078-0432.CCR-10-0250
10. Takeuchi M, Doi T, Obayashi K, Hirai A, Yoneda K, Tanaka F, et al. Soluble PD-L1 with PD-1-binding capacity exists in the plasma of patients with non-small cell lung cancer. *Immunol Lett.* (2018) 196:155–60. doi: 10.1016/j.imlet.2018.01.007
11. Ding Y, Sun C, Li J, Hu L, Li M, Liu J, et al. The prognostic significance of soluble programmed death ligand 1 expression in cancers: a systematic review and meta-analysis. *Scand J Immunol.* (2017) 86:361–7. doi: 10.1111/sji.12596
12. Enninga EAL, Harrington SM, Creedon DJ, Ruano R, Markovic SN, Dong H, et al. Immune checkpoint molecules soluble program death ligand 1 and galectin-9 are increased in pregnancy. *Am J Reprod Immunol.* (2018) 79(2). doi: 10.1111/aji.12795
13. Amancha PK, Hong JJ, Rogers K, Ansari AA, Villinger F. *In vivo* blockade of the programmed cell death-1 pathway using soluble recombinant PD-1-Fc enhances CD4+ and CD8+ T cell responses but has limited clinical benefit. *J Immunol.* (2013) 191:6060–70. doi: 10.4049/jimmunol.1302044
14. Bartee MY, Dunlap KM, Bartee E. Tumor-localized secretion of soluble PD1 enhances oncolytic virotherapy. *Cancer Res.* (2017) 77:2952–63. doi: 10.1158/0008-5472.CAN-16-1638
15. Sorensen SF, Demuth C, Weber B, Sorensen BS, Meldgaard P. Increase in soluble PD-1 is associated with prolonged survival in patients with advanced EGFR-mutated non-small cell lung cancer treated with erlotinib. *Lung Cancer* (2016) 100:77–84. doi: 10.1016/j.lungcan.2016.08.001
16. Niwa S, Mezawa H, Kobayashi N, Ida H, Urashima M. Inverse association between maternal 25OHD level and cord GLP-1/GIP concentrations. *Pediatr Res.* (2016) 79:536–42. doi: 10.1038/pr.2015.253
17. Andorsky DJ, Yamada RE, Said J, Pinkus GS, Betting DJ, Timmerman JM. Programmed death ligand 1 is expressed by non-hodgkin lymphomas and inhibits the activity of tumor-associated T cells. *Clin Cancer Res.* (2011) 17:4232–44. doi: 10.1158/1078-0432.CCR-10-2660
18. Sullivan KE, Cutilli J, Piliero LM, Ghavimi-Alagha D, Starr SE, Campbell DE, et al. Measurement of cytokine secretion, intracellular protein expression, and mRNA in resting and stimulated peripheral blood mononuclear cells. *Clin Diagn Lab Immunol.* (2000) 7:920 4.
19. Cuzick J. A wilcoxon-type test for trend. *Stat Med.* (1985) 4:87–90. doi: 10.1002/sim.4780040112
20. Kharkova OA, Grjibovski AM, Krettek A, Nieboer E, Odland JO. Effect of smoking behavior before and during pregnancy on selected birth outcomes among singleton full-term pregnancy: a murmansk county birth registry study. *Int J Environ Res Public Health* (2017) 14:E867. doi: 10.3390/ijerph14080867
21. Zdravkovic T, Genbacev O, McMaster MT, Fisher SJ. The adverse effects of maternal smoking on the human placenta: a review. *Placenta* (2005) 26 (Suppl. A):S81–6. doi: 10.1016/j.placenta.2005.02.003
22. Tian M, Zhang Y, Liu Z, Sun G, Mor G, Liao A. The PD-1/PD-L1 inhibitory pathway is altered in pre-eclampsia and regulates T cell responses in pre-eclamptic rats. *Sci Rep.* (2016) 6:27683. doi: 10.1038/srep27683
23. Dong H, Strome SE, Salomao DR, Tamura H, Hirano F, Flies DB, et al. Tumor-associated B7-H1 promotes T-cell apoptosis: a potential mechanism of immune evasion. *Nat Med.* (2002) 8:793–800. doi: 10.1038/nm730
24. Moller W, Barth W, Pohlit W, Rust M, Siekmeier R, Stahlhofen W, et al. Smoking impairs alveolar macrophage activation after inert dust exposure. *Toxicol Lett.* (1996) 88:131–7. doi: 10.1016/0378-4274(96)03728-9
25. Hodge S, Hodge G, Ahern J, Jersmann H, Holmes M, Reynolds PN. Smoking alters alveolar macrophage recognition and phagocytic ability: implications in chronic obstructive pulmonary disease. *Am J Respir Cell Mol Biol.* (2007) 37:748–55. doi: 10.1165/rcmb.2007-0025OC

5

Evaluating the Safety of West Nile Virus Immunity During Congenital Zika Virus Infection in Mice

Joshua A. Acklin[1,2], *Javier D. Cattle*[1,3], *Arianna S. Moss*[1], *Julia A. Brown*[1,2], *Gregory A. Foster*[4], *David Krysztof*[4], *Susan L. Stramer*[4] *and Jean K. Lim*[1*]

[1] *Department of Microbiology, Icahn School of Medicine at Mount Sinai, New York, NY, United States,* [2] *Graduate School of Biomedical Sciences, Icahn School of Medicine at Mount Sinai, New York, NY, United States,* [3] *Department of Epidemiology, Mailman School of Public Health, Columbia University, New York, NY, United States,* [4] *Scientific Affairs, American Red Cross, Gaithersburg, MD, United States*

***Correspondence:**
Jean K. Lim
jean.lim@mssm.edu

Antibody-dependent enhancement (ADE) is a phenomenon that occurs when cross-reactive antibodies generated from a previous flaviviral infection increase the pathogenesis of a related virus. Zika virus (ZIKV) is the most recent flavivirus introduced to the Western Hemisphere and has become a significant public health threat due to the unanticipated impact on the developing fetus. West Nile virus (WNV) is the primary flavivirus that circulates in North America, and we and others have shown that antibodies against WNV are cross-reactive to ZIKV. Thus, there is concern that WNV immunity could increase the risk of severe ZIKV infection, particularly during pregnancy. In this study, we examined the extent to which WNV antibodies could impact ZIKV pathogenesis in a murine pregnancy model. To test this, we passively transferred WNV antibodies into pregnant *Stat2*$^{-/-}$ mice on E6.5 prior to infection with ZIKV. Evaluation of pregnant dams showed weight loss following ZIKV infection; however, no differences in maternal weights or viral loads in the maternal brain, spleen, or spinal cord were observed in the presence of WNV antibodies. Resorption rates, and other fetal parameters, including fetal and placental size, were similarly unaffected. Further, the presence of WNV antibodies did not significantly alter the viral load or the inflammatory response in the placenta or the fetus in response to ZIKV. Our data suggest that pre-existing WNV immunity may not significantly impact the pathogenesis of ZIKV infection during pregnancy. Our findings are promising for the safety of implementing WNV vaccines in the continental US.

Keywords: flavivirus, congenital Zika syndrome, antibody dependent enhancement, vaccines, placenta

INTRODUCTION

Antibody-dependent enhancement (ADE) is a phenomenon by which antibodies elicited from a previous infection facilitate viral entry into a susceptible cell through the engagement of Fc gamma receptors (FcγRs) (1, 2). The most established example of ADE in humans occurs between the four serotypes of dengue virus (DENV), a mosquito-transmitted flavivirus that is estimated to cause ~390 million infections annually around the globe (3, 4). Studies show that while primary infections with DENV are typically mild, secondary infections with a heterotypic DENV serotype are more frequently severe, with increased incidence of dengue hemorrhagic fever (DHF) and dengue shock syndrome (DSS) (5, 6). ADE between the DENV serotypes is poised to occur due to the unique degree of cross-reactivity between the antigenic envelope proteins, and the fact that the four serotypes co-circulate (7–12). While high concentrations of cross-reactive antibodies may offer protection in the short term, these same antibodies can promote pathogenesis through ADE if secondary infection occurs during a time when the concentration of antibodies falls below the neutralization threshold (13, 14). Observing ADE in human populations is difficult and requires prospective studies in flavivirus endemic areas (15). In the case of dengue, while the phenomenon of severe secondary infections has been observed for decades, the correlation between antibody titers and severe disease was only directly demonstrated recently (16). A major question in the field that remains is whether this occurs with other flaviviruses in humans. In the absence of human data, *in vitro* and *in vivo* models can offer clues into this possibility. The data generated by such studies hold broad implications for the development of any flavivirus vaccine (17).

In 2016, Zika virus (ZIKV), a flavivirus closely related to DENV, received global attention after it was found to be the cause of a large outbreak that started in Brazil and spread to nearly every South and Central American country. While ZIKV has historically been associated with mild disease, this recent outbreak was much more severe (18–23). The most concerning disease outcomes were observed in pregnant women, where the virus impacted the developing fetus, resulting in spontaneous abortions and fetal abnormalities such as microcephaly (24). Based on confirmed ZIKV infections, the CDC estimates that 10% of pregnancies resulted in some form of fetal abnormality; this number increased to 15% when evaluating infections that occured during the first trimester (22, 25). Additionally, two recent studies showed that children that were exposed to ZIKV *in utero* were at greater risk of developing neurological deficits and developmental delays in their early years of life despite no overt signs of ZIKV-related damage at birth (26, 27). It remains unclear what factors may have led to the increased pathogenesis of ZIKV in the most recent outbreaks, but one possibility is the involvement of ADE. Given that antibodies against DENV can both bind to and enhance ZIKV *in vitro* and *in vivo*, and since DENV is endemic in ZIKV outbreak regions, pre-existing immunity to DENV could have been a contributing factor to the severity of the recent ZIKV outbreak (28–35). We have previously reported that passive transfer of DENV reactive antibodies can potently enhance ZIKV infection in pregnant mice. Enhanced infection resulted in heightened maternal weight loss, fetal developmental delays, damage to the developing placenta, and finally increased resorption. We further showed the dependency on antibodies as this process was maintained with purified DENV reactive IgG and reversed with FcγR blocking (32).

In the United States, DENV does not regularly circulate as it does in South and Central America. However, West Nile virus (WNV), another closely related flavivirus, causes annual outbreaks of neurological disease, primarily meningitis, encephalitis, and acute flaccid paralysis (36). WNV is estimated to have infected at least 7 million people since its introduction into the Western Hemisphere in 1999 (37, 38). There is a great need for a WNV vaccine for human use, and should one be approved, WNV seropositivity would increase significantly. This is concerning because we and others have demonstrated that antibodies elicited by WNV are cross-reactive to ZIKV, suggesting that preexisting WNV immunity has the potential to impact ZIKV pathogenesis (31, 39, 40). In fact, during the 2016 outbreak, mosquito transmission of ZIKV occurred in both Texas and Florida, demonstrating the potential for ZIKV to expand into WNV-endemic areas (41). This risk is expected to increase as global temperatures rise (42). In this manuscript, we seek to understand the extent to which pre-existing WNV immunity impacts ZIKV outcomes during pregnancy using a *Stat2*$^{-/-}$ mouse model of ZIKV ADE.

MATERIALS AND METHODS

Generation of Human Immune Plasma

WNV-infected blood donors were identified through screening 52,355,427 blood donations in the United States between August 2003-December 2011. Initial screening was conducted through WNV nucleic acid testing (NAT). Blood donors were identified as WNV-infected if the initial WNV NAT was reactive, repeat WNV NAT was also reactive, and WNV-specific IgM and/or IgG antibody testing results were positive on the initial blood donation or upon follow up testing. Testing for WNV antibodies was conducted by Abbott Laboratories (2003-2004; Abbott Park IL) or Focus Diagnostics (2003-2011; San Juan Capistrano CA). We received plasma from 471 WNV-infected blood donors that met these criteria. Among these, we included only those samples where positive reactivity for WNV-specific IgG on the index sample was documented (n = 146). DENV-immune plasma samples were collected as previously described (31). Random blood donor plasma samples (n = 54) that were negative for all infectious pathogens were used as negative controls. All plasma samples were individually tested for reactivity to ZIKV E protein by ELISA as previously described (31). 15 individual donors with the highest reactivity to ZIKV E protein from the DENV or WNV cohorts were pooled and used for these experiments. All control plasma failed to react to ZIKV E protein, and 15 random donors were pooled and used for the CTRL-immune plasma condition.

Neutralization Assays

Neutralization titers were determined by co-incubating serially diluted, heat-inactivated pooled immune plasma with 10 50% tissue culture infectious doses ($TCID_{50}$) of WNV Kunjin isolate (CH16532), DENV-1 (BC89/94), or ZIKV (PRVABC-59) in DMEM with 2% FBS. After shaking at room temperature for 1 hour, the virus-antibody mixture was added to a monolayer of Vero cells in 96 well format. Following a two-day incubation at

37°C, cells were detached from the plate using trypsin/EDTA, fixed with 4% PFA, permeabilized with PBS containing 0.2% BSA and 0.05% saponin, and stained with 4G2 antibody (1 µg/ml) for 1 hour at room temperature. After washing, cells were incubated with goat anti-mouse IgG conjugated to phycoerythrin (1µg/ml, Invitrogen) for 1 hour at room temperature. The percentage of infected cells was determined by flow cytometry using a FACS Caliber and analyzed using FlowJo2 software version 10.1.r7. The 50% inhibitory doses (IC_{50}) of each plasma pool was calculated by using the four-parameter logarithmic regression in GraphPad Prism.

In Vitro Antibody-Dependent Enhancement of ZIKV Infection

Antibody-dependent enhancement of ZIKV infection was measured using a flow cytometry-based assay. Briefly, serial dilutions of either non-reactive (CTRL), DENV-immune or WNV-immune human plasma were pre-incubated with ZIKV strain PRVABC-59 at an MOI of 1 for 1 hour at 37°C. Immune complexes were then co-incubated with K562 cells (5×10^4) in 96 well U-bottom plates in RPMI 1640 media supplemented with 10% FBS, 2 mM L-glutamine, 10 µg/ml penicillin, and 10µg/ml streptomycin. After incubation for 48 hours at 37°C, cells were fixed with 4% PFA, permeabilized with PBS containing 0.2% BSA and 0.05% saponin, and stained with 4G2 antibody (1 µg/ml) for 1 hour at room temperature. After washing, cells were incubated with goat anti-mouse IgG conjugated to phycoerythrin (1µg/ml, Invitrogen) for 1hr at room temperature. The percentage of infected cells was determined by flow cytometry using a FACS Caliber and analyzed using FlowJo2 software version 10.1.r7. The data were then fit to a Gaussian distribution utilizing the non-linear regression functionality of GraphPad Prism, and the enhancing concentration at which 50% of maximum enhancement was reached (EC_{50}) was determined utilizing the Gaussian fit.

ZIKV Infection of *Stat2*$^{-/-}$ Mice

Mouse studies were carried out in an animal Biosafety Level 2+ facility under a protocol approved by the Icahn School of Medicine at Mount Sinai Animal Care and Use Committee. Breeding pairs were formed using *Stat2*$^{-/-}$ mice (provided by Christian Schindler; 8-10 week old nulliparous females and >8 week old non-virgin males). Females were then separated after plugs were detected (defined as E0.5) and infected at E6.5. Pregnant *Stat2*$^{-/-}$ mice were injected intraperitoneally with 20 µl of CTRL-, WNV- or DENV- immune plasma two hours prior to intradermal infection with 5×10^3 PFU ZIKV (strain PRVABC-59, GenBank: KU501215.1). ZIKV was obtained originally from the CDC, passaged once in Vero cells, and sequence verified. Mice were monitored daily for weight loss. Fetal and maternal tissues were harvested at E13.5 for analysis.

ZIKV Quantification

Total RNA was isolated from tissue homogenates using Direct-zol RNA MiniPrep Plus (Zymo Research) according to manufacturer's protocol, and 1 µg of RNA was reverse transcribed into cDNA using the High Capacity Reverse Transcription Kit (Applied Biosciences) with random hexamer primers. The following ZIKV-specific primers (5′-TTGGTCATGATACTGCTGATTGC-3′ and 5′-CCYTCCACRAAGTCYCTATTGC-3′) were used for qRT-PCR (43), and detection of amplification was determined *via* PerfeCTa SYBR Green fast mix (Quanta) following the manufacturer's protocol. PCR amplification was conducted in 384-well format using the Roche LightCycler 480 System. RNA quantification was determined by fitting to an *in vitro*-transcribed RNA standard.

Cytokine and Chemokine Protein Quantification

Tissue homogenates were evaluated for 23 cytokines/chemokines by multiplexed ELISA for the following analytes: IL-17A, IL-22, IL-10, IL-2, IL-4, IFNγ, IL-21, TNFα, IL-5, IL-6, Cxcl16, Ccl4/MIP-1β, Ccl3/MIP-1α, IL-12(p70), Ccl11, IL-1β, Cxcl1/GROα, Cxcl2/GROβ, Ccl5/RANTES, Ccl7/MCP-3, Ccl2/MCP-1, Ccl12, and Cxcl10/IP-10 as previously described (44). Samples were analyzed on a Luminex MAGPIX platform. For each bead region, >50 beads were collected per analyte. The median fluorescence intensity was recorded and used to extrapolate pg/ml based on a 5P regression fitting of a standard curve of each analyte. Heat maps for median fold induction were generated in R by logarithmic base 2 transformation of the median cytokine level in the ZIKV-infected conditions divided by the median cytokine level of uninfected controls. Hierarchical clustering was performed using the hclust function in R, which stratifies based on Euclidean distance.

Histological and Tissue Analysis

Tissues were fixed in 10% neutral-buffered formalin before embedding into paraffin and cutting into 5 µm sections. Deparaffinization and antigen retrieval was performed as previously described (31). Slides were stained with hematoxylin (Gill's formula, Vector Laboratories H3401) and eosin Y (Sigma Aldrich E4009) according to manufacturer's instructions. For vimentin staining, slides were blocked in Tris-buffered saline containing 0.01% Tween-20 (TBST) and 2.5% normal goat serum for 40 minutes at room temperature. After washing, slides were incubated with rabbit monoclonal anti-vimentin antibody (1:1000, clone EPR3776, Abcam) for 1 hour at 4°C, then washed and incubated with goat anti-rabbit Alexa Fluor 488 before mounting with Vectashield hard-set mounting medium with DAPI (Vector Laboratories). Full-slice images were taken with an AxioImager Z2 microscope (Zeiss) and Zen 2012 software.

In situ hybridization using RNAscope® (ACDBio) was performed on 5 µm paraffin-embedded sections. Slides were baked at 55°C for twenty minutes for deparaffinization. Slides were then washed twice with xylene, twice in ethanol, and dried at 60°C. Slides were then incubated with hydrogen peroxide for 10 minutes at RT, and then rinsed in diH2O. Antigen retrieval was performed as per the manufacturer's guidelines, and slides were washed with water, transferred into 100% ethanol for three minutes and air dried. Sections were treated with RNAscope Protease Plus at 40°C for 30 minutes and washed with diH2O. Fluorescence *in situ* hybridization was subsequently performed according to the manufacturer's protocol (ACD# 323110) with RNAscope Probe V-ZIKVsph2015 (ACD #467871; binds sense

RNA) as previously described (Cao et al., 2017). Slides were mounted with Vectashield hard-set mounting medium with DAPI (Vector Laboratories). Full-slice images were taken with an AxioImager Z2 microscope (Zeiss) and Zen 2012 software. Images were rendered in FIJI for final visualization.

Quantification and Statistical Analysis

For all statistical significance indications in this manuscript, **** indicates a p-value ≤ 0.0001, *** indicates a p-value ≤ 0.001, ** indicates a p-value ≤ 0.01, and * indicates a p-value ≤ 0.05. NS indicates non significance. All sample sizes, replicate numbers, statistical tests and significance can be found in the figures and figure legends of this manuscript. Graphical representations were rendered in GraphPad Prism 8.0.1.

RESULTS

In Vitro Characterization of WNV Antibodies Elicited Through Natural Infection

To study how WNV antibodies could impact ZIKV pathogenesis, we utilized a cohort of individuals that were naturally infected with WNV identified through routine screening of the blood supply in the United States (31). To confirm antibody reactivity to WNV, we conducted a neutralization assay using the Kunjin isolate of WNV (WNV^{KUN}), which is 97.7% identical at the amino acid level to the NY99 strain that was introduced to the US (45). In brief, plasma from 15 WNV-seropositive blood donors were pooled and tested for the ability to neutralize WNV^{KUN} using a flow-cytometry based microneutralization assay. Compared to plasma from geographically-matched WNV-uninfected control (CTRL) individuals, immune plasma from WNV-infected individuals showed a strong capacity to neutralize WNV (IC_{50} = 1:5,770), while the CTRL plasma showed no activity (**Figure 1A**). Given that WNV antibodies have previously been shown to cross-react with ZIKV, we next sought to assess the ability of WNV immune plasma to neutralize and enhance ZIKV (31, 40). For comparison, we used DENV immune plasma, which is known to neutralize and enhance ZIKV both *in vitro* and *in vivo* (31–34). To directly compare WNV plasma potential with DENV immune plasma, we first needed to characterize the neutralization capacity of our DENV plasma against DENV. As shown in **Figure 1A**, DENV plasma potently neutralizes DENV-1, while non-reactive CTRL plasma is incapable. Indeed, the neutralization potential of DENV plasma against DENV-1 (IC_{50} = 1:10,021) is comparable to that of WNV plasma to neutralize WNV. Therefore, any differences in the potential to neutralize and enhance ZIKV are a result of antigenic cross-reactivity, and not of differing concentrations of virus-specific antibodies. We next conducted neutralization assays against ZIKV, utilizing our CTRL, WNV, and DENV plasma. Consistent with the relative antigenic distance from ZIKV, DENV immune plasma showed ~10-fold increased capacity to neutralize ZIKV (IC_{50} = 1:4,320) compared to WNV immune plasma (**Figure 1B**) (46, 47).

Having shown the neutralizing potential of the WNV and DENV plasma against ZIKV, we next asked to what extent these samples could enhance ZIKV. WNV, DENV or CTRL plasma were serially-diluted and co-incubated with ZIKV. These virus-antibody complexes were then used to infect K562 cell, which are only susceptible to ZIKV infection through antibody-mediated entry (48). After 2 days, we evaluated infection using flow cytometry to determine fold enhancement in the presence of varying concentrations of antibodies. Enhancement potential was quantified by fitting data to a Gaussian curve, and calculating the enhancing concentration at which 50% of maximum enhancement was achieved (EC_{50}). While WNV antibodies could enhance infection (EC_{50} = 390), DENV antibodies were more potent (EC_{50} = 3,470), showing ~10 fold increase in potency relative to WNV (**Figure 1C**). Together, these results demonstrate that WNV antibodies can modulate ZIKV infection *in vitro*, but to a lesser extent compared to DENV antibodies.

Impact of WNV Antibodies on the Pathogenesis of ZIKV in Pregnant Mice

Given that WNV antibodies can both bind and enhance ZIKV *in vitro*, we next evaluated how WNV antibodies could alter the course of ZIKV disease during pregnancy. To do this, we utilized ZIKV-infected pregnant $Stat2^{-/-}$ mice, a model we have

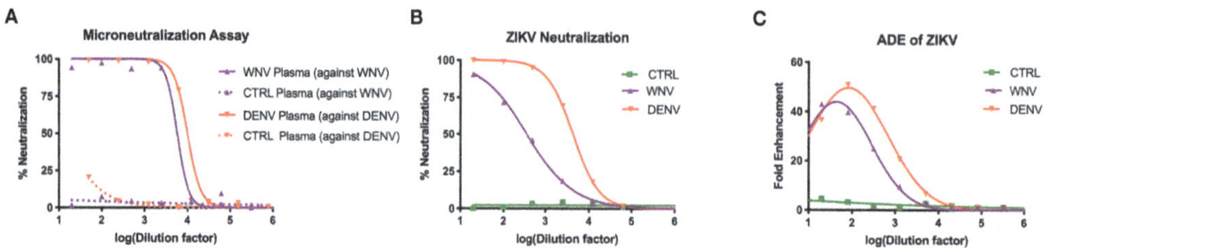

FIGURE 1 | Neutralization and enhancement potential of WNV immune plasma. **(A)** The capacity of plasma from WNV-infected individuals to neutralize WNV (Kunjin isolate) was compared to the capacity of plasma from DENV-infected individuals to neutralize DENV (serotype 1) in Vero cells. Non-reactive CTRL plasma was used as a negative control for each. Neutralization is represented by the percent reduction in infection compared to virus alone. **(B)** Neutralization of ZIKV (strain PRVABC-59) by WNV, DENV, and CTRL immune plasma in Vero cells is shown. **(C)** Enhancement of ZIKV by WNV, DENV, and CTRL immune plasma was tested in K562 cells. Enhancement was determined based on percent infection over the virus alone condition. All assays were completed in technical triplicate.

previously employed to evaluate the enhancement of ZIKV infection in the presence of DENV antibodies (32). Pregnant *Stat2*$^{-/-}$ mice were infected on E6.5 with 5,000 PFU of the PRVABC-59 strain of ZIKV, a clinical strain from the 2015 outbreak in Puerto Rico. Two hours prior to infection, mice were injected intraperitoneally with either WNV-immune plasma, DENV-immune plasma or CTRL plasma. Uninfected control mice were also treated with either WNV (n = 2) or CTRL (n = 2) plasma. No differences were observed for maternal weights or any fetal parameters between the uninfected groups (**Figure S1**) and thus were combined into a single group. Maternal weights were monitored through E13.5, at which point maternal organs and uterine horns were evaluated. We found that while all ZIKV-infected mice lost weight over the course of pregnancy compared to uninfected mice, no significant differences were observed in the presence or absence of WNV antibodies (**Figure 2A**). Pregnant mice that received DENV plasma prior to infection steadily lost weight over the course of pregnancy, consistent with our previous findings (32). Evaluation of viremia revealed a significant increase in mice that received DENV plasma at 3 days post infection, but not in mice that received WNV plasma, compared to CTRL (**Figure 2B**). However, viral loads in maternal brains, spleens, and spinal cords revealed no significant differences in the presence of WNV antibodies or DENV antibodies by qRT-PCR (**Figures 2C–E**). While the presence of DENV antibodies in ZIKV-infected mice elevated the broad inflammatory response significantly, no striking differences existed between mice that received WNV antibodies or CTRL (**Figure 2F**).

Impact of WNV Antibodies on ZIKV Induced Fetal Tissue Damage

We next investigated how the presence of WNV antibodies altered fetal outcomes during pregnancy in this model. We evaluated uterine horns and individual fetal-placental pairs for morphological differences upon infection to determine if the presence of WNV antibodies impacted ZIKV associated fetal damage (**Figure 3A**). Uterine horns from ZIKV infected dams, irrespective of plasma group, were darker in color and morphologically damaged compared to those from uninfected dams, with DENV plasma showing the most damage, CTRL plasma showing the least, and WNV plasma showing an intermediate phenotype. This observation was supported by quantifying the resorption rates between groups. Although the resorption rates among ZIKV-infected dams treated with WNV plasma revealed a trend towards an increase in resorption, this was not statistically significant compared to mice that received CTRL antibodies ($p > 0.99$; **Figure 3B**). This was in contrast to the mice that received DENV antibodies, where a significant increase in the resorption rate was observed (**Figure 3B**). We next evaluated fetuses and placentas for developmental defects compared to uninfected fetuses. Due to the high resorption rate, we were unable to include fetuses from dams that received the DENV antibodies in subsequent analyses and instead limited our comparisons to fetuses from pregnant dams that received WNV and CTRL antibodies. While fetuses from infected dams were significantly smaller than fetuses from uninfected dams, there were no significant differences in fetal size, fetal mass, placental length or placental mass between mice that received WNV plasma or CTRL plasma (**Figures 3C–F**).

In our previous reports, we showed that much of the damage caused by cross-reactive DENV antibodies was the result of higher viral loads in the placenta, which led to greater inflammation and placental damage (32). Therefore, we next asked whether viral replication differed in the fetal tissue in the presence of WNV antibodies by qRT-PCR. While all placentas from infected mice had viral loads in the placentas, there were no differences in viral load in mice that received WNV antibodies compared to mice that received non-specific CTRL antibodies (**Figure 4A**). Evaluation of viral loads in the fetal heads showed the same trend, with no significant differences between the two groups (**Figure 4B**).

We also asked whether the presence of WNV antibodies could alter the inflammatory landscape in the placentas and fetal heads during ZIKV infection. We examined fetal and placental homogenates from mice that received either WNV or CTRL antibodies for chemokine and cytokine production by multiplex ELISA. Examination across 21 cytokines showed no significant differences in the inflammatory milieu in either the placentas or the fetal heads obtained from ZIKV-infected pregnant dams that received WNV or CTRL antibodies (**Figure 4C**).

Pathogenesis of ZIKV in the Placenta in the Presence of WNV Antibodies

Our previous study evaluating ADE caused by the presence of DENV antibodies implicated increased damage to the labyrinth zone of the placenta during ZIKV infection. Therefore, we wondered whether WNV antibodies had any impact on placental structure in ZIKV-infected mice. Harvested placentas across numerous pregnancies were evaluated for overall pathological changes by H&E staining (**Figure 5A**, left) as well as the density and structure of the labyrinth zone using Vimentin staining (**Figure 5A**, right). In all cases, we found a pronounced reduction in the size and density of the labyrinth zone due to ZIKV infection; however, there were no obvious differences in the placentas harvested from mice that received WNV plasma or CTRL plasma (**Figure 5A**). The extent of viral infection between mice that received CTRL or WNV antibodies was similar, consistent with the qRT-PCR results, and infection was limited to the decidual-placental interface (**Figure 5B**, red arrows) as examined by fluorescence RNA *in situ* hybridization. This is consistent with our previous findings during ZIKV infections in the absence of cross-reactive antibodies in this model (32). Together, our findings show no significant impact of WNV antibodies on the pathogenesis of ZIKV during pregnancy.

DISCUSSION

Our study is the first to examine the potential for WNV antibodies to enhance ZIKV infection in the context of pregnancy. We found no significant evidence that WNV

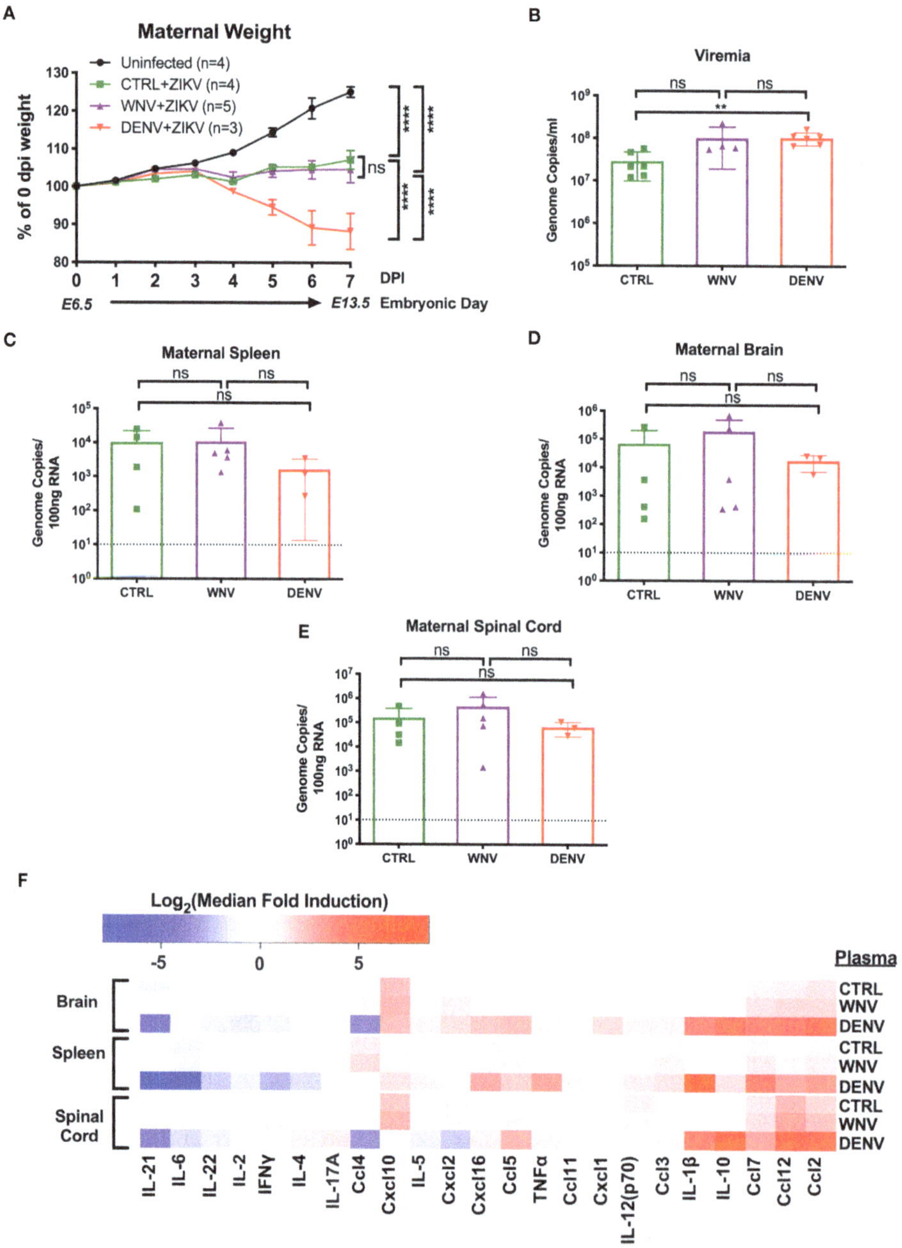

FIGURE 2 | Impact of WNV antibodies on ZIKV infected dams. ZIKV-infected *Stat2*$^{-/-}$ dams that received 20μl of either CTRL (n=4), WNV (n=5) or DENV (n=3) plasma were compared to uninfected dams that also received WNV or CTRL plasma (n=4; See **Figure S1**). **(A)** Maternal weights between infection at E6.5 and tissue collection at E13.5 are shown as a percentage of starting weight at E6.5. Significance was determined by two-way ANOVA, and error bars represents SD. **(B)** Viremia was determined at 3 days post infection in ZIKV-infected dams by qRT-PCR. Mice included in this subfigure are from an unmatched cohort of CTRL (n=6), WNV (n=4), and DENV (n=6) mice. Viral loads in dams from **(A)** were determined in the maternal spleens **(C)**, brains **(D)**, and spinal cords **(E)** by qRT-PCR. For **(C–E)**, dotted lines indicate the limit of detection, and mean values with SD are depicted with the overlaid bar plots. Significance was determined by Mann-Whitney U-test. **(F)** Tissue homogenates from brain, spleen and spinal cords from ZIKV-infected mice in **(A)** were evaluated for inflammatory markers by multiplex ELISA. Data are shown as a $\log_2$ transformed median fold induction over the median pg/ml expression in the uninfected condition. ns, not significant; $^{**}p < 0.01$, $^{****}p < 0.0001$.

antibodies mediate enhancement of ZIKV in pregnant mice. In the absence of thorough prospective human studies on the influence of WNV immunity on ZIKV infections, we hope that these data provide the first insights into the safety of introducing greater WNV immunity into ZIKV endemic regions and regions at risk of ZIKV expansion. This finding has major implications for WNV vaccine development and begins to address larger questions about the process of ADE.

ADE is known to be a function of antigenic distance, with a 'sweet spot' level of antigenic relatedness resulting in the

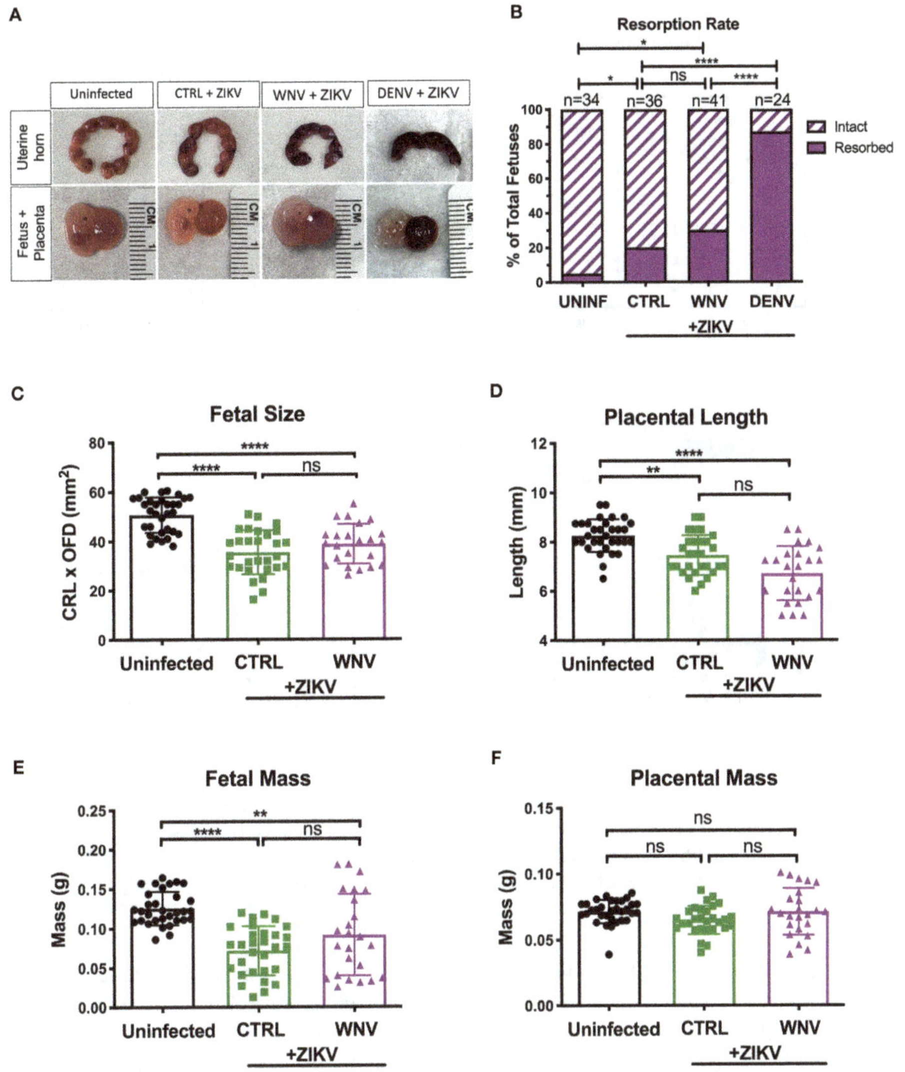

FIGURE 3 | Impact of WNV antibodies on ZIKV-infected fetuses. Uterine horns were harvested and morphologically examined at E13.5 from ZIKV-infected or uninfected dams (**A**, top). Fetal and placental pairs were isolated from each harvested conceptus, and representative images are shown (**A**, bottom). The resorption rate across all pregnancies are represented by the proportion of resorbed and intact fetuses **(B)**; uninfected mice (n=34), CTRL (n=36), WNV (n=41), and DENV (n=24). Significance between groups was determined by χ^2 analysis. Intact fetuses and placentas were measured for fetal size **(C)** by multiplying the crown-to-rump length (CRL) by the occipital-frontal diameter (OFD), placental length **(D)**, represented by diameter, fetal mass **(E)**, and placental mass **(F)**. Significance for **(C–F)** was determined by a one-way ANOVA, with a Kruskal-Wallis post-test for multiple comparisons between uninfected mice (n=32), CTRL (n=29) and WNV (n=24). Bar plot overlays for **(C–F)** depict mean and SD. Resorbed and partially resorbed fetuses were excluded from the analysis in **(C–F)**. ns, not significant; *$p < 0.05$, **$p < 0.01$, ****$p < 0.0001$.

possibility of enhancement. In general, higher relatedness will result in greater antigenic affinity and neutralization, while lower relatedness will result in less binding and weak or no enhancement potential. Based on ADE observed between the DENV serotypes, ~68% identity at the amino acid level for the E proteins appears to be sufficient for enhancement to be observed (49). ZIKV and the four serotypes of DENV are on average 55% similar at the antigenic E level, and *in vitro/in vivo* data suggest that enhancement *can* occur between the two viruses (50). Consistent with this notion, a recently published study showed that antibodies against ZIKV could enhance infection in children subsequently infected with DENV (51–53). However, studies that have evaluated the impact of DENV immunity on ZIKV pathogenesis in humans have largely shown that DENV immunity is protective, with one study showing a concentration dependent loss of protection against ZIKV at intermediate DENV antibody levels (54). It is possible that these seemingly conflicting data, where enhancement occurs in one direction but not the other, are the result of a wider window of severe symptomology for DENV infections compared to ZIKV infections. Alternatively, perhaps the order in which infection occurs generates antibodies against antigenic epitopes that are

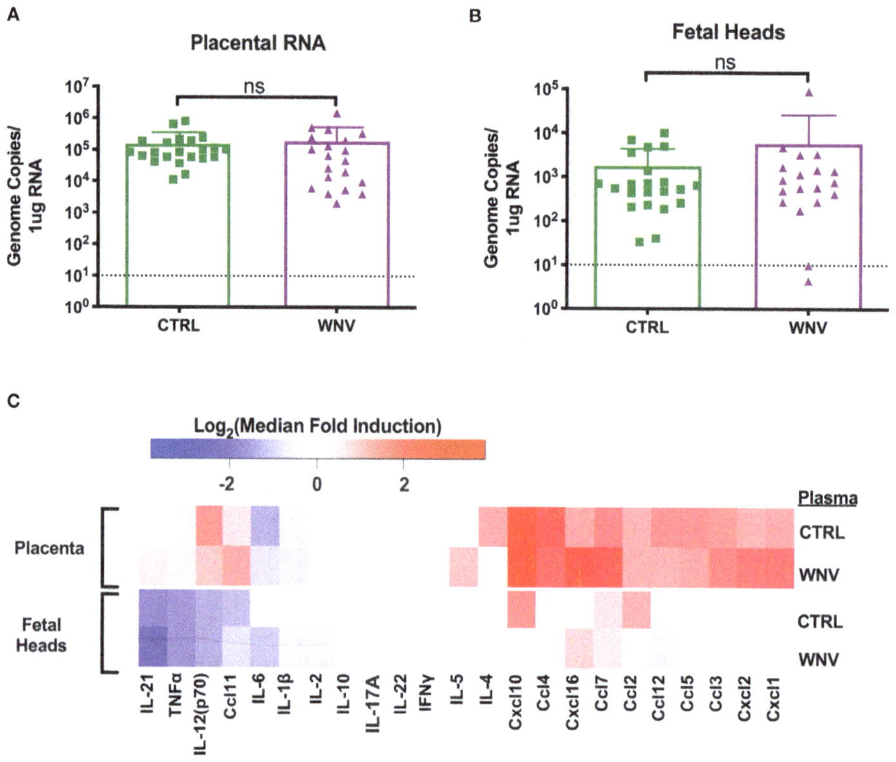

FIGURE 4 | Molecular characterization of ZIKV infection in the fetus and placenta. RNA was extracted from **(A)** placentas (CTRL n=22; WNV n=20) and **(B)** fetal heads (CTRL n=22; WNV= 19) to examine viral loads by qRT-PCR. Significance was determined by Mann-Whitney U-test, and the dashed lines represent the limit of detection. Overlaid bar plots depict mean and SD. **(C)** Tissue homogenates from placentas and fetal heads were evaluated for inflammatory markers by multiplex ELISA. Data are shown as a $\log_2$ transformed median fold induction over the median pg/ml expression in the uninfected condition. ns, not significant.

more or less potently neutralizing or enhancing. WNV is slightly more antigenically distant from ZIKV (~54% amino acid identity to the E protein) (49). Our study showed that WNV antibodies could enhance ZIKV at the *in vitro* level, but not at the *in vivo* level in ZIKV-infected pregnant mice. Given that the mouse model is a very sensitive model for detecting ADE, our results suggest that WNV is unlikely to alter ZIKV pathogenesis in humans, at least in the context of pregnancy. However, carefully designed prospective human studies need to test this hypothesis considering that the antigenic relatedness of these two viruses suggests that ADE could be possible. Further, the role of ZIKV specific antibodies impacting the pathogenesis of WNV has yet to be examined.

Our data also provide further evidence for how enhancement might influence ZIKV pathogenesis in pregnancy. In our report on DENV enhancement of ZIKV in this model, we identified that the placenta was the primary target for enhanced ZIKV damage (32). We found that enhancing antibodies expanded the tropism of ZIKV from the decidual-placental interface into the cytotrophoblast layer, which correlated with an increase in cytokine production, as well as in the disruption of the placental labyrinth zone. The labyrinth zone is a bed of fetal derived endothelium essential for maternal-fetal blood and nutrient transfer, and thus we hypothesized that the disruption of this zone was responsible for the fetal abnormalities noted (55). In this work, we did not find any evidence of enhancement by increased pathogenesis, inflammation or viral load. Infection was limited to the decidual interface, demonstrating cross-reactive antibodies which are not capable of increasing the infectious range of ZIKV in the placenta. It is not clear if ZIKV gains access to this compartment through direct Fc-mediated endocytosis, or if this is the result of increased access to the compartment during inflammatory responses. However, we believe that based on our data, infection of this zone is critical for the ZIKV mediated pathology observed in enhanced infections.

Our study has several limitations. One major limitation is that we only assessed a single concentration of WNV antibodies in this study (20μl/mouse). This concentration was chosen because it is the concentration where DENV antibodies can potently enhance ZIKV. However, as we showed that the enhancement potential for DENV antibodies for ZIKV is ~1 log greater than that of WNV antibodies *in vitro* (**Figure 1C**), it is possible that WNV antibodies would require ~10-fold higher concentration to achieve enhancement. Our previous data suggest that increasing the antibody concentration 10-fold would also increase mortality non-specifically due to the non-physiological concentration of circulating antibodies (31). One possibility for why DENV plasma enhances while WNV plasma does not in our

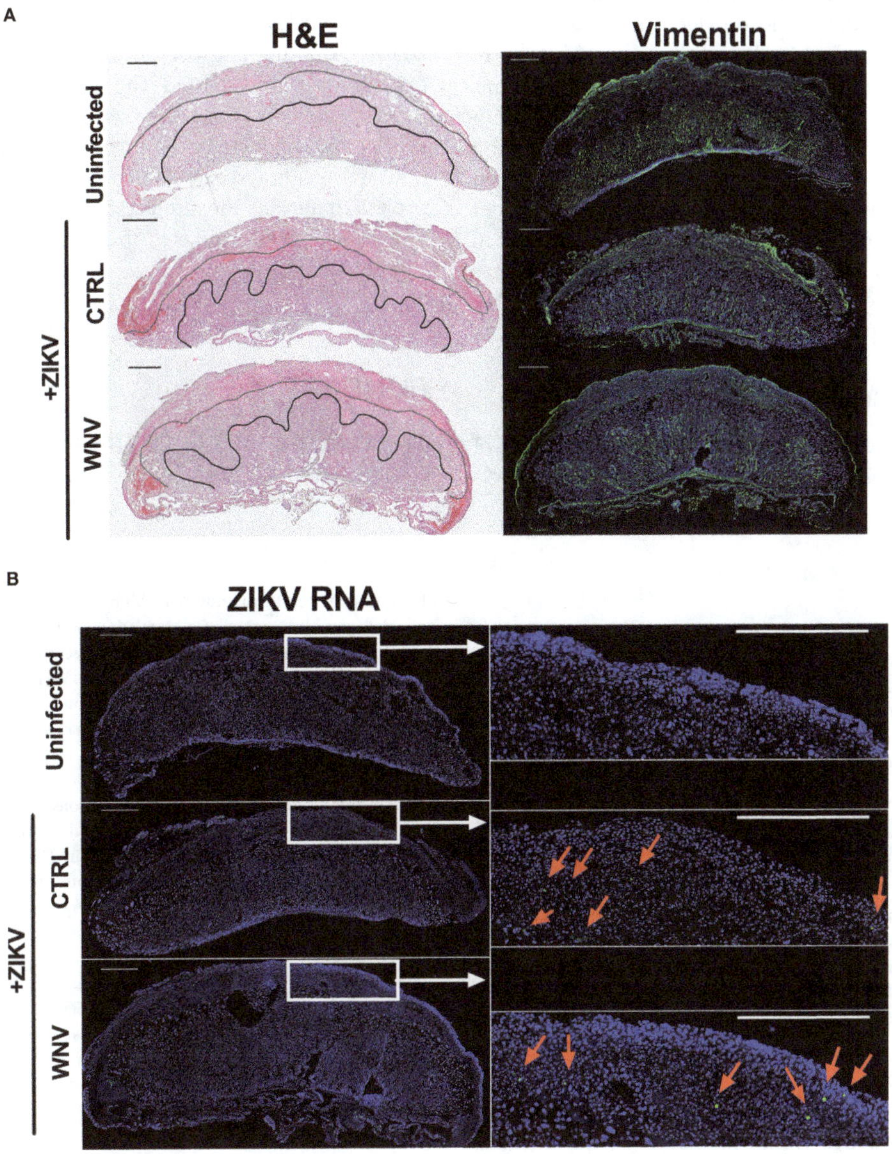

FIGURE 5 | ZIKV-induced damage in the developing placenta. Placentas harvested at E13.5 from uninfected of ZIKV-infected dams that received either WNV or CTRL plasma were examined for **(A)** the disruption of the placental labyrinth zone by both hematoxylin and eosin (H&E) staining (left) and immunofluorescence staining for vimentin (right), which marks fetal endothelium (green). DAPI is shown in blue. **(B)** Placentas were evaluated for ZIKV RNA localization by *in situ* hybridization. Tiled images of representative whole placentas are shown on the left, with tiles from white boxed regions shown on the right for ease of comparison (scale = 500μm). ZIKV-infected cells (green) are highlighted with red arrows and DAPI is shown in blue.

experiments is because the concentration of WNV-specific antibodies is lower in the pooled WNV plasma than the concentration of DENV-specific antibodies in the DENV plasma. To address this, we quantified the number of WNV specific IC_{50}'s we injected per mouse of WNV plasma and compared that to the number of DENV specific IC_{50}'s injected per mouse of DENV plasma. We found that we were using a comparable concentration of IC_{50}'s (<2-fold difference). Therefore, we find it unlikely that the differences observed between the WNV and DENV groups in our mouse studies are a result of differing amounts of WNV and DENV specific IgG. Instead, these data suggest that the differences we have observed are due to the relative antigenic cross-reactivity to ZIKV.

An additional limitation of this study is the use of *Stat2*$^{-/-}$ mice. ZIKV NS5 is known to bind and degrade human STAT2, but not mouse Stat2, resulting in a species barrier (56). To overcome this, the human STAT2 knock-in mouse model has recently been described for ZIKV infection in non-pregnant adult mice. Our future work will aim to utilize the human *STAT2* knock-in model for studying ADE in the context of pregnancy (34), which may be more translatable to human disease.

Ultimately, the goal of studying ADE should be to model the relative risk that immunity to any one virus poses to the severity of another. Understanding this would provide risk assessments for severe outbreak zones, vaccine development, and identification of patients at risk for severe disease sequelae. As one could imagine, this model will likely be complex and multifactorial - with antibody concentration already having been identified to be a major risk factor for ADE. Antigenic distance, neutralization capacity, antibody durability, antibody subclass, infection order and many other factors are still under investigation for their role in predisposing enhanced infection (57). This current study has begun to address the role of cross reactivity, and we hope that our findings will be helpful in building this risk model.

ETHICS STATEMENT

The animal study was reviewed and approved by Icahn School of Medicine at Mount Sinai Animal Care and Use Committee.

AUTHOR CONTRIBUTIONS

JA conceptualized the project, conducted the experiments, data analysis, drafting and editing of the manuscript. JC conducted experiments and edited the manuscript. AM conducted experiments and edited the manuscript. JB conceptualized the project and conducted experiments. GF, DK, and SS contributed critical reagents and edited the manuscript. JL conceptualized the project, managed the project and edited the manuscript. All authors contributed to the article and approved the submitted version.

FUNDING

This work was funded by NIAID grant R01AI150837 and NHLBI F31HL149295.

REFERENCES

1. Takada A, Kawaoka Y. Antibody-dependent Enhancement of Viral Infection: Molecular Mechanisms and In Vivo Implications. *Rev Med Virol* (2003) 13:387–98. doi: 10.1002/rmv.405
2. Taylor A, Foo SS, Bruzzone R, Dinh LV, King NJ, Mahalingam S. Fc Receptors in Antibody-Dependent Enhancement of Viral Infections. *Immunol Rev* (2015) 268:340–64. doi: 10.1111/imr.12367
3. Narayan R, Tripathi S. Intrinsic ADE: The Dark Side of Antibody Dependent Enhancement During Dengue Infection. *Front Cell Infect Microbiol* (2020) 10:580096. doi: 10.3389/fcimb.2020.580096
4. Gyawali N, Bradbury RS, Taylor-Robinson AW. The Epidemiology of Dengue Infection: Harnessing Past Experience and Current Knowledge to Support Implementation of Future Control Strategies. *J Vector Borne Dis* (2016) 53:293–304.
5. Soo KM, Khalid B, Ching SM, Chee HY. Meta-Analysis of Dengue Severity During Infection by Different Dengue Virus Serotypes in Primary and Secondary Infections. *PLoS One* (2016) 11:e0154760. doi: 10.1371/journal.pone.0154760
6. Halstead SB. Dengue Antibody-Dependent Enhancement: Knowns and Unknowns. *Microbiol Spectr* (2014) 2. doi: 10.1128/microbiolspec.AID-0022-2014
7. Toh YX, Gan V, Balakrishnan T, Zuest R, Poidinger M, Wilson S, et al. Dengue Serotype Cross-Reactive, Anti-E Protein Antibodies Confound Specific Immune Memory for 1 Year After Infection. *Front Immunol* (2014) 5:388. doi: 10.3389/fimmu.2014.00388
8. Zidane N, Dussart P, Bremand L, Bedouelle H. Cross-reactivities Between Human IgMs and the Four Serotypes of Dengue Virus as Probed With Artificial Homodimers of domain-III From the Envelope Proteins. *BMC Infect Dis* (2013) 13:302. doi: 10.1186/1471-2334-13-302
9. Moi ML, Takasaki T, Kurane I. Human Antibody Response to Dengue Virus: Implications for Dengue Vaccine Design. *Trop Med Health* (2016) 44:1. doi: 10.1186/s41182-016-0004-y
10. Khan E, Prakoso D, Imtiaz K, Malik F, Farooqi JQ, Long MT, et al. The Clinical Features of Co-circulating Dengue Viruses and the Absence of Dengue Hemorrhagic Fever in Pakistan. *Front Public Health* (2020) 8:1–10. doi: 10.3389/fpubh.2020.00287
11. Hamel R, Surasombatpattana P, Wichit S, Dauvé A, Donato C, Pompon J, et al. Phylogenetic Analysis Revealed the Co-Circulation of Four Dengue Virus Serotypes in Southern Thailand. *PLoS One* (2019) 14:e0221179. doi: 10.1371/journal.pone.0221179
12. Racherla RG, Pamireddy ML, Mohan A, Mudhigeti N, Mahalakshmi PA, Nallapireddy U, et al. Co-circulation of Four Dengue Serotypes at South Eastern Andhra Pradesh, India: A Prospective Study. *Indian J Med Microbiol* (2018) 36:236–40. doi: 10.4103/ijmm.IJMM_18_109
13. Moi ML, Takasaki T, Saijo M, Kurane I. Determination of Antibody Concentration as the Main Parameter in a Dengue Virus Antibody-Dependent Enhancement Assay Using Fcγr-Expressing BHK Cells. *Arch Virol* (2014) 159:103–16. doi: 10.1007/s00705-013-1787-3
14. Ripoll DR, Wallqvist A, Chaudhury S. Molecular Simulations Reveal the Role of Antibody Fine Specificity and Viral Maturation State on Antibody-Dependent Enhancement of Infection in Dengue Virus. *Front Cell Infect Microbiol* (2019) 9:200. doi: 10.3389/fcimb.2019.00200
15. Katzelnick LC, Harris E. The Use of Longitudinal Cohorts for Studies of Dengue Viral Pathogenesis and Protection. *Curr Opin Virol* (2018) 29:51–61. doi: 10.1016/j.coviro.2018.03.004
16. Katzelnick LC, Gresh L, Halloran ME, Mercado JC, Kuan G, Gordon A, et al. Antibody-dependent Enhancement of Severe Dengue Disease in Humans. *Science* (2017) 358:929–32. doi: 10.1126/science.aan6836
17. Fischer C, de Oliveira-Filho EF, Drexler JF. Viral Emergence and Immune Interplay in Flavivirus Vaccines. *Lancet Infect Dis* (2020) 20:15–7. doi: 10.1016/S1473-3099(19)30697-8
18. Lazear HM, Diamond MS. Zika Virus: New Clinical Syndromes and Its Emergence in the Western Hemisphere. *J Virol* (2016) 90:4864–75. doi: 10.1128/JVI.00252-16
19. Brasil P, Pereira JP Jr., Moreira ME, Ribeiro Nogueira RM, Damasceno L, Wakimoto M, et al. Zika Virus Infection in Pregnant Women in Rio De Janeiro. *N Engl J Med* (2016) 375:2321–34. doi: 10.1056/NEJMoa1602412
20. Coyne CB, Lazear HM. Zika Virus - Reigniting the TORCH. *Nat Rev Microbiol* (2016) 14:707–15. doi: 10.1038/nrmicro.2016.125
21. Honein MA, Dawson AL, Petersen EE, Jones AM, Lee EH, Yazdy MM, et al. Birth Defects Among Fetuses and Infants of US Women With Evidence of Possible Zika Virus Infection During Pregnancy. *JAMA* (2017) 317:59–68. doi: 10.1001/jama.2016.19006
22. Reynolds MR, Jones AM, Petersen EE, Lee EH, Rice ME, Bingham A, et al. Vital Signs: Update on Zika Virus-Associated Birth Defects and Evaluation of All U.s. Infants With Congenital Zika Virus Exposure - U.S. Zika Pregnancy Registry, 2016. *MMWR Morb Mortal Wkly Rep* (2017) 66:366–73. doi: 10.15585/mmwr.mm6613e1

23. Schaub B, Vouga M, Najioullah F, Gueneret M, Monthieux A, Harte C, et al. Analysis of Blood From Zika Virus-Infected Fetuses: A Prospective Case Series. *Lancet Infect Dis* (2017) 17:520–7. doi: 10.1016/S1473-3099(17)30102-0
24. Wheeler AC. Development of Infants With Congenital Zika Syndrome: What Do We Know and What can We Expect? *Pediatrics* (2018) 141:S154–s160. doi: 10.1542/peds.2017-2038D
25. Shapiro-Mendoza CK, Rice ME, Galang RR, Fulton AC, VanMaldeghem K, Prado MV, et al. Pregnancy Outcomes After Maternal Zika Virus Infection During Pregnancy - U.s. *Territories* (2017). *MMWR Morb Mortal Wkly Rep* (2017) 66(23):615–21. doi: 10.15585/mmwr.mm6623e1
26. Mulkey SB, Arroyave-Wessel M, Peyton C, Bulas DI, Fourzali Y, Jiang J, et al. Neurodevelopmental Abnormalities in Children With In Utero Zika Virus Exposure Without Congenital Zika Syndrome. *JAMA Pediatr* (2020) 174:269–76. doi: 10.1001/jamapediatrics.2019.5204
27. Pereira H, Dos Santos SP, Amâncio A, de Oliveira-Szejnfeld PS, Flor EO, de Sales Tavares J, et al. Neurological Outcomes of Congenital Zika Syndrome in Toddlers and Preschoolers: A Case Series. *Lancet Child Adolesc Health* (2020) 4:378–87. doi: 10.1016/S2352-4642(20)30041-9
28. Barba-Spaeth G, Dejnirattisai W, Rouvinski A, Vaney MC, Medits I, Sharma A, et al. Structural Basis of Potent Zika-dengue Virus Antibody Cross-Neutralization. *Nature* (2016) 536:48–53. doi: 10.1038/nature18938
29. Kostyuchenko VA, Lim EX, Zhang S, Fibriansah G, Ng TS, Ooi JS, et al. Structure of the Thermally Stable Zika Virus. *Nature* (2016) 533:425–8. doi: 10.1038/nature17994
30. Sirohi D, Chen Z, Sun L, Klose T, Pierson TC, Rossmann MG, et al. The 3.8 Å Resolution cryo-EM Structure of Zika Virus. *Science* (2016) 352:467–70. doi: 10.1126/science.aaf5316
31. Bardina SV, Bunduc P, Tripathi S, Duehr J, Frere JJ, Brown JA, et al. Enhancement of Zika Virus Pathogenesis by Preexisting Antiflavivirus Immunity. *Science* (2017) 356:175–80. doi: 10.1126/science.aal4365
32. Brown JA, Singh G, Acklin JA, Lee S, Duehr JE, Chokola AN, et al. Dengue Virus Immunity Increases Zika Virus-Induced Damage During Pregnancy. *Immunity* (2019) 50:751–762.e5. doi: 10.1016/j.immuni.2019.01.005
33. Zimmerman MG, Quicke KM, O'Neal JT, Arora N, Machiah D, Priyamvada L, et al. Cross-Reactive Dengue Virus Antibodies Augment Zika Virus Infection of Human Placental Macrophages. *Cell Host Microbe* (2018) 24:731–742.e6. doi: 10.1016/j.chom.2018.10.008
34. Rathore APS, Saron WAA, Lim T, Jahan N, St John AL. Maternal Immunity and Antibodies to Dengue Virus Promote Infection and Zika Virus-Induced Microcephaly in Fetuses. *Sci Adv* (2019) 5:eaav3208. doi: 10.1126/sciadv.aav3208
35. Li M, Zhao L, Zhang C, Wang X, Hong W, Sun J, et al. Dengue Immune Sera Enhance Zika Virus Infection in Human Peripheral Blood Monocytes Through Fc Gamma Receptors. *PLoS One* (2018) 13:e0200478. doi: 10.1371/journal.pone.0200478
36. Petersen LR, Brault AC, Nasci RS. West Nile Virus: Review of the Literature. *JAMA* (2013) 310:308–15. doi: 10.1001/jama.2013.8042
37. Murray KO, Mertens E, Despres P. West Nile Virus and its Emergence in the United States of America. *Vet Res* (2010) 41:67. doi: 10.1051/vetres/2010039
38. Ronca SE, Murray KO, Nolan MS. Cumulative Incidence of West Nile Virus Infection, Continental United States, 1999-2016. *Emerg Infect Dis* (2019) 25:325–7. doi: 10.3201/eid2502.180765
39. Keasey SL, Pugh CL, Jensen SMR, Smith JL, Hontz RD, Durbin AP, et al. Antibody Responses to Zika Virus Infections in Environments of Flavivirus Endemicity. *Clin Vaccine Immunol* (2017) 24:e00036–17. doi: 10.1128/CVI.00036-17
40. Willis E, Hensley SE. Characterization of Zika Virus Binding and Enhancement Potential of a Large Panel of Flavivirus Murine Monoclonal Antibodies. *Virology* (2017) 508:1–6. doi: 10.1016/j.virol.2017.04.031
41. Adams LE, Martin SW, Lindsey NP, Lehman JA, Rivera A, Kolsin J, et al. Epidemiology of Dengue, Chikungunya, and Zika Virus Disease in U.S. States and Territories, 2017. *Am J Trop Med Hyg* (2019) 101:884–90. doi: 10.4269/ajtmh.19-0309
42. Messina JP, Brady OJ, Golding N, Kraemer MUG, Wint GRW, Ray SE, et al. The Current and Future Global Distribution and Population at Risk of Dengue. *Nat Microbiol* (2019) 4:1508–15. doi: 10.1038/s41564-019-0476-8
43. Schwarz MC, Sourisseau M, Espino MM, Gray ES, Chambers MT, Tortorella D, et al. Rescue of the 1947 Zika Virus Prototype Strain With a Cytomegalovirus Promoter-Driven cDNA Clone. *mSphere* (2016) 1:e00246–16. doi: 10.1128/mSphere.00246-16
44. Aguado LC, Schmid S, Sachs D, Shim JV, Lim JK, tenOever BR. Microrna Function is Limited to Cytokine Control in the Acute Response to Virus Infection. *Cell Host Microbe* (2015) 18:714–22. doi: 10.1016/j.chom.2015.11.003
45. Daffis S, Lazear HM, Liu WJ, Audsley M, Engle M, Khromykh AA, et al. The Naturally Attenuated Kunjin Strain of West Nile Virus Shows Enhanced Sensitivity to the Host Type I Interferon Response. *J Virol* (2011) 85:5664–8. doi: 10.1128/JVI.00232-11
46. Heinz FX, Stiasny K. The Antigenic Structure of Zika Virus and Its Relation to Other Flaviviruses: Implications for Infection and Immunoprophylaxis. *Microbiol Mol Biol Rev* (2017) 81. doi: 10.1128/MMBR.00055-16
47. Gupta SK, Singh S, Nischal A, Pant KK, Seth PK. Molecular-based Identification and Phylogeny of Genomic and Proteomic Sequences of Mosquito-Borne Flavivirus. *Genes Genomics* (2014) 36:31–43. doi: 10.1007/s13258-013-0137-x
48. Castanha PMS, Nascimento EJM, Braga C, Cordeiro MT, de Carvalho OV, de Mendonça LR, et al. Dengue Virus-Specific Antibodies Enhance Brazilian Zika Virus Infection. *J Infect Dis* (2017) 215:781–5. doi: 10.1093/infdis/jiw638
49. Xu X, Vaughan K, Weiskopf D, Grifoni A, Diamond MS, Sette A, et al. Identifying Candidate Targets of Immune Responses in Zika Virus Based on Homology to Epitopes in Other Flavivirus Species. *PLoS Curr* (2016) 8. doi: 10.1371/currents.outbreaks.9aa2e1fb61b0f632f58a098773008c4b
50. Wen J, Shresta S. Antigenic Cross-Reactivity Between Zika and Dengue Viruses: Is it Time to Develop a Universal Vaccine? *Curr Opin Immunol* (2019) 59:1–8. doi: 10.1016/j.coi.2019.02.001
51. Katzelnick LC, Narvaez C, Arguello S, Lopez Mercado B, Collado D, Ampie O, et al. Zika Virus Infection Enhances Future Risk of Severe Dengue Disease. *Science* (2020) 369:1123–8. doi: 10.1126/science.abb6143
52. Gordon A, Gresh L, Ojeda S, Katzelnick LC, Sanchez N, Mercado JC, et al. Prior Dengue Virus Infection and Risk of Zika: A Pediatric Cohort in Nicaragua. *PLoS Med* (2019) 16:e1002726. doi: 10.1371/journal.pmed.1002726
53. Rodriguez-Barraquer I, Costa F, Nascimento EJM, Nery NJ, Castanha PMS, Sacramento GA, et al. Impact of Preexisting Dengue Immunity on Zika Virus Emergence in a Dengue Endemic Region. *Science* (2019) 363:607–10. doi: 10.1126/science.aav6618
54. Terzian ACB, Schanoski AS, Mota MTO, da Silva RA, Estofolete CF, Colombo TE, et al. Viral Load and Cytokine Response Profile Does Not Support Antibody-Dependent Enhancement in Dengue-Primed Zika Virus-Infected Patients. *Clin Infect Dis* (2017) 65:1260–5. doi: 10.1093/cid/cix558
55. Woods L, Perez-Garcia V, Hemberger M. Regulation of Placental Development and Its Impact on Fetal Growth—New Insights From Mouse Models. *Front Endocrinol* (2018) 9:1–18. doi: 10.3389/fendo.2018.00570
56. Grant A, Ponia SS, Tripathi S, Balasubramaniam V, Miorin L, Sourisseau M, et al. Zika Virus Targets Human STAT2 to Inhibit Type I Interferon Signaling. *Cell Host Microbe* (2016) 19:882–90. doi: 10.1016/j.chom.2016.05.009
57. Guzman MG, Vazquez S. The Complexity of Antibody-Dependent Enhancement of Dengue Virus Infection. *Viruses* (2010) 2:2649–62. doi: 10.3390/v2122649

6

Therapeutic Potential of Regulatory T Cells in Preeclampsia—Opportunities and Challenges

Sarah A. Robertson[1], Ella S. Green[1], Alison S. Care[1], Lachlan M. Moldenhauer[1], Jelmer R. Prins[2], M. Louise Hull[1,3], Simon C. Barry[1] and Gustaaf Dekker[1]*

[1] Robinson Research Institute and Adelaide Medical School, University of Adelaide, Adelaide, SA, Australia, [2] University Medical Center Groningen, Groningen, Netherlands, [3] Women's and Children's Hospital, Adelaide, SA, Australia

***Correspondence:**
Sarah A. Robertson
sarah.robertson@adelaide.edu.au

Inflammation is a central feature and is implicated as a causal factor in preeclampsia and other hypertensive disorders of pregnancy. Inflammatory mediators and leukocytes, which are elevated in peripheral blood and gestational tissues, contribute to the uterine vascular anomalies and compromised placental function that characterize particularly the severe, early onset form of disease. Regulatory T (Treg) cells are central mediators of pregnancy tolerance and direct other immune cells to counteract inflammation and promote robust placentation. Treg cells are commonly perturbed in preeclampsia, and there is evidence Treg cell insufficiency predates onset of symptoms. A causal role is implied by mouse studies showing sufficient numbers of functionally competent Treg cells must be present in the uterus from conception, to support maternal vascular adaptation and prevent later placental inflammatory pathology. Treg cells may therefore provide a tractable target for both preventative strategies and treatment interventions in preeclampsia. Steps to boost Treg cell activity require investigation and could be incorporated into pregnancy planning and preconception care. Pharmacological interventions developed to target Treg cells in autoimmune conditions warrant consideration for evaluation, utilizing rigorous clinical trial methodology, and ensuring safety is paramount. Emerging cell therapy tools involving *in vitro* Treg cell generation and/or expansion may in time become relevant. The success of preventative and therapeutic approaches will depend on resolving several challenges including developing informative diagnostic tests for Treg cell activity applicable before conception or during early pregnancy, selection of relevant patient subgroups, and identification of appropriate windows of gestation for intervention.

Keywords: pregnancy, preeclampsia, placenta, embryo implantation, maternal vascular adaptation, inflammation, Treg cells, immune tolerance

INTRODUCTION

Preeclampsia and related hypertensive disorders complicate 3–5% of pregnancies. They are a leading cause of maternal deaths and perinatal morbidity and mortality (1) and are enormously expensive to health care systems, with an estimated cost in the US of \$2.18 billion for the first 12 months of life alone (2). Preterm birth and fetal intrauterine growth restriction (IUGR) are common sequalae, causing developmental challenges for the neonate that adversely impact cardiovascular, metabolic, and neurodevelopmental health (3). Preeclampsia also has long-term consequences for maternal cardiovascular health (4). Despite extensive research, the pathophysiological origins of preeclampsia remain unclear and effective preventative interventions are lacking. Current clinical management is aimed at alleviating symptoms and delaying delivery, rather than preventing occurrence by modifying the underlying cause (5, 6).

An emerging view is that critical initiating events before pregnancy and in the conception and implantation phase determine preeclampsia susceptibility, eliciting changes in placental development much earlier in gestation than when symptoms appear (7–9). This is particularly the case for the severe, early onset form of preeclampsia where failed maternal vascular adaptation to pregnancy is implicated—but also likely contributes to later onset disease (10, 11). There is strong evidence that failure of the maternal immune response to adapt correctly in early pregnancy underpins the placental and cardiovascular anomalies that become evident in later gestation. Disturbance in the immune response appears to be central and causal of later placental and hypertensive symptoms (8, 12, 13).

The adaptive immune response, with its typical features of immunological priming and memory, appears integral to the pathophysiological origin of the condition. Preeclampsia is more common in first pregnancies, particularly after limited sexual contact with the conceiving partner due to short sexual cohabitation, use of barrier contraceptive methods or assisted reproduction (14–16). Prior pregnancy with the same partner offers protection, but this is partner-specific and is lost with a new partner, implying alloantigen specificity (17). Assisted reproduction with donor oocytes, where there is no prior contact with the donor's alloantigens, is associated with a 4.3-fold increase in preeclampsia compared to natural conception (18). The risk is also increased with donor sperm but this is reduced with multiple exposures to the same donor (19). Pregnancy-induced memory in T cells (20) and in uterine NK cells (21) likely contributes to the protective benefit of prior pregnancy, and mechanisms by which seminal fluid may also induce memory are emerging (22). Recognizing this protective role for the adaptive immune response offers scope for new approaches to tackle this prevalent condition.

All women show evidence of altered immunity and elevated inflammatory activation in pregnancy. Immune adaptation for pregnancy commences during the pre-implantation phase when conception and implantation evoke a controlled inflammatory response in the female reproductive tract, which must be rapidly resolved by specific cytokines and pro-tolerogenic mechanisms into an anti-inflammatory milieu, in order for pregnancy to progress (23). In preeclampsia there are excessive pro-inflammatory mediators and inappropriate activation of effector immune cells, detectable in peripheral blood and gestational tissues from the first trimester (24, 25), implying incomplete or insufficient establishment of anti-inflammatory mechanisms (**Figure 1**).

In healthy pregnancy, inflammation associated with conception and implantation is rapidly resolved, and then remains suppressed by anti-inflammatory protective mechanisms, amongst which the specialized subset of $CD4^+$ T lymphocytes called regulatory T cells (Treg cells), are pivotal (26–28). Through their critical roles in constraining inflammation, suppressing effector immunity, and modulating vascular function, Treg cells are emerging along with uNK cells and macrophages as key coordinators of implantation and early placental development (23, 29–31).

In preeclampsia, Tregs in the maternal peripheral blood and decidua are fewer in number (26, 28, 32) and their suppressive function is impaired (33, 34), while pro-inflammatory Th17 cells (27), $CD8^+$ effector T cells and trophoblast apoptosis (28) are increased. The underlying reasons are unclear, but number and functional capacity of Treg cells are known to vary between individuals and are influenced by agents and exposures identified as pre-pregnancy antecedents of preeclampsia and other adverse pregnancy outcomes. Risk factors for impaired Treg activity include elevated inflammatory load associated with obesity and metabolic dysfunction (35), autoimmune conditions and systemic inflammatory exposures (36, 37), nutritional deficiencies (38, 39), and age (40). Their abundance and phenotype in the uterus are furthermore regulated by relevant clinical factors including prior pregnancy, disparity between male and female partner alloantigens, and seminal fluid contact (23). Other obstetric disorders including fetal growth restriction, gestational diabetes, and spontaneous preterm birth also have an inflammatory etiology, but amongst these conditions, the causal link between Treg cell dysregulation and preeclampsia is most clear.

In this review, we make the case that interventions to boost the number, functional competence and stability of Treg cells may offer realistic preventative and therapeutic strategies to protect against preeclampsia in at-risk women. Several pharmacological agents and cell therapy approaches to target Treg cells are in clinical trials or under development for auto-immune disorders and organ transplantation (37, 41, 42). We argue that as Treg therapies move closer to reality in other clinical settings, these interventions warrant evaluation for their potential utility in preeclampsia and related obstetric disorders with an immune etiology.

TREG CELLS—ESSENTIAL FOR MATERNAL ADAPTATION TO PREGNANCY

Several mechanisms of active immune tolerance arise in early pregnancy to dampen inflammation and suppress allo-reactive immune responses that otherwise threaten conceptus survival. These include attenuated expression of polymorphic MHC molecules on placental tissues, trophoblast production of anti-inflammatory and pro-tolerogenic cytokines and hormones, and epigenetic modulation of decidual cell chemokine expression to

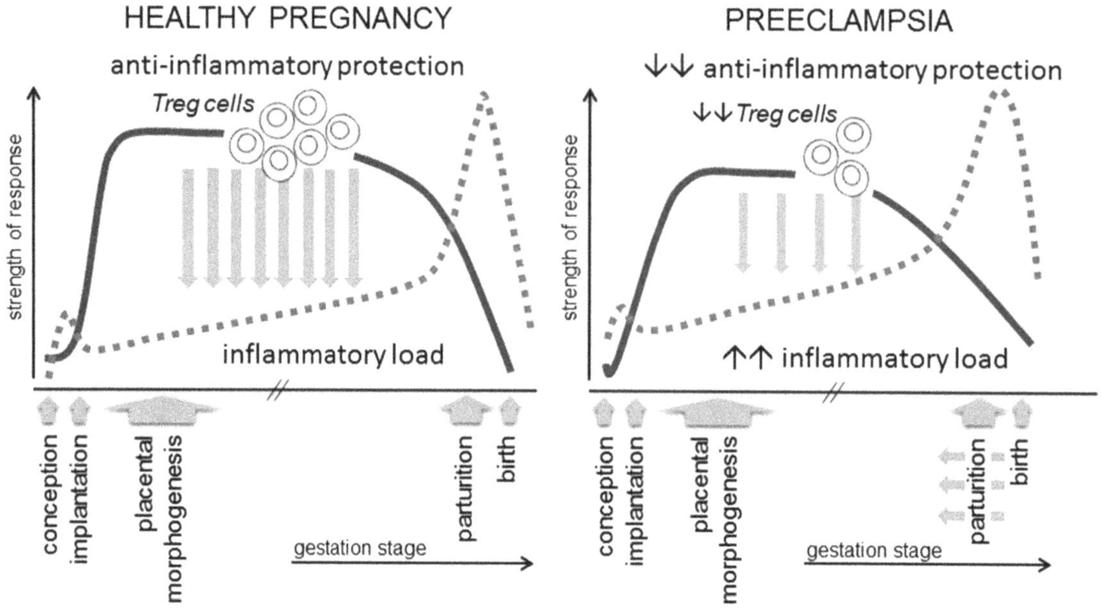

FIGURE 1 | A robust immune response is essential for healthy pregnancy. Regulatory T cells (Treg cells) are a critical and rate-limiting element of the anti-inflammatory protection required to suppress inflammation and prevent adverse effects of anti-fetal effector immune responses. Treg cells arise as a consequence of an inflammation-like response during the peri-conception phase, and their abundance, suppressive function and stability are influenced by events prior to and during early pregnancy. Insufficient numbers, reduced suppressive function or instability are linked with preeclampsia and IUGR, potentially mediated by insufficient Treg cell capacity to support normal placental development and to suppress the elevated inflammatory load typical of this condition.

prevent effector T cells (Teff) cells accumulating at the maternal-placental interface (43–45).

Amongst the various mechanisms of maternal tolerance, CD4$^+$ Treg cells are essential for embryo implantation and early placental development (46, 47). Their capacity to constrain and resolve the inflammation elicited during embryo implantation, and suppress generation of immune effector cells in local lymph nodes, is pivotal to controlling inflammation and promoting immune tolerance over the course of gestation, until an inflammatory shift emerges again at parturition (**Figure 1**). This function is consistent with essential roles for Treg cells in immune homeostasis throughout the body, where they prevent autoimmunity to self-antigens, suppress Teff cells reacting to non-dangerous foreign antigens, regulate and limit excessive inflammation (48–50), and have important roles in tissue repair and homeostasis (51).

Different subsets of T cells with regulatory functions exist. CD4$^+$ Treg cells, CD8$^+$ Treg cells, gamma/delta T cells, Tr1 cells, and NKT cells can all exert suppressive functions and appear to operate collaboratively to control immune responses. CD4$^+$ Treg cells are of particular interest because of their strong association with preeclampsia, and their potential for therapeutic manipulation (41). CD4$^+$ Treg cells comprise about 1–3% of total T helper cells in humans and 3–10% in mice, and are defined by their expression of the master transcription factor Forkhead Box P3 (FOXP3). As well as FOXP3, CD4$^+$ Treg cells constitutively express surface molecules including the IL2 receptor α-chain (CD25), the immune checkpoint receptor cytotoxic T-lymphocyte protein 4 (CTLA4), and glucocorticoid-induced tumor necrosis factor receptor (GITR), and in humans are CD127$^-$ or CD127^{low} (49, 52).

There are two types of CD4$^+$ Treg cells (referred to hereon as "Treg cells"). Thymus-derived Treg cells (tTreg cells) emerge from the thymus after self antigen-driven selection as functional suppressor T cells. Peripheral Treg cells (pTreg cells) differentiate from naïve CD4$^+$ precursors after contact with antigens in peripheral lymph nodes or tissues (52). Differentiation of naïve CD4$^+$ T cells into pTreg cells requires cognate antigen to be presented by antigen-presenting cells (APCs) such as pro-tolerogenic dendritic cells (tDCs) in the presence of IL2 and TGFB. The CD4 cells are thereby induced to express FOXP3 and become committed to suppressive function (53). These cells then promote a cycle of *de novo* Treg cell generation and drive the development of long-lasting immunologic memory, which is reinforced by persistent antigen exposure (54). Like pTreg, tTregs can also be induced to proliferate and acquire greater suppressive function by antigen contact in the periphery (51, 55, 56). In humans, tTregs and pTregs are not readily distinguishable but in mice, tTregs express neuropilin 1 (Nrp1) while pTregs are generally Nrp1 low or negative (52).

pTreg cells and tTreg cells exert anti-inflammatory and immune suppressive activity by secreting a range of soluble factors including IL10 and TGFB, as well as through cell contact-dependent mechanisms. Importantly, Treg cell suppressive function inhibits proliferation and cytokine release from pro-inflammatory CD4$^+$ Teff cells, T helper 1 (Th1) and T helper

17 (Th17) cells, which typically produce pro-inflammatory IFNG and IL17, respectively. Activated Treg cells interact with DCs through CTLA4, to cause down-regulation of DC co-stimulatory molecules CD80 and CD86, which drive Teff cell activation (49).

ALTERED TREG CELLS ACCOMPANY AND MAY PRECEDE PREECLAMPSIA ONSET IN WOMEN

In women, T cells comprise 10–20% of decidual immune cells in the first trimester (57). Many decidual T cells are $CD8^+$, including regulatory subsets (58, 59). Amongst the $CD4^+$ T cells, around 10–30% express FOXP3, which is a substantial enrichment compared to peripheral blood (60–62). The Tregs comprise of both tTregs and pTregs and exhibit heterogeneous phenotypes that vary across the menstrual cycle and phase of pregnancy (32, 63, 64).

There is substantial evidence that many pregnant women with preeclampsia have fewer and less functionally competent Treg cells, accompanied by increased Teff cell activity, particularly Th1 and Th17 cells in decidual tissue and peripheral blood (26–28, 34, 65, 66). In a recent meta-analysis, a total of 17 independent primary studies were evaluated, and all but 2 showed consistent evidence of association between both severe, early-onset and late onset preeclampsia with fewer Treg cells in the third trimester (67). As well as reduced numbers, the suppressive function of Treg cells is often compromised in preeclampsia (33, 34, 68). The decrease in Treg cells may be proportional to the severity of disease (26), although relationship with time of disease onset and co-incidence of fetal growth restriction have not been consistently documented. There is evidence of an altered balance in Treg cell subsets in preeclampsia, with reports of fewer peripheral blood naïve $HLADR^{neg}$ $CD45RA^+$ Treg cells (68, 69) and fewer $CD45RA^+CD31^+$ recent thymic emigrant Tregs (64) in peripheral blood. Decidual Treg populations may be differentially affected, given decidual tDCs exhibit a reduced capacity to induce pTreg in preeclampsia (32).

Treg cell changes become evident in peripheral blood and gestational tissues shortly after conception and accumulate in decidua reaching their highest levels in early to mid-gestation, before decreasing as term approaches (28, 61, 70). A recent study utilizing chorionic villous sampling (CVS) at week 10–12 of gestation, showed that women who progress to preeclampsia demonstrate dysregulated expression of decidual and immune cell genes from this early time (71). In another study, elevated expression of IL6 which counteracts Treg stability and promotes Th17 generation (72), as well as reduced numbers of alternatively activated M2 macrophage and T cell markers, were detected in CVS tissues of women who later develop preeclampsia associated with fetal growth restriction (IUGR) (73). Although longitudinal studies to track Treg cells over the course of gestation are not yet reported in women with preeclampsia, there is good evidence that low abundance of circulating Treg cells in the first trimester is predictive of miscarriage before 12 weeks (74). Collectively, these observations underpin a working hypothesis that disturbed immune adaptation in early pregnancy precedes impaired placental development, setting the scene for later emergence of preeclampsia and related complications of pregnancy (8, 10, 29, 75).

This fits an emerging paradigm which positions early pregnancy as the origin of disorders of deep placentation that underpin early onset, severe preeclampsia, and also contribute to IUGR, preterm labor, premature rupture of membranes, and late spontaneous abortion (11, 76, 77). So-called shallow placentation arises from insufficient trophoblast invasion and failure to adequately remodel spiral arteries and to achieve high capacity maternal blood flow, which further compromises placental development and function, and leads to IUGR (1, 7, 8).

Treg cells are emerging as key regulators in the decidual leukocyte network which controls implantation and placental development. Through interactive cross-regulation, growth factor secretion and extracellular matrix remodeling, this network controls the decidual immune environment which facilitates trophoblast invasion and cytotrophoblast shell development, and enables remodeling of the decidual vasculature to support placental development (10, 78).

Inappropriate function or insufficient numbers of Treg cells in the decidua are linked with inadequate extravillous trophoblast invasion, and poor spiral artery remodeling, in turn destabilizing placental development and resulting in "shallow" placentation (12, 79). There is also a clear link between Treg deficiency and both recurrent implantation failure and recurrent pregnancy loss, where more severe forms of impaired uterine receptivity arrest trophoblast invasion and early placental development (80, 81). Thus, it is not difficult to envisage how insufficient Treg cells in the preconception and peri-conception phase could be a key upstream trigger for the sequence of events leading to impaired vessel remodeling and shallow placentation, which ultimately cause the overt symptoms of preeclampsia in later gestation (**Figure 2**).

TREG CELL REGULATION OF THE DECIDUAL IMMUNE ENVIRONMENT

Mouse models have been instrumental for defining mechanisms through which Treg cells exert anti-inflammatory activity to influence the decidual environment and early placental development. Kinetic studies show that Treg cells accumulate in the uterine decidua from very early in pregnancy, and that these originate after naïve T cell activation and proliferation in local lymph nodes, causing numbers to expand through the first half of gestation (20, 46). After recruitment into the implantation site, Treg cells comprise around 30% of decidual T cells in the mouse (46).

Extensive experiments wherein Treg cells are selectively depleted, or overwhelmed by exacerbated Teff cell responses, show an essential role for Treg cells in preventing generation of destructive immunity to fetal alloantigens (82–85). Without sufficient Treg cells, an aggressive Th1 and Th17 mediated-response causes fetal loss in allogeneic but not syngeneic pregnancy (46).

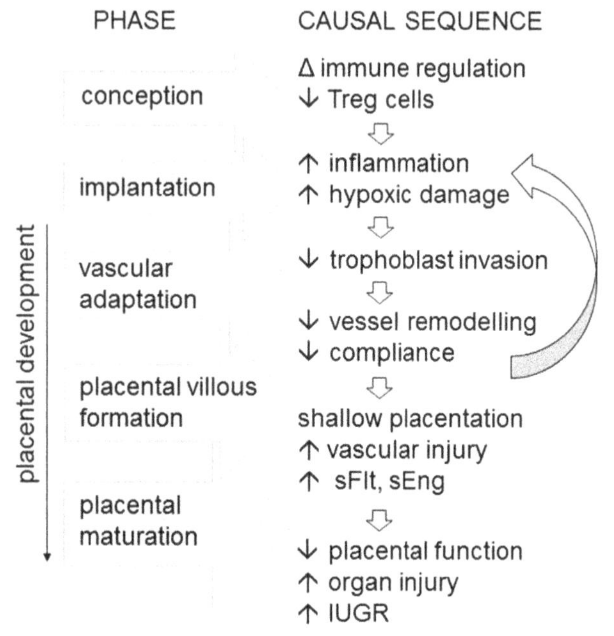

FIGURE 2 | Immune imbalance associated with insufficient or incompetent Treg cells are implicated as an upstream cause of preeclampsia, particularly in severe, early onset disease. In a working model of the sequence of pathophysiological events, fewer Treg cells generated at conception impact the decidual environment at implantation, to limit trophoblast invasion, constrain maternal vascular adaptation, and vessel compliance. The resulting "shallow" placentation causes vascular inflammatory injury accompanied by elevated soluble Fms-like tyrosine kinase (sFlt) and soluble endoglin (eEng), reducing placental function, and causing maternal organ injury and *in utero* growth restriction (IUGR) of the fetus.

Depending on the severity and timing of manipulation, Treg depletion can manifest as implantation failure, miscarriage or fetal growth restriction. Several studies show the pre- and peri-implantation phase is highly vulnerable. Administration of anti-CD25 Ab before or shortly after mating causes complete implantation failure (86–88). Depleting $FOXP3^+$ cells from *FOXP3-Dtr* mice during early placentation increases later fetal resorption (85, 89), but depletion in mid-gestation only moderately reduces fetal viability (20), unless mice receive a second hit inflammatory challenge such that Treg depletion exacerbates the adverse impact (90–92). Mice deficient in T cells due to *Rag1*-null mutation are highly vulnerable to inflammation-induced fetal loss, but this is reversed by administering $CD4^+$ T cells that differentiate to Tregs after transfer (90). Midgestation depletion of $CD25^+$ cells using anti-CD25 mAb has a less severe impact than in early pregnancy, but this may be because Teff cells are also removed (86, 93). Additionally, other tolerogenic mechanisms including IL10 secretion by uNK cells (94) may compensate for Treg deficiency once placental development is complete.

Mouse models with a high rate of spontaneous fetal loss also demonstrate a critical role for Tregs in embryo implantation. CBA/J females mated with DBA/2J males have fewer decidual Tregs and elevated Th1 cells (87, 95). Adoptive transfer of Tregs from donor CBA/J females mated with Balb/c males boosts decidual Tregs and corrects fetal loss (87), but only if Treg transfer occurs before embryo implantation (87). These findings confirm that Tregs are most essential in the uterus during the peri-implantation period, consistent with a central role in orchestrating the transition to an anti-inflammatory mileu required for placental development (**Figure 1**).

Treg cells co-localize in clusters with uNK cells and other leukocytes in the human decidua basalis (78), where they exhibit activity expected to potently influence the local immune environment by enforcing an anti-inflammatory phenotype in other leukocyte lineages. In particular Tregs regulate uNK phenotype, through releasing TGFB and IL10 to control DC release of uNK viability factor IL15 (96), and suppress uNK cytolytic activity (91, 97). This may be particularly important in first pregnancy, given that uNK cells acquire memory and assume a more differentiated "trained" phenotype in subsequent pregnancies (21). Whether there is an interaction between antigen-experienced Tregs and trained uNK cells, remains to be investigated.

Treg cells also regulate M2 macrophages (98), mast cells (99), and tDCs, releasing heme oxygenase-1 which maintains immature DCs (100) and promotes indoleamine 2,3-dioxygenase (IDO) production to impair Th1 cell survival (101, 102). M2 macrophages and tDCs promote further Treg generation (98, 100) and produce an array of cytokines that reinforce a pro-tolerogenic decidual environment, including TGFB, CSF2 (GMCSF), IL4, IL10, CSF3 (GCSF), and prostaglandin E (103). Decidual Tregs also express other hallmark mediators of Teff suppression CD25, CTLA4, and PD-L1 (61, 91, 104–106).

Uterine NK cells and DCs are implicated as key regulators of decidual transformation (107–109) so through regulating uterine DC and uNK phenotype, Tregs would indirectly influence the extent and quality of the decidual response. Furthermore, trophoblasts engage with Tregs in a reciprocal interaction to modulate the secretory profile of both lineages (110). Together, these coordinated interactions allow Tregs to constrain inflammation and limit oxidative stress caused by trophoblast invasion during early placental development (13, 25, 111).

TREG CELLS INFLUENCE MATERNAL VASCULAR REMODELING AND EARLY PLACENTAL DEVELOPMENT

Treg cells are emerging as critical participants in the process of maternal vascular remodeling, through their modulating effects on the decidual leukocyte network (**Figure 3**). There is extensive evidence to demonstrate key roles for uNK cells (30, 112), macrophages (31), and mast cells (99) in decidual vessel transformation, and in collaborating with invading trophoblasts to restructure the endothelial surface and smooth muscle wall (7, 13, 104). As detailed above, Treg cells exert potent anti-inflammatory actions on uNK cells (91, 97), M2 macrophages (98), mast cells (99), and tDCs (100), thereby influencing the vascular remodeling process.

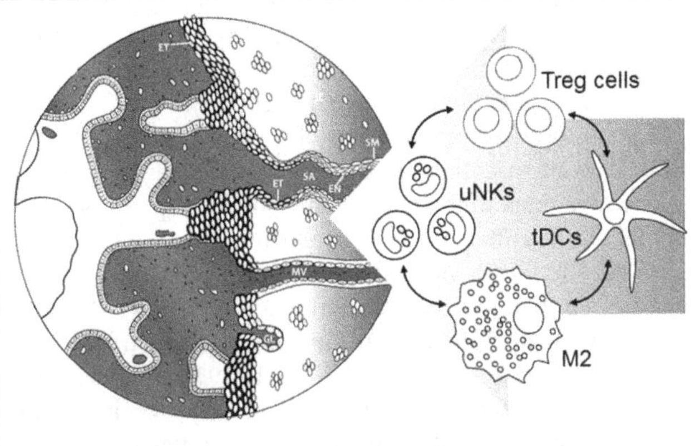

FIGURE 3 | Events during early placental development require immune cells in the decidua to support maternal blood vessel (MV) adaptation and spiral artery (SA) transformation. Treg cells interact with uNK cells, M2 macrophages, and tDCs to suppress inflammation and provide secretory factors regulating extravillous trophoblast (ET) invasion, and functional changes in endothelial cells (EN) and surrounding smooth muscle (SM). Severe early-onset preeclampsia is accompanied by insufficient Treg cells, which in turn would be expected to contribute directly and indirectly through immune cell networks to impair vascular adaptations required for robust placental development. Left hand part of Figure is adapted from Steegers et al. (1).

This is unsurprising given growing evidence that Treg cells play important roles in modulating cardiovascular function, and vascular homeostasis throughout the body (113). In hypertensive mouse models, Treg cell infusion reduces blood pressure and vascular damage, and reverses hypertensive sequelae (114, 115). Treg cell-derived cytokines, particularly IL10 and TGFB, suppress inflammatory endothelial cell activation and inhibit development of atherosclerosis (113).

Rodent models of preeclampsia support a critical function for Treg cells in the pathophysiological events underlying abnormal placental development, through coordinated interactions with uNK cells, DCs, and macrophages (**Figure 3**). Experiments in mice deficient in T cells and/or NK cells show that T cells interact with uNK cells to influence the maternal hemodynamic response to pregnancy (116, 117). When cause-and-effect relationships are explored by antibody-mediated or genetic modulation of T cell subsets, Treg cells are implicated as having causal roles in the maternal and fetal symptoms of preeclampsia models.

Treg-deficient mice consistently show impaired uterine spiral arterial modification, reduced placental blood flow, and fetal growth restriction (85, 89, 118). Depletion of FOXP3$^+$ Tregs in early pregnancy causes later dysfunction in uterine arteries accompanied by increased endothelin-1 production (89). Peripheral Treg cells are particularly implicated, as indicated by experiments in mice with a null mutation in the CNS1 gene which is a *FOXP3* enhancer element essential for pTreg cell but dispensable for tTreg generation. CNS1 is only present in eutherian mammals, suggesting its introduction into the FOXP3 locus to enable pTreg generation, in turn facilitated evolution of placentation (85). In CNS1-null mice, impaired remodeling of material spiral arteries underpins defective placental development (85). Compromised trophoblast invasion and failed transformation of spiral arteries is also seen in mice where neutrophil depletion causes insufficiency of pro-angiogenic, neutrophil-induced Treg cells (118).

In the reduced uterine perfusion pressure (RUPP) model of preeclampsia in rats, reduced uterine artery flow is induced by clip placement on the abdominal aorta and right and left uterine artery arcades at day 14 of gestation, resulting in placental ischemia and oxidative stress. The model replicates human preeclampsia symptoms with hypertension accompanied by increased circulating VEGF, sEng, Flt1, and placental growth factor (PlGF), plus elevated inflammatory cytokines and IUGR. A substantial ($\sim$50%) reduction in decidual and placental Treg cells, and elevation in total CD4$^+$ T cells and Th17 cells, is a consequence of the RUPP intervention. Remarkably, the preeclampsia symptoms induced in this model are T cell dependent since the RUPP intervention does not cause hypertension and IUGR in T cell deficient athymic rats, and disease can be induced by passive transfer of Th17 effector CD4$^+$ T cells (119). Treg cell deficiency is a key driver of hypertension and IUGR and these symptoms are mitigated when Treg cells from pregnant control donor rats are administered shortly after the RUPP procedure (120). Treatment strategies applied to boost endogenous Treg cells, including IL10 administration (121) or low dose CD28 superagonist (120), also reduce hypertension and IUGR.

Rodent models show that the protective effects of Treg cells are crucial from the early implantation phase, when vascular adaptation and early placental development begin. Several studies using different approaches to deplete Treg cells at various time points show the peri-implantation phase is most severely affected, with extensive Treg cell depletion at embryo implantation causing complete implantation failure (46, 86, 87). Experiments in the abortion-prone CBA/J x DBA/2 mouse model indicate transferred Treg cells can rescue the underlying placental defect, but only if Treg cells are transferred from healthy pregnant mice at or before the time of embryo implantation (87). Treg cell replacement influences other immune cells in the decidua, including mast cells, to repair placental and vascular defects and prevent sFlt elevation and fetal loss (99). Consistent with a critical role for peri-implantation Treg cells, a genetic model of preeclampsia involving overexpression of human angiotensinogen and renin in rats showed greater responsiveness to Treg cell therapy when it was applied in early gestation (122).

Even subtle disturbances to the T cell response in early pregnancy may impact later pregnancy progression. This may be the consequence of an altered environment during T cell activation, as we have recently demonstrated for CD8$^+$ T cells in pregnancy (123). Other studies in mice show that reduced numbers or altered function of Treg cells at conception can disrupt fetal-placental development without immediate adverse effects, but with a legacy that becomes apparent in mid- or late gestation, particularly when a "second-hit" inflammatory challenge is applied (106, 124).

THE TREG CELL RESPONSE IS DETERMINED IN THE PRE- AND PERI-CONCEPTION PHASE

The conditions under which the Treg cell populations of pregnancy originate are likely to be critical to the reduced quantity and impaired quality of the Treg response in preeclampsia. Uterine recruitment of Tregs in readiness for possible embryo implantation commences in the proliferative phase of each cycle, with an estrogen-driven increase peaking around ovulation (125). $CD4^+$ $FOXP3^+$ cells, thought to be pTregs based on expression of the Helios marker, are a major subset amongst the expanding Treg populations in blood and decidua in early human pregnancy (32). $Helios^+$ Treg cells appear to be preferentially recruited into the decidua in the first trimester (63). Amongst peripheral blood tTregs the population of $CD45RA^+CD31^+$ cells, which have recently emigrated from the thymus, expand prominently in the first trimester and differentiate into $CD45RA^-CD31^-$ memory Tregs (64).

The majority of decidual T cells in women have a memory phenotype ($CD45RA^-$ or $CD45RO^+$) (59, 126) and show evidence of fetal antigen specificity (62), which indicates antigen exposure must occur to elicit the full Treg cell response. HLA-C is the only polymorphic HLA expressed by human placental trophoblasts, and fetal-maternal HLA-C mismatch is associated with a greater expansion in decidual Tregs (127). Many decidual Tregs show fetal HLA-C antigen specificity (62, 128), but whether other reproductive or tissue antigens are involved has not been investigated.

In preeclampsia, Treg cell deficiency is most pronounced in pTreg cells (32), as well as $CD45RA^+CD31^+$ recent thymic emigrant tTregs less able to acquire a memory phenotype (64). This implies there may be an underlying problem with antigen priming. Consistent with this, dysfunctional DCs with reduced HLA-G and ILT4 (32), and/or insufficent PD-L1 (129), have been reported in preeclampsia.

Contact with fetal alloantigens must occur under conditions that favor antigen presentation and stable Treg cell (not Teff cell) development. These conditions occur in two waves in the reproductive process. Paternally-derived transplantation antigens shared by the fetus are first and most frequently contacted during transmission of seminal fluid at coitus, at conception and in pre-conception cycles (22). Seminal fluid primes the activation of pTregs that are specific for paternal transplantation antigens which will later be expressed by fetal and placental cells. Additionally, once pregnancy is established and maternal blood comes into contact with the syncytiotrophoblast surface, placental exosomes are released into maternal blood, providing a second wave of alloantigen exposure (130, 131).

Again, mouse models have been informative in tracing the origins and regulation of Treg cells and point to specific events as critical for generation of the Treg cell pool in early pregnancy (132). The two stages of T cell activation can be tracked through the first half of gestation using T cell transgenic mice (93). The strength of seminal fluid as the initial priming event is first seen as a burst of T cell proliferation in the peri-conception phase, evident in cells recovered from the uterus-draining para-aortic lymph nodes (dLN) on day 3.5 post-coitus (pc), followed by a steady progressive increase during the post-implantation phase once placental morphogenesis is complete (93).

The first wave of proliferation of Treg cells can be detected within days of insemination in the lymph nodes draining the reproductive tract, in the peripheral blood, and spleen (46, 133). Seminal fluid contains paternal alloantigens and high levels of TGFB, and elicits an inflammation-like response in female reproductive tract tissues. DCs and macrophages recruited into female tissues take up seminal fluid alloantigens, traffic to the dLN and present antigen to naive T cells (93). Treg expansion is maximized in allogeneic compared with syngeneic matings, demonstrating a contribution of male alloantigens (134), but endogenous antigens might also contribute to the activation and expansion of Tregs in early pregnancy (135). Amongst the responding pTregs, paternal antigen-reactive pTreg cells are selectively enriched (133, 136). Data from mice with a mutation in the CNS1 gene show elevated fetal loss when pTreg alone are deficient, suggesting that pTreg cells have non-redundant functions important for viviparous pregnancy (85).

A population of tTreg cells of thymic origin also expand systemically prior to conception. These cells are recruited into the uterus after proliferation in the dLN during the estrous stage of the reproductive cycle in mice, in response to rising estrogen at ovulation (125, 137). After mating, factors in seminal fluid induce tTreg to proliferate and express elevated FOXP3 and CTLA4, both markers of suppressive competence, accompanied by demethylation of the Treg-specific demethylation region (TSDR) in the *FOXP3* locus (138). This expansion of tTreg cells occurs in parallel with the seminal fluid antigen-driven expansion of pTreg cells. This population may well have different functional qualities to pTreg, although these are still to be defined.

After recirculation via peripheral blood, Treg cells are recruited into the fetal-maternal interface in response to chemokines secreted by uterine epithelial cells including CCL19 (133), and may be stimulated to undergo further rounds of proliferation locally in the uterine tissue (46). The resulting expansion of the Treg cell pool induces a state of hypo-responsiveness to paternal alloantigens, concurrent with embryo implantation when the conceptus first contacts maternal tissues (136, 139). The kinetics of Treg cell induction in the peri-conception phase ensures sufficient abundance of Treg cells in the endometrium at embryo implantation, when their function is most critical (86, 87, 140). Continued release of paternally-inherited alloantigen from trophoblasts over the course of pregnancy sustains the T cell response until post-partum (20, 93). After birth, a population of paternal alloantigen-reactive Tregs are sustained, and in the event of a subsequent mating with a male expressing the same alloantigens, there is accelerated expansion of Treg cells driven by proliferation of fetal-specific Treg cells retained from the prior pregnancy (20).

Mouse studies imply that the immune response initiated at seminal fluid priming is a crucial initiating step and highly vulnerable phase for Treg cell tolerance to be established. In particular, responding pTreg cells require appropriate environmental signals including the cytokines IL2 and TGFB, to ensure naïve T cells differentiate into Treg cells and not Th1 or Th17 effector T cells (93, 133). Both the size of the Treg cell pool and the suppressive competence of pTreg cells will be determined by the strength of the antigenic challenge, and the nature of the cytokine context in which antigen contact occurs—parameters which are determined by seminal fluid composition as well as female tract factors. Since newly generated pTreg cells that have only recently commenced FOXP3 expression appear more vulnerable to phenotype switching and lineage instability (141), the extent to which pTreg cells primed at coitus will commit to a secure Treg fate will be substantially influenced by the conception environment. Relevant factors impacting this environment would include MHC disparity between male and female partners, the abundance and phenotype of DCs involved in antigen presentation, and bioavailability of local cytokines, hormones and other positive and negative regulators including microRNAs and the local microbiome (23).

Similar events occur in women, where the cervical immune response to seminal fluid mirrors the mouse response, causing elevated cytokine production, recruitment of leukocytes and T cell activation (22, 142), consistent with prior seminal fluid contact contributing to priming the paternal antigen-specific Treg cell response of pregnancy (62). It is yet to be proven that seminal fluid induces pTreg cells in women, and other factors must contribute to uterine Treg accumulation since IVF pregnancy can be established without seminal plasma contact. Expansion of uterine Tregs after conception may be further facilitated by human chorionic gonadotropin (hCG) secreted by invading placental trophoblasts (143). This builds on the hormone-driven expansion of Treg cells in the follicular phase of the menstrual cycle, correlating with progressively elevating serum E2 levels (125). However, the *in vivo* cervical response and an array of *in vitro* studies demonstrating that seminal fluid skews DC cells to an tDC phenotype and induces Treg cells *in vitro*, is consistent with a key role for seminal fluid in women (22, 144, 145). A priming effect of seminal fluid contact in women also explains the benefit of cumulative seminal fluid contact with the conceiving partner in protecting from preeclampsia (17, 146).

IS INSUFFICIENT PRIMING A CAUSE OF TREG CELL DEFICIENCY IN PREECLAMPSIA?

An important question is why some women have fewer Treg cells and/or impaired Treg function at the outset of pregnancy. The nature and significance of factors that cause variation in the uterine Treg cell response are unclear and require investigation. As detailed above, antigen priming in the appropriate environmental context is a critical factor in the strength and quality of any peripheral tissue Treg cell response. In the reproductive tissues, the strength and quality of antigen and immune-regulatory signals in the female reproductive mucosa during priming would be paramount, as well as the number and timing of prior exposures to the conceiving partner's seminal fluid and any previous pregnancies with that partner (25).

This raises the possibility that some women develop preeclampsia after conceiving without adequate prior priming to male partner alloantigens. It seems likely that pTregs reacting with paternal alloantigens would be more vulnerable than tTregs to variations in population size, antigen experience and memory, functional competence, and stability. Because newly generated pTregs are particularly susceptible to phenotype-switching and lineage instability (141), the priming environment would be a key determinant of a secure fate amongst pTreg with male partner alloantigen specificity. Recent evidence in mice that seminal fluid contact regulates tTreg cells, inducing proliferation and reinforcing a suppressive phenotype through epigenetic modulation, suggests tTreg as well as pTreg are impacted (138).

Priming may be dysregulated due to seminal fluid composition or female responsiveness to seminal fluid signals (22, 25). It has been shown that recurrent miscarriage patients produce more $CD4^{+}IL17^{+}$ and $CD4^{+}IFNG^{+}$ cells and fewer $CD4^{+}CD25^{+}FOXP3^{+}$ Tregs, compared to fertile controls, when $CD4^{+}$ T cells are cultured with DCs and partner's seminal fluid antigens (147). The balance of immune-regulatory agents in seminal fluid, particularly pro-tolerogenic TGFB, varies between men, and within men over time (148). The anti-tolerogenic cytokine IFNG, which drives generation of Th1 immunity, fluctuates substantially and can become elevated in seminal fluid in the event of infection or other inflammatory conditions (149). IFNG interferes with synthesis of CSF2 required to drive the T cell proliferative response at conception (150, 151), skews Th0 differentiation toward Th17 cells (48, 152), and increases Treg susceptibility to transdifferentiate into Th17 cells (153).

CLINICAL AND LIFESTYLE FACTORS IMPACTING THE TREG CELL RESPONSE

A suboptimal Treg cell adaptation for pregnancy could also occur in women due to intrinsic Treg deficiency. The specific factors determining between individual variation in Treg numbers and functional capacity are yet to be fully defined. An interaction between genetic, epigenetic, and environmental factors seems likely, based on data from animal models and limited studies in population cohorts (154). The thymic output of tTreg, and peripheral tissue induction of pTreg cells, are independently regulated and can be affected by a range of metabolic and nutritional parameters, inflammatory exposures, autoimmune conditions, and age (35–40). Common health conditions that affect the immune system including intestinal microbial dysbiosis and dietary deficiencies, particularly vitamin A and vitamin D, have been associated with poor adaptive immunity and may be a common cause of compromised Treg activity (38). Exposure to sunlight (55) and exercise (56) are also recently identified to support Treg homeostasis, but how these are linked to variation in human Treg parameters are yet to be defined.

In hyper-inflammatory conditions caused by autoimmune, infectious or metabolic disorders some pTreg cells exhibit phenotypic plasticity and instability, with increased disposition to shift phenotype, or lose *FOXP3* expression and become reprogrammed into a Teff fate (154). Studies in mice and humans demonstrate that $FOXP3^{+}$ T cells can be induced by inflammatory stimuli to express IL17 and IFNG characteristic of Teff cells (155, 156), and may then transdifferentiate into effector Th17-like cells, known as "exTregs," which can amplify inflammatory pathology (157).

Epigenetic regulation of *FOXP3* through demethylation of the TSDR region is a key factor in the resilience of Tregs to inflammatory stress, that controls whether T cells can express sufficient *FOXP3* to overrule Teff functions and maintain a Treg suppressive phenotype (158). Increased TSDR methylation and associated underexpression of *FOXP3* is a feature of some autoimmune conditions (159).

There is little information on whether Treg cells exhibit signaling defects, lineage instability or methylation changes in preeclampsia. Given the evidence of elevated Th1 and Th17 cells counteracting the decrease in Treg number and function in preeclampsia, defects in both Treg cell induction and/or stability seem plausible, and would explain the concurrent reduction in Treg cell suppressive function (34, 68). Although large populations have not been examined, exploratory studies in preeclampsia suggest an elevated incidence of gene variants within the promoter region of *FOXP3* that may affect expression levels and hence Treg stability (160, 161). Elevated IL6 trans-signaling, which is known to promote Treg instability and transdifferentiation, has been described in women with recurrent miscarriage (162). IL6 is associated with reduced TGFB output and IL2-mediated STAT5 signaling (163), and is a possible candidate contributing to impaired Treg capacity in preeclampsia, given that elevated expression of IL6 is seen in gestational tissues of women who later develop the condition (73).

POTENTIAL INTERVENTIONS TO TARGET TREG CELLS IN PREGNANCY

Recognition that excessive inflammation secondary to insufficient anti-inflammatory protection is a key driver of preeclampsia gives rise to the prospect of targeting the immune response to prevent or suppress progression of the disease. In particular, Treg cells provide an attractive target, because of (1) the clear link between compromised Treg cells and preeclampsia; (2) a logical mechanistic pathway placing insufficient Treg cells as an upstream event in the placental and systemic pathophysiological sequalae; (3) compelling evidence from preclinical rodent models showing that insufficient Treg cells can elicit preeclampsia-like symptoms, while boosting Treg cells mitigates symptoms, and (4) encouraging progress in development of Treg cell therapies for other autoimmune and inflammatory conditions.

Interventions to boost Treg cell populations and their suppressive competence are under development and show promise in autoimmunity and tissue transplantation (41, 42), and more recently have been considered for cardiovascular disease (113). Treg cell therapies relevant to preeclampsia could take one of three alternative approaches: (1) lifestyle and health advice during preconception planning to assist immune adaptation to pregnancy; (2) neutraceutical, pharmacological, or other strategies to increase Treg cell numbers and/or function in an antigen non-specific, systemic manner, or (3) cell therapy treatments that involve *ex vivo* generation and/or expanding Treg cells in a highly-individualized process. These clearly represent different degrees of technical challenge, invasiveness, cost and risk. While lifestyle adjustments or dietary supplements are generally safe and tractable, cell therapies are labor-intensive, expensive, and higher risk.

The evidence base for approaches to target Tregs in other clinical settings is building (41, 42), but to date little consideration has been given to applications in reproductive conditions. To advance new treatments targeting Treg cells for preeclampsia prevention and mitigation, research on several fronts is required. Most immediate goals should be to develop appropriate diagnostics, and to investigate and validate pre-pregnancy planning interventions to boost Treg cells. There should also be careful consideration of the rationale for initiating clinical studies, using robust clinical trial methodology, to evaluate pharmacological and/or cell therapy treatments for application when Treg deficiencies are not responsive to lower intervention approaches.

Diagnosis of Treg Cell Deficiency

To progress understanding of Treg cell insufficiency in preeclampsia, and to develop therapeutic options targeting these, it is essential that effective diagnostic tools are developed and validated. These should detect common and informative defects in Treg cell parameters that define competency for healthy pregnancy, and ideally be applied to peripheral blood if preference to endometrial biopsies. Treg tests should be appropriate for routine use during pregnancy planning or early after conception, to provide a therapeutic window for early treatment interventions to prevent progression to miscarriage or later obstetric conditions. To date little work has been done to investigate Treg cell deficiency before conception, or in early pregnancy, in the blood or endometrium of women who go on to develop preeclampsia. Ongoing studies to address the pre-pregnancy origins of preeclampsia may begin to address this (9).

A recent meta-analysis of Treg cell parameters quantified in preeclampsia highlights the considerable variability in markers that different groups have measured to date (67). A useful step will be to develop a consensus definition of minimum essential Treg markers to facilitate harmonization across future studies, and to determine the best stage in preconception cycles or early pregnancy for analysis (164). Given the significance of tTreg cells vs. pTreg cells, and of naïve vs. memory cells in preeclampsia (68, 69), extensive marker panels to discriminate these subsets in flow cytometry-based tests will be most informative. Along with standard markers CD4, CD25, CD127, and FOXP3, markers that reflect memory, suppressive capacity, and activation status amongst Treg cells should be measured. These may include GITR which is emerging as a superior marker of active, functional Tregs (165), plus CTLA4, CD45RO, HLADR, and potentially intracellular cytokines or transcription factors which appear particularly informative in the preeclampsia setting (27, 34).

Ideally, Treg cell assays should also inform on suppressive competence in a paternal antigen-specific manner. Assessment of suppressive function by *in vitro*-based assays and/or analysis of *FOXP3* methylation status has been the gold standard for assessment of suppressive potential, but new markers such GITR, CD154, and PI16 may supersede these tests and be more amenable to a clinical diagnostic setting (165–167). With increasing availability of tetramer-based diagnostic tools for identifying TCR specificity, identification of partner alloantigen-reactive Treg cells may in time become feasible.

Optimal Timing for Interventions

A major challenge for developing strategies to target Treg cells in pregnancy is timing—how and when would Treg cell deficiency be diagnosed, and how would this relate to the window of opportunity for intervention? With evidence that Treg cells are most critical during the implantation and early placentation phase of pregnancy, interventions in cycles prior to conception, or as soon as possible after conception would likely be most advantageous. The timing would need to align with hormone-driven regulation across the menstrual cycle, and might leverage events controlling estrogen and progesterone-regulated expansion of the Treg pool (125). Interventions would need to be coupled with Treg screening of high risk women during pre-pregnancy planning or early after conception to allow the best chance to identify patient subgroups that could be amenable to therapy.

Treg Cells and Preconception Care

A tractable approach worthy of further investigation is advice on immune system health and boosting immune priming during preconception planning. In nulliparous women, the available evidence suggests on average, 3–6 months of sexual cohabitation without using barrier contraceptives is required for sufficient seminal fluid priming to minimize the chance of preeclampsia (15). Consistent with this, in a recent study of 340 women, women in the highest 10th percentile of exposure to partner's seminal fluid had a 70% reduced odds of preeclampsia relative to women in the lowest 25th percentile (168). Thus, advising nulliparous women to avoid use of barrier contraceptive methods and to consider increasing vaginal coitus prior to conceiving may reduce preeclampsia risk. A key question is the impact of different non-barrier approaches to facilitating immune priming, such as oral contraceptive pill or intrauterine device, which both deliver immune-modulating hormones. Further studies are required to evaluate the impact on preeclampsia rates of preconception advice on seminal fluid contact and contraceptive choice, and to investigate whether a partner-specific Treg cell response is involved.

Detecting and correcting any immune imbalance due to clinical, nutritional and/or, lifestyle factors is also likely to be effective for pregnancy planning and reducing susceptibility to preeclampsia. Elevated inflammatory load due to chronic infection, smoking, diabetic and pre-diabetic conditions, obesity and/or microbiome dysbiosis in women would be expected to adversely affect intrinsic Treg cell parameters and responsiveness to priming (35, 169), while in men these conditions may increase seminal fluid IFNG and reduce capacity to elicit a healthy female response (149). A range of autoimmune conditions known to impact reproductive function likely have a shared underlying etiology and correcting the immune disorder with validated approaches would reasonably yield dividends for pregnancy health (170). Microbiome disorders, and vitamin and micronutrient deficiencies also affect Treg cells, and treating these might have utility in boosting Treg cell activity in the reproductive setting, as has been shown for some other immune disorders (38). It will be important for future studies to trial the efficacy of alternative approaches to pre-pregnancy care, in order to determine the most effective interventions.

Pharmaceutical Interventions to Expand Treg Cells for Pregnancy

High-risk women with a previous pre-eclamptic pregnancy are an obvious target for preconception care to boost immune tolerance. However, duration of sexual cohabitation is unlikely to be limiting in this patient group, and couple-intrinsic issues such as insufficient HLA disparity between partners, or HLA incompatibility resulting in low immunogenicity of male alloantigens, could theoretically interfere with priming and expansion of the Treg cell pool. In selected women with a demonstrated intrinsic Treg deficiency, approaches that target Treg cells might warrant consideration.

Agents of potential utility to induce Treg cell-mediated tolerance in women include cytokines and other biological agents. Two cytokines that been used clinically to attempt to enhance embryo implantation and placentation, CSF3 (171) and CSF2 (172), act on myeloid immune cells and promote recruitment and function of tDCs in the reproductive tract mucosa. Mouse studies are consistent with their fertility-promoting effects being mediated via tDC-mediated induction of Treg cells (151, 173), but their effect on T cells has not been studied in women. IL10 and several microRNAs that act to expand the Treg cell pool and increase functional competence, and are known to be induced naturally in the female tract response to seminal fluid, are also worthy of investigation (106, 174).

Several existing drugs deployed in pregnancy may act at least partly through Treg cells. Studies in mice suggest that progesterone mediates suppression of the Teff cell response, affecting $CD4^+$ T cell and Treg cell phenotype (175, 176). Progesterone effectively suppresses the generation of Th1 cells and Th17 cells and induces Treg cell differentiation (177–179). Treg cells induced by progesterone have increased capacity to suppress the activation and expansion of Teff cells (177, 178). This fits with evidence of progesterone-regulated increases in uterine Treg cell populations in mice and in women (125, 137). Physiological levels of progesterone increase the functional population of $CD4^+FOXP3^+$ cells in pseudopregnant mice and increase the splenic $CD4^+FOXP3^+$ cell proportions in mid gestation (180). Progesterone also acts to selectively repress *IFNG* gene expression in $CD4^+$ T cells (181), allowing enhanced induction of Treg cells and suppression of Th1 and Th17 differentiation (84, 182). A Cochrane meta-analysis demonstrated a benefit of progesterone for reducing recurrent miscarriage in women (183), but whether this impacts Treg cells is unknown. Furthermore, the outcomes in this setting are confounded by the large proportion of losses related to embryo chromosomal abnormalities, rather than immune dysregulation in the endometrium (184). There is no proven clinical benefit of progesterone in preeclampsia, and a Cochrane review did not find sufficient evidence to support its clinical use to prevent preeclampsia when administration was commenced between 16 and 28 weeks gestation in 4 clinical trials (185). Administration in early pregnancy would likely be required to improve Treg cells at the relevant developmental phase, but the effect of early administration of progesterone on susceptibility to preeclampsia has not been assessed.

Although immune suppressive glucocorticoid drugs conventionally used in autoimmune conditions are sometimes administered in assisted reproduction settings, these suppress both Treg cells and Teff cells, and carry risks when used in pregnancy (186). Intravenous immunoglobulins (IVIg) and Intralipid have also been empirically used in artificial reproductive technology settings to enhance implantation and in recurrent miscarriage clinics to reduce miscarriage rates (187). IVIg did not demonstrate an improvement in livebirth outcomes in 8 small studies in 303 women who suffered recurrent miscarriage (188). Although there is some evidence to suggest that intralipid infusions are associated with immune suppression and alter NK cell activity (189), their effects on Treg cell parameters has not been measured and their clinical benefit for implantation disorders or miscarriage is unproven in clinical trials. The impact of administering intralipid and IVIg infusion in early pregnancy on the development of early or late onset preeclampsia has not been assessed.

There are several drugs under development for autoimmune diseases, including immune checkpoint regulators and other immune-active biologics, that may afford greater selectivity for Treg cells than the immune modulating treatments described above (42). These approaches may be worthy of cautious evaluation in reproductive conditions. Drugs targeting immune checkpoint regulators CTLA4 and PD-1 offer enormous potential, and studies in preclinical models offer encouragement. A recent study in rats where preeclampsia-like symptoms are induced by L-NAME administration showed treatment with PD-L1-Fc protein was effective in reversing Treg/Th17 imbalance and mitigating placental damage (129). Substantial promise for a CD28 superagonist treatment was demonstrated in a rat model of preeclampsia induced by overexpression of human angiotensinogen. Administration of CD28 superagonist was highly effective in increasing Treg cells and alleviating maternal hypertension, proteinuria and IUGR, particularly when treatment was applied from the pre-implantation phase (122). Low dose IL2 has been used to expand Tregs in several conditions, including in abortion-prone mice where protection against fetal loss was achieved (135).

Other relevant agents include humanized antibodies against T cell markers such as anti-CD3, anti-CD52, and anti-CD45 RO/RA which reestablish immune tolerance by selectively depleting Teff cells and retaining Treg cells (37). Other approaches utilize cytokine specific monoclonal antibodies to promote Treg cells—these include anti-TNFA which is approved for use in rheumatoid arthritis and Crohn's Disease, or protolerogenic cytokines such as TGFB and IL10 (37).

Epigenetic regulation of *FOXP3* to impart elevated suppressive function and stability in Tregs is another candidate approach. Inhibitors of DNA methyltransferases such as 5-aza-2′-deoxycytidine (Aza), or factors involved in DNA methylation such as Ten-eleven translocation (TET) protein, have been utilized *in vitro* to drive hypomethylation of the *FOXP3* locus, resulting in strong, stable *FOXP3* expression in Treg cells (190–192). In mouse models, administration of DNMT inhibitors enhances Treg number, *FOXP3* expression and suppressive capacity which assists in reducing inflammation associated with LPS-induced lung injury (193), and prolongs cardiac allograft survival (194). Histone deacetylase (HDACs) inhibitors have also been shown to boost Treg cells and improve suppressive function, resulting in decreased inflammatory bowel disease and increase tissue graft survival in mice (195). These agents carry risks as well as potential, so any application in a reproductive setting would need to be carefully evaluated, initially in preclinical studies.

Cell Therapy Interventions to Boost Treg Cells for Pregnancy

Cell therapy provides a challenging but highly personalized and thus potentially more effective approach to tackling Treg-mediated conditions (37). Cell therapy involves either (i) isolating *in vivo* differentiated Treg cells and expanding them *ex vivo* or (ii) generating and expanding pTreg cells *in vitro*, before subsequent reinfusion. These approaches are in development for transplantation and severe autoimmune disease, but would currently be difficult to justify for a non-life-threatening pregnancy condition. However, given that in preeclampsia the Teff response is not overwhelming, once Treg cell therapy becomes a reality it may prove to be more amenable than other conditions where an extreme immune deviation is beyond rescue (37, 41).

A substantial benefit of cell therapy is that antigen-specific Treg cells can be manipulated without systemic effects on the immune response, with lower risk of off target effects in the mother and fetus than with pharmacological approaches. Studies in type 1 diabetes and other diseases show that T cell receptor (TCR) reactivity with relevant antigens in the target tissue improve Treg cell recruitment and capacity to persist and execute effective suppression, with a low chance of non-specific immune suppression (41, 196). This is a challenge for many disease conditions that might be considered for Treg cell therapy, when Treg cells reactive to tissue-specific antigens are rare. However, the relevant antigens in pregnancy are paternal alloantigens where the starting frequency is much higher. A large proportion of naturally-occurring naïve $CD4^+$ T cells, pTreg cells and tTreg cells react with allo-antigens and could readily be expanded amongst polyclonal populations. Furthermore, because of their capacity to suppress immune responses in an antigen non-specific manner (bystander suppression) and their capacity to skew T cell responses to other tissue antigens toward tolerance (infectious tolerance), it is possible to regulate the immune response in a whole organ using Treg cells reactive with a single antigen (37, 41). In pregnancy, this means that Treg cells reactive with just one or a subset of paternally-inherited fetal alloantigens, or perhaps even a male minor histocompatibility antigen such as H-Y, could reasonably be effective in suppressing immune responses to a wide range of placental and fetal antigens.

Enormous potential is offered by new gene modification developments in generating alloantigen-specific Treg cells using chimeric antigen receptor technology. This approach overcomes the challenge of the low frequency of antigen-reactive T cells occurring naturally in peripheral blood, by genetically manipulating Treg cells with self-specificity to express either a TCR complex, or a chimeric antigen receptor (CAR) reactive to specific antigens. Use of CAR technology can reliably generate potent, functionally competent, and stable alloantigen-specific human Treg cells that have utility in a wide range of human autoimmune diseases (197). Ongoing clinical trials are showing exciting results in Crohn's disease and are likely to soon be applied in the tissue transplant setting (198). There is a prospect that in time, obstetric disorders may be amongst the range of diseases to benefit from CAR T cell therapy—but again, this must wait until relevant reproductive antigens are identified, and can be targeted in a patient-specific manner.

CONCLUSIONS

Immune imbalance or "maladaptation" has been implicated as central and causal in disease development in preeclampsia, and Treg cells are identified as a pivotal immune cell lineage. Their unique combination of anti-inflammatory, and immune modulatory properties affords Treg cells a potent capacity to support maternal vascular adaptation and placental development, suppress inflammation and sustain maternal tolerance of the fetus. The effects of Treg cells appear most critical at the time of pregnancy establishment and during early placental morphogenesis. Insufficient or dysfunctional Tregs provides a mechanism through which environmental, metabolic, and genetic factors can converge to increase disease risk (154), likely interacting with clinical factors such as prior pregnancy and immune compatibility between partners, which are known to be important pre-pregnancy antecedents of preeclampsia (10).

Given the rapid advances in Treg cell immunology including informative diagnostics based on flow cytometry of peripheral blood, and development of a range of low and high intervention treatments, the prospect of targeting Treg cells in at-risk women to treat early placental disturbances and effectively mitigate preeclampsia onset, warrants evaluation. It will be important to focus on developing diagnostics and interventions for application before or during early pregnancy, to divert the course of disease development before placental or fetal injury occurs. Proof-of-concept experiments in rodent models of preeclampsia already demonstrate the utility of biological agents PF-L1 Fc (129), CD28 superligand (122), and low dose IL2 (135) to boost Treg cell numbers and stability.

Experimental evaluation of any strategy to increase Tregs in a human reproductive setting must take a highly cautious approach and be founded in robust clinical trial design principles. It is critical that safety for mothers and infants is paramount, and the different risk-benefit ratio of reproductive and obstetric conditions, compared to life-threatening immune diseases, is recognized. Possible adverse consequences of artificially boosting maternal Treg cells, including reduced pathogen defense (199) or even reduced immune surveillance against malignancy (200) would need to be considered. Notwithstanding the substantial work to be done to evaluate alternative approaches and identify responsive patient groups, there is an imperative to invest in developing immune therapy options with the goal to reduce the morbidity and mortality associated with preeclampsia.

AUTHOR CONTRIBUTIONS

SR, EG, AC, and LM assembled and interpreted the relevant literature and prepared manuscript drafts and Figures. JP, MH, SB, and GD provided expert knowledge on content and revised manuscript drafts.

FUNDING

This research is funded by NHMRC Project Grant APP1099461 to SR and SB.

REFERENCES

1. Steegers EA, von Dadelszen P, Duvekot JJ, Pijnenborg R. Pre-eclampsia. *Lancet.* (2010) 376:631–44. doi: 10.1016/S0140-6736(10)60279-6
2. Stevens W, Shih T, Incerti D, Ton TGN, Lee HC, Peneva D, et al. Short-term costs of preeclampsia to the United States health care system. *Am J Obstet Gynecol.* (2017) 2017:32. doi: 10.1016/j.ajog.2017.04.032
3. Saigal S, Doyle LW. An overview of mortality and sequelae of preterm birth from infancy to adulthood. *Lancet.* (2008) 371:261–9. doi: 10.1016/S0140-6736(08)60136-1
4. Duley L. The global impact of pre-eclampsia and eclampsia. *Semin Perinatol.* (2009) 33:130–7. doi: 10.1053/j.semperi.2009.02.010
5. Turanov AA, Lo A, Hassler MR, Makris A, Ashar-Patel A, Alterman JF, et al. RNAi modulation of placental sFLT1 for the treatment of preeclampsia. *Nat Biotechnol.* (2018) 2018:4297. doi: 10.1038/nbt.4297
6. Robertson SA. Preventing preeclampsia by silencing sFLT1? *N Engl J Med.* (2019) 36:12. doi: 10.1056/NEJMcibr1817501
7. Huppertz B. Placental origins of preeclampsia: challenging the current hypothesis. *Hypertension.* (2008) 51:970–5. doi: 10.1161/HYPERTENSIONAHA.107.107607
8. Redman CW, Sargent IL. Immunology of pre-eclampsia. *Am J Reprod Immunol.* (2010) 63:534–43. doi: 10.1111/j.1600-0897.2010.00831.x
9. Wen SW, Xie RH, Tan H, Walker MC, Smith GN, Retnakaran R. Preeclampsia and gestational diabetes mellitus: pre-conception origins? *Med Hypotheses.* (2012) 79:120–5. doi: 10.1016/j.mehy.2012.04.019
10. Roberts JM, Redman CW. Global Pregnancy Collaboration symposium: prepregnancy and very early pregnancy antecedents of adverse pregnancy outcomes: overview and recommendations. *Placenta.* (2017) 60:1039. doi: 10.1016/j.placenta.2017.07.012

11. Brosens I, Pijnenborg R, Vercruysse L, Romero R. The "Great Obstetrical Syndromes" are associated with disorders of deep placentation. *Am J Obstet Gynecol.* (2011) 204:193–201. doi: 10.1016/j.ajog.2010.08.009
12. Harmon AC, Cornelius DC, Amaral LM, Faulkner JL, Cunningham MW Jr, Wallace K, et al.The role of inflammation in the pathology of preeclampsia. *Clin Sci.* (2016) 130:409–19. doi: 10.1042/CS20150702
13. Saito S, Shiozaki A, Nakashima A, Sakai M, Sasaki Y. The role of the immune system in preeclampsia. *Mol Aspects Med.* (2007) 28:192–209. doi: 10.1016/j.mam.2007.02.006
14. Wang JX, Knottnerus AM, Schuit G, Norman RJ, Chan A, Dekker GA. Surgically obtained sperm, and risk of gestational hypertension and pre-eclampsia. *Lancet.* (2002) 359:673–4. doi: 10.1016/S0140-6736(02)07804-2
15. Kho EM, McCowan LM, North RA, Roberts CT, Chan E, Black MA, et al. Duration of sexual relationship and its effect on preeclampsia and small for gestational age perinatal outcome. *J Reprod Immunol.* (2009) 82:66–73. doi: 10.1016/j.jri.2009.04.011
16. Klonoff-Cohen HS, Savitz DA, Celafo RC, McCann MF. An epidemiologic study of contraception and preeclampsia. *JAMA.* (1989) 262:3143–7. doi: 10.1001/jama.1989.03430220066032
17. Dekker G. The partner's role in the etiology of preeclampsia. *J Reprod Immunol.* (2002) 57:203–15. doi: 10.1016/S0165-0378(02)00039-6
18. Masoudian P, Nasr A, de Nanassy J, Fung-Kee-Fung K, Bainbridge SA, DemellawyDE. Oocyte donation pregnancies and the risk of preeclampsia or gestational hypertension: a systematic review and metaanalysis. *Am J Obstet Gynecol.* (2016) 214:328–39. doi: 10.1016/j.ajog.2015.11.020
19. Kyrou D, Kolibianakis EM, Devroey P, Fatemi HM. Is the use of donor sperm associated with a higher incidence of preeclampsia in women who achieve pregnancy after intrauterine insemination? *Fertil Steril.* (2010) 93:1124–7. doi: 10.1016/j.fertnstert.2008.12.021
20. Rowe JH, Ertelt JM, Xin L, Way SS. Pregnancy imprints regulatory memory that sustains anergy to fetal antigen. *Nature.* (2012) 490:102–6. doi: 10.1038/nature11462
21. Gamliel M, Goldman-Wohl D, Isaacson B, Gur C, Stein N, Yamin R, et al. Trained memory of human uterine NK cells enhances their function in subsequent pregnancies. *Immunity.* (2018) 48:951–962 e5. doi: 10.1016/j.immuni.2018.03.030
22. Robertson SA, Sharkey DJ. Seminal fluid and fertility in women. *Fertil Steril.* (2016) 106:511–9. doi: 10.1016/j.fertnstert.2016.07.1101
23. Robertson SA, Care AS, Moldenhauer LM. Regulatory T cells in embryo implantation and the immune response to pregnancy. *J Clin Invest.* (2018) 128:4224–35. doi: 10.1172/JCI122182
24. Redman CW, Sacks GP, Sargent IL. Preeclampsia: an excessive maternal inflammatory response to pregnancy. *Am J Obstet Gynecol.* (1999) 180:499–506. doi: 10.1016/S0002-9378(99)70239-5
25. Saito S, Sakai M, Sasaki Y, Nakashima A, Shiozaki A. Inadequate tolerance induction may induce pre-eclampsia. *J Reprod Immunol.* (2007) 76:30–9. doi: 10.1016/j.jri.2007.08.002
26. Sasaki Y, Darmochwal-Kolarz D, Suzuki D, Sakai M, Ito M, Shima T, et al. Proportion of peripheral blood and decidual CD4(+) CD25(bright) regulatory T cells in pre-eclampsia. *Clin Exp Immunol.* (2007) 149:139–45. doi: 10.1111/j.1365-2249.2007.03397.x
27. Santner-Nanan B, Peek MJ, Khanam R, Richarts L, Zhu E, Fazekas de St Groth B, Nanan R. Systemic increase in the ratio between Foxp3+ and IL-17-producing CD4+ T cells in healthy pregnancy but not in preeclampsia. *J Immunol.* (2009) 2009:1154. doi: 10.4049/jimmunol.0901154
28. Quinn KH, Lacoursiere DY, Cui L, Bui J, Parast MM. The unique pathophysiology of early-onset severe preeclampsia: role of decidual T regulatory cells. *J Reprod Immunol.* (2011) 91:76–82. doi: 10.1016/j.jri.2011.05.006
29. LaMarca B, Cornelius DC, Harmon AC, Amaral LM, Cunningham MW, Faulkner JL, et al. Identifying immune mechanisms mediating the hypertension during preeclampsia. *Am J Physiol Regul Integr Comp Physiol.* (2016) 311:R1–9. doi: 10.1152/ajpregu.00052.2016
30. Hanna J, Goldman-Wohl D, Hamani Y, Avraham I, Greenfield C, Natanson-Yaron S, et al. Decidual NK cells regulate key developmental processes at the human fetal-maternal interface. *Nat Med.* (2006) 12:1065–74. doi: 10.1038/nm1452
31. Lash GE, Pitman H, Morgan HL, Innes BA, Agwu CN, Bulmer JN. Decidual macrophages: key regulators of vascular remodeling in human pregnancy. *J Leukoc Biol.* (2016) 100:315–25. doi: 10.1189/jlb.1A0815-351R
32. Hsu P, Santner-Nanan B, Dahlstrom JE, Fadia M, Chandra A, Peek M, et al. Altered decidual DC-SIGN+ antigen-presenting cells and impaired regulatory T-cell induction in preeclampsia. *Am J Pathol.* (2012) 181:2149–60. doi: 10.1016/j.ajpath.2012.08.032
33. Darmochwal-Kolarz D, Kludka-Sternik M, Tabarkiewicz J, Kolarz B, Rolinski J, Leszczynska-Gorzelak B, et al. The predominance of Th17 lymphocytes and decreased number and function of Treg cells in preeclampsia. *J Reprod Immunol.* (2012) 93:75–81. doi: 10.1016/j.jri.2012.01.006
34. Steinborn A, Schmitt E, Kisielewicz A, Rechenberg S, Seissler N, Mahnke K, et al. Pregnancy-associated diseases are characterized by the composition of the systemic regulatory T cell (Treg) pool with distinct subsets of Tregs. *Clin Exp Immunol.* (2012) 167:84–98. doi: 10.1111/j.1365-2249.2011.04493.x
35. Carbone F, La Rocca C, De Candia P, Procaccini C, Colamatteo A, Micillo T, et al.Metabolic control of immune tolerance in health and autoimmunity. *Semin Immunol.* (2016) 28:491–504. doi: 10.1016/j.smim.2016.09.006
36. Murai M, Krause P, Cheroutre H, Kronenberg M. Regulatory T-cell stability and plasticity in mucosal and systemic immune systems. *Mucosal Immunol.* (2010) 3:443–9. doi: 10.1038/mi.2010.27
37. Bluestone JA, Trotta E, Xu D. The therapeutic potential of regulatory T cells for the treatment of autoimmune disease. *Expert Opin Ther Targets.* (2015) 19:1091–103. doi: 10.1517/14728222.2015.1037282
38. Issazadeh-Navikas S, Teimer R, Bockermann R. Influence of dietary components on regulatory T cells. *Mol Med.* (2012) 18:95–110. doi: 10.2119/molmed.2011.00311
39. Kim W, Lee H. Advances in nutritional research on regulatory T-cells. *Nutrients.* (2013) 5:4305–15. doi: 10.3390/nu5114305
40. Jagger A, Shimojima Y, Goronzy JJ, Weyand CM. Regulatory T cells and the immune aging process: a mini-review. *Gerontology.* (2014) 60:130–7. doi: 10.1159/000355303
41. Allan SE, Broady R, Gregori S, Himmel ME, Locke N, Roncarolo MG, et al. CD4+ T-regulatory cells: toward therapy for human diseases. *Immunol Rev.* (2008) 223:391–421. doi: 10.1111/j.1600-065X.2008.00634.x
42. Furukawa A, Wisel SA, Tang Q. Impact of immune-modulatory drugs on regulatory T cell. *Transplantation.* (2016) 100:2288–300. doi: 10.1097/TP.0000000000001379
43. Trowsdale J, Betz AG. Mother's little helpers: mechanisms of maternal-fetal tolerance. *Nat Immunol.* (2006) 7:241–6. doi: 10.1038/ni1317
44. Guleria I, Sayegh MH. Maternal acceptance of the fetus: true human tolerance. *J Immunol.* (2007) 178:3345–51. doi: 10.4049/jimmunol.178.6.3345
45. Nancy P, Tagliani E, Tay CS, Asp P, Levy DE, Erlebacher A. Chemokine gene silencing in decidual stromal cells limits T cell access to the maternal-fetal interface. *Science.* (2012) 336:1317–21. doi: 10.1126/science.1220030
46. Aluvihare VR, Kallikourdis M, Betz AG. Regulatory T cells mediate maternal tolerance to the fetus. *Nat Immunol.* (2004) 5:266–71. doi: 10.1038/ni1037
47. Guerin LR, Prins JR, Robertson SA. Regulatory T-cells and immune tolerance in pregnancy: a new target for infertility treatment? *Hum Reprod Update.* (2009) 15:517–35. doi: 10.1093/humupd/dmp004
48. Bettelli E, Carrier Y, Gao W, Korn T, Strom TB, Oukka M, et al. Reciprocal developmental pathways for the generation of pathogenic effector TH17 and regulatory T cells. *Nature.* (2006) 441:235–8. doi: 10.1038/nature04753
49. Sakaguchi S, Yamaguchi T, Nomura T, Ono M. Regulatory T cells and immune tolerance. *Cell.* (2008) 133:775–87. doi: 10.1016/j.cell.2008.05.009
50. Rudensky AY. Regulatory T cells and Foxp3. *Immunol Rev.* (2011) 241:260–8. doi: 10.1111/j.1600-065X.2011.01018.x
51. Arpaia N, Green JA, Moltedo B, Arvey A, Hemmers S, Yuan S, et al. A distinct function of regulatory T cells in tissue protection. *Cell.* (2015) 162:1078–89. doi: 10.1016/j.cell.2015.08.021
52. Josefowicz SZ, Lu LF, Rudensky AY. Regulatory T cells: mechanisms of differentiation and function. *Annu Rev Immunol.* (2012) 30:531–64. doi: 10.1146/annurev.immunol.25.022106.141623
53. Chen W, Jin W, Hardegen N, Lei KJ, Li L, Marinos N, et al. Conversion of peripheral CD4+CD25- naive T cells to CD4+CD25+ regulatory T cells

by TGF-beta induction of transcription factor Foxp3. *J Exp Med.* (2003) 198:1875–86. doi: 10.1084/jem.20030152

54. Waldmann H, Adams E, Fairchild P, Cobbold S. Infectious tolerance and the long-term acceptance of transplanted tissue. *Immunol Rev.* (2006) 212:301–13. doi: 10.1111/j.0105-2896.2006.00406.x
55. Yamazaki S, Nishioka A, Kasuya S, Ohkura N, Hemmi H, Kaisho T, et al. Homeostasis of thymus-derived Foxp3+ regulatory T cells is controlled by ultraviolet B exposure in the skin. *J Immunol.* (2014) 193:5488–97. doi: 10.4049/jimmunol.1400985
56. Burzyn D, Kuswanto W, Kolodin D, Shadrach JL, Cerletti M, Jang Y, et al. A special population of regulatory T cells potentiates muscle repair. *Cell.* (2013) 155:1282–95. doi: 10.1016/j.cell.2013.10.054
57. Williams PJ, Searle RF, Robson SC, Innes BA, Bulmer JN. Decidual leucocyte populations in early to late gestation normal human pregnancy. *J Reprod Immunol.* (2009) 82:24–31. doi: 10.1016/j.jri.2009.08.001
58. Shao L, Jacobs AR, Johnson VV, Mayer L. Activation of CD8+ regulatory T cells by human placental trophoblasts. *J Immunol.* (2005) 174:7539–47. doi: 10.4049/jimmunol.174.12.7539
59. Tilburgs T, Schonkeren D, Eikmans M, Nagtzaam NM, Datema G, Swings GM, et al. Human decidual tissue contains differentiated CD8+ effector-memory T cells with unique properties. *J Immunol.* (2010) 185:4470–7. doi: 10.4049/jimmunol.0903597
60. Dimova T, Nagaeva O, Stenqvist AC, Hedlund M, Kjellberg L, Strand M, et al. Maternal Foxp3 expressing CD4+ CD25+ and CD4+ CD25- regulatory T-cell populations are enriched in human early normal pregnancy decidua: a phenotypic study of paired decidual and peripheral blood samples. *Am J Reprod Immunol.* (2011) 66(Suppl 1):44–56. doi: 10.1111/j.1600-0897.2011.01046.x
61. Mjosberg J, Berg G, Jenmalm MC, Ernerudh J. FOXP3+ regulatory T cells and T helper 1, T helper 2, and T helper 17 cells in human early pregnancy decidua. *Biol Reprod.* (2010) 82:698–705. doi: 10.1095/biolreprod.109.081208
62. Tilburgs T, Roelen DL, van der Mast BJ, de Groot-Swings GM, Kleijburg C, Scherjon S, et al. Evidence for a selective migration of fetus-specific CD4+CD25bright regulatory T cells from the peripheral blood to the decidua in human pregnancy. *J Immunol.* (2008) 180:5737–45. doi: 10.4049/jimmunol.180.8.5737
63. Inada K, Shima T, Ito M, Ushijima A, Saito S. Helios-positive functional regulatory T cells are decreased in decidua of miscarriage cases with normal fetal chromosomal content. *J Reprod Immunol.* (2015) 107:10–9. doi: 10.1016/j.jri.2014.09.053
64. Wagner MI, Jost M, Spratte J, Schaier M, Mahnke K, Meuer S, et al. Differentiation of ICOS+ and ICOS- recent thymic emigrant regulatory T cells (RTE T regs) during normal pregnancy, pre-eclampsia and HELLP syndrome. *Clin Exp Immunol.* (2016) 183:129–42. doi: 10.1111/cei.12693
65. Sargent IL, Borzychowski AM, Redman CWG. Immunoregulation in normal pregnancy and pre-eclampsia: an overview. *Reprod BioMed Online.* (2006) 13:680–6. doi: 10.1016/S1472-6483(10)60659-1
66. Hudic I, Fatusic Z. Progesterone - induced blocking factor (PIBF) and Th(1)/Th(2) cytokine in women with threatened spontaneous abortion. *J Perinat Med.* (2009) 37:338–42. doi: 10.1515/jpm.2009.061
67. Rahimzadeh M, Norouzian M, Arabpour F, Naderi N. Regulatory T-cells and preeclampsia: an overview of literature. *Expert Rev Clin Immunol.* (2016) 12:209–27. doi: 10.1586/1744666X.2016.1105740
68. Steinborn A, Haensch GM, Mahnke K, Schmitt E, Toermer A, Meuer S, et al. Distinct subsets of regulatory T cells during pregnancy: is the imbalance of these subsets involved in the pathogenesis of preeclampsia? *Clin Immunol.* (2008) 129:401–12. doi: 10.1016/j.clim.2008.07.032
69. Toldi G, Vasarhelyi ZE, Rigo J Jr, Orban C, Tamassy Z, Bajnok A, et al. Prevalence of regulatory T-cell subtypes in preeclampsia. *Am J Reprod Immunol.* (2015) 74:110–5. doi: 10.1111/aji.12380
70. Mjosberg J, Svensson J, Johansson E, Hellstrom L, Casas R, Jenmalm MC, et al. Systemic reduction of functionally suppressive CD4dimCD25highFoxp3+ Tregs in human second trimester pregnancy is induced by progesterone and 17beta-estradiol. *J Immunol.* (2009) 183:759–69. doi: 10.4049/jimmunol.0803654
71. Rabaglino MB, Post Uiterweer ED, Jeyabalan A, Hogge WA, Conrad KP. Bioinformatics approach reveals evidence for impaired endometrial maturation before and during early pregnancy in women who developed preeclampsia. *Hypertension.* (2015) 65:421–9. doi: 10.1161/HYPERTENSIONAHA.114.04481
72. Prins JR, Gomez-Lopez N, Robertson SA. Interleukin-6 in pregnancy and gestational disorders. *J Reprod Immunol.* (2012) 95:1–14. doi: 10.1016/j.jri.2012.05.004
73. Prins JR, Faas MM, Melgert BN, Huitema S, Timmer A, Hylkema MN, et al. Altered expression of immune-associated genes in first-trimester human decidua of pregnancies later complicated with hypertension or foetal growth restriction. *Placenta.* (2012) 33:453–5. doi: 10.1016/j.placenta.2012.02.010
74. Winger EE, Reed JL. Low circulating CD4(+) CD25(+) Foxp3(+) T regulatory cell levels predict miscarriage risk in newly pregnant women with a history of failure. *Am J Reprod Immunol.* (2011) 66:320–8. doi: 10.1111/j.1600-0897.2011.00992.x
75. Ahn H, Park J, Gilman-Sachs A, Kwak-Kim J. Immunologic characteristics of preeclampsia, a comprehensive review. *Am J Reprod Immunol.* (2011) 65:377–94. doi: 10.1111/j.1600-0897.2010.00913.x
76. Romero R, Kusanovic JP, Chaiworapongsa T, Hassan SS. Placental bed disorders in preterm labor, preterm PROM, spontaneous abortion and abruptio placentae. *Best Pract Res Clin Obstet Gynaecol.* (2011) 25:313–27. doi: 10.1016/j.bpobgyn.2011.02.006
77. Romero R, Dey SK, Fisher SJ. Preterm labor: one syndrome, many causes. *Science.* (2014) 345:760–5. doi: 10.1126/science.1251816
78. Zhang J, Dunk C, Croy AB, Lye SJ. To serve and to protect: the role of decidual innate immune cells on human pregnancy. *Cell Tissue Res.* (2016) 363:249–65. doi: 10.1007/s00441-015-2315-4
79. Nevers T, Kalkunte S, Sharma S. Uterine regulatory T cells, IL-10 and hypertension. *Am J Reprod Immunol.* (2011) 66(Suppl 1):88–92. doi: 10.1111/j.1600-0897.2011.01040.x
80. Jasper MJ, Tremellen KP, Robertson SA. Primary unexplained infertility is associated with reduced expression of the T-regulatory cell transcription factor Foxp3 in endometrial tissue. *Mol Hum Reprod.* (2006) 12:301–8. doi: 10.1093/molehr/gal032
81. Kwak-Kim J, Bao S, Lee SK, Kim JW, Gilman-Sachs A. Immunological modes of pregnancy loss: inflammation, immune effectors, and stress. *Am J Reprod Immunol.* (2014) 72:129–40. doi: 10.1111/aji.12234
82. Zenclussen AC, Fest S, Joachim R, Klapp BF, Arck PC. Introducing a mouse model for pre-eclampsia: adoptive transfer of activated Th1 cells leads to pre-eclampsia-like symptoms exclusively in pregnant mice. *Eur J Immunol.* (2004) 34:377–87. doi: 10.1002/eji.200324469
83. Wegorzewska M, Nijagal A, Wong CM, Le T, Lescano N, Tang Q, et al. Fetal intervention increases maternal T cell awareness of the foreign conceptus and can lead to immune-mediated fetal demise. *J Immunol.* (2014) 192:1938–45. doi: 10.4049/jimmunol.1302403
84. Xin L, Ertelt JM, Rowe JH, Jiang TT, Kinder JM, Chaturvedi V, et al. Cutting edge: committed Th1 CD4+ T cell differentiation blocks pregnancy-induced Foxp3 expression with antigen-specific fetal loss. *J Immunol.* (2014) 192:2970–4. doi: 10.4049/jimmunol.1302678
85. Samstein RM, Josefowicz SZ, Arvey A, Treuting PM, Rudensky AY. Extrathymic generation of regulatory T cells in placental mammals mitigates maternal-fetal conflict. *Cell.* (2012) 150:29–38. doi: 10.1016/j.cell.2012.05.031
86. Shima T, Sasaki Y, Itoh M, Nakashima A, Ishii N, Sugamura K, et al. Regulatory T cells are necessary for implantation and maintenance of early pregnancy but not late pregnancy in allogeneic mice. *J Reprod Immunol.* (2010) 85:121–9. doi: 10.1016/j.jri.2010.02.006
87. Zenclussen AC, Gerlof K, Zenclussen ML, Sollwedel A, Bertoja AZ, Ritter T, et al. Abnormal T-cell reactivity against paternal antigens in spontaneous abortion: adoptive transfer of pregnancy-induced CD4+CD25+ T regulatory cells prevents fetal rejection in a murine abortion model. *Am J Pathol.* (2005) 166:811–22. doi: 10.1016/S0002-9440(10)62302-4
88. Darrasse-Jeze G, Klatzmann D, Charlotte F, Salomon BL, Cohen JL. CD4+CD25+ regulatory/suppressor T cells prevent allogeneic fetus rejection in mice. *Immunol Lett.* (2006) 102:106–9. doi: 10.1016/j.imlet.2005.07.002
89. Care AS, Bourque SL, Morton JS, Hjartarson EP, Robertson SA, Davidge ST. Reduction in regulatory T cells in early pregnancy causes uterine artery dysfunction in mice. *Hypertension.* (2018) 72:177–87. doi: 10.1161/HYPERTENSIONAHA.118.10858

90. Bizargity P, Del Rio R, Phillippe M, Teuscher C, Bonney EA. Resistance to lipopolysaccharide-induced preterm delivery mediated by regulatory T cell function in mice. *Biol Reprod.* (2009) 80:874–81. doi: 10.1095/biolreprod.108.074294
91. Li L, Tu J, Jiang Y, Zhou J, Schust DJ. Regulatory T cells decrease invariant natural killer T cell-mediated pregnancy loss in mice. *Mucosal Immunol.* (2017) 10:613–23. doi: 10.1038/mi.2016.84
92. Lin Y, Liu X, Shan B, Wu J, Sharma S, Sun Y. Prevention of CpG-induced pregnancy disruption by adoptive transfer of in vitro-induced regulatory T cells. *PLoS ONE.* (2014) 9:e94702. doi: 10.1371/journal.pone.0094702
93. Moldenhauer LM, Diener KR, Thring DM, Brown MP, Hayball JD, Robertson SA. Cross-presentation of male seminal fluid antigens elicits T cell activation to initiate the female immune response to pregnancy. *J Immunol.* (2009) 182:8080–93. doi: 10.4049/jimmunol.0804018
94. Murphy SP, Fast LD, Hanna NN, Sharma S. Uterine NK cells mediate inflammation-induced fetal demise in IL-10-null mice. *J Immunol.* (2005) 175:4084–90. doi: 10.4049/jimmunol.175.6.4084
95. Thuere C, Zenclussen ML, Schumacher A, Langwisch S, Schulte-Wrede U, Teles A, et al. Kinetics of regulatory T cells during murine pregnancy. *Am J Reprod Immunol.* (2007) 58:514–23. doi: 10.1111/j.1600-0897.2007.00538.x
96. Terme M, Chaput N, Combadiere B, Ma A, Ohteki T, Zitvogel L. Regulatory T cells control dendritic cell/NK cell cross-talk in lymph nodes at the steady state by inhibiting CD4+ self-reactive T cells. *J Immunol.* (2008) 180:4679–86. doi: 10.4049/jimmunol.180.7.4679
97. Ghiringhelli F, Menard C, Terme M, Flament C, Taieb J, Chaput N, et al. CD4+CD25+ regulatory T cells inhibit natural killer cell functions in a transforming growth factor-beta-dependent manner. *J Exp Med.* (2005) 202:1075–85. doi: 10.1084/jem.20051511
98. Vacca P, Cantoni C, Vitale M, Prato C, Canegallo F, Fenoglio D, et al. Crosstalk between decidual NK and CD14+ myelomonocytic cells results in induction of Tregs and immunosuppression. *Proc Natl Acad Sci USA.* (2010) 107:11918–23. doi: 10.1073/pnas.1001749107
99. Woidacki K, Meyer N, Schumacher A, Goldschmidt A, Maurer M, Zenclussen AC. Transfer of regulatory T cells into abortion-prone mice promotes the expansion of uterine mast cells and normalizes early pregnancy angiogenesis. *Sci Rep.* (2015) 5:13938. doi: 10.1038/srep13938
100. Schumacher A, Wafula PO, Teles A, El-Mousleh T, Linzke N, Zenclussen ML, et al. Blockage of heme oxygenase-1 abrogates the protective effect of regulatory T cells on murine pregnancy and promotes the maturation of dendritic cells. *PLoS ONE.* (2012) 7:e42301. doi: 10.1371/journal.pone.0042301
101. Fallarino F, Grohmann U, Hwang KW, Orabona C, Vacca C, Bianchi R, et al. Modulation of tryptophan catabolism by regulatory T cells. *Nat Immunol.* (2003) 4:1206–12. doi: 10.1038/ni1003
102. Munn DH, Zhou M, Attwood JT, Bondarev I, Conway SJ, Marshall B, et al. Prevention of allogeneic fetal rejection by tryptophan catabolism. *Science.* (1998) 281:1191–3. doi: 10.1126/science.281.5380.1191
103. Blois SM, Kammerer U, Alba Soto C, Tometten MC, Shaikly V, Barrientos G, et al. Dendritic cells: key to fetal tolerance? *Biol Reprod.* (2007) 77:590–8. doi: 10.1095/biolreprod.107.060632
104. Zhang Y, Liu Z, Tian M, Hu X, Wang L, Ji J, et al. The altered PD-1/PD-L1 pathway delivers the 'one-two punch' effects to promote the Treg/Th17 imbalance in pre-eclampsia. *Cell Mol Immunol.* (2017) 2017:70. doi:10.1038/cmi.2017.70
105. Blois SM, Ilarregui JM, Tometten M, Garcia M, Orsal AS, Cordo-Russo R, et al. A pivotal role for galectin-1 in fetomaternal tolerance. *Nat Med.* (2007) 13:1450–7. doi: 10.1038/nm1680
106. Prins JR, Zhang B, Schjenken JE, Guerin LR, Barry SC, Robertson SA. Unstable Foxp3+ regulatory T cells and altered dendritic cells are associated with lipopolysaccharide-induced fetal loss in pregnant interleukin 10-deficient mice. *Biol Reprod.* (2015) 93:95. doi: 10.1095/biolreprod.115.128694
107. Plaks V, Birnberg T, Berkutzki T, Sela S, BenYashar A, Kalchenko V, et al. Uterine DCs are crucial for decidua formation during embryo implantation in mice. *J Clin Invest.* (2008) 118:3954–65. doi: 10.1172/JCI36682
108. Tirado-Gonzalez I, Barrientos G, Freitag N, Otto T, Thijssen VL, Moschansky P, et al. Uterine NK cells are critical in shaping DC immunogenic functions compatible with pregnancy progression. *PLoS ONE.* (2012) 7:e46755. doi: 10.1371/journal.pone.0046755
109. Blois SM, Klapp BF, Barrientos G. Decidualization and angiogenesis in early pregnancy: unravelling the functions of DC and NK cells. *J Reprod Immunol.* (2011) 88:86–92. doi: 10.1016/j.jri.2010.11.002
110. Du MR, Guo PF, Piao HL, Wang SC, Sun C, Jin LP, et al. Embryonic trophoblasts induce decidual regulatory T cell differentiation and maternal-fetal tolerance through thymic stromal lymphopoietin instructing dendritic cells. *J Immunol.* (2014) 192:1502–11. doi: 10.4049/jimmunol.1203425
111. Redman CW, Sargent IL. Placental stress and pre-eclampsia: a revised view. *Placenta.* (2009) 30(Suppl A):S38–42. doi: 10.1016/j.placenta.2008.11.021
112. Ashkar AA, Di Santo JP, Croy BA. Interferon gamma contributes to initiation of uterine vascular modification, decidual integrity, and uterine natural killer cell maturation during normal murine pregnancy. *J Exp Med.* (2000) 192:259–70. doi: 10.1084/jem.192.2.259
113. Yamashita T, Sasaki N, Kasahara K, Hirata K. Anti-inflammatory and immune-modulatory therapies for preventing atherosclerotic cardiovascular disease. *J Cardiol.* (2015) 66:1–8. doi: 10.1016/j.jjcc.2015.02.002
114. Matrougui K, Abd Elmageed Z, Kassan M, Choi S, Nair D, Gonzalez-Villalobos RA, et al. Natural regulatory T cells control coronary arteriolar endothelial dysfunction in hypertensive mice. *Am J Pathol.* (2011) 178:434–41. doi: 10.1016/j.ajpath.2010.11.034
115. Maganto-Garcia E, Bu DX, Tarrio ML, Alcaide P, Newton G, Griffin GK, et al. Foxp3+-inducible regulatory T cells suppress endothelial activation and leukocyte recruitment. *J Immunol.* (2011) 187:3521–9. doi: 10.4049/jimmunol.1003947
116. Croy BA, Burke SD, Barrette VF, Zhang J, Hatta K, Smith GN, et al. Identification of the primary outcomes that result from deficient spiral arterial modification in pregnant mice. *Pregnancy Hypertens.* (2011) 1:87–94. doi: 10.1016/j.preghy.2010.10.002
117. Burke SD, Barrette VF, Carter AL, Gravel J, Adams MA, Croy BA. Cardiovascular adaptations of pregnancy in T and B cell-deficient mice. *Biol Reprod.* (2011) 85:605–14. doi: 10.1095/biolreprod.111.092668
118. Nadkarni S, Smith J, Sferruzzi-Perri AN, Ledwozyw A, Kishore M, Haas R, et al. Neutrophils induce proangiogenic T cells with a regulatory phenotype in pregnancy. *Proc Natl Acad Sci USA.* (2016) 113:E8415–24. doi: 10.1073/pnas.1611944114
119. Cornelius DC, Amaral LM, Wallace K, Campbell N, Thomas AJ, Scott J, et al. Reduced uterine perfusion pressure T-helper 17 cells cause pathophysiology associated with preeclampsia during pregnancy. *Am J Physiol Regul Integr Comp Physiol.* (2016) 311:R1192–9. doi: 10.1152/ajpregu.00117.2016
120. Cornelius DC, Amaral LM, Harmon A, Wallace K, Thomas AJ, Campbell N, et al. An increased population of regulatory T cells improves the pathophysiology of placental ischemia in a rat model of preeclampsia. *Am J Physiol Regul Integr Comp Physiol.* (2015) 309:R884–91. doi: 10.1152/ajpregu.00154.2015
121. Harmon A, Cornelius D, Amaral L, Paige A, Herse F, Ibrahim T, et al. IL-10 supplementation increases Tregs and decreases hypertension in the RUPP rat model of preeclampsia. *Hypertens Pregnancy.* (2015) 34:291–306. doi: 10.3109/10641955.2015.1032054
122. Przybyl L, Ibrahim T, Haase N, Golic M, Rugor J, Luft FC, et al. Regulatory T cells ameliorate intrauterine growth retardation in a transgenic rat model for preeclampsia. *Hypertension.* (2015) 65:1298–306. doi: 10.1161/HYPERTENSIONAHA.114.04892
123. Moldenhauer LM, Diener KR, Hayball JD, Robertson SA. An immunogenic phenotype in paternal antigen-specific CD8+ T cells at embryo implantation elicits later fetal loss in mice. *Immunol Cell Biol.* (2017) 2017:41.doi: 10.1038/icb.2017.41
124. Robertson SA, Moldenhauer LM. Immunological determinants of implantation success. *Int J Dev Biol.* (2014) 58:205–17. doi: 10.1387/ijdb.140096sr
125. Arruvito L, Sanz M, Banham AH, Fainboim L. Expansion of CD4+CD25+and FOXP3+ regulatory T cells during the follicular phase of the menstrual cycle: implications for human reproduction. *J Immunol.* (2007) 178:2572–8. doi: 10.4049/jimmunol.178.4.2572
126. Saito S, Nishikawa K, Morii T, Narita N, Enomoto M, Ito A, et al. A study of CD45RO, CD45RA and CD29 antigen expression on human decidual

T cells in an early stage of pregnancy. *Immunol Lett.* (1994) 40:193–7. doi: 10.1016/0165-2478(93)00019-A
127. Tilburgs T, Scherjon SA, van der Mast BJ, Haasnoot GW, Versteeg VDV-M, Roelen D, et al. Fetal-maternal HLA-C mismatch is associated with decidual T cell activation and induction of functional T regulatory cells. *J Reprod Immunol.* (2009) 82:148–57. doi: 10.1016/j.jri.2009.05.003
128. Mjosberg J, Berg G, Ernerudh J, Ekerfelt C. CD4+ CD25+ regulatory T cells in human pregnancy: development of a Treg-MLC-ELISPOT suppression assay and indications of paternal specific Tregs. *Immunology.* (2007) 120:456–66. doi: 10.1111/j.1365-2567.2006.02529.x
129. Tian M, Zhang Y, Liu Z, Sun G, Mor G, Liao A. The PD-1/PD-L1 inhibitory pathway is altered in pre-eclampsia and regulates T cell responses in pre-eclamptic rats. *Sci Rep.* (2016) 6:27683. doi: 10.1038/srep27683
130. Petroff MG. Review: fetal antigens–identity, origins, and influences on the maternal immune system. *Placenta.* (2011) 32(Suppl 2):S176–81. doi: 10.1016/j.placenta.2010.12.014
131. Chamley LW, Chen Q, Ding J, Stone PR, Abumaree M. Trophoblast deportation: just a waste disposal system or antigen sharing? *J Reprod Immunol.* (2011) 88:99–105. doi: 10.1016/j.jri.2011.01.002
132. Moldenhauer LM, Hayball JD, Robertson SA. Utilising T cell receptor transgenic mice to define mechanisms of maternal T cell tolerance in pregnancy. *J Reprod Immunol.* (2010) 87:1–13. doi: 10.1016/j.jri.2010.05.007
133. Guerin LR, Moldenhauer LM, Prins JR, Bromfield JJ, Hayball JD, Robertson SA. Seminal fluid regulates accumulation of FOXP3+ regulatory T cells in the preimplantation mouse uterus through expanding the FOXP3+ cell pool and CCL19-mediated recruitment. *Biol Reprod.* (2011) 85:397–408. doi: 10.1095/biolreprod.110.088591
134. Zhao JX, Zeng YY, Liu Y. Fetal alloantigen is responsible for the expansion of the CD4(+)CD25(+) regulatory T cell pool during pregnancy. *J Reprod Immunol.* (2007) 75:71–81. doi: 10.1016/j.jri.2007.06.052
135. Chen T, Darrasse-Jeze G, Bergot AS, Courau T, Churlaud G, Valdivia K, et al. Self-specific memory regulatory T cells protect embryos at implantation in mice. *J Immunol.* (2013) 191:2273–81. doi: 10.4049/jimmunol.120 2413
136. Shima T, Inada K, Nakashima A, Ushijima A, Ito M, Yoshino O, et al. Paternal antigen-specific proliferating regulatory T cells are increased in uterine-draining lymph nodes just before implantation and in pregnant uterus just after implantation by seminal plasma-priming in allogeneic mouse pregnancy. *J Reprod Immunol.* (2015) 108:72–82. doi: 10.1016/j.jri.2015.02.005
137. Kallikourdis M, Betz AG. Periodic accumulation of regulatory T cells in the uterus: preparation for the implantation of a semi-allogeneic fetus? *PLoS ONE.* (2007) 2:e382. doi: 10.1371/journal.pone.0000382
138. Moldenhauer LM, Schjenken JE, Hope CM, Green ES, Zhang B, Eldi P, et al. Thymus-derived regulatory T cells exhibit Foxp3 epigenetic modification and phenotype attenuation after mating in mice. *J Immunol.* (2019) 4:253. doi: 10.3389/fimmu.2013.00253
139. Robertson SA, Guerin LR, Bromfield JJ, Branson KM, Ahlström AC, AS Care. Seminal fluid drives expansion of the CD4+CD25+ T regulatory cell pool and induces tolerance to paternal alloantigens in mice. *Biol Reprod.* (2009) 80:1036–45. doi: 10.1095/biolreprod.108.074658
140. Johansson M, Bromfield JJ, Jasper MJ, Robertson SA. Semen activates the female immune response during early pregnancy in mice. *Immunology.* (2004) 112:290–300. doi: 10.1111/j.1365-2567.2004.01876.x
141. Hori S. Lineage stability and phenotypic plasticity of Foxp3(+) regulatory T cells. *Immunol Rev.* (2014) 259:159–72. doi: 10.1111/imr.12175
142. Sharkey DJ, Tremellen KP, Jasper MJ, Gemzell-Danielsson K, Robertson SA. Seminal fluid induces leukocyte recruitment and cytokine and chemokine mRNA expression in the human cervix after coitus. *J Immunol.* (2012) 188:2445–54. doi: 10.4049/jimmunol.11 02736
143. Schumacher A, Heinze K, Witte J, Poloski E, Linzke N, Woidacki K, et al. Human chorionic gonadotropin as a central regulator of pregnancy immune tolerance. *J Immunol.* (2013) 190:2650–8. doi: 10.4049/jimmunol.1202698
144. Balandya E, Wieland-Alter W, Sanders K, Lahey T. Human seminal plasma fosters CD4(+) regulatory T-cell phenotype and transforming growth factor-beta1 expression. *Am J Reprod Immunol.* (2012) 68:322–30. doi: 10.1111/j.1600-0897.2012.01176.x
145. Meuleman T, Snaterse G, van Beelen E, Anholts JD, Pilgram GS, van der Westerlaken LA, et al. The immunomodulating effect of seminal plasma on T cells. *J Reprod Immunol.* (2015) 110:109–16. doi: 10.1016/j.jri.2015.01.012
146. Triche EW, Harland KK, Field EH, Rubenstein LM, Saftlas AF. Maternal-fetal HLA sharing and preeclampsia: variation in effects by seminal fluid exposure in a case-control study of nulliparous women in Iowa. *J Reprod Immunol.* (2014) 101–102:111–9. doi: 10.1016/j.jri.2013.06.004
147. Liu C, Wang XZ, Sun XB. Assessment of sperm antigen specific T regulatory cells in women with recurrent miscarriage. *Early Hum Dev.* (2012) 2012:003.doi: 10.1016/j.earlhumdev.2012.08.003
148. Sharkey DJ, Tremellen KP, Briggs NE, Dekker GA, Robertson SA. Seminal plasma transforming growth factor-beta, activin A and follistatin fluctuate within men over time. *Hum Reprod.* (2016) 31:2183–91. doi: 10.1093/humrep/dew185
149. Sharkey DJ, Tremellen KP, Briggs NE, Dekker GA, Robertson SA. Seminal plasma pro-inflammatory cytokines interferon-gamma (IFNG) and C-X-C motif chemokine ligand 8 (CXCL8) fluctuate over time within men. *Hum Reprod.* (2017) 2017:1–9. doi: 10.1093/humrep/dex106
150. Sharkey DJ, Glynn DJ, Schjenken JE, Tremellen KP, Robertson SA. Interferon-gamma inhibits seminal plasma induction of colony-stimulating factor 2 in mouse and human reproductive tract epithelial cells. *Biol Reprod.* (2018) 99:514–26. doi: 10.1093/biolre/ioy071
151. Moldenhauer LM, Keenihan SN, Hayball JD, Robertson SA. GM-CSF is an essential regulator of T cell activation competence in uterine dendritic cells during early pregnancy in mice. *J Immunol.* (2010) 185:7085–96. doi: 10.4049/jimmunol.1001374
152. Kryczek I, Bruce AT, Gudjonsson JE, Johnston A, Aphale A, Vatan L, et al. Induction of IL-17+ T cell trafficking and development by IFN-gamma: mechanism and pathological relevance in psoriasis. *J Immunol.* (2008) 181:4733–41. doi: 10.4049/jimmunol.181.7.4733
153. Zhao J, Zhao J, Perlman S. Differential effects of IL-12 on Tregs and non-Treg T cells: roles of IFN-γ, IL-2 and IL-2R. *PLoS ONE.* (2012) 7:e46241. doi: 10.1371/journal.pone.0046241
154. Sadlon T, Brown CY, Bandara V, Hope CM, Schjenken JE, Pederson SM, et al. Unravelling the molecular basis for regulatory T-cell plasticity and loss of function in disease. *Clin Trans Immunol.* (2018) 7:e1011. doi: 10.1002/cti2.1011
155. Voo KS, Wang YH, Santori FR, Boggiano C, Wang YH, Arima K, et al. Identification of IL-17-producing FOXP3+ regulatory T cells in humans. *Proc Natl Acad Sci USA.* (2009) 106:4793–8. doi: 10.1073/pnas.090 0408106
156. Feng T, Cao AT, Weaver CT, Elson CO, Cong Y. Interleukin-12 converts Foxp3+ regulatory T cells to interferon-gamma-producing Foxp3+ T cells that inhibit colitis. *Gastroenterology.* (2011) 140:2031–43. doi: 10.1053/j.gastro.2011.03.009
157. Komatsu N, Okamoto K, Sawa S, Nakashima T, Oh-hora M, Kodama T, et al. Pathogenic conversion of Foxp3+ T cells into TH17 cells in autoimmune arthritis. *Nat Med.* (2014) 20:62–8. doi: 10.1038/nm.3432
158. Beyer M, Thabet Y, Muller RU, Sadlon T, Classen S, Lahl K, et al. Repression of the genome organizer SATB1 in regulatory T cells is required for suppressive function and inhibition of effector differentiation. *Nat Immunol.* (2011) 12:898–907. doi: 10.1038/ni.2084
159. Ngalamika O, Liang G, Zhao M, Yu X, Yang Y, Yin H, et al. Peripheral whole blood FOXP3 TSDR methylation: a potential marker in severity assessment of autoimmune diseases and chronic infections. *Immunol Invest.* (2015) 44:126–36. doi: 10.3109/08820139.2014.938165
160. Chen X, Gan T, Liao Z, Chen S, Xiao J. Foxp3 (-/ATT) polymorphism contributes to the susceptibility of preeclampsia. *PLoS ONE.* (2013) 8:e59696. doi: 10.1371/journal.pone.0059696
161. Norouzian M, Rahimzadeh M, Rajaee M, Arabpour F, Naderi N. FoxP3 gene promoter polymorphism affects susceptibility to preeclampsia. *Hum Immunol.* (2016) 77:1232–8. doi: 10.1016/j.humimm.2016.09.001
162. Arruvito L, Billordo A, Capucchio M, Prada ME, Fainboim L. IL-6 trans-signaling and the frequency of CD4+FOXP3+ cells in women with reproductive failure. *J Reprod Immunol.* (2009) 82:158–65. doi: 10.1016/j.jri.2009.04.010
163. Arruvito L, Sotelo AI, Billordo A, Fainboim L. A physiological role for inducible FOXP3(+) Treg cells. Lessons from women with reproductive

failure. *Clin Immunol.* (2010) 136:432–41. doi: 10.1016/j.clim.2010.05.002

164. Prins JR, Holvast F, van 't Hooft J, Bos AF, Ganzevoort JW, Scherjon SA, et al. Development of a core outcome set for immunomodulation in pregnancy (COSIMPREG): a protocol for a systematic review and Delphi study. *BMJ Open.* (2018) 8:e021619. doi: 10.1136/bmjopen-2018-021619
165. Petrillo MG, Ronchetti S, Ricci E, Alunno A, Gerli R, Nocentini G, et al. GITR+ regulatory T cells in the treatment of autoimmune diseases. *Autoimmun Rev.* (2015) 14:117–26. doi: 10.1016/j.autrev.2014.10.011
166. Hill D, Eastaff-Leung N, Bresatz-Atkins S, Warner N, Ruitenberg J, Krumbiegel D, et al. Inhibition of activation induced CD154 on CD4+ CD25- cells: a valid surrogate for human Treg suppressor function. *Immunol Cell Biol.* (2012) 90:812–21. doi: 10.1038/icb.2012.18
167. Nicholson IC, Mavrangelos C, Bird DR, Bresatz-Atkins S, Eastaff-Leung NG, Grose R, et al. PI16 is expressed by a subset of human memory Treg with enhanced migration to CCL17 and CCL20. *Cell Immunol.* (2012) 275:12–8. doi: 10.1016/j.cellimm.2012.04.002
168. Saftlas AF, Rubenstein L, Prater K, Harland KK, Field E, Triche EW. Cumulative exposure to paternal seminal fluid prior to conception and subsequent risk of preeclampsia. *J Reprod Immunol.* (2014) 101–102:104–10. doi: 10.1016/j.jri.2013.07.006
169. Brown HM, Green ES, Tan TCY, Gonzalez MB, Rumbold AR, Hull ML, Norman RJ, et al. Periconception onset diabetes is associated with embryopathy and fetal growth retardation, reproductive tract hyperglycosylation and impaired immune adaptation to pregnancy. *Sci Rep.* (2018) 8:2114. doi: 10.1038/s41598-018-19263-8
170. Gleicher N, el-Roeiy A. The reproductive autoimmune failure syndrome. *Am J Obstet Gynecol.* (1988) 159:223–7. doi: 10.1016/0002-9378(88)90525-X
171. Scarpellini F, Sbracia M. Use of granulocyte colony-stimulating factor for the treatment of unexplained recurrent miscarriage: a randomised controlled trial. *Hum Reprod.* (2009) 24:2703–8. doi: 10.1093/humrep/dep240
172. Ziebe S, Loft A, Povlsen BB, Erb K, Agerholm I, Aasted M, et al. A randomized clinical trial to evaluate the effect of granulocyte-macrophage colony-stimulating factor (GM-CSF) in embryo culture medium for in vitro fertilization. *Fertil Steril.* (2013) 99:1600–9. doi: 10.1016/j.fertnstert.2012.12.043
173. Rahmati M, Petitbarat M, Dubanchet S, Bensussan A, Chaouat G, Ledee N. Colony Stimulating Factors 1:2, 3 and early pregnancy steps: from bench to bedside. *J Reprod Immunol.* (2015) 109:1–6. doi: 10.1016/j.jri.2015.01.005
174. Schjenken JE, Zhang B, Chan HY, Sharkey DJ, Fullston T, Robertson SA. miRNA regulation of immune tolerance in early pregnancy. *Am J Reprod Immunol.* (2016) 75:272–80. doi: 10.1111/aji.12490
175. Szekeres-Bartho J. Progesterone-mediated immunomodulation in pregnancy: its relevance to leukocyte immunotherapy of recurrent miscarriage. *Immunotherapy.* (2009) 1:873–82. doi: 10.2217/imt.09.54
176. Druckmann R, Druckmann M-A. Progesterone and the immunology of pregnancy. *J Steroid Biochem Mol Biol.* (2005) 97:389–96. doi: 10.1016/j.jsbmb.2005.08.010
177. Lee JH, Ulrich B, Cho J, Park J, Kim CH. Progesterone promotes differentiation of human cord blood fetal T cells into T regulatory cells but suppresses their differentiation into Th17 cells. *J Immunol.* (2011) 187:1778–87. doi: 10.4049/jimmunol.1003919
178. Lee JH, Lydon JP, Kim CH. Progesterone suppresses the mTOR pathway and promotes generation of induced regulatory T cells with increased stability. *Eur J Immunol.* (2012) 42:2683–96. doi: 10.1002/eji.201142317
179. Piccinni M-P, Scaletti C, Maggi E, Romagnani S. Role of hormone-controlled Th1- and Th2-type cytokines in successful pregnancy. *J Neuroimmunol.* (2000) 109:30–3. doi: 10.1016/S0165-5728(00)00299-X
180. Mao G, Wang J, Kang Y, Tai P, Wen J, Zou Q, et al. Progesterone increases systemic and local uterine proportions of CD4+CD25+ Treg cells during midterm pregnancy in mice. *Endocrinology.* (2010) 151:5477–88. doi: 10.1210/en.2010-0426
181. Hughes GC, Clark EA, Wong AH. The intracellular progesterone receptor regulates CD4+ T cells and T cell-dependent antibody responses. *J Leukoc Biol.* (2013) 93:369–75. doi: 10.1189/jlb.1012491
182. Thangamani S, Kim M, Son Y, Huang X, Kim H, Lee JH, et al. Cutting edge: progesterone directly upregulates vitamin D receptor gene expression for efficient regulation of T cells by calcitriol. *J Immunol.* (2015) 194:883–6. doi: 10.4049/jimmunol.1401923
183. Haas DM, Hathaway TJ, Ramsey PS. Progestogen for preventing miscarriage in women with recurrent miscarriage of unclear etiology. *Cochrane Database Syst Rev.* (2018) 10:CD003511.doi: 10.1002/14651858.CD003511.pub4
184. Ogasawara M, Aoki K, Okada S, Suzumori K. Embryonic karyotype of abortuses in relation to the number of previous miscarriages. *Fertil Steril.* (2000) 73:300–4. doi: 10.1016/S0015-0282(99)00495-1
185. Meher S, Duley L. Progesterone for preventing pre-eclampsia and its complications. *Cochrane Database Syst Rev.* (2006) 4:CD006175. doi: 10.1002/14651858.CD006175
186. Robertson SA, Jin M, Yu D, Moldenhauer LM, Davies MJ, Hull ML, et al. Corticosteroid therapy in assisted reproduction - immune suppression is a faulty premise. *Hum Reprod.* (2016) 31:2164–73. doi: 10.1093/humrep/dew186
187. Coulam CB, Acacio B. Does immunotherapy for treatment of reproductive failure enhance live births? *Am J Reprod Immunol.* (2012) 67:296–304. doi: 10.1111/j.1600-0897.2012.01111.x
188. Wong LF, Porter TF, Scott JR. Immunotherapy for recurrent miscarriage. *Cochrane Database Syst Rev.* (2014) 10:CD000112. doi: 10.1002/14651858.CD000112.pub3
189. Roussev RG, Acacio B, Ng SC, Coulam CB. Duration of intralipid's suppressive effect on NK cell's functional activity. *Am J Reprod Immunol.* (2008) 60:258–63. doi: 10.1111/j.1600-0897.2008.00621.x
190. Lal G, Zhang N, van der Touw W, Ding Y, Ju W, Bottinger EP, et al. Epigenetic regulation of Foxp3 expression in regulatory T cells by DNA methylation. *J Immunol.* (2009) 182:259–73. doi: 10.4049/jimmunol.182.1.259
191. Lu CH, Wu CJ, Chan CC, Nguyen DT, Lin KR, Lin SJ, et al. DNA methyltransferase inhibitor promotes human CD4(+)CD25(h)FOXP3(+) regulatory T lymphocyte induction under suboptimal TCR stimulation. *Front Immunol.* (2016) 7:488. doi: 10.3389/fimmu.2016.00488
192. Someya K, Nakatsukasa H, Ito M, Kondo T, Tateda KIAkanuma T, et al. Improvement of Foxp3 stability through CNS2 demethylation by TET enzyme induction and activation. *Int Immunol.* (2017) 29:365–75. doi: 10.1093/intimm/dxx049
193. Singer BD, Mock JR, Aggarwal NRGaribaldi BT, Sidhaye VK, Florez MA, et al. Regulatory T cell DNA methyltransferase inhibition accelerates resolution of lung inflammation. *Am J Respir Cell Mol Biol.* (2015) 52:641–52. doi: 10.1165/rcmb.2014-0327OC
194. Cheng C, Wang S, Ye P, Huang X, Liu Z, Wu J, et al. 'Default' generated neonatal regulatory T cells are hypomethylated at conserved non-coding sequence 2 and promote long-term cardiac allograft survival. *Immunology.* (2014) 143:618–30. doi: 10.1111/imm.12343
195. Tao R, de Zoeten EF, Ozkaynak E, Chen C, Wang L, Porrett PM, et al. Deacetylase inhibition promotes the generation and function of regulatory T cells. *Nat Med.* (2007) 13:1299–307. doi: 10.1038/nm1652
196. Tang Q, Henriksen KJ, Bi M, Finger EB, Szot G, Ye J, et al. *In vitro*-expanded antigen-specific regulatory T cells suppress autoimmune diabetes. *J Exp Med.* (2004) 199:1455–65. doi: 10.1084/jem.20040139
197. MacDonald KG, Hoeppli RE, Huang Q, Gillies J, Luciani DS, Orban PC, et al. Alloantigen-specific regulatory T cells generated with a

chimeric antigen receptor. *J Clin Invest.* (2016) 126:1413–24. doi: 10.1172/JCI82771

198. Boardman D, Maher J, Lechler R, Smyth L, Lombardi G. Antigen-specificity using chimeric antigen receptors: the future of regulatory T-cell therapy? *Biochem Soc Trans.* (2016) 44:342–8. doi: 10.1042/BST20150247
199. Rowe JH, Ertelt JM, Xin L, Way S. Regulatory T cells and the immune pathogenesis of prenatal infection. *Reproduction.* (2013) 2013:262. doi: 10.1530/REP-13-0262
200. Tanaka A, Sakaguchi S. Regulatory T cells in cancer immunotherapy. *Cell Res.* (2017) 27:109–18. doi: 10.1038/cr.2016.151

7

Immediate Pre-Partum SARS-CoV-2 Status and Immune Profiling of Breastmilk

Laura Sánchez García[1†], Natalia Gómez-Torres[2†], Fernando Cabañas[3], Raquel González-Sánchez[4], Manuela López-Azorín[4], M. Teresa Moral-Pumarega[5], Diana Escuder-Vieco[5], Esther Cabañes-Alonso[6], Irma Castro[2], Claudio Alba[2], Juan Miguel Rodríguez Gómez[2] and Adelina Pellicer[1]*

[1] Neonatology Department, Biomedical Research Foundation-IDIPAZ, La Paz University Hospital, Madrid, Spain, [2] Nutrition and Food Science Department, Complutense University, Madrid, Spain, [3] Neonatology Department, Quironsalud Madrid University Hospital and Quironsalud San José Hospital, Biomedical Research Foundation-IDIPAZ, La Paz University Hospital, Madrid, Spain, [4] Neonatology Department, Quironsalud Madrid University Hospital and Quironsalud San José Hospital, Madrid, Spain, [5] Neonatology Department, 12 Octubre University Hospital, Madrid, Spain, [6] Neonatology Department and Regional Human Milk Bank, 12 Octubre University Hospital, Madrid, Spain

***Correspondence:**
Laura Sánchez García
laurasg_alcobendas@yahoo.es

†These authors have contributed equally to this work and share first authorship

Objetive: To address the prevalence of SARS-CoV-2 and the evolutionary profile of immune compounds in breastmilk of positive mothers according to time and disease state.

Methods: Forty-five women with term pregnancies with confirmed non-severe SARS-CoV-2 infection (case group), and 96 SARS-CoV-2 negative women in identical conditions (control group) were approached, using consecutive sample. Weekly (1st to 5th week postpartum) reverse transcription polymerase chain reaction (RT-PCR) in nasopharyngeal swabs (cases) and breastmilk (cases and controls) were obtained. Concentration of cytokines, chemokines, and growth factors in breastmilk (cases and controls) were determined at 1st and 5th week post-partum.

Results: Thirty-seven (study group) and 45 (control group) women were enrolled. Symptomatic infection occurred in 56.8% of women in the study group (48% fever, 48% anosmia, 43% cough). SARS-CoV-2 RNA was not found in breastmilk samples. Concentrations of cytokines (IFN-γ, IL-1ra, IL-4, IL-6, IL-9, IL-13, and TNF-α) chemokines (eotaxin, IP-10, MIP-1α, and RANTES) and growth factors (FGF, GM-CSF, IL7, and PDGF-BB) were higher in breastmilk of the study compared with the control group at 1st week postpartum. Immune compounds concentrations decreased on time, particularly in the control group milk samples. Time of nasopharyngeal swab to become negative influenced the immune compound concentration pattern. Severity of disease (symptomatic or asymptomatic infection) did not affect the immunological profile in breast milk.

Conclusions: This study confirms no viral RNA and a distinct immunological profile in breastmilk according to mother's SARS-CoV-2 status. Additional studies should address whether these findings indicate efficient reaction against SARS-CoV-2 infection, which might be suitable to protect the recipient child.

Keywords: COVID-19, vertical infectious disease transmission, breastfeeding, immunologic factors, immune system

INTRODUCTION

During the first months of COVID-19 pandemic, some concerns arose about the safety of breastfeeding because of the potential risk of viral transmission. However, most of the human milk samples assayed for SARS-CoV-2 RNA Reverse Transcription Polymerase Chain Reaction (RT-PCR) have yielded negative results (1–5), whereas no evidence of SARS-CoV-2 transmission through human milk has been provided yet (6, 7).

With regard to the efficacy of breastmilk to provide protecting anti-SARS-CoV-2 antibodies (3, 8, 9), most studies carried so far have addressed their presence. However, information regarding the impact of COVID-19 on other immune compounds, such as cytokines, chemokines, and growth factors, is lacking. These immune factors act in the prevention of infantile infection and can modulate the immunological development of the infant (10–15). In fact, their abundance in human milk is often inversely related to their scarcity in the infant's gut, characterized by a deficit of mucosal-related anti-inflammatory mechanisms, a limited production of secretory IgA, and a poor innate effector cell function (15).

Activation of inflammatory signaling pathway is a critical mediator in the pathophysiology of COVID-19 (16–18), and maternal environmental factors, including viral infections and previous antigenic exposures, are known to affect immunological composition of human milk (19–23). Therefore, a deeper insight on the impact of SARS-CoV-2 infection on the composition of breastmilk is needed.

This research aims to address questions related on the safety and the efficacy of breastmilk feeding of neonates born to mothers with non-severe SARS-CoV-2 infection, through the systematic assessment of: (a) the prevalence of viral RNA in breastmilk according to SARS-CoV-2 status, (b) the impact of SARS-CoV-2 infection on the milk profile of cytokines, chemokines, and growth factors, and (c) the evolution of their concentrations during the first five weeks of lactation.

METHODS

This multicenter, prospective case-control study was conducted in Madrid, between April and July 2020. Since March 2020, maternity hospitals tested pregnant woman for SARS-CoV-2 infection by routine nasopharyngeal RT-PCR as screening prior delivery. Given the high incidence of COVID-19 disease at the start of the study, the Spanish Ministry of Health considered a patient had confirmed SARS-CoV-2 infection whenever the RT-PCR was positive, regardless of clinical features. Four level 3 institutions of the health system of the Madrid region (Spain) (La Paz University Hospital, 12 de Octubre University Hospital, Quironsalud Madrid University Hospital and Quironsalud San José Hospital) participated in this study. The protocol was approved by the reference Clinical Research Ethics Committee. Informed consent was obtained from mothers before enrolment. Every mother-infant's information was treated anonymously.

Eligibility Criteria

Women with term pregnancies with confirmed SARS-CoV-2 infection at the time of delivery, who were in good clinical condition and had a decision to breastfeed were considered eligible for the study (study group). For each positive case, two consecutive women with term pregnancies, in identical conditions, who were SARS-CoV-2 negative were approached (control group). Prospective data recording of participant mothers (age, underlying pathology, type of delivery, time of positive SARS-CoV-2 RT-PCR and related clinical features/treatment) and their infants (gestational age, birth weight, neonatal diagnoses) were obtained.

Study Procedures

During the first month after delivery, breastmilk (case and control groups) and nasopharyngeal swabs (case group) were collected by the participant mothers, who were instructed on accomplishment and storage of samples. Breastmilk samples were collected every 72 h from delivery after careful hand, breast, and nipple hygiene, with the mouth and nose covered by a mask. Milk was collected either by pump or manual extraction, and kept in individual sterile container for each aliquot. After milk extraction, breast pump was cleaned with soap and water, and disinfected by alcohol or immersion in boiling water. Case group mothers self-performed weekly nasopharyngeal smear using swab kits and the corresponding RT-PCR transport medium. Control group mothers underwent a serological study prior to hospital discharge. Blood samples were centrifuged and stored for analysis. Presence of IgG and IgM antibodies against SARS-CoV-2 was assessed using the IgG+IgM Combo Detection Kit (SD Biosensor, Korea).

All biological samples were identified by a study code and date of extraction, immediately frozen at −20°C, periodically collected at home by a specialized transport system and shipped on dry ice (−78.5°C) to the Nutrition and Food Science Department, Complutense University of Madrid where the samples were analyzed. To eliminate or minimize potential lab biases, all the samples were submitted to a single freeze–thaw cycle and were analyzed by the same researchers. After hospital discharge, follow up of the infants was done by serial phone calls during the first month of age.

RT-PCR Assays

RNA extraction from the nasopharyngeal and milk samples (200 µl) was carried out using the KINGFISHER FLEX 96 extraction robot (ThermoFisher), the MagMax_Core_Flex extraction program and the MagMAX Viral/Pathogen II Nucleic Acid Isolation kit (Applied Biosistems, ThermoFisher). For the detection of SARS-CoV-2, the TaqPath COVID-19 CE-IVD RT-PCR kit (Applied Biosystems, Thermo Fisher Scientific) was used in a 384-well format with the QuantStudio 7 Flex System equipment (Applied Biosystems). All procedures were performed following the manufacturer's instructions.

Immunoassays in Breastmilk Samples

Concentration and frequency of detection of 30 soluble immune factors in the milk samples were determined by magnetic bead-based multiplex immunoassays using a Bioplex 200 instrument (Bio-Rad, Hercules, CA, USA) and the pro-human cytokine 27-plex assay (Bio-Rad). The immune factors included in this study were interleukin (IL) 1β, IL1ra, IL2, IL4, IL5, IL6, IL7, IL8, IL9, IL10, IL12(p70), IL13, IL15, and IL17, interferon-gamma (IFN-γ), granulocyte colony stimulating factor (G-CSF), granulocyte-macrophage colony stimulating factor (GM-CSF), monocyte chemoattractant protein-1 (MCP-1), macrophage inflammatory protein 1α and 1β (MIP-1α, MIP-1β), eotaxin, basic fibroblast growth factor (Basic FGF), tumor necrosis factor-alpha (TNF-α), inferon γ-induced protein (IP-10), platelet-derived growth factor-BB (PDGF-BB), regulated on activation normal T-cells expressed and secreted (RANTES), and vascular endothelial growth factor (VEGF). In addition, levels of transforming growth factor-beta 2 (TGF-β2), epidermal growth factor (EGF), and growth-related oncogene-α (Groα) were measured, respectively, by the human TGF-β2, human EGF, and human GRO alpha (CXCL1) ELISA kits (RayBiotech, Norcross, GA, USA).

To avoid interferences, the fatty layer and the somatic cells were removed from the milk samples. Briefly, sample aliquots (1 ml) were centrifuged at 11,000g for 15 min at 4°C, the intermediate aqueous phase was collected and stored at −20°C until analysis. Every assay was run in duplicate according to the manufacturer's instructions using the same reagents' batches and equipment; standard curves were performed for each analyte in every assay. All the concentrations were expressed as nanograms per liter (ng/L), except IP-10, VEGF, TGFβ2, EGF, and Groα, which were expressed as micrograms per liter (μg/L).

Statistical Analysis

Demographic data with normal distribution were presented as the mean and standard deviation (SD). Regarding immune factors, normality of data distribution was examined through visual inspection of histograms and Shapiro-Wilks tests, both evidencing a non-normal distribution for all tested parameters ($\rho < 0.05$). Accordingly, nonparametric statistical analyses were performed, and data were expressed as the median and interquartile range (IQR). Immune factor concentrations were logarithmically transformed prior to statistical analysis. Differences in the relative abundance of the immune compounds were compared by Wilcoxon rank test and Mann-Whitney *U* test. To compare multiple comparisons, Bonferroni-adjusted *post hoc* significance levels were performed. Fisher's exact probability test was performed to compare the frequency of detection of different immunological compounds. Significance was declared at $\rho < 0.05$ for all analyses. All analyses were performed with the R software version 4.0.3 (R-project, http://www.r-project.org). For the purpose of this report, immune factor concentration on one of the milk samples obtained during week 1 (day 3 to day 6) and week 5 (beyond day 28) postpartum were used for comparisons.

RESULTS

During the study period a total of 141 term-pregnant women who fulfilled eligibility criteria were approached. Of them, 37 study group and 45 control group women were included in the final analyses. Details on participants' chart flow and reasons for exclusion are described in **Figure 1**.

No differences in maternal age [33.9 (5.4) *vs* 34.5 (5.1) years, p=0.612], previous maternal health problems prevalence (19% *vs* 13%, p= 0.493, only 1 case of obesity in study group), rates of vaginal delivery (73% *vs* 89%, p= 0.064), gestational age at birth [39.1 (1.8) *vs* 39.1 (1.6) weeks, p= 0.852], or birth weight [3187 (543) *vs* 3240 (469) grams, p= 0.639] between study and control group were found.

By hospital protocol, nasopharyngeal PCR was performed at 24 h and at 36 to 48 h from birth on infants of positive SARS-COV-2 mothers, resulting negative in all cases. None of infants of mothers in study and control group presented clinical signs of SARS-COV-2 infection in the first month of life.

Among the study group, 21 (56.8%) women presented mild SARS-CoV-2 infection related symptoms, consisting of fever (48%), anosmia (48%), cough (43%), ageusia (14%), odynophagia (10%), myalgia (10%), diarrhea (10%), or headache (5%). Nineteen (51.3%) received medication (anticoagulation, antibiotics, hydroxychloroquine, oxygen therapy) around labor. Serological analyses of control women were negative.

RT-PCR Assays

Nasopharyngeal RT-PCR tests were serially conducted in 30 of the 37 SARS-CoV-2–positive women [four samples (1 per week), n=25; three samples (weeks 1–3), n=5; no samples, n=7]. Nasopharyngeal RT-PCR tests attained negative results at week 2 (n=7, 23.3%), at week 3 (n=9, 30%), and at week 4 (n=9, 30%) postpartum and remained positive at the last sample that was tested in 5 (16.6%) participants (3 at week 3, and 2 at week 4).

All human milk samples analyzed were negative for SARS-CoV-2 RNA as assessed by RT-PCR.

Immunological Assays in Breastmilk Samples

All of the 30 immunological factors that were searched for in breastmilk could be detected in, at least, some of the milk samples. IFN-γ, IL-8, IL-12(p70), IL-17, IP-10, MIP-1β, TNF-α, VEGF, TGFβ2, EGF, and GROα displayed the highest frequencies of detection (100% of the samples), closely followed by eotaxin, G-CSF, IL-1β, IL-1ra, IL-2, IL-4, IL-6, IL-7, IL-9, and RANTES, which were detected in >95% of the samples. In contrast, IL-5 and IL-15 were the least frequently detected compounds (≤70% of the samples).

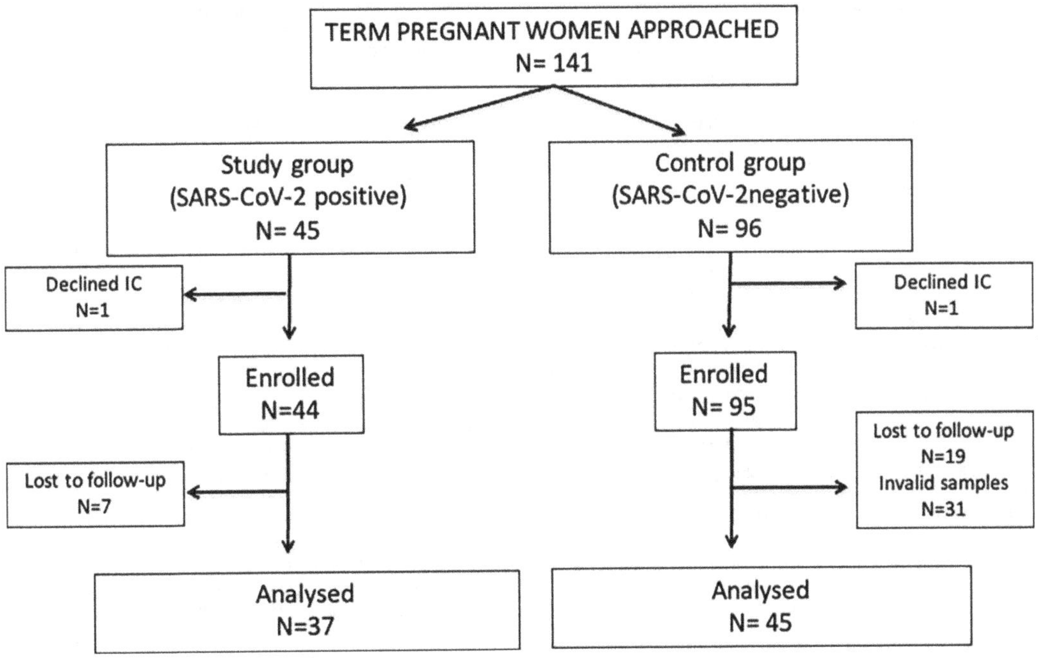

FIGURE 1 | Flow diagram of participants. IC, informed consent; Invalid samples, non-availability of all samples to be compared, inadequate sample identification or conservation.

No differences were observed between samples collected in week 1 or week 5 postpartum, with the exception of GM-CSF, which frequency of detection in week 1 (79%) was lower than that in week 5 (90%) (p=0.047).

Breastmilk Cytokine Pattern

Table 1 displays concentration of cytokines in breastmilk samples. IFN-γ, IL-1ra, IL-4, IL-6, IL-9, IL-13, and TNF-α showed higher concentrations in study than in the control group at both sampling times. In addition, IL-1β and IL-2 at week 5 postpartum were higher in breastmilk samples of the study group.

Evolution of cytokine concentration on breastmilk samples over time showed no differences in the study group women, with the exception of IFN-γ, IL1ra, IL4, IL9 that significantly decreased between week 1 and week 5 postpartum. In the control group women, all the tested cytokines decreased over time, with the exception of IL10, IL12, and IL13 that remained stable. Time of nasopharyngeal swab to become negative influenced the cytokines pattern in breastmilk (**Figure 2**).

Breastmilk Chemokine Pattern

Table 2 displays concentration of chemokines in breastmilk samples. Eotaxin, IP-10, MIP-1α, and RANTES showed higher breastmilk concentration among the study group than in the control group at week 1 postpartum; at week 5, the concentration of chemokines, except for GRO-α, was significantly higher in breastmilk samples of the study group than in the control group.

Concentration of chemokines decreased over time, it being statistically significant for most of them in the study group and for all tested chemokines in the control group. Time of nasopharyngeal swab to become negative influenced the chemokines pattern in breastmilk (**Figure 3**).

Breastmilk Growth Factor Pattern

Table 3 displays concentration of growth factors in breastmilk samples. Overall, concentrations of growth factors were higher in the breastmilk samples of the study group compared with the control group women. The differences were statistically significant for basic FGF, GM-CSF, IL7, and PDGF-BB at week 1 postpartum, and for all of them, with the exception of IL-5 and EGF, in the samples collected at week 5.

Most growth factor concentrations remained stable over time in study group; in contrast, concentrations of basic FGF, G-CSF, VEGF, TGF-β2, and EGF significantly decreased from week 1 to week 5 postpartum in the control group breastmilk samples. Time of nasopharyngeal swab to become negative influenced the growth factor pattern in breastmilk (**Figure 4**).

Breastmilk Immunological Pattern According to Disease State

Concentration of immune factors in breastmilk samples in the SARS-CoV-2–positive women depending on the presence or not of COVID-19-related symptoms did not show relevant differences, neither in the first sampling time (lower IL-12 in symptomatic than in asymptomatic women, $p<0.01$) nor in the second (higher IL-15 ($p<0.01$) and lower GM-CSF ($p<0.03$) in symptomatic women).

TABLE 1 | Concentration (ng/l) of cytokines in milk samples of study and control group women over time.

	Week 1 postpartum			Week 5 postpartum				
	STUDY GROUP (n = 36)	CONTROL GROUP (n = 45)		STUDY GROUP (n = 37)	CONTROL GROUP (n = 45)			
Immune Factors	Median (IQR)	Median (IQR)	p^a	Median (IQR)	Median (IQR)	^bp	^cp	^dp
IFN- γ	160.5 (78.8-301.8)	50.4 (23.7-117.7)	0.003	135.8 (18.3-151.6)	11.8 (4.3-23)	<0.001	<0.001	<0.001
IL-1β	3.2 (1.5-5.0)	2.1 (1.4-3.7)	0.273	2.7 (1.8-3.3)	1.0 (0.7-1.4)	<0.001	0.117	<0.001
IL-1ra	5966.4 (1642.5-62227.1)	1444.3 (676.2-3939.5)	0.023	5896.3 (662.9-5979.4)	443.6 (271.9-852.4)	<0.001	0.004	<0.001
IL-2	5.8 (3.8-7.8)	4.2 (3.0-6.1)	0.164	4.7 (2.4-6.7)	3.1 (2.3-3.8)	0.014	0.300	0.002
IL-4	3.9 (1.3-3.7)	1.0 (0.6-2.1)	0.001	2.6 (1.6-2.7)	0.5 (0.3-0.7)	<0.001	0.007	<0.001
IL-6	208.5 (28.5-223.7)	17.7 (7.5-46.2)	<0.001	207.1 (21.1-212.1)	3.6 (2.3-10.9)	<0.001	0.075	<0.001
IL-9	29.8 (14.8-40.8)	13.1 (8.6-20.0)	0.005	27.3 (11.1-29.7)	5.4 (3.9-8.4)	<0.001	0.041	< 0.001
IL-10	3.3 (1.8-4.8)	3.7 (2.0-4.7)	0.795	2.9 (1.9-4.2)	3.3 (2.7-4.3)	0.363	0.279	0.565
IL-12 (p70)	3.9 (3.0-4.5)	3.8 (3.4-4.3)	0.890	3.4 (2.8-4.1)	3.8 (3.4-4.1)	0.052	0.505	0.712
IL-13	1.4 (0.9-1.9)	0.9 (0.7-1.3)	0.007	1.4 (0.8-1.9)	0.9 (0.7-1.3)	0.043	0.260	0.756
IL-15	94.3 (59.9-164.7)	99.2 (82.6-137.2)	0.921	90.7 (67.5-149.9)	90.7 (49.1-128.3)	0.560	0.734	0.039
IL-17	13.2 (5.4-15.9)	11.3 (10.4-16.7)	0.436	11.8 (5.0-15.3)	9.7 (8.1-12.5)	0.567	0.915	0.007
TNF-α	106.3 (67.9-130.2)	35.5 (25.9-75.8)	0.001	92.2 (73.0-112.4)	17.7 (11.5-50.8)	<0.001	0.314	<0.001

[a]*p: Mann-Whitney U test was used to evaluate differences in concentration of cytokines between milk samples from STUDY GROUP and CONTROL GROUP collected in week 1 postpartum.*

[b]*p: Mann-Whitney U was used to evaluate differences in concentration of cytokines between milk samples STUDY GROUP and CONTROL GROUP collected in week 5 postpartum.*

[c]*p: Wilcoxon signed rank test was used to evaluate differences in the concentration of cytokines of the milk samples of STUDY GROUP between week 1 and week 5 postpartum.*

[d]*p: Wilcoxon signed rank test was used to evaluate differences in the concentration of cytokines of the milk samples of CONTROL GROUP between week 1 and week 5 postpartum.*

DISCUSSION

This study confirms that in the asymptomatic or non-severe infected pregnant woman, breastmilk samples do not carry SARS-CoV-2 RNA. These results coincide with those found in previous studies (1–3, 7, 24–26), although a very low rate of positive milk samples (4) or isolated case reports (27–31) have also been published. This information is crucial as neonatal infection by SARS-CoV-2 is uncommon and usually asymptomatic (32–34). The lack of viral RNA in breastmilk supports its safety, and it is in accord with recent epidemiological data, as several small observational studies reported on the absence of infection in infants fed by breastmilk of SARS-CoV-2 positive woman (35, 36) or inadvertently fed with SARS-CoV-2 RNA-positive milk (29).

SARS-CoV-2 RNA seems to be widespread on surfaces from COVID-19 patient rooms (37) and, also, on the breast skin of lactating mothers (3). This suggests that milk samples may become contaminated with viral RNA when a mother and/or

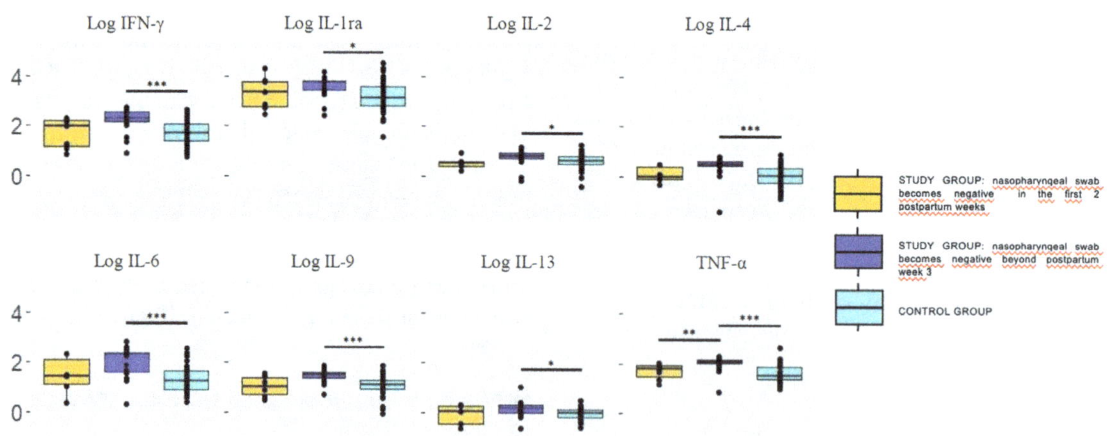

FIGURE 2 | Concentration (log) of cytokines in breastmilk of study group women according to the moment in which the nasopharyngeal test becomes negative (pooling samples obtained at weeks 1 and 5). Cytokine concentrations were significantly higher in breastmilk samples of mothers whose RT-PCR remained positive at postpartum week 3 (dark blue box) compared with the control group. Trends also pointed toward higher concentrations in the former compared with those who became negative sooner, within the first 2 postpartum weeks (yellow box). The values are expressed as log_{10} of the concentrations (ng/L). Statistical differences on pairwise *post hoc* comparisons between the study and control groups are indicated with an asterisk (*p < 0.05; **p ≤ 0.01; ***p ≤ 0.001, Wilcoxon rank test, Bonferroni *post hoc* test).

TABLE 2 | Concentration* of chemokines in milk samples of study group and control group women over time.

	Week 1 postpartum			Week 5 postpartum				
	STUDY GROUP (n = 36)	CONTROL GROUP (n = 45)		STUDY GROUP (n = 37)	CONTROL GROUP (n = 45)			
Immune Factors	**Median (IQR)**	**Median (IQR)**	^{a}p	**Median (IQR)**	**Median (IQR)**	^{b}p	^{c}p	^{d}p
Eotaxin	24.2 (14.6-32.9)	14.5 (4.3-23.3)	0.020	16.9 (10.4-21)	3.1 (1.8-5.3)	<0.001	<0.001	<0.001
IL-8	1919.0 (299.7-2606.6)	584.2 (234.7-1916.7)	0.137	1921.4 (213.4-2021.5)	47.7 (20.5-167.7)	<0.001	0.001	<0.001
IP-10	18.2 (7.2-53)	10.5 (4.1-18.5)	0.025	21.9 (10.0-58.3)	2.8 (1.2-11.8)	<0.001	0.750	0.002
MCP-1	2078.4 (650.8-2738.4)	892.7 (544.1-2601.7)	0.221	2010.2 (730.6-2288.2)	123.1 (53.4-732.4)	<0.001	0.027	<0.001
MIP-1α	43.9 (10.3-47.1)	13.4 (5.3-41.9)	0.040	43.4 (26.1-44.0)	2.5 (1.0-6.7)	<0.001	0.041	<0.001
MIP-1β	212.7 (81.2-344.9)	112.9 (38.3-293.6)	0.270	191.6 (88.2-204.3)	10.5 (7.3-44.3)	<0.001	0.054	<0.001
RANTES	84.5 (48.7-115.0)	44.3 (26.2-84.1)	0.032	81.0 (61.1-142.1)	18.5 (14-39.8)	<0.001	0.427	0.011
GRO-α	7.4 (4.8-8.9)	7.9 (6.6-8.5)	0.314	7.3 (4.7-8.7)	7.3 (6.0-8.1)	0.856	<0.001	<0.001

*Concentrations are expressed as ng/L, with the exception of IP-10 and GRO-α (expressed as μg/L).

^{a}p: Mann-Whitney U test was used to evaluate differences in concentration of chemokines between milk samples of STUDY GROUP and CONTROL GROUP collected in week 1 postpartum.

^{b}p: Mann-Whitney U test was used to evaluate differences in concentration of chemokines between milk samples of STUDY GROUP and CONTROL GROUP collected in week 5 postpartum.

^{c}p: Wilcoxon signed rank test was used to evaluate differences in the concentration of chemokines of milk the samples of STUDY GROUP between week 1 and week 5 postpartum.

^{d}p: Wilcoxon signed rank test was used to evaluate differences in the concentration of chemokines of the milk samples of CONTROL GROUP between week 1 and week 5 postpartum.

her neonate are positive; therefore, caution should be extreme to avoid contaminations when performing SARS-CoV-2 assessments of human milk. In addition, it must be highlighted that RT-PCR assays can only detect viral RNA but not viable infectious viruses. A detailed virological assessment of some COVID-19 cases showed that, although high concentrations of viral RNA were found both in pharyngeal and fecal samples, the virus itself could be readily isolated from throat or lung samples but not from the fecal ones (38). A study involving 64 milk samples from 18 women who had confirmed SARS-CoV-2 supported this affirmation. Only one sample had a detectable level of viral RNA but no replication-competent virus was detectable in any sample, including the sample that was positive for SARS-CoV-2 RNA (2). To date, no study has described presence of infectious SARS-CoV-2 in colostrum and milk.

The second objective of this study was the profiling of cytokines, chemokines, and growth factors in the milk samples. Overall, the concentrations of most of the immune factors analyzed were higher in the samples of positive women than in those of negative ones. This activation of innate and adaptative immune response constitutes the first line of defense against viral infections (16–18, 39).

A study involving the assessment of immunological compounds in milk produced by healthy women, found a higher co-occurrence

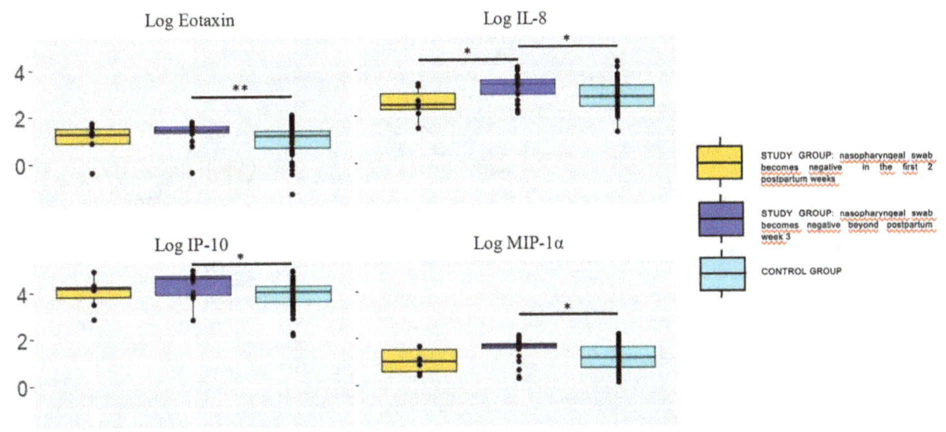

FIGURE 3 | Concentration (log) of chemokines in breastmilk of study group women according to the moment in which the nasopharyngeal test becomes negative (pooling samples obtained at weeks 1 and 5). Chemokyne concentrations were significantly higher in breastmilk samples of mothers whose RT-PCR remained positive at postpartum week 3 (dark blue box) compared with the control group. Trends also pointed toward higher concentrations in the former compared with those who became negative sooner, within the first 2 postpartum weeks (yellow box). The values are expressed as $\log_{10}$ of the concentrations (ng/L), with the exception of IP-10 (μg/L). Statistical differences on pairwise *post hoc* comparisons between the study and control groups are indicated with an asterisk (*p < 0.05; **p ≤ 0.01; ***p ≤ 0.001, Wilcoxon rank test, Bonferroni *post hoc* test).

TABLE 3 | Concentration* of growth factors in milk samples from study group and control group women over time.

	Week 1 postpartum			Week 5 postpartum				
	STUDY GROUP (n = 36)	CONTROL GROUP (n = 45)		STUDY GROUP (n = 37)	CONTROL GROUP (n = 45)			
Immune Factors	Median (IQR)	Median (IQR)	^{a}p	Median (IQR)	Median (IQR)	^{b}p	^{c}p	^{d}p
Basic FGF	64.0 (28.6-73.3)	22.5 (16.4-46.3)	<0.001	59.4 (55.1-64.3)	12.8 (9.6-21.7)	<0.001	0.394	<0.001
G-CSF	178.6 (116.1-287.1)	104.3 (68.1-224.6)	0.227	147.8 (121.9-203.5)	32.4 (12-110.9)	<0.001	0.245	<0.001
GM-CSF	13.5 (12.9-14.6)	1.4 (0.8-2.7)	<0.001	13.6 (7.8-16.1)	2 (0.8-11)	0.006	0.086	0.016
IL-5	17.4 (7.9-24.3)	23.7 (10.9-36.9)	0.321	21.1 (14.8-35.7)	20.8 (9.8-29.5)	0.540	0.275	0.612
IL-7	114.7 (33.3-147.7)	27.5 (19.3-33.4)	<0.001	113.9 (53.2-135.0)	28.2 (21.1-52.3)	<0.001	0.225	0.052
PDGF-BB	54.8 (28.7-70.7)	23.6 (14.9-31.5)	<0.001	40.9 (35.7-67.5)	23.6 (13.3-34.8)	<0.001	0.458	0.786
VEGF	11.5 (4.5-16.4)	7.6 (3.8-11.2)	0.090	10.4 (3.7-11.5)	2.7 (1.8-3.4)	<0.001	0.007	<0.001
TGF-β2	2.5 (1.7-3.0)	2.1 (1.7-2.5)	0.164	2.7 (1.7-3.0)	1.9 (1.7-2.1)	0.003	0.014	<0.001
EGF	5.6 (4.5-6.6)	5.4 (4.9-5.9)	0.768	5.4 (4.3-6.0)	5 (4.3-5.5)	0.120	<0.001	<0.001

*Concentrations are expressed as ng/L, with the exception of VEGF, TFG-β2 and EFG (expressed as μg/L).

^{a}p: Mann-Whitney U test was used to evaluate differences in concentration of growth factors between milk samples of STUDY GROUP and CONTROL GROUP collected in week 1 postpartum.

^{b}p: Mann-Whitney U test was used to evaluate differences in concentration of growth factors between t milk samples of STUDY GROUP and CONTROL GROUP collected in week 5 postpartum.

^{c}p: Wilcoxon signed rank test was used to evaluate differences in the concentration of growth factors of the milk samples of STUDY GROUP between week 1 and week 5 postpartum.

^{d}p: Wilcoxon signed rank test was used to evaluate differences in the concentration of growth factors of the milk samples of CONTROL GROUP between week 1 and week 5postpartum.

of immune factors and higher TNFα to IL10 ratios in milk samples from healthy women with a higher level of exposure to microorganisms (40). In our study, the same was observed in the milk of SARS-CoV-2-positive women, a finding which is consistent with a wider plasticity of the immune responses.

Concentrations of most of the immune factors analyzed remained stable over time in SARS-CoV-2-positive women milk samples. In contrast, most of these compounds significantly decreased from the first to the fifth week postpartum in negative women. Previous studies have reported notably higher concentrations of several cytokines, chemokines, growth factors, and immunoglobulins in colostrum than in mature milk (13, 41–44). Although this could simply be a physiological response from the mother to infection and not enough proof for it to be protective, our findings could also suggest that, in the presence of a viral infection, the immunological profile of human milk may be adapted to provide additional infant's protection against the maternal infection. Evidences for an immunological cross-talk between mothers and their breast-fed infants during infections, including severe viral respiratory infections, have already been provided (45, 46). In our study, positive women were either asymptomatic or suffered mild disease, therefore the evolutive profile of immunological compounds in breastmilk was related to the time when RT-PCR swabs became negative, as a marker of disease state. Mothers who later became negative for nasopharyngeal RT-PCR presented persistently higher levels of

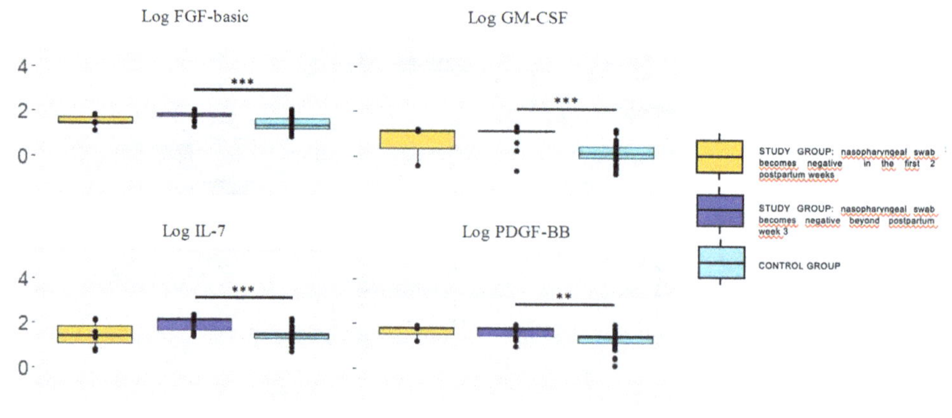

FIGURE 4 | Concentration (log) of growth factors in breastmilk of study group women according to the moment in which the nasopharyngeal test becomes negative (pooling samples obtained at week 1 and 5). Growth factors concentrations were significantly higher in breastmilk samples of mothers whose RT-PCR remained positive at postpartum week 3 (dark blue box) compared with the control group. Trends also pointed toward higher concentrations in the former compared with those who became negative sooner, within the first two postpartum weeks (yellow box). The values are expressed as $\log_{10}$ of the concentrations (ng/L). Statistical differences on pairwise *post hoc* comparisons between the study and control groups are indicated with an asterisk (*p < 0.05; **p ≤ 0.01; ***p ≤ 0.001, Wilcoxon rank test, Bonferroni *post hoc* test).

several immunological factors. This immunological profile has been described in COVID19 pathophysiology related to the severity of the infection (16–18, 39). Of note, all the newborns in the study and control group remained free of clinical signs of SARS-COV-2 infection in the first month of life.

In this study, VEGF, TGF-β2 and EGF were the most abundant growth factors found in the milk samples, independently of the SARS-CoV-2 status or the sampling time, the concentration being 50- to 100-fold higher, coinciding with those detected in healthy women as reported in a previous study (40). These three immune compounds play critical roles in infants' health and development, including protection against infectious diseases, modulation of inflammatory processes, and establishment of food tolerance (12, 40, 47–49).

This study has several limitations. There is a lack of comparison between serum and milk immune factors profile, and the antibody levels were not assayed. The distinct profile in immune compounds in breast milk of SARS-CoV-2 positive women could not be translated into effective gastrointestinal absorption and in a functional form to impact the infant immune system. Follow-up losses in the control group could eventually modify the results. Finally, the analysis of the immune compounds was limited to two milk samples, with an interval of approximately 1 month. We took this decision after confirmation of the lack of viral RNA in any of the milk samples over time. Therefore, we considered that the observation period was adequate to see eventual evolution of the immune compounds related to mother's infection status. On the other hand, a strength of this work is the huge variety of compounds that have been analyzed, and the systematic approach to both SARS-CoV-2 documented infection and control women.

In summary, the results of this study provide additional evidence to the safety of breastfeeding in SARS-CoV-2 infected women, as RNA was not detected in any of the milk samples tested throughout the observation period. Our results also suggest that the immune system of the infected women reacted efficiently against SARS-CoV-2 as a distinct pattern of cytokines, chemokines, and growth factors was observed in the milk samples of infected women, that persisted over time. However, this cannot be directly extrapolated to a beneficial effect in the infant. More studies are required to elucidate if this pattern only reflects the inflammatory status of the mother or if it may be linked to the development of an integration of the mother-infant immune systems, being especially suitable to protect recipient child.

ETHICS STATEMENT

The studies involving human participants were reviewed and approved by Ethical committee of clinical research of La Paz University Hospital. Written informed consent to participate in this study was provided by the participants' legal guardian/next of kin.

AUTHOR CONTRIBUTIONS

LS conceptualized and designed the study, participated in patient's enrolment, data gathering and analysis, drafted the initial manuscript, and reviewed and approved the final version. AP and JR conceptualized and designed the study, and participated in data analyses, drafted the initial manuscript, and reviewed and approved the final version. FC conceptualized and designed the study, and reviewed and approved the final version of the manuscript. RG-S, ML-A, MM-P, DE-V and EC-A participated in patient's enrolment and data gathering, and reviewed and approved the final version of the manuscript. NG-T and IC participated in sampling management and analysis, drafted the initial manuscript, and reviewed and approved the final version. CA participated in statistical and data analyses. All authors contributed to the article and approved the submitted version.

FUNDING

This work was supported by Instituto de Salud San Carlos III [COV20/01046]; Ministerio de Ciencia, Innovación y Universidades (Spain) by Irma Castro predoctoral contract [BES-2017-080713] and RETICS "Maternal and Child Health and Development Network" (SAMID Network), funded by the PN I+D+i 2013-2016 (Spain), ISCIII-Sub-Directorate General for Research Assessment and Promotion and the European Regional Development Fund (ERDF) [RD16/0022].

REFERENCES

1. Marín Gabriel MA, Cuadrado I, Álvarez Fernández B, González Carrasco E, Alonso Díaz C, Neo-COVID-19 Research Group, et al. Multicenter Spanish Study Found No Incidences of Viral Transmission in Infants Born to Mothers With COVID-19. *Acta Paediatr* (2020) 109(11):2302–8. doi: 10.1111/apa.15474
2. Chambers CD, Krogstad P, Bertrand K, Contreras D, Tobin NH, Bode L, et al. Evaluation of SARS-CoV-2 in Breastmilk From 18 Infected Women. *JAMA* (2020) 324(13):1347–8. doi: 10.1001/jama.2020.15580
3. Pace RM, Williams JE, Järvinen KM, Belfort MB, Dw Pace C, Lackey KA, et al. COVID-19 and Human Milk: SARS-CoV-2, Antibodies, and Neutralizing Capacity. (2020). doi: 10.1101/2020.09.16.20196071. medRxiv.
4. Bertino E, Moro GE, De Renzi G, Viberti G, Cavallo RCollaborative Research Group on SARS-CoV-2 in Human Milk, et al. Detection of SARS-CoV-2 in Milk From COVID-19 Positive Mothers and Follow-Up of Their Infants. *Front Pediatr* (2020) 27:8:597699. doi: 10.3389/fped.2020.597699
5. Cheema R, Partridge E, Kair LR, Kuhn-Riordon K, Silva AI, Bettinelli ME, et al. Protecting Breastfeeding During the COVID-19 Pandemic. *Am J Perinatol* (2020). doi: 10.1055/s-0040-1714277
6. Centeno-Tablante E, Medina-Rivera M, Finkelstein JL, Rayco-Solon P, García-Casal MN, Rogers L, et al. Transmission of SARS-CoV-2 Through Breast Milk and Breastfeeding: A Living Systematic Review. *Ann N Y Acad Sci* (2021) 1484(1):32–54. doi: 10.1111/nyas.14477
7. Martins-Filho PR, Santos VS, Santos HPJr. To Breastfeed or Not to Breastfeed? Lack of Evidence on the Presence of SARS-CoV-2 in

Breastmilk of Pregnant Women With COVID-19. *Rev Panam Salud Publica* (2020) 44:e59. doi: 10.26633/RPSP.2020.59

8. Demers-Mathieu V, Do DM, Mathijssen GB, Sela DA, Seppo A, Järvinen KM, et al. Difference in Levels of SARS-CoV-2 S1 and S2 Subunits- and Nucleocapsid Protein-Reactive SIgM/IgM, IgG and SIgA/IgA Antibodies in Human Milk. *J Perinatol* (2020). doi: 10.1038/s41372-020-00805-w
9. Fox A, Marino J, Amanat F, Krammer F, Hanh-Holbrook J, Zolla-Pazner S, et al. Robust and Specific Secretory IgA Against SARS-CoV-2 Detected in Human Milk. *iScience* (2020) 23(11):101735. doi: 10.1016/j.isci.2020.101735
10. Garofalo RP, Goldman AS. Cytokines, Chemokines, and Colony-Stimulating Factors in Human Milk: The 1997 Update. *Biol Neonate* (1998) 4(2):134–42. doi: 10.1159/000014019
11. Field CJ. The Immunological Components of Human Milk and Their Effect on Immune Development in Infants. *J Nutr* (2005) 135:1–4. doi: 10.1093/jn/135.1.1
12. Dvorak B. Milk Epidermal Growth Factor and Gut Protection. *J Pediatr* (2010) 156(2 Suppl):S31–5. doi: 10.1016/j.jpeds.2009.11.018
13. Garofalo RP. Cytokines in Human Milk. *J Pediatr* (2010) 156:S36–40. doi: 10.1016/j.jpeds.2009.11.019
14. Dawod B, Marshall JS. Cytokines and Soluble Receptors in Breast Milk as Enhancers of Oral Tolerance Development. *Front Immunol* (2019) 10:16. doi: 10.3389/fimmu.2019.00016
15. Ruiz L, Fernández L, Rodríguez JM. *Immune Factors in Human Milk. In Human Milk: Sampling and Measurement of Energy-Yielding Nutrients and Other Macromolecules*. M McGuire, D O'Connor, editors. London: Academic Press (2020).
16. Azkur AK, Akdis M, Azkur D, Sokolowska M, van de Veen W, Brüggen MC. Immune Response to SARS-CoV-2 and Mechanisms of Immunopathological Changes in COVID-19. *Allergy* (2020) 75(7):1564–81. doi: 10.1111/all.14364
17. Chatterjee SK, Saha S, Munoz MNM. Molecular Pathogenesis, Immunopathogenesis and Novel Therapeutic Strategy Against COVID-19. *Front Mol Biosci* (2020) 7:196. doi: 10.3389/fmolb.2020.00196
18. Choudhary S, Sharma K, Silakari O. The Interplay Between Inflammatory Pathways and COVID-19: A Critical Review on Pathogenesis and Therapeutic Options. *Microb Pathog* (2020) 150:104673. doi: 10.1016/j.micpath.2020.104673
19. Farquhar C, Mbori-Ngacha DA, Redman MW, Bosire RK, Lohman BL, Piantadosi AL, et al. CC and CXC Chemokines in Breastmilk are Associated With Mother-to-Child HIV-1 Transmission. *Curr HIV Res* (2005) 3:361–9. doi: 10.2174/157016205774370393
20. Bosire R, Guthrie BL, Lohman-Payne B, Mabuka J, Majiwa M, Wariua G, et al. Longitudinal Comparison of Chemokines in Breastmilk Early Postpartum Among HIV-1-Infected and Uninfected Kenyan Women. *Breastfeed Med Off J Acad Breastfeed Med* (2007) 2:129–38. doi: 10.1089/bfm.2007.0009
21. Walter J, Ghosh MK, Kuhn L, Semrau K, Sinkala M, Kankasa C, et al. High Concentrations of Interleukin 15 in Breast Milk are Associated With Protection Against Postnatal HIV Transmission. *J Infect Dis* (2009) 200:1498–502. doi: 10.1086/644603
22. de Quental OB, França EL, Honório-França AC, Morais TC, Daboin BEG, Bezerra IMP, et al. Zika Virus Alters the Viscosity and Cytokines Profile in Human Colostrum. *J Immunol Res* (2019) 2019:9020519. doi: 10.1155/2019/9020519
23. Rabe T, Lazar K, Cambronero C, Goelz R, Hamprecht K. Human Cytomegalovirus (HCMV) Reactivation in the Mammary Gland Induces a Proinflammatory Cytokine Shift in Breast Milk. *Microorganisms* (2020) 8 (2):289. doi: 10.3390/microorganisms8020289
24. Lackey KA, Pace RM, Williams JE, Bode L, Donovan SM, Järvinen KM, et al. SARS-CoV-2 and Human Milk: What Is the Evidence? *Matern Child Nutr* (2020) 16(4):e13032. doi: 10.1111/mcn.13032
25. Yang N, Che S, Zhang J, Wang X, Tang YCOVID-19 Evidence and Recommendations Working Group, et al. Breastfeeding of Infants Born to Mothers With COVID-19: A Rapid Review. *Ann Transl Med* (2020) 8 (10):618. doi: 10.21037/atm-20-3299
26. Chen L, Li Q, Zheng D, Jiang H, Wei Y, Zou L, et al. Clinical Characteristics of Pregnant Women With Covid-19 in Wuhan, China. *N Engl J Med* (2020) 382 (25):e100. doi: 10.1056/NEJMc2009226
27. Groß R, Conzelmann C, Müller JA, Stenger S, Steinhart K, Kirchhoff F, et al. Detection of SARS-CoV-2 in Human Breastmilk. *Lancet* (2020) 395 (10239):1757–8. doi: 10.1016/S0140-6736(20)31181-8
28. Hinojosa-Velasco A, de Oca PVB, García-Sosa LE, Mendoza-Durán JG, Pérez-Méndez MJ, Dávila-González E, et al. A Case Report of Newborn Infant With Severe COVID-19 in Mexico: Detection of SARS-CoV-2 in Human Breast Milk and Stool. *Int J Infect Dis* (2020) 100:21–4. doi: 10.1016/j.ijid.2020.08.055
29. Lugli L, Bedetti L, Lucaccioni L, Gennari W, Leone C, Ancora G, et al. An Uninfected Preterm Newborn Inadvertently Fed SARS-CoV-2-Positive Breast Milk. *Pediatrics* (2020) 146(6):e2020004960. doi: 10.1542/peds.2020-004960
30. Costa S, Posteraro B, Marchetti S, Tamburrini E, Carducci B, Lanzone A, et al. Excretion of SARS-CoV-2 in Human Breast Milk. *Clin Microbiol Infect* (2020) 26(10):1430–2. doi: 10.1016/j.cmi.2020.05.027
31. De Rose DU, Piersigilli F, Ronchetti MP, Santisi A, Bersani I. Study Group of Neonatal Infectious Diseases of The Italian Society of Neonatology (SIN), et al. Novel Corornavirus Disease (COVID-19) in Newborns and Infants: What We Know So Far. *Ital J Pediatr* (2020) 46(1):56. doi: 10.1186/s13052-020-0820-x
32. Fernández Colomer B, Sánchez-Luna M, de Alba Romero C, Alarcón A, Baña Souto A, Camba Longueira F, et al. Neonatal Infection Due to SARS-CoV-2: An Epidemiological Study in Spain. *Front Pediatr* (2020) 8:580584.
33. White A, Mukherjee P, Stremming J, Sherlock LG, Reynolds RM, Smith D, et al. Neonates Hospitalized With Community-Acquired SARS-CoV-2 in a Colorado Neonatal Intensive Care Unit. *Neonatology* (2020) 117(5):641–5. doi: 10.1159/000508962
34. Wei M, Yuan J, Liu Y, Fu T, Yu X, Zhang ZJ. Novel Coronavirus Infection in Hospitalized Infants Under 1 Year of Age in China. *JAMA* (2020) 323 (14):1313–4. doi: 10.1001/jama.2020.2131
35. Walker KF, O'Donoghue K, Grace N, Dorling J, Comeaud JL, Li W, et al. Maternal Transmission of SARS-COV-2 to the Neonate, and Possible Routes for Such Transmission: A Systematic Review and Critical Analysis. *BJOG* (2020) 127(11):1324–36. doi: 10.1111/1471-0528.16362
36. Pereira A, Cruz-Melguizo S, Adrien M, Fuentes L, Marin E, Forti Z, et al. Breastfeeding Mothers With COVID-19 Infection: A Case Series. *Int Breastfeed J* (2020) 15(1):69. doi: 10.1186/s13006-020-00314-8
37. Marotz C, Belda-Ferre P, Ali F, Das P, Huang S, Cantrel K, et al. Microbial Context Predicts SARS-CoV-2 Prevalence in Patients and the Hospital Built Environment. (2020). doi: 10.1101/2020.11.19.20234229. medRxiv.
38. Wölfel R, Corman VM, Guggemos W, Seilmaier M, Zange S, Müller MA, et al. Virological Assessment of Hospitalized Patients With COVID-2019. *Nature* (2020) 581(7809):465–9. doi: 10.1038/s41586-020-2196-x
39. Tay MZ, Poh CM, Rénia L, MacAry PA, Ng LFP. The Trinity of COVID-19: Immunity, Inflammation and Intervention. *Nat Rev Immunol* (2020) 20 (6):363–74. doi: 10.1038/s41577-020-0311-8
40. Ruiz L, Espinosa-Martos I, García-Carral C, Manzano S, McGuire MK, Meehan CL, et al. What's Normal? Immune Profiling of Human Milk From Healthy Women Living in Different Geographical and Socioeconomic Settings. *Front Immunol* (2017) 8:696. doi: 10.3389/fimmu.2017.00696
41. Chollet-Hinton LS, Stuebe AM, Casbas-Hernandez P, Chetwynd E, Troester MA. Temporal Trends in the Inflammatory Cytokine Profile of Human Breastmilk. *Breastfeed Med* (2014) 9(10):530–7. doi: 10.1089/bfm.2014.0043
42. Moles L, Manzano S, Fernández L, Montilla A, Corzo N, Ares S, et al. Bacteriological, Biochemical, and Immunological Properties of Colostrum and Mature Milk From Mothers of Extremely Preterm Infants. *J Pediatr Gastroenterol Nutr* (2015) 60(1):120–6. doi: 10.1097/MPG.0000000000000560
43. Collado MC, Santaella M, Mira-Pascual L, Martínez-Arias E, Khodayar-Pardo P, Ros G, et al. Longitudinal Study of Cytokine Expression, Lipid Profile and Neuronal Growth Factors in Human Breast Milk From Term and Preterm Deliveries. *Nutrients* (2015) 7(10):8577–91. doi: 10.3390/nu7105415
44. Trend S, Strunk T, Lloyd ML, Heen Kok C, Metcalfe J, Geddes DT, et al. Levels of Innate Immune Factors in Preterm and Term Mother's Breast Milk During the 1st Month Postpartum. *Br J Nutr* (2016) 115(7):1178–93. doi: 10.1017/S0007114516000234
45. Bryan DL, Hart PH, Forsyth KD, Gibson RA. Immunomodulatory Constituents of Human Milk Change in Response to Infant Bronchiolitis. *Pediatr Allergy Immunol* (2007) 18(6):495–502. doi: 10.1111/j.1399-3038.2007.00565.x
46. Riskin A, Almog M, Peri R, Halasz K, Srugo I, Kessel A. Changes in Immunomodulatory Constituents of Human Milk in Response to Active Infection in the Nursing Infant. *Pediatr Res* (2012) 71(2):220–5. doi: 10.1038/pr.2011.34

47. Veldhoen M, Hocking RJ, Atkins CJ, Locksley RM, Stockinger B. TGFbeta in the Context of an Inflammatory Cytokine Milieu Supports *De Novo* Differentiation of IL-17-Producing T Cells. *Immunity* (2006) 24:179–89. doi: 10.1016/j.immuni.2006.01.001
48. Verhasselt V. Neonatal Tolerance Under Breastfeeding Influence: The Presence of Allergen and Transforming Growth Factor-β in Breast Milk Protects the Progeny From Allergic Asthma. *J Pediatr* (2010) 156:S16–20. doi: 10.1016/j.jpeds.2009.11.015
49. Penttila IA. Milk-Derived Transforming Growth Factor-β and the Infant Immune Response. *J Pediatr* (2010) 156:S21–5. doi: 10.1016/j.jpeds.2009.11.016

8

New Paradigm in the Role of Regulatory T Cells During Pregnancy

*Sayaka Tsuda, Akitoshi Nakashima, Tomoko Shima and Shigeru Saito**

Department of Obstetrics and Gynecology, University of Toyama, Toyama, Japan

***Correspondence:**
Shigeru Saito
s30saito@med.u-toyama.ac.jp

Semi-allogenic fetuses are not rejected by the maternal immune system because feto-maternal tolerance induced by $CD4^{+}CD25^{+}FoxP3^{+}$ regulatory T (Treg) cells is established during pregnancy. Paternal antigen-specific Treg cells accumulate during pregnancy, and seminal plasma priming plays an important role in expanding paternal antigen-specific Treg cells in mouse models. Although paternal-antigen specific Treg cells have not been identified in humans, recent studies suggest that antigen-specific Treg cells exist and expand at the feto-maternal interface in humans. Studies have also revealed that reduction of decidual functional Treg cells occurs during miscarriage with normal fetal chromosomal content, whereas insufficient clonal expansion of decidual Treg cells is observed in preeclampsia. In this review, we will discuss the recent advances in the investigation of mechanisms underlying Treg cell-dependent maintenance of feto-maternal tolerance.

Keywords: miscarriage, preeclampsia, pregnancy, regulatory T cells, seminal plasma

INTRODUCTION

Feto-maternal tolerance protects the fetal tissues from rejection and leads to a successful pregnancy (1–7). After implantation of the blastocyst in the uterine endometrium, trophoblasts start to invade the endometrial tissue, and uterine spiral artery. Maternal lymphocytes such as $CD4^{+}$ T cells, $CD8^{+}$ T cells, and $CD16^{-}CD56^{bright}$ natural killer (NK) cells express activation markers on their surfaces, suggesting that maternal lymphocytes recognize trophoblasts or fetuses (8). Interaction with maternal immune regulation and trophoblast-derived tolerogenic molecules induces a tolerogenic environment at the feto-maternal interface. Considering the maternal immune system, regulatory T cells (Treg cells) play an essential role in the maintenance of allogenic pregnancy (9–12). $CD4^{+}CD25^{+}Foxp3^{+}$ regulatory T (Treg) cells regulate the T cell response. Treg cells are necessary to sustain tissue homeostasis and establish immune tolerance (13), and are also related to tumor growth and organ transplantation tolerance (14). Previous studies in mouse models have demonstrated that paternal antigen-specific Treg cells are expanded systemically and locally during pregnancy (15–17). Seminal plasma primes the induction of paternal antigen-specific Treg cells (17, 18). Treg cells also increase systemically and locally during human pregnancies (12, 19), whereas paternal antigen-specific Treg cells have not been identified in humans. Recent studies show that target-specific, clonally expanded Treg cells are expanded at the feto-maternal interface in human pregnancies (20). In the first part of this review, we discuss mechanisms by which Treg cells induce feto-maternal tolerance and highlight antigen-specific Treg cells by introducing recent important findings. Following that, we will attempt to analyze the relationship between maldistribution and dysfunction of Treg cells and implantation failure, recurrent pregnancy loss, and preeclampsia in humans.

Maternal Immune Cells at the Feto-Maternal Interface

Maternal immune cells in the reproductive tissues first come into contact with paternal antigens when seminal fluid is ejaculated into the vagina during intercourse. Seminal fluid is composed of seminal plasma and sperm. Maternal immune cells recognize paternal antigens which are contained in the seminal plasma. Sperm reach the fallopian tube and fertilize the oocyte present there. After fertilization, the blastocyst migrates to the uterus while undergoing cell cleavage and finally attaches to the decidua. During the implantation period, the blastocyst adheres to and starts invading the uterine endometrium. In human pregnancy, the cells of the trophoblast differentiate into villous and extravillous trophoblasts (EVTs), forming the placenta. EVTs invade the decidua and myometrium. Subsequent to implantation, EVTs further penetrate the maternal spiral artery and finally replace the vascular lumen (21, 22). The feto-maternal interface is thereby formed, and EVTs and maternal immune cells contact each other (23). EVTs escape from maternal immune cells by controlling the major histocompatibility complex (MHC) and expressing immune suppressive molecules. The maternal immune system also dynamically changes to induce tolerance against fetal tissues (**Figure 1**).

Villous trophoblasts lack the surface expression of MHC class I and class II. EVTs do not express polymorphic HLA-A, B, whereas they express HLA-C and non-polymorphic HLA-E, G, and F (24–29). Maternal $CD8^+$ T cells and NK cells can directly recognize paternal HLA-C, and $CD4^+$ T cells can indirectly recognize it. On the other hand, HLA- E and G protect EVTs from NK-cell mediated cytotoxicity (30, 31). HLA-G positive EVTs regulate T cell activation through the induction of tolerogenic dendritic cells (DCs) (32) and directly cause the expansion of Treg cells (33). Furthermore, trophoblasts suppress maternal immune cells via the expression of indoleamine 2,3-dioxygenase (IDO) (34, 35), the secretion of inhibitory cytokines, such as IL-10 and TGF-β (36), and the expression of programmed death ligand (PD-L I) (37).

Considering maternal immune cells in the decidua, Treg cells and $CD56^{bright}CD16^-$uterine NK (uNK) cells play an important role in the maintenance of feto-maternal tolerance (3, 4, 38–41) (**Figure 1**). Treg cells, which are discussed in detail at a later part, can recognize fetal antigens via maternal antigen presenting cells (APCs) and induce tolerance in an antigen-specific manner. Compared with ordinary peripheral blood (pb) NK cells that have high cytotoxicity, uNK cells ($CD56^{bright}CD16^-$ NK cells) produce many cytokines and their cytotoxic activities are low (42). Rather, uNK cells play an important role in uterine angiogenesis and spiral artery remodeling (23, 38, 43–46). The expression patterns of cell surface NK receptors in uNK cells differ from those of pbNK cells. For example, killer immunoglobulin-like receptor (KIR) and natural killer group 2 (NKG2) receptors are expressed at high levels on uNK cells (47). When the NKG2A receptor recognizes HLA-E on EVTs, an inhibitory signal suppresses the cytotoxicity of uNK cells (26). When KIR2DL on uNK cells interacts with HLA-G, the uNK cell activity is suppressed (30, 33).

$CD8^+$ cytotoxic T cells can recognize the fetal antigen directly via HLA-C on EVTs and indirectly via maternal APCs (**Figure 1**). A previous report showed that fetal antigen-specific $CD8^+$ cytotoxic T cells (CTLs) are detected in maternal peripheral blood during human pregnancies (48, 49). Viral antigen-specific decidual CTLs that can cross-react against allo-antigens are also reported (50, 51). CTLs in the decidua have distinct phenotypes and functions compared with those in peripheral blood. T-cell immunoglobulin mucin-3 (Tim-3) and programmed cell death-1 (PD-1) are negative immune regulatory molecules. The expression of $Tim\text{-}3^+PD\text{-}1^+CD8^+$ T cells was higher in the human decidua than in peripheral blood. EVTs promote enrichment of $Tim\text{-}3^+PD\text{-}1^+CD8^+$ T cells in an HLA-C dependent manner, suggesting that decidual $CD8^+$ T cells would not attack trophoblasts. Furthermore, maternal $Tim\text{-}3^+PD\text{-}1^+CD8^+$ T cells recognize PD-L I expressed on EVTs, resulting in trophoblast antigen-specific tolerance (52). Highly differentiated resident memory $CD8^+$ T cells are observed in the decidua. This subset shows a lower expression of perforin and granzyme B (53). These reports suggest that antigen-specific CTLs exist at the feto-maternal interface, but their cytotoxic activity is controlled by the placental tissue (53).

How Do Paternal Antigen-Specific Treg Cells Function in Allogenic Pregnancy?

Previous studies suggest that Treg cells play an essential role in the induction of paternal antigen-specific tolerance in allogenic pregnancy in mice. Paternal MHC-specific tolerance during allogenic pregnancy was demonstrated by Tafuri et al. where a paternal MHC-bearing tumor graft was not rejected during pregnancy with the conceptus MHC being identical to the tumor graft, but was rejected in the postpartum period (54).

Aluvihare et al. (11) demonstrated that Treg cells are necessary for allogenic pregnancy in mice, but not necessary for syngeneic pregnancy. When T cell-depleted BALB/C nu/nu female mice were mated with C57BL/6 male mice (allogenic pregnancy) after transfer of total lymphocytes, pregnancies were normally maintained. On the other hand, mating after transfer of Treg cell-depleted lymphocytes resulted in fetal loss, suggesting that Treg cells are essential for the maintenance of allogenic pregnancies (11). Adoptive transfer of $CD4^+CD25^+$ Treg cells from mice with an allogenic pregnancy prevented fetal rejection in an abortion-prone mouse model during allogenic pregnancy, if the transfer was conducted before day 4.5 of gestation (9). Furthermore, depletion of Treg cells using anti-CD25 monoclonal antibodies induced implantation failure and abortion in allogenic pregnancies, but did not induce any pregnancy complications during the late stages of pregnancy (10). These findings suggest that Treg cells induce allo-antigen-specific tolerance and are necessary from implantation through early pregnancy periods in mice.

Where and how do fetal antigen-specific Treg cells expand during pregnancy? Previous studies have demonstrated the existence of fetal antigen-specific Treg cells and their distribution in mouse models (**Table 1**). Kahn and Baltimore showed that the H-Y-specific suppressive capability of Treg cells in splenocytes

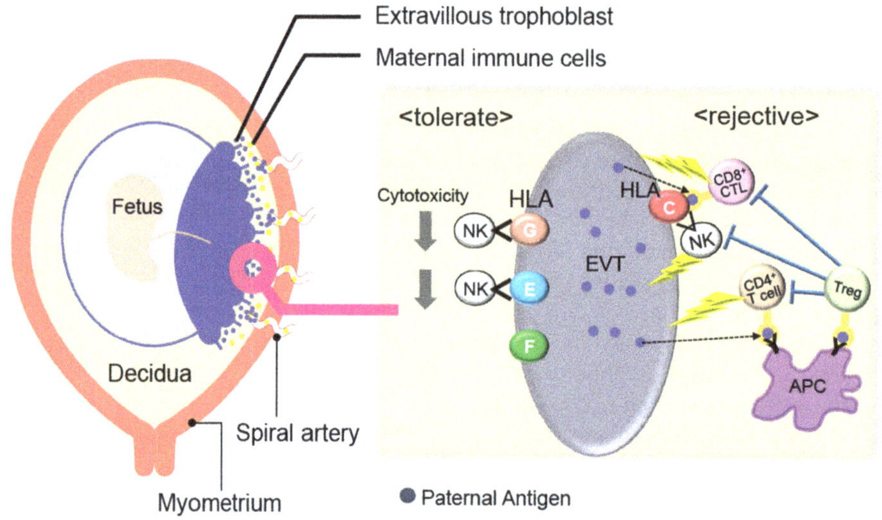

FIGURE 1 | Immunological balance at the feto-maternal interface during early pregnancy. EVTs did not express polymorphic HLA-A, B whereas HLA-C and non-polymorphic HLA-E, G, and F were expressed. Maternal $CD8^+$ T cells and NK cells can directly recognize paternal HLA-C and $CD4^+$ T cells can indirectly recognize it. HLA- E and G protect EVTs from NK-cell mediated cytotoxicity. Treg cells can recognize fetal antigens via maternal antigen presenting cells (APCs) and induce tolerance in an antigen-specific manner. EVT, Extravillous trophoblast; NK, natural killer cell; Treg; regulatory T cell; APC, antigen-presenting cell.

escalated more during pregnancy than before pregnancy (15). Rowe et al. demonstrated that Treg cells specific for the 2W1S antigen, which is derived from the mouse MHC-Eα chain, expanded in the systemic lymph nodes during the 1st pregnancy and rapidly re-accumulated during the 2nd pregnancy (16). Furthermore, Shima et al. reported the local distribution of paternal antigen-specific Treg cells during the implantation period and after pregnancy (**Figure 2**). DBA/2 mice have the Mls 1a super antigen, which is recognized by Vβ6 of the T cell receptor β chain. When BALB/C female mice were mated with DBA/2 male mice, CD4+CD25+Vβ6+ Treg cells, which can be regarded as Mls 1a-specific Treg cells, increased in the uterine-draining lymph nodes one day before implantation. This phenomenon was not observed when BALB/C female mice were mated with seminal vesicle-excised DBA/2 male mice. The local fetal antigen-specific Treg cells might be expanded at the draining lymph nodes by seminal plasma-priming and migrate to the uterus after pregnancy. After implantation, the Vβ6+ Treg cell population in the uterus increased day by day during pregnancy, but that in peripheral lymph nodes and spleen did not (17). Therefore, accumulation of paternal antigen-specific Treg cells is regulated in an organ-specific manner.

Paternal Antigen-Specific Treg Cells in Human Pregnancies

During pregnancy in humans, the systemic and local expansion of the Treg cell pool is observed from the 1st trimester and reaches a maximum in the 2nd trimester (12, 19). Although fetal antigen-specific regulatory T cells and their systemic and local expansion were observed in a mouse model, direct detection of fetal antigen-specific Treg cells is difficult in humans due to heterogenic MHC expression and limited knowledge concerning the physiological target peptide of Treg cells (55). However, the existence of fetal antigen-specific Treg cells in human pregnancies was indirectly suggested in some reports.

Decidual Treg cells, but not peripheral blood Treg cells, showed higher suppression toward self-fetal cord blood than 3rd party cord blood, suggesting that fetal antigen-specific Treg cells might exist at the feto-maternal interface during human pregnancy (56). Among human Treg cell subsets, $CD4^+CD45RA^-FoxP3^{high}$ comprises effector Treg cells which are memory type T cells with a high suppressive capability, and $CD4^+CD45RA^+FoxP3^{low}$ comprises naïve Treg cells with a relatively lower suppressive capability (57, 58). Effector Treg cells are the most dominant among Treg cells in both peripheral blood and decidua in the late gestation stage of human pregnancies (59). To demonstrate if expansion of the effector Treg cell pool is a reflection of clonal expansion of antigen-specific Treg cells, we conducted single-cell-based T cell receptor (TCR) repertoire analysis of $CD4^+CD25^+CD45RA^-CD127^{low}$ effector Treg cells in human pregnancies (**Figure 3**). Our study was the first to reveal that clonally expanded effector Treg cells were observed only in the decidua, but not in the peripheral blood (**Figure 4A**). Clonally expanded effector Treg cells were higher in the 3rd trimester than in the 1st trimester (**Figure 4A**). On the other hand, the common clonotypic effector Treg cells between the decidua and peripheral blood were rarely observed (20). Therefore, decidual effector Treg cells might recognize some antigens expressed at the feto-maternal interface and proliferate upon antigen stimulation. However, effector Treg cells in the peripheral blood expand nonspecifically. Interestingly, the same clonotypic decidual effector Treg cells repeatedly appeared in previous and subsequent pregnancies in three cases: two ended with paired normal term deliveries and the third ended with paired miscarriages (20). TCRβ varies, with over

TABLE 1 | Paternal antigen-specific Treg cells in mouse models.

Target Antigen	PA-specific Treg cells	Method	Existence of PA-antigen specific Treg cells	References
H-Y antigen derived peptide (Dby)	MHC classII I-A^b H-Y ($Dby_{608-622}$)restricted Treg cells	MLR	Systemic	(15)
I-A^b restricted $2W1S_{52-68}$ peptide	MHC classII I-Ab $2W1S_{52-68}$ restricted Treg cells	Direct detection by tetramer	Syetemic	(16)
Mls 1a superantigen	CD4+CD25+Vβ6+ Treg cells (Vβ6 of the T cell receptor β chain recognize Mls 1a superantigen	Direct detection by anti-Vβ6 antibody	Uterine-draining lymph nodes, Uterus	(17)

PA-specific Treg cells, Paternal antigen-specific Treg cells; MLR, Mixed lymphocyte reaction.

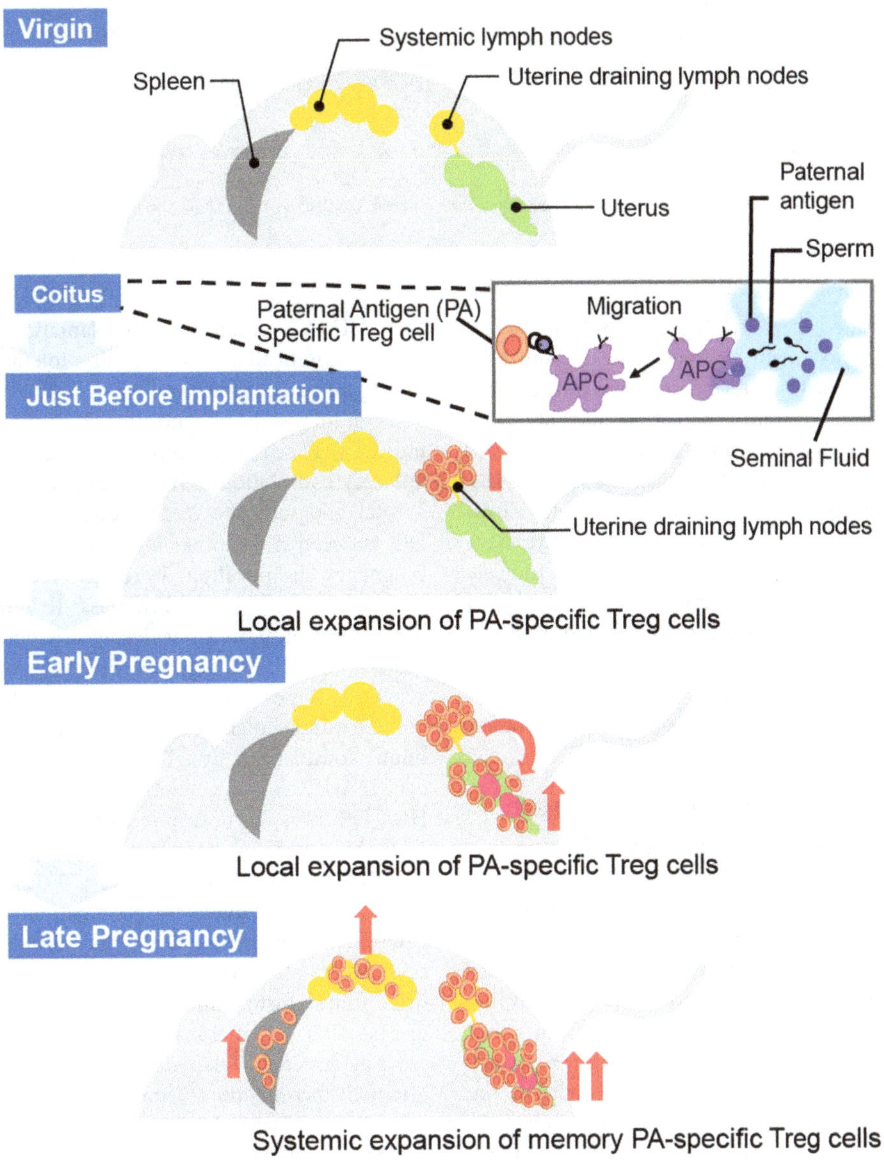

FIGURE 2 | Distribution of paternal antigen-specific Treg cells in mice. When a female mouse is mated with an allogenic male mouse, paternal antigen-specific Treg cells increase in the uterine-draining lymph nodes one day before implantation due to seminal plasma priming. After implantation, the paternal antigen-specific Treg cells population in the uterus increases day by day during the course of the pregnancy, but not in the peripheral lymph nodes and the spleen. APC, antigen-presenting cell.

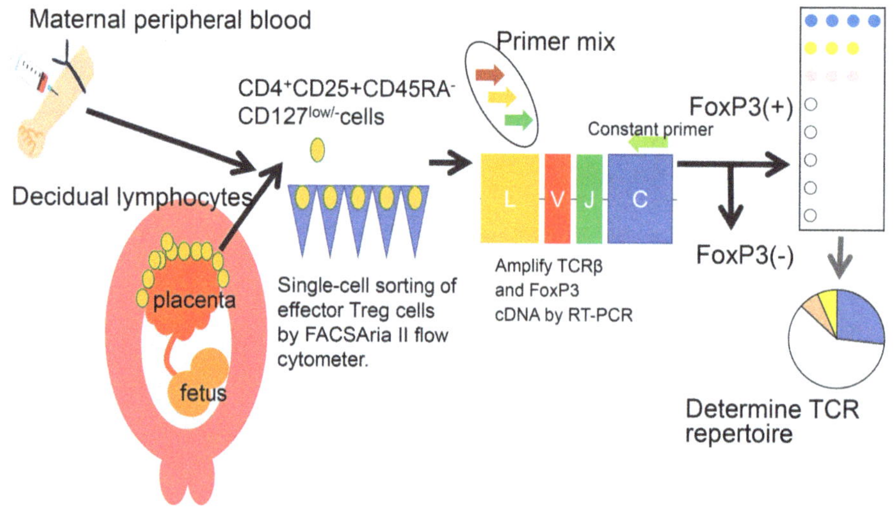

FIGURE 3 | Single-cell based TCR repertoire analysis method. To study the clonality of effector Treg cells, a single-cell based T cell receptor (TCR) repertoire analysis method was used. Paired samples of maternal peripheral blood mononuclear cells and decidual lymphocytes were obtained. CD4+CD25+CD45RA-CD127low/- effector Treg cells were single-cell sorted. The cDNAs of complementarity determining lesion 3 (CDR3) in TCRβ chain and FoxP3 were amplified by RT-PCR. The nucleotides and amino acid sequences of CDR3 were analyzed.

2×10^7 patterns estimated in young humans (60), thus these same clonotypic Treg cells might be repeatedly recruited by the same antigens at the feto-maternal interface rather than by accidental coincidence. Furthermore, clonal populations of decidual effector Treg cells were lower in the 3rd trimester in preeclampsia cases than in normal pregnancies (**Figure 4B**). However, while the effector Treg cell pool was reduced, clonal populations were not reduced in 1st trimester miscarriage cases (20) (**Figure 4B**). Taken together, these data indicate that fetal antigen-specific Treg cells might be recruited and expand in a fetal antigen-specific manner at the feto-maternal interface, and polyclonally expand in systemic circulation during human pregnancy. Clonally expanded decidual Treg cells might be important in the maintenance of feto-maternal tolerance, especially in the 3rd trimester.

Which Peptides Are Recognized by Treg Cells at the Feto-Maternal Interface?

Paternal MHC and minor antigen-derived peptide-specific Treg cells were identified in mouse models as previously described (15–17). A recent study showed that non-inherited maternal antigen (NIMA)-specific Treg cells enforce tolerance in a mouse model (61). NIMAs are peptides derived from polymorphic genes such as MHC and are expressed in the mother but not in offspring. Microchimerism, developed during pregnancy and breast feeding, enables transfer of maternal cells to the offspring. Microchimeric maternal cells persist for a long time and tolerance for NIMAs persists during this time. Kinder et al. demonstrated that the paternal MHC-derived antigen was identical to the NIMA, and the rapid expansion of NIMA-specific Treg cells contributed to successful pregnancy (61). NIMA-matched organ transplantation presents a lower risk of rejection than NIMA-mismatched transplantation in humans (62–65). Thus, theoretically, NIMA-specific tolerance might be induced during human pregnancy.

In humans, a polymorphic HLA-C mismatch pregnancy indicates T cell activation and Treg cell expansion (66). In an oocyte donation (OD) pregnancy, in which the fetus is a total allograft, the match level of HLA-A, B, C, DR, and DQ between the mother and offspring was higher, and fewer pregnancy complications were observed (67). Trophoblasts lack surface expression of HLA-class II molecules, but contain them intracellularly. Considering microchimerism between the mother and fetus, peptides derived from HLA-class II can act as epitopes presented by maternal APCs. Trophoblasts contain intracellular HLA-class II and release HLA-DR molecules upon stimulation by IFN-γ (68). Cell surface expression of HLA-DR in syncytiotrophoblasts and the presence of HLA-DR in syncytiotrophoblast-derived extracellular vesicles were observed in preeclampsia (69). Seminal plasma also contains soluble HLA molecules (70–72). Additionally, human EVTs express minor histocompatibility antigens, such as HY, HA, and ACC (73). HY antigen-specific $CD8^+$ T cells were observed during human pregnancy (48). Even these minor histocompatibility antigens mediate graft-vs.-host disease after organ transplantation (73); however, fetal tissues are not rejected. Taken together, allogenic-HLA-derived, and minor histocompatibility antigen-derived peptides presented by maternal APCs might be recognized by $CD4^+$ conventional T cells and Treg cells. The main target antigens of decidual $CD4^+$ conventional T cells, CTLs, and Treg cells are yet unclear. Further investigation is required to reveal the antigen-specificity of each T cell type and their regulation at the feto-maternal interface.

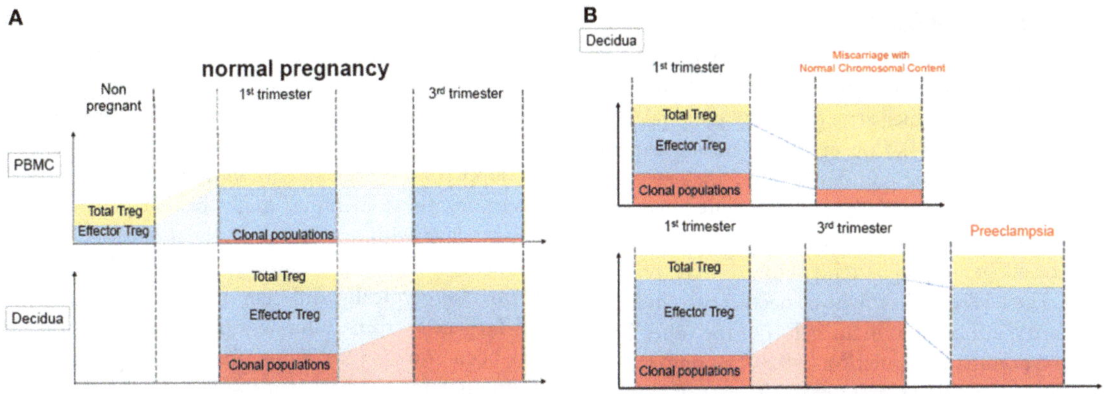

FIGURE 4 | Distribution of clonally expanded effector Treg cells in humans. **(A)** Frequencies of total Treg cells, effector Treg cells and clonal populations of effector Treg cells in normal pregnancy. The systemic and local expansion of the Treg cells and effector Treg cells pool is observed during pregnancies in humans. Clonally expanded effector Treg cells increase in decidua, but not in peripheral blood. Clonal populations of effector Treg cells more increase in 3rd trimester than 1st trimester. **(B)** Clonally expanded decidual effector Treg cells in miscarriage and preeclampsia. In decidua, effector Treg cells pool decreased in miscarriage with normal chromosomal content than 1st trimester normal pregnancy, whereas the frequency of clonal populations of effector Treg cells does not significantly decrease. On the other hand, clonal populations of decidual effector Treg cells decreased preeclampsia than 3rd trimester normal pregnancies.

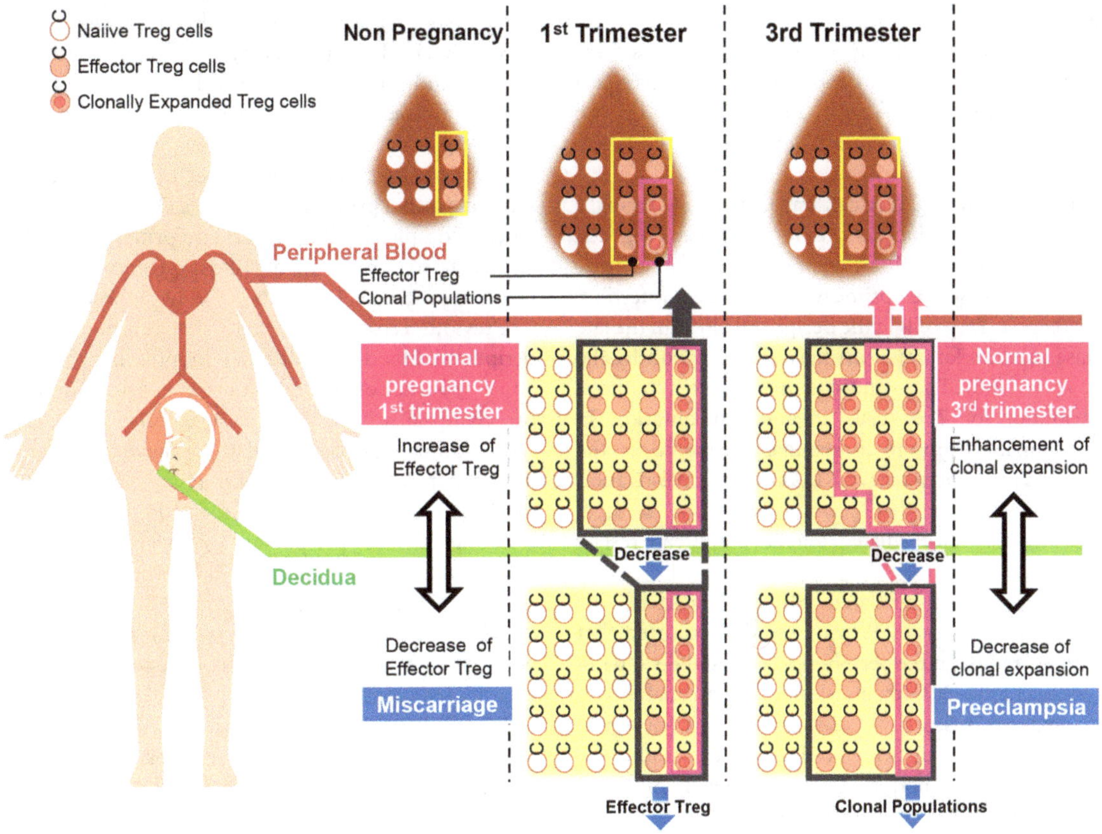

FIGURE 5 | Pathological change in Treg cells during pregnancy in humans. During pregnancy, Treg cell pools both in the peripheral blood and decidua expand. Clonally expanded effector Treg cells are observed only in the decidua, but not in the peripheral blood. Clonally expanded effector Treg cells are higher in the 3rd trimester than in the 1st trimester. In miscarriage cases with normal chromosomal fetal content, the number of decidual effector Treg cells decreases. On the other hand, clonal populations of decidual effector Treg cells decrease in cases of preeclampsia.

What Is the Origin of Treg Cells at the Feto-Maternal Interface?

There are two types of Treg cells in terms of origin: naturally occurring Treg (nTreg) cells, which originate in the thymus, and inducible Treg (iTreg) cells, which arise from conventional CD4$^+$ T cells in peripheral tissues (74). Conserved noncoding sequence 1 (CNS1) is a FoxP3 enhancer and is necessary for developing iTreg cells. Interestingly, only placental mammals have CNS-1, while marsupials and monotremes do not. CNS-1 knockout female mice with allogenic pregnancies showed increased fetal resorption (75). Thus, iTreg cells might be necessary to maintain allogenic pregnancy in placental mammals. On the other hand, nTreg cells are the dominant population (~95%) among decidual Treg cells in the 1st trimester of human pregnancy, and the proportion of nTreg cells is similar between normal pregnancy and miscarriage (76). However, decidual iTreg cells significantly decreased in preeclampsia (77). To maintain human pregnancy, nTreg cells might be important in early stage pregnancy, and iTreg cells might also be important in late-stage gestation. Further study is necessary to confirm this possibility.

Pregnancy Complications and Treg Cells in Humans

Maldistribution and functional impairment of Treg cells were reported in implantation failure, miscarriage, and preeclampsia in humans. Contrarily, Treg cells are necessary in the implantation period and early gestation, but not in late gestation in mice (10).

Multiple factors, including Treg cell impairment, are thought to be related to implantation failure in humans. Treg cell transcription factor FoxP3 mRNA expression in the uterine endometrium is decreased in primary unexplained infertility (78, 79). A decrease in Treg cells in the peripheral blood in the late follicular phase predicts failure of artificial insemination by the donor (AID) sperm (80). These findings support the hypothesis that maldistribution of Treg cells impairs implantation in humans. Additionally, exposure to seminal plasma raises the success rate of IVF-ET pregnancy (81). Further investigation can validate the evidence that priming with the seminal plasma results in Treg cell-mediated tolerance and can rescue implantation failure.

Disturbance of Treg cell-mediated tolerance might be one of the etiologies of miscarriage. Previous studies reported that Treg cells were decreased in the peripheral blood and decidua in miscarriage cases (12, 82–84). Impaired suppressive capability of Treg cells in recurrent miscarriage cases has also been observed (85–88). Effector Treg cells and nTreg cells were decreased in the case of miscarriage with a normal karyotyped fetus compared to that in the 1st trimester of a normal pregnancy or in the case of miscarriage with an abnormal karyotyped fetus (76, 89). On the other hand, the clonally expanded population of Treg cells showed no significant difference between these groups (20) (**Figure 5**). These findings suggest that the number of nTreg cells and effector Treg cells is more important than antigen-specific Treg cell recruitment during the 1st trimester. The total Treg cell volume that regulates excessive inflammation might be important for the maintenance of the early gestation phase of pregnancy. A previous report demonstrated that high dose immunoglobulin therapy improved the live birth rate for refractory recurrent miscarriage cases with four or more consecutive miscarriages (90). Other studies also showed the effectiveness of anti-TNF-alfa inhibitor therapy (91). These medications have the potential to suppress immune activity in an antigen-nonspecific manner; therefore, these therapies might benefit patients with recurrent miscarriage with a reduced decidual effector Treg cell pool. In humans, peripheral blood Treg cells and decidual Treg cells form clonotypically different populations, and the migration of Treg cells from systemic circulation to the decidua has not yet been shown (20). Thus, these findings might explain why immunization therapy using white blood cells from the patient's partner is not effective for treating recurrent miscarriage (92).

Preeclampsia, which is defined as hypertension concomitant with proteinuria or placental dysfunction occurring in mid to late gestation, is a major cause of maternal and fetal morbidity and mortality. Chronic inflammation due to activation of neutrophils and NK cells, elevation of pro-inflammatory cytokines, and dysfunction of Treg cells is also thought to contribute to the pathogenesis of preeclampsia (93). Epidemiological findings provide the hypothesis that failure in maintaining paternal antigen-specific tolerance is related to the development of preeclampsia. First pregnancy, pregnancy following a partner change, and a pregnancy interval of more than ten years raise the risk of preeclampsia (94–96). Long-term condom usage and AID pregnancy also elevate the risk of preeclampsia, suggesting insufficient paternal antigen-specific tolerance mediated by seminal plasma priming (70, 97, 98). OD pregnancy, in which the fetus is completely allogenic and no priming effect has occurred, is associated with a high risk of preeclampsia (6, 98). Basic research on Treg cells supports this hypothesis.

Previous reports show that Treg cell pools decrease in the peripheral blood and decidua in preeclampsia (77, 99–108). Some reports demonstrate functionally impaired Treg cells in preeclampsia, where Treg cell apoptosis can be easily induced (109). Other reports showed that effector Treg cells decreased in the peripheral blood (108). Hsu et al. demonstrated that the function of decidual APCs was impaired in preeclampsia, resulting in fewer peripherally induced Treg cells (iTreg cells) than in normal pregnancies (77). Elevation of soluble endoglin (sEND), which is a co-receptor of TGFβ, results in the capture of circulating TGFβ, resulting in a systemic decrease of the Treg cell pool. It might also disturb the conversion of conventional Treg cells to iTreg cells (6).

So far, it has not been clarified whether a decreased total volume of Treg cells or decreased paternal antigen-specific Treg cells are related to the pathogenesis of preeclampsia. Our study reported for the first time that clonal expansion of decidual Treg cells was impaired in preeclampsia, suggesting that paternal antigen-specific tolerance might be insufficient. The frequencies of clonal populations of decidual effector Treg cells were 20.9% (15.4–28.1%) in the 3rd trimester during normal pregnancy and 9.3% (4.4–14.5%) in pregnancies with preeclampsia (**Figure 5**). Both early onset and late onset preeclampsia showed the same tendency (20). Our result is compatible with epidemiological evidence that inadequate paternal antigen-specific tolerance raises the risk of preeclampsia. Paternal antigen-specific Treg cells are more important in the late gestation period of pregnancy than in early gestation (**Figure 3**). Decidual iTreg cells and clonal populations of decidual effector Treg cells decreased in preeclampsia (20, 77). The main population of decidual effector Treg cells during early pregnancy was that of nTreg (76), and the clonal population of decidual effector Treg cells did not decrease. These findings suggest that clonally expanded Treg cells might be iTreg cells. This point requires clarification in the future.

In terms of the clinical applications of these findings, oocyte donation after HLA matching with maternal or paternal HLA might reduce the risk of preeclampsia. Encouraging seminal plasma exposure might play a protective role for high risk patients.

CONCLUSION

Treg cell-mediated feto-maternal tolerance is important in the maintenance of allogenic pregnancy. Paternal antigen-specific Treg cells are expanded systemically and locally during mouse pregnancy. Seminal plasma priming induces paternal antigen-specific Treg cells. Although paternal antigen-specific Treg cells have not been identified in humans, clonal expansion of decidual effector Treg cells implies that antigen-specific tolerance by Treg cells might be induced during human pregnancy. A reduced amount of decidual Treg cells might be related to the pathogenesis of miscarriage, and the failure of decidual Treg cell clonal expansion might be related to the pathogenesis of preeclampsia in humans.

AUTHOR CONTRIBUTIONS

SS, ST, TS, and AN conception and design, drafting manuscript and revision of the manuscript for important intellectual content.

FUNDING

This work was supported by grants from Ministry of Education, Culture, Sports, Science, and Technology in Japan [KAKENHI Grant Number 15H04980 (SS), 17K11221(TS)].

ACKNOWLEDGMENTS

We would like to thank Editage (www.editage.jp) for English language editing.

REFERENCES

1. Saito S, Shima T, Nakashima A, Shiozaki A, Ito M, Sasaki Y. What is the role of regulatory T cells in the success of implantation and early pregnancy? *J Assist Reprod Genet.* (2007) 24:379–86. doi: 10.1007/s10815-007-9140-y
2. Erlebacher A. Mechanisms of T cell tolerance towards the allogeneic fetus. *Nat Rev Immunol.* (2013) 13:23–33. doi: 10.1038/nri3361
3. Robertson SA, Prins JR, Sharkey DJ, Moldenhauer LM. Seminal fluid and the generation of regulatory T cells for embryo implantation. *Am J Reprod Immunol.* (2013) 69:315–30. doi: 10.1111/aji.12107
4. Zenclussen AC. Adaptive immune responses during pregnancy. *Am J Reprod Immunol.* (2013) 69:291–303. doi: 10.1111/aji.12097
5. PrabhuDas M, Bonney E, Caron K, Dey SCA, Fazleabas A, et al. Immune mechanisms at the maternal-fetal interface: perspectives and challenges. *Nat Immunol.* (2015) 16:328–34. doi: 10.1038/ni.3131
6. Saito S, Nakabayashi Y, Nakashima A, Shima T, Yoshino O. A new era in reproductive medicine: consequences of third-party oocyte donation for maternal and fetal health. *Semin Immunopathol.* (2016) 38:687–97. doi: 10.1007/s00281-016-0577-x
7. Saito S, Shima T, Nakashima A, Inada K, Yoshino O. Role of paternal antigen-specific treg cells in successful implantation. *Am J Reprod Immunol.* (2016) 75:310–6. doi: 10.1111/aji.12469
8. Saito S, Nishikawa K, Morii T, Narita N, Enomoto M, Ichijo M. Expression of activation antigens CD69, HLA-DR, interleukin-2 receptor-alpha (IL-2R alpha) and IL-2R beta on T cells of human decidua at an early stage of pregnancy. *Immunology.* (1992) 75:710–2.
9. Zenclussen AC, Gerlof K, Zenclussen ML, Sollwedel A, Bertoja AZ, Ritter T, et al. Abnormal T-cell reactivity against paternal antigens in spontaneous abortion: adoptive transfer of pregnancy-induced CD_4^+ CD_{25}^+ T regulatory cells prevents fetal rejection in a murine abortion model. *Am J Pathol.* (2005) 166:811–22. doi: 10.1016/S0002-9440(10)62302-4
10. Shima T, Sasaki Y, Itoh M, Nakashima A, Ishii N, Sugamura K, et al. Regulatory T cells are necessary for implantation and maintenance of early pregnancy but not late pregnancy in allogeneic mice. *J Reprod Immunol.* (2010) 85:121–9. doi: 10.1016/j.jri.2010.02.006
11. Aluvihare VR, Kallikourdis M, Betz AG. Regulatory T cells mediate maternal tolerance to the fetus. *Nat Immunol.* (2004) 5:266–71. doi: 10.1038/ni1037
12. Sasaki Y, Sakai M, Miyazaki S, Higuma S, Shiozaki A, Saito S. Decidual and peripheral blood CD4+CD25+ regulatory T cells in early pregnancy subjects and spontaneous abortion cases. *Mol Hum Reprod.* (2004) 10:347–53. doi: 10.1093/molehr/gah044
13. Sakaguchi S, Sakaguchi N, Asano M, Itoh M, Toda M. Immunologic self-tolerance maintained by activated T cells expressing IL-2 receptor alpha-chains (CD25). Breakdown of a single mechanism of self-tolerance causes various autoimmune diseases. *J Immunol.* (1995) 155:1151–64.
14. Sakaguchi S, Yamaguchi T, Nomura T, Ono M. Regulatory T cells and immune tolerance. *Cell.* (2008) 133:775–87. doi: 10.1016/j.cell.2008.05.009
15. Kahn DA, Baltimore D. Pregnancy induces a fetal antigen-specific maternal T regulatory cell response that contributes to tolerance. *Proc Natl Acad Sci USA.* (2010) 107:9299–304. doi: 10.1073/pnas.1003909107
16. Rowe JH, Ertelt JM, Xin L, Way SS. Pregnancy imprints regulatory memory that sustains anergy to fetal antigen. *Nature.* (2012) 490:102–6. doi: 10.1038/nature11462
17. Shima T, Inada K, Nakashima A, Ushijima A, Ito M, Yoshino O, et al. Paternal antigen-specific proliferating regulatory T cells are increased in uterine-draining lymph nodes just before implantation and in pregnant uterus just after implantation by seminal plasma-priming in allogeneic mouse pregnancy. *J Reprod Immunol.* (2015) 108:72–82. doi: 10.1016/j.jri.2015.02.005
18. Robertson SA, Guerin LR, Bromfield JJ, Branson KM, Ahlstrom AC, Care AS. Seminal fluid drives expansion of the CD_4^+ CD_{25}^+ T regulatory cell pool and induces tolerance to paternal alloantigens in mice. *Biol Reprod.* (2009) 80:1036–45. doi: 10.1095/biolreprod.108.074658
19. Somerset DA, Zheng Y, Kilby MD, Sansom DM, Drayson MT. Normal human pregnancy is associated with an elevation in the immune suppressive CD_{25}^+ CD_4^+ regulatory T-cell subset. *Immunology.* (2004) 112:38–43. doi: 10.1111/j.1365-2567.2004.01869.x

20. Tsuda S, Zhang X, Hamana H, Shima T, Ushijima A, Tsuda K, et al. Clonally expanded decidual effector regulatory T cells increase in late gestation of normal pregnancy, but not in preeclampsia, in humans. *Front Immunol.* (2018) 9:1934. doi: 10.3389/fimmu.2018.01934
21. Fisher SJ, Damsky CH. Human cytotrophoblast invasion. *Semin Cell Biol.* (1993) 4:183–8. doi: 10.1006/scel.1993.1022
22. Fisher SJ. Why is placentation abnormal in preeclampsia? *Am J Obstet Gynecol.* (2015) 213:S115–22. doi: 10.1016/j.ajog.2015.08.042
23. Wallace AE, Fraser R, Cartwright JE. Extravillous trophoblast and decidual natural killer cells: a remodelling partnership. *Hum Reprod Update.* (2012) 18:458–71. doi: 10.1093/humupd/dms015
24. Kovats S, Main EK, Librach C, Stubblebine M, Fisher SJ, DeMars R. A class I antigen, HLA-G, expressed in human trophoblasts. *Science.* (1990) 248:220–3. doi: 10.1126/science.2326636
25. McMaster MT, Librach CL, Zhou Y, Lim KH, Janatpour MJ, DeMars R, et al. Human placental HLA-G expression is restricted to differentiated cytotrophoblasts. *J Immunol.* (1995) 154:3771–8.
26. King A, Allan DS, Bowen M, Powis SJ, Joseph S, Verma S, et al. HLA-E is expressed on trophoblast and interacts with CD94/NKG2 receptors on decidual NK cells. *Eur J Immunol.* (2000) 30:1623–31. doi: 10.1002/1521-4141(200006)30:6<1623::AID-IMMU1623>3.0.CO;2-M
27. King A, Burrows TD, Hiby SE, Bowen JM, Joseph S, Verma S, et al. Surface expression of HLA-C antigen by human extravillous trophoblast. *Placenta.* (2000) 21:376–87. doi: 10.1053/plac.1999.0496
28. Barakonyi A, Kovacs KT, Miko E, Szereday L, Varga P, Szekeres-Bartho J. Recognition of nonclassical HLA class I antigens by gamma delta T cells during pregnancy. *J Immunol.* (2002) 168:2683–8. doi: 10.4049/jimmunol.168.6.2683
29. Ishitani A, Sageshima N, Lee N, Dorofeeva N, Hatake K, Marquardt H, et al. Protein expression and peptide binding suggest unique and interacting functional roles for HLA-E, F, and G in maternal-placental immune recognition. *J Immunol.* (2003) 171:1376–84. doi: 10.4049/jimmunol.171.3.1376
30. Rajagopalan S, Long EO. A human histocompatibility leukocyte antigen (HLA)-G-specific receptor expressed on all natural killer cells. *J Exp Med.* (1999) 189:1093–100. doi: 10.1084/jem.189.7.1093
31. Li C, Houser BL, Nicotra ML, Strominger JL. HLA-G homodimer-induced cytokine secretion through HLA-G receptors on human decidual macrophages and natural killer cells. *Proc Natl Acad Sci USA.* (2009) 106:5767–72. doi: 10.1073/pnas.0901173106
32. Ristich V, Liang S, Zhang W, Wu J, Horuzsko A. Tolerization of dendritic cells by HLA-G. *Eur J Immunol.* (2005) 35:1133–42. doi: 10.1002/eji.200425741
33. Tilburgs T, Crespo AC, van der Zwan A, Rybalov B, Raj T, Stranger B, et al. Human HLA-G+ extravillous trophoblasts: Immune-activating cells that interact with decidual leukocytes. *Proc Natl Acad Sci USA.* (2015) 112:7219–24. doi: 10.1073/pnas.1507977112
34. Munn DH, Zhou M, Attwood JT, Bondarev I, Conway SJ, Marshall B, et al. Prevention of allogeneic fetal rejection by tryptophan catabolism. *Science.* (1998) 281:1191–3. doi: 10.1126/science.281.5380.1191
35. Chang RQ, Li DJ, Li MQ. The role of indoleamine-2,3-dioxygenase in normal and pathological pregnancies. *Am J Reprod Immunol.* (2018) 79:e12786. doi: 10.1111/aji.12786
36. Guzeloglu-Kayisli O, Kayisli UA, Taylor HS. The role of growth factors and cytokines during implantation: endocrine and paracrine interactions. *Semin Reprod Med.* (2009) 27:62–79. doi: 10.1055/s-0028-1108011
37. Nagamatsu T, Schust DJ, Sugimoto J, Barrier BF. Human decidual stromal cells suppress cytokine secretion by allogenic $CD4^+$ T cells via PD-1 ligand interactions. *Hum Reprod.* (2009) 24:3160–71. doi: 10.1093/humrep/dep308
38. King A, Wooding P, Gardner L, Loke YW. Expression of perforin, granzyme A and TIA-1 by human uterine CD56+ NK cells implies they are activated and capable of effector functions. *Hum Reprod.* (1993) 8:2061–7. doi: 10.1093/oxfordjournals.humrep.a137982
39. Higuma-Myojo S, Sasaki Y, Miyazaki S, Sakai M, Siozaki A, Miwa N, et al. Cytokine profile of natural killer cells in early human pregnancy. *Am J Reprod Immunol.* (2005) 54:21–9. doi: 10.1111/j.1600-0897.2005.00279.x
40. Saito S, Nakashima A, Myojo-Higuma S, Shiozaki A. The balance between cytotoxic NK cells and regulatory NK cells in human pregnancy. *J Reprod Immunol.* (2008) 77:14–22. doi: 10.1016/j.jri.2007.04.007
41. Moffett A, Colucci F. Uterine NK cells: active regulators at the maternal-fetal interface. *J Clin Invest.* (2014) 124:1872–9. doi: 10.1172/JCI68107
42. Saito S, Nishikawa K, Morii T, Enomoto M, Narita N, Motoyoshi K, et al. Cytokine production by CD16-CD56bright natural killer cells in the human early pregnancy decidua. *Int Immunol.* (1993) 5:559–63. doi: 10.1093/intimm/5.5.559
43. King A, Birkby C, Loke YW. Early human decidual cells exhibit NK activity against the K562 cell line but not against first trimester trophoblast. *Cell Immunol.* (1989) 118:337–44. doi: 10.1016/0008-8749(89)90382-1
44. Hanna J, Goldman-Wohl D, Hamani Y, Avraham I, Greenfield C, Natanson-Yaron S, et al. Decidual NK cells regulate key developmental processes at the human fetal-maternal interface. *Nat Med.* (2006) 12:1065–74. doi: 10.1038/nm1452
45. Lash GE, Schiessl B, Kirkley M, Innes BA, Cooper A, Searle RF, et al. Expression of angiogenic growth factors by uterine natural killer cells during early pregnancy. *J Leukoc Biol.* (2006) 80:572–80. doi: 10.1189/jlb.0406250
46. Pollheimer J, Vondra S, Baltayeva J, Beristain AG, Knofler M. Regulation of placental extravillous trophoblasts by the maternal uterine environment. *Front Immunol.* (2018) 9:2597. doi: 10.3389/fimmu.2018.02597
47. Cerdeira AS, Rajakumar A, Royle CM, Lo A, Husain Z, Thadhani RI, et al. Conversion of peripheral blood NK cells to a decidual NK-like phenotype by a cocktail of defined factors. *J Immunol.* (2013) 190:3939–48. doi: 10.4049/jimmunol.1202582
48. Lissauer D, Piper K, Goodyear O, Kilby MD, Moss PA. Fetal-specific CD8+ cytotoxic T cell responses develop during normal human pregnancy and exhibit broad functional capacity. *J Immunol.* (2012) 189:1072–80. doi: 10.4049/jimmunol.1200544
49. Tilburgs T, Strominger JL. CD8+ effector T cells at the fetal-maternal interface, balancing fetal tolerance and antiviral immunity. *Am J Reprod Immunol.* (2013) 69:395–407. doi: 10.1111/aji.12094
50. van Egmond A, van der Keur C, Swings GM, Scherjon SA, Claas FH. The possible role of virus-specific CD8(+) memory T cells in decidual tissue. *J Reprod Immunol.* (2016) 113:1–8. doi: 10.1016/j.jri.2015.09.073
51. van der Zwan A, van der Meer-Prins EMW, van Miert P, van den Heuvel H, Anholts JDH, Roelen DL, et al. Cross-reactivity of virus-specific CD8+ T cells against allogeneic HLA-C: possible implications for pregnancy outcome. *Front Immunol.* (2018) 9:2880. doi: 10.3389/fimmu.2018.02880
52. Wang SC, Li YH, Piao HL, Hong XW, Zhang D, Xu YY, et al. PD-1 and Tim-3 pathways are associated with regulatory $CD8^+$ T-cell function in decidua and maintenance of normal pregnancy. *Cell Death Dis.* (2015) 6:e1738. doi: 10.1038/cddis.2015.112
53. Tilburgs T, Schonkeren D, Eikmans M, Nagtzaam NM, Datema G, Swings GM, et al. Human decidual tissue contains differentiated $CD8^+$ effector-memory T cells with unique properties. *J Immunol.* (2010) 185:4470–77. doi: 10.4049/jimmunol.0903597
54. Tafuri A, Alferink J, Moller P, Hammerling GJ, Arnold B. T cell awareness of paternal alloantigens during pregnancy. *Science.* (1995) 270:630–3. doi: 10.1126/science.270.5236.630
55. Bacher P, Scheffold A. New technologies for monitoring human antigen-specific T cells and regulatory T cells by flow-cytometry. *Curr Opin Pharmacol.* (2015) 23:17–24. doi: 10.1016/j.coph.2015.04.005
56. Tilburgs T, Roelen DL, van der Mast BJ, de Groot-Swings GM, Kleijburg C, Scherjon SA, et al. Evidence for a selective migration of fetus-specific CD_4^+ CD_{25}^{bright} regulatory T cells from the peripheral blood to the decidua in human pregnancy. *J Immunol.* (2008) 180:5737–45. doi: 10.4049/jimmunol.180.8.5737
57. Miyara M, Yoshioka Y, Kitoh A, Shima T, Wing K, Niwa A, et al. Functional delineation and differentiation dynamics of human $CD4^+$ T cells

expressing the FoxP3 transcription factor. *Immunity.* (2009) 30:899–911. doi: 10.1016/j.immuni.2009.03.019

58. Miyara M, Chader D, Sage E, Sugiyama D, Nishikawa H, Bouvry D, et al. Sialyl Lewis x (CD15s) identifies highly differentiated and most suppressive FOXP3high regulatory T cells in humans. *Proc Natl Acad Sci USA.* (2015) 112:7225–30. doi: 10.1073/pnas.1508224112
59. Loewendorf AI, Nguyen TA, Yesayan MN, Kahn DA. Normal human pregnancy results in maternal immune activation in the periphery and at the uteroplacental interface. *PLoS ONE.* (2014) 9:e96723. doi: 10.1371/journal.pone.0096723
60. Qi Q, Liu Y, Cheng Y, Glanville J, Zhang D, Lee JY, et al. Diversity and clonal selection in the human T-cell repertoire. *Proc Natl Acad Sci USA.* (2014) 111:13139–44. doi: 10.1073/pnas.1409155111
61. Kinder JM, Jiang TT, Ertelt JM, Xin L, Strong BS, Shaaban AF, et al. Cross-generational reproductive fitness enforced by microchimeric maternal cells. *Cell.* (2015) 162:505–15. doi: 10.1016/j.cell.2015.07.006
62. Burlingham WJ, Grailer AP, Heisey DM, Claas FH, Norman D, Mohanakumar T, et al. The effect of tolerance to noninherited maternal HLA antigens on the survival of renal transplants from sibling donors. *N Engl J Med.* (1998) 339:1657–64. doi: 10.1056/NEJM199812033392302
63. van Rood JJ, Claas F. Both self and non-inherited maternal HLA antigens influence the immune response. *Immunol Today.* (2000) 21:269–73. doi: 10.1016/S0167-5699(00)01628-5
64. van Rood JJ, Loberiza FRJr, Zhang MJ, Oudshoorn M, Claas F, Cairo MS, et al. Effect of tolerance to noninherited maternal antigens on the occurrence of graft-versus-host disease after bone marrow transplantation from a parent or an HLA-haploidentical sibling. *Blood.* (2002) 99:1572–7. doi: 10.1182/blood.V99.5.1572
65. Nijagal A, Fleck S, MacKenzie TC. Maternal microchimerism in patients with biliary atresia: implications for allograft tolerance. *Chimerism.* (2012) 3:37–9. doi: 10.4161/chim.20152
66. Tilburgs T, Scherjon SA, van der Mast BJ, Haasnoot GW, Versteeg VDV-MM, Roelen DL, et al. Fetal-maternal HLA-C mismatch is associated with decidual T cell activation and induction of functional T regulatory cells. *J Reprod Immunol.* (2009) 82:148–57. doi: 10.1016/j.jri.2009.05.003
67. Lashley LE, Haasnoot GW, Spruyt-Gerritse M, Claas FH. Selective advantage of HLA matching in successful uncomplicated oocyte donation pregnancies. *J Reprod Immunol.* (2015) 112:29–33. doi: 10.1016/j.jri.2015.05.006
68. Ranella A, Vassiliadis S, Mastora C, Valentina M, Dionyssopoulou E, Athanassakis I. Constitutive intracellular expression of human leukocyte antigen (HLA)-DO and HLA-DR but not HLA-DM in trophoblast cells. *Hum Immunol.* (2005) 66:43–55. doi: 10.1016/j.humimm.2004.10.002
69. Tersigni C, Redman CW, Dragovic R, Tannetta D, Scambia G, Di Simone N, et al. HLA-DR is aberrantly expressed at fetomaternal interface in pre-eclampsia. *J Reprod Immunol.* (2018) 129:48–52. doi: 10.1016/j.jri.2018.06.024
70. Koelman CA, Coumans AB, Nijman HW, Doxiadis II, Dekker GA, Claas FH. Correlation between oral sex and a low incidence of preeclampsia: a role for soluble HLA in seminal fluid? *J Reprod Immunol.* (2000) 46:155–66. doi: 10.1016/S0165-0378(99)00062-5
71. Larsen MH, Bzorek M, Pass MB, Larsen LG, Nielsen MW, Svendsen SG, et al. Human leukocyte antigen-G in the male reproductive system and in seminal plasma. *Mol Hum Reprod.* (2011) 17:727–38. doi: 10.1093/molehr/gar052
72. Craenmehr MH, Heidt S, Eikmans M, Claas FH. What is wrong with the regulatory T cells and foetomaternal tolerance in women with recurrent miscarriages? *Hla.* (2016) 87:69–78. doi: 10.1111/tan.12737
73. Linscheid C, Petroff MG. Minor histocompatibility antigens and the maternal immune response to the fetus during pregnancy. *Am J Reprod Immunol.* (2013) 69:304–14. doi: 10.1111/aji.12075
74. Chen W, Jin W, Hardegen N, Lei KJ, Li L, Marinos N, et al. Conversion of peripheral CD4+CD25- naive T cells to CD4+CD25+ regulatory T cells by TGF-beta induction of transcription factor Foxp3. *J Exp Med.* (2003) 198:1875–86. doi: 10.1084/jem.20030152
75. Samstein RM, Josefowicz SZ, Arvey A, Treuting PM, Rudensky AY. Extrathymic generation of regulatory T cells in placental mammals mitigates maternal-fetal conflict. *Cell.* (2012) 150:29–38. doi: 10.1016/j.cell.2012.05.031
76. Inada K, Shima T, Ito M, Ushijima A, Saito S. Helios-positive functional regulatory T cells are decreased in decidua of miscarriage cases with normal fetal chromosomal content. *J Reprod Immunol.* (2015) 107:10–9. doi: 10.1016/j.jri.2014.09.053
77. Hsu P, Santner-Nanan B, Dahlstrom JE, Fadia M, Chandra A, Peek M, et al. Altered decidual DC-SIGN+ antigen-presenting cells and impaired regulatory T-cell induction in preeclampsia. *Am J Pathol.* (2012) 181:2149–60. doi: 10.1016/j.ajpath.2012.08.032
78. Zhou J, Wang Z, Zhao X, Wang J, Sun H, Hu Y. An increase of Treg cells in the peripheral blood is associated with a better in vitro fertilization treatment outcome. *Am J Reprod Immunol.* (2012) 68:100–6. doi: 10.1111/j.1600-0897.2012.01153.x
79. Jasper MJ, Tremellen KP, Robertson SA. Primary unexplained infertility is associated with reduced expression of the Tregulatory cell transcription factor Foxp3 in endometrial tissue. *Mol Hum Reprod.* (2006) 12:301–8. doi: 10.1093/molehr/gal032
80. Lu Y, Zhang F, Zhang Y, Zeng B, Hu L, Liao A. Quantitative reduction of peripheral CD_4^+ CD_{25}^+ $FOXP_3^+$ regulatory T cells in reproductive failure after artificial insemination by donor sperm. *Am J Reprod Immunol.* (2013) 69:188–93. doi: 10.1111/aji.12041
81. Tremellen KP, Valbuena D, Landeras J, Ballesteros A, Martinez J, Mendoza S, et al. The effect of intercourse on pregnancy rates during assisted human reproduction. *Hum Reprod.* (2000) 15:2653–8. doi: 10.1093/humrep/15.12.2653
82. Yang H, Qiu L, Chen G, Ye Z, Lu C, Lin Q. Proportional change of CD_4^+ CD_{25}^+ regulatory T cells in decidua and peripheral blood in unexplained recurrent spontaneous abortion patients. *Fertil Steril.* (2008) 89:656–61. doi: 10.1016/j.fertnstert.2007.03.037
83. Mei S, Tan J, Chen H, Chen Y, Zhang J. Changes of CD_4^+ CD_{25}^{high} regulatory T cells and FOXP3 expression in unexplained recurrent spontaneous abortion patients. *Fertil Steril.* (2010) 94:2244–7. doi: 10.1016/j.fertnstert.2009.11.020
84. Wang WJ, Hao CF, Yi L, Yin GJ, Bao SH, Qiu LH, et al. Increased prevalence of T helper 17 (Th17) cells in peripheral blood and decidua in unexplained recurrent spontaneous abortion patients. *J Reprod Immunol.* (2010) 84:164–70. doi: 10.1016/j.jri.2009.12.003
85. Jin LP, Chen QY, Zhang T, Guo PF, Li DJ. The CD4+CD25 bright regulatory T cells and CTLA-4 expression in peripheral and decidual lymphocytes are down-regulated in human miscarriage. *Clin Immunol.* (2009) 133:402–10. doi: 10.1016/j.clim.2009.08.009
86. Wang WJ, Hao CF, Qu QL, Wang X, Qiu LH, Lin QD. The deregulation of regulatory T cells on interleukin-17-producing T helper cells in patients with unexplained early recurrent miscarriage. *Hum Reprod.* (2010) 25:2591–6. doi: 10.1093/humrep/deq198
87. Liu C, Wang XZ, Sun XB. Assessment of sperm antigen specific T regulatory cells in women with recurrent miscarriage. *Early Hum Dev.* (2013) 89:95–100. doi: 10.1016/j.earlhumdev.2012.08.003
88. Arruvito L, Sotelo AI, Billordo A, Fainboim L. A physiological role for inducible FOXP3(+) Treg cells. Lessons from women with reproductive failure. *Clin Immunol.* (2010) 136:432–41. doi: 10.1016/j.clim.2010.05.002
89. Inada K, Shima T, Nakashima A, Aoki K, Ito M, Saito S. Characterization of regulatory T cells in decidua of miscarriage cases with abnormal or normal fetal chromosomal content. *J Reprod Immunol.* (2013) 97:104–11. doi: 10.1016/j.jri.2012.12.001
90. Yamada H, Takeda M, Maezawa Y, Ebina Y, Hazama R, Tanimura K, et al. A high dose intravenous immunoglobulin therapy for women with four or more recurrent spontaneous abortions. *ISRN Obstet Gynecol.* (2012) 2012:512732. doi: 10.5402/2012/512732
91. Winger EE, Reed JL. Treatment with tumor necrosis factor inhibitors and intravenous immunoglobulin improves live birth rates in women with recurrent spontaneous abortion. *Am J Reprod Immunol.* (2008) 60:8–16. doi: 10.1111/j.1600-0897.2008.00585.x
92. Wong LF, Porter TF, Scott JR. Immunotherapy for recurrent miscarriage. *Cochrane Database Syst Rev.* (2014) Cd000112. doi: 10.1002/14651858.CD000112.pub3

93. Redman CW, Sacks GP, Sargent IL. Preeclampsia: an excessive maternal inflammatory response to pregnancy. *Am J Obstet Gynecol.* (1999) 180(Pt 1):499–506.
94. Robillard PY, Hulsey TC, Alexander GR, Keenan A, de Caunes F, Papiernik E. Paternity patterns and risk of preeclampsia in the last pregnancy in multiparae. *J Reprod Immunol.* (1993) 24:1–12.
95. Trupin LS, Simon LP, Eskenazi B. Change in paternity: a risk factor for preeclampsia in multiparas. *Epidemiology.* (1996) 7:240–4.
96. Skjaerven R, Wilcox AJ, Lie RT. The interval between pregnancies and the risk of preeclampsia. *N Engl J Med.* (2002) 346:33–8. doi: 10.1056/NEJMoa011379
97. Klonoff-Cohen HS, Savitz DA, Cefalo RC, McCann MF. An epidemiologic study of contraception and preeclampsia. *JAMA.* (1989) 262:3143–7.
98. Salha O, Sharma V, Dada T, Nugent D, Rutherford AJ, Tomlinson AJ, et al. The influence of donated gametes on the incidence of hypertensive disorders of pregnancy. *Hum Reprod.* (1999) 14:2268–73.
99. Darmochwal-Kolarz D, Saito S, Rolinski J, Tabarkiewicz J, Kolarz B, Leszczynska-Gorzelak B, et al. Activated T lymphocytes in pre-eclampsia. *Am J Reprod Immunol.* (2007) 58:39–45. doi: 10.1111/j.1600-0897.2007.00489.x
100. Sasaki Y, Darmochwal-Kolarz D, Suzuki D, Sakai M, Ito M, Shima T, et al. Proportion of peripheral blood and decidual CD4(+) CD25(bright) regulatory T cells in pre-eclampsia. *Clin Exp Immunol.* (2007) 149:139–45. doi: 10.1111/j.1365-2249.2007.03397.x
101. Toldi G, Svec P, Vasarhelyi B, Meszaros G, Rigo J, Tulassay T, et al. Decreased number of FoxP3+ regulatory T cells in preeclampsia. *Acta Obstet Gynecol Scand.* (2008) 87:1229–33. doi: 10.1080/00016340802389470
102. Miko E, Szereday L, Barakonyi A, Jarkovich A, Varga P, Szekeres-Bartho A. Immunoactivation in preeclampsia: Vδ2+ and regulatory T cells during the inflammatory stage of disease. *J Reprod Immunol.* (2009) 80:100–8. doi: 10.1016/j.jri.2009.01.003
103. Santner-Nanan B, Peek MJ, Khanam R, Richarts L, Zhu E, Fazekas de St Groth B, et al. Systemic increase in the ratio between Foxp3+ and IL-17-producing CD4+ T cells in healthy pregnancy but not in preeclampsia. *J Immunol.* (2009) 183:7023–30. doi: 10.4049/jimmunol.0901154
104. Toldi G, Rigo J Jr, Stenczer B, Vasarhelyi B, Molvarec A. Increased prevalence of IL-17-producing peripheral blood lymphocytes in pre-eclampsia. *Am J Reprod Immunol.* (2011) 66:223–9. doi: 10.1111/j.1600-0897.2011.00987.x
105. Darmochwal-Kolarz D, Kludka-Sternik M, Tabarkiewicz J, Kolarz B, Rolinski J, Leszczynska-Gorzelak B, et al. The predominance of Th17 lymphocytes and decreased number and function of Treg cells in preeclampsia. *J Reprod Immunol.* (2012) 93:75–81. doi: 10.1016/j.jri.2012.01.006
106. Zeng B, Kwak-Kim J, Liu Y, Liao AH. Treg cells are negatively correlated with increased memory B cells in pre-eclampsia while maintaining suppressive function on autologous B-cell proliferation. *Am J Reprod Immunol.* (2013) 70:454–63. doi: 10.1111/aji.12154
107. Moreno-Eutimio MA, Tovar-Rodriguez JM, Vargas-Avila K, Nieto-Velazquez NG, Frias-De-Leon MG, Sierra-Martinez M, et al. Increased serum levels of inflammatory mediators and low frequency of regulatory T cells in the peripheral blood of preeclamptic Mexican women. *Biomed Res Int.* (2014) 2014:413249. doi: 10.1155/2014/413249
108. Toldi G, Vasarhelyi ZE, Rigo J Jr, Orban C, Tamassy Z, Bajnok A, et al. Prevalence of Regulatory T-Cell Subtypes in Preeclampsia. *Am J Reprod Immunol.* (2015) 74:110–15. doi: 10.1111/aji.12380
109. Darmochwal-Kolarz D, Saito S, Tabarkiewicz J, Kolarz B, Rolinski J, Leszczynska-Gorzelak B, et al. Apoptosis signaling is altered in CD4(+)CD25(+)FoxP3(+) T regulatory lymphocytes in pre-eclampsia. *Int J Mol Sci.* (2012) 13:6548–60. doi: 10.3390/ijms13066548

9

The Placental Response to Guinea Pig Cytomegalovirus Depends Upon the Timing of Maternal Infection

Zachary W. Berkebile[1], *Dira S. Putri*[1], *Juan E. Abrahante*[2], *Davis M. Seelig*[3], *Mark R. Schleiss*[1] *and Craig J. Bierle*[1*]

[1] Department of Pediatrics, Division of Pediatric Infectious Diseases, University of Minnesota, Minneapolis, MN, United States, [2] Informatics Institute, University of Minnesota, Minneapolis, MN, United States, [3] Department of Veterinary Clinical Sciences, University of Minnesota, Minneapolis, MN, United States

***Correspondence:**
Craig J. Bierle
cjbierle@umn.edu

Human cytomegalovirus (HCMV) infects the placenta, and these placental infections can cause fetal injury and/or demise. The timing of maternal HCMV infection during pregnancy is a determinant of fetal outcomes, but how development affects the placenta's susceptibility to infection, the likelihood of placental injury post-infection, and the frequency of transplacental HCMV transmission remains unclear. In this study, guinea pig cytomegalovirus (GPCMV) was used to model primary maternal infection and compare the effects of infection at two different times on the placenta. When guinea pigs were infected with GPCMV at either 21- or 35-days gestation (dGA), maternal and placental viral loads, as determined by droplet digital PCR, were not significantly affected by the timing of maternal infection. However, when the transcriptomes of gestational age-matched GPCMV-infected and control placentas were compared, significant infection-associated changes in gene expression were only observed after maternal infection at 35 dGA. Notably, transcripts associated with immune activation (e.g. *Cxcl10*, *Ido1*, *Tgtp1*, and *Tlr8*) were upregulated in the infected placenta. A GPCMV-specific *in situ* hybridization assay detected rare infected cells in the main placenta after maternal infection at either time, and maternal infection at 35 dGA also caused large areas of GPCMV-infected cells in the junctional zone. As GPCMV infection after mid-gestation is known to cause high rates of stillbirth and/or fetal growth restriction, our results suggest that the placenta becomes sensitized to infection-associated injury late in gestation, conferring an increased risk of adverse pregnancy outcomes after cytomegalovirus infection.

Keywords: cytomegalovirus, congenital infection, inflammation, placenta, fetal membranes, guinea pig

INTRODUCTION

Congenital cytomegalovirus infection (cCMV), a leading cause of sensorineural hearing loss and neurocognitive disability in children, occurs in roughly 1 in 200 pregnancies (1–3). cCMV is also a cause of intrauterine growth restriction, preterm birth, and fetal demise (4–8). The timing of maternal human cytomegalovirus (HCMV) infection during pregnancy affects the rate of congenital transmission and fetal outcomes post-infection (9–18). Neurologic sequelae are most frequently observed in congenitally infected children when maternal infection occurs in the first trimester (14–17). Maternal infection late in pregnancy is associated with the highest rates of intrauterine growth restriction (IUGR) and congenital infection (9–13, 15, 18).

HCMV infects the placenta and these placental infections can cause fetal injury, including spontaneous abortion and neonatal demise, even in the absence of detectable viral transmission to the fetus (4, 5, 19–22). HCMV-associated placental pathology includes chronic villitis, cytomegalic cells, and areas of necrosis and calcification (19, 22–24). HCMV was detected in 15% of fetal remains and/or placenta after stillbirth and infection was found to be associated with fetal thrombotic vasculopathy (4). In a cohort of women with a prenatal diagnosis of fetal growth restriction, the detection of HCMV antigen in the placenta correlated with higher rates of villitis and more severe growth restriction than cases of IUGR without HCMV involvement (21). While HCMV appears to cause a hypoxia-like condition in infected placenta, how HCMV causes placental dysfunction remains poorly understood (22).

HCMV and other viruses may injure the placenta either directly by causing cytopathic effects in infected cells or by activating the maternal or fetal immune system and triggering placental immunopathology (25). Dysmature villi were frequently observed in HCMV-infected placentas, suggesting that infection can interfere with early placental development (19). Trophoblast progenitor cells can be infected by HCMV, and HCMV infection both limits the capacity of trophoblast progenitors to differentiate *in vitro* and disrupts the formation of anchoring villi in first trimester placental explants (26–28). The inflammatory response to viral infection during pregnancy can also cause placental dysfunction and adverse pregnancy outcomes (29). For example, type I interferon signaling triggered by Zika virus can cause abnormal placental development in mice and syncytial knot formation in villous explants (30). cCMV causes a proinflammatory cytokine bias in the placenta and amniotic fluid, but whether this host response disrupts normal placental function has yet to be determined (31, 32).

As the species-specificity of HCMV precludes its study in animals, guinea pig cytomegalovirus (GPCMV) has become the most widely used experimental model of cCMV (33, 34). Guinea pigs deliver precocious pups after gestational periods that average 65 days. Similarities between guinea pigs and humans include hemomonochorial placentas that invade deeply into the decidua and the prenatal development of major organs and the immune system (35–37). These similarities between human and guinea pig placentation and development make the rodent a uniquely powerful comparative model for understanding the developmental origins of health and disease (35). GPCMV infection studies have revealed that placental and fetal infection occur sequentially after maternal inoculation (34, 38–41). If maternal infection occurs early in pregnancy, infectious virus may not be detected in pup organs and evidence of prior fetal infection can be limited to the presence of infection-associated histologic lesions in pup organs (41–43). Maternal GPCMV infection after mid-gestation has been found to cause high rates of stillbirth and IUGR in pups (42–44).

In this study, we investigated whether the susceptibility and antiviral responses of the placenta to GPCMV infection varied across gestation. Time mated guinea pigs were infected either at 21 days gestation (dGA, "early") or at 35 dGA ("late"). No significant differences in maternal or placental viral loads were noted between the two groups at 21 days post-infection (dpi). However, infection after mid-gestation caused more frequent fetal membrane infections and significant changes in placental gene expression that were not observed after infection at the earlier time point. Furthermore, *in situ* hybridization revealed that GPCMV infection primarily localized to the junctional zone after maternal infection at the later time. Our observations lead us to propose that GPCMV-associated stillbirth and IUGR are the result of developmentally regulated changes in the placenta that predispose the organ to infection-associated injury late in gestation.

MATERIALS AND METHODS

Cells and Virus

A minimally tissue culture adapted stock of GPCMV 22122 (ATCC VR-682), prepared as previously described by passaging guinea pig salivary gland homogenate twice on JH4 guinea pig lung fibroblasts (ATCC CCL-158), was used for this study (33, 45, 46). JH4 cells were purchased from ATCC and propagated according to their specifications excepting that the growth media was supplemented with sodium bicarbonate (47). GPCMV stocks were prepared as previously described and titered on JH4 cells (48). For animal studies, virus was aliquoted into single-use units, flash-frozen, and stored at -80°C. These aliquots were routinely re-titered as guinea pigs were infected to confirm that the stock did not deteriorate during storage.

Ethics Statement

All animal procedures were conducted in accordance with protocols approved by the Institutional Animal Care and Use Committee (IACUC) at the University of Minnesota, Minneapolis (Protocol ID: 1810-36403A). Experimental protocols and endpoints were developed in strict accordance to the National Institutes of Health Office of Laboratory Animal Welfare (Animal Welfare Assurance #A3456-01), Public Health Service Policy on Humane Care and Use of Laboratory Animals, and United States Department of Agriculture Animal Welfare Act guidelines and regulations (USDA Registration # 41-R-0005) with the oversight and approval of the IACUC. Outbred Hartley guinea pigs were initially purchased from Elm Hill Laboratories (Chelmsford, MA). Breeding pairs of strain 2 and strain 13 guinea pigs were generously shared by MS and the U.S. Army Medical Research Institute of Infectious Diseases, respectively. Guinea pigs were housed in a facility maintained by the University of Minnesota Research Animal Resources, who were accredited through the Association for Assessment and Accreditation of Laboratory Animal Care, International (AAALAC). All procedures were conducted by trained personnel under the supervision of veterinary staff.

Animal Pathogenicity Study

The GPCMV serostatus of all animals received from an external source was tested by ELISA within one week of receipt and again after one month of housing at the University of Minnesota (49). Only GPCMV seronegative animals were used for infection studies. Female guinea pigs were bred at two to three months of age. After the delivery of their first litter, the animals were bred a second time during postpartum estrus to establish timed pregnancies by housing with a male for three days postpartum. These second pregnancies were confirmed by progesterone ELISA (DRG International); only animals with plasma progesterone concentrations exceeding 15 ng/ml by 20 days postpartum were included in this study (50).

At either 21 (range 18 to 23) or 35 (range 33 to 35) dGA guinea pigs were injected subcutaneously into the scruff of the neck with 0.5 ml of PBS containing $2x10^5$ PFU of GPCMV or PBS alone. Blood and plasma were collected from dams every seven days post-infection (dpi) until they were euthanized at 14, 21, or 28 dpi. After euthanasia, blood and plasma were collected from the dams and amniotic fluid was collected from the pups. Pup tissue samples were divided and frozen for DNA extraction, stabilized in RNAlater (ThermoFisher) for RNA extraction, embedded in optimal cutting temperature (O.C.T.) compound (Fisher Scientific), or immersion-fixed using Shandon Formal-Fixx (ThermoFisher) and embedded in paraffin.

Viral Load Quantification by Droplet Digital PCR

After DNA was extracted from whole blood, tissue, and amniotic fluid, GPCMV genomes were quantified by droplet digital PCR (ddPCR) using primers and probes specific to *GP54* using the Bio-Rad QX200 system as previously described (46). ddPCR results were analyzed using the QuantaSoft™ Analysis Pro software (Bio-Rad); GPCMV viral loads are presented as the number of copies genome per ml of fluid or mg of tissue.

RNA Sequencing

RNA was extracted from guinea pig placentas that had been stabilized in RNAlater (ThermoFisher) and stored at -20°C using the RNAeasy Mini Kit (Qiagen). ~30 mg pieces of placenta were combined with 0.6 ml of β-mercaptoethanol-containing RLT buffer and Lysing Matrix D (MP Biomedicals) and pulsed at 6 m/s for 30 seconds in a FastPrep 24 (MP Biomedicals). RNA was extracted from 0.45 ml of the resulting homogenate using the manufacturer's standard protocol, including the optional on-column DNase I digest (Qiagen), Total RNA integrity was assessed by capillary electrophoresis using an Agilent TapeStation; all samples used for library creation had RNA integrity numbers that exceeded 7.0.

Dual indexed TruSeq stranded mRNA libraries were prepared and sequenced using a NextSeq 550 high-output 75-bp single-end run (mean of $22.4x10^6$ reads/sample). FastQ reads were trimmed using Trimmomatic (v 0.33) enabled with the optional "-q" option; 3bp sliding-window trimming from 3' end requiring minimum Q30 (51). Quality control on raw sequence data for each sample was performed with FastQC. Read mapping was performed *via* Hisat2 (v2.1.0) using the "Cavpor3.0" genome (GCF_000151735.1) as reference (52). Gene quantification was done *via* Cuffquant for FPKM values and Feature Counts for raw read counts (53, 54). Differentially expressed genes were identified using the edgeR (negative binomial) feature in CLCGWB (Qiagen) using raw read counts (55). The generated list was filtered based on a minimum 2X Absolute Fold Change and False Discovery Rate corrected $p < 0.05$. Raw and processed RNA-Seq data have been deposited in NCBI's Gene Expression Omnibus and are accessible through GEO Series accession number GSE169358 (56). Normalized gene expression data (FPKM) was uploaded to ClustVis for data visualization and heat map analysis (57). Gene Ontology (GO) analysis was performed by uploading a list of differentially expressed transcripts to g:Profiler (58). Results from this GO analysis were visualized using Cytoscape, Enrichment Map, ClusterMaker2, and WordCloud (59–63).

Real-Time Droplet Digital PCR Analyses

RNA was extracted from placenta as described above. A two-step reverse transcriptase ddPCR (RT-ddPCR) protocol was used to quantify transcript abundance (46). cDNA was synthesized from total RNA using the Maxima™ H Minus cDNA Synthesis Master Mix (ThermoFisher). PCR primers targeting guinea pig transcripts were designed using the Primer Quest tool and were ordered from Integrated DNA Technologies (**Table S2**). ddPCR reactions were prepared using the EvaGreen Digital PCR Supermix (Bio-Rad) using a primer concentration of 250 nM and cycled using the following thermal conditions: 95°C for 5 min; 40 cycles of 95°C for 30 s and 60°C for 30s; 4°C for 5 min; 90°C for 5 min; hold at 4°C. The ddPCR data were analyzed with QuantaSoft™ Analysis Pro software (Bio-Rad). Absolute quantification of gene expression was presented as copies per nanogram of total RNA.

In Situ Hybridization

5-µm sections of paraffin-embedded placenta were mounted onto Superfrost Plus slides (ThermoFisher). After air drying the tissue sections overnight, the slides were baked at 60°C for 1 hr. Tissue was deparaffinized and pretreated using the recommended protocol for RNAscope® 2.5 Assays (ACD Document #322452). For target retrieval, samples were incubated at 99°C for 15 minutes, and the slides were treated with RNAscope Protease Plus for 30 minutes. Slides were stained using either the RNAscope 2.5 HD Detection Reagent - RED (ACD Document # 322360-USM) or the RNAscope 2.5 HD Duplex Reagent (322500-USM) and the RNAscope Probe V-CavHV-2-gp3. Stained slides were scanned using a Huron TissueScope LE and the number of *gp3+* foci and areas of *gp3*-staining were counted and calculated using NIS-Elements BR (Nikon).

RESULTS

The Timing of Maternal GPCMV Infection Affects the Rate of Fetal Membrane Infection but Not Placental Viral Loads

To study how the timing of maternal GPCMV infection affects viral loads in the placenta, extraplacental membranes, and fetus, guinea pigs were time mated during postpartum estrus and infected at either 21 or 35 days gestation (dGA) (**Figure 1**). HCMV infection during the first trimester causes most cases of neurologic disability in congenitally infected children, and infecting guinea pigs at 21 dGA exposes the pup and placenta to virus during a comparable period of late embryonic/early fetal development (14–17, 65). GPCMV infection after mid-gestation has been found to often cause fetal growth restriction and/or stillbirth (42–44). As high rates of ischemic injury and virus-specific focal necrosis and inflammation had been reported 21 days after maternal infection at 30 dGA, we elected to infect animals at 35 dGA and analyze matched pups and placentas at 21 dpi, before expected still- or preterm birth, to identify mechanisms that could cause these adverse pregnancy outcomes (39).

Five groups of animals were used in this study. Three groups of Hartley guinea pigs were infected at 21 dGA and euthanized at either 14, 21, or 28 dpi. The remaining two groups were inbred strain 2 females bred with strain 13 males to create hybrid pregnancies (2X13) and were infected with GPCMV at either at 21 or 35 dGA and euthanized at 21 dpi (66). This study compared GPCMV pathogenesis between the outbred and inbred guinea pigs and examined the effect of maternal infection at the two different times on the placenta. Most prior GPCMV research has been done in Hartley guinea pigs, and the few studies that compared GPCMV infection between inbred and outbred guinea pigs have yielded conflicting results as to whether strain 2 or strain 13 animals are more susceptible to infection than Hartley guinea pigs (67–69).

Guinea pigs were infected with $2X10^5$ PFU of GPCMV or mock-infected by subcutaneous injection. While Hartley dams were on-average larger than strain 2 females, no differences in maternal weight gain were noted between GPCMV-infected and control dams (**Figure S1**). Maternal blood and serum were collected weekly until each animal's predetermined endpoint. GPCMV viral load was quantified using a droplet digital PCR (ddPCR) assay targeting *GP54* (46). When maternal viremia at 7 dpi and viral loads in spleen were quantified, infection was confirmed in all dams and no significant differences were noted between the five groups (**Table S1** and **Figure S2A**).

The placentas from the two groups of guinea pigs that were infected at 21 dGA and euthanized at 21 dpi were compared, and significantly higher viral loads were detected in the strain 2X13 placentas than in their Hartley counterparts (Mann–Whitney U test, P<0.0001) (**Figure 2A**). No other significant differences in placental viral load were noted in the remaining groups. When viral loads were assessed in the extraplacental membranes, GPCMV was detected in both the amnion and visceral yolk sac (**Table 1** and **Figure S2B**) (46). A significant correlation (Pearson r=0.5056, $p<0.001$) in GPCMV viral loads was observed in the amnion and yolk sac of individual fetuses (**Figure 2B**). The highest frequencies of fetal membrane infection and the highest viral loads in the membranes were observed in the dams infected at 35 dGA. GPCMV was only detected in a handful of amniotic fluid samples collected from guinea pigs infected at 35 dGA, consistent with previous observations that GPCMV generally does not accumulate in amniotic fluid (43, 46, 69).

Fetal infection was assayed by quantifying viral loads in the brain. GPCMV was most often detected at 14 dpi and occasionally at later times post-infection. As the brain is less frequently infected by GPCMV than other fetal tissues, these results may underreport the actual rate of congenital GPCMV infection in this experiment and/or indicate that fetal infections resolved *in utero* (42, 43). The fetuses of GPCMV infected dams trended smaller than their mock-infected counterparts in most cases (**Table S1** and **Figure S2C**). However, due in part to unexpectedly large variation in litter sizes, this study was underpowered to determine whether GPCMV caused fetal growth restriction. Guinea pigs bred during postpartum estrus had significantly larger litters than expected, including many large litters of 6-8 pups, and fetal weights correlate with litter size after mid-gestation (37).

To summarize, our animal studies found that maternal infection at 35 dGA resulted in higher rates of fetal membrane

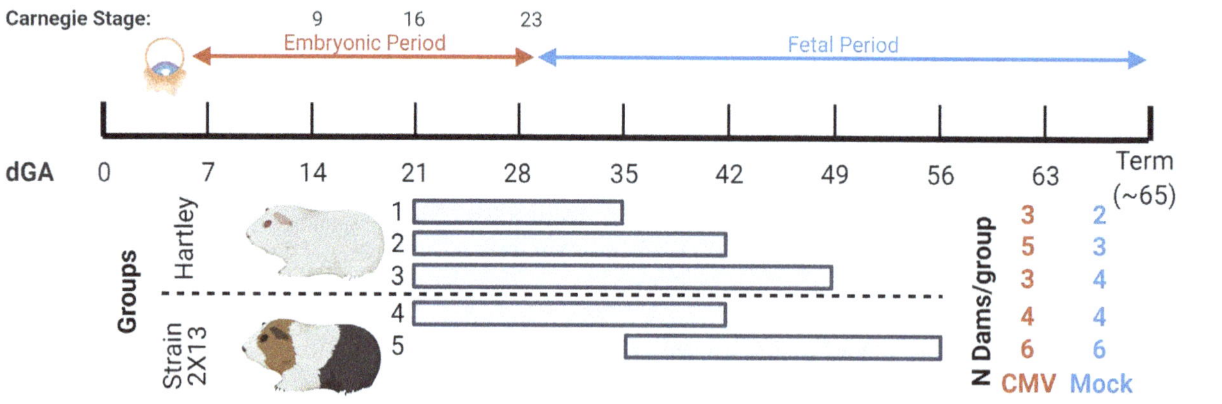

FIGURE 1 | Summary of GPCMV infections in time mated guinea pigs. The ~65-day gestational period of guinea pigs is diagramed. Implantation occurs at 5-6 dGA and the embryonic period ends at 29 dGA. Reference Carnegie stages for guinea pig development are indicated (64). Five groups of GPCMV-infected and control guinea pigs were used in this study, including outbred Hartley guinea pigs and inbred strain 2 females that were bred to strain 13 males (producing semi-allogenic, hybrid pregnancies). Guinea pigs were infected either at 21 dGA (embryonic period) or at 35 dGA (fetal period). The number of GPCMV- and mock-infected dams for each group is shown. Figure created with BioRender.com.

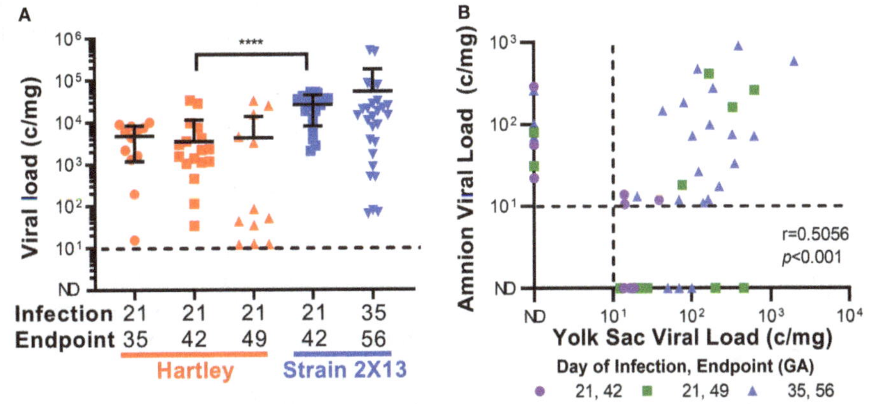

FIGURE 2 | GPCMV viral loads after maternal infection during pregnancy. Time mated guinea pigs were infected at either 21 or 35 dGA with $2X10^5$ PFU of GPCMV and euthanized 14, 21, or 28 days later. DNA was extracted from tissues and GPCMV viral loads were determined using a ddPCR assay specific to *GP54*. The limit of detection for this assay is indicated by the dashed line. **(A)** Viral load in placentas. Significantly higher viral loads (Mann-Whitney test, **** $p < 0.0001$) were observed in the placentas of strain 2X13 hybrids than in the placentas of Hartley guinea pigs. **(B)** Viral loads in infected fetal membranes. The number of GPCMV genome copies detected in the amnion and visceral yolk sac of individual fetuses was significantly correlated (Pearson r=0.5056, $p < 0.001$).

TABLE 1 | Summary of GPCMV viral load data.

Strain	dGA of infection, endpoint	Placenta		Amnion		Yolk Sac		Fetus[3]	AF[4]
		CMV+[1]	MVL[2]	CMV+[1]	MVL[2]	CMV+[1]	MVL[2]	CMV+[1]	CMV+[1]
Hartley	21,35	12/12	$5.7x10^3$	0/10	N/A	0/10	N/A	9/10	0/10
	21,42	17/29	$6.0x10^3$	4/29	$1.5x10^1$	4/28	$2.0x10^1$	9/29	0/29
	21,49	12/19	$6.8x10^3$	6/19	$1.6x10^2$	11/19	$1.8x10^2$	9/19	0/18
2X13	21,42	18/19	$2.8x10^4$	2/18	$1.7x10^2$	2/18	$1.7x10^1$	0/18	0/18
	35,56	27/27	$5.4x10^4$	18/24	$1.8x10^2$	22/24	$2.5x10^2$	4/27	4/21

[1]*Samples containing detectable GPCMV DNA/total number of samples.*
[2]*Mean viral load (MVL) expressed as copies/ml for infected blood and amniotic fluid or copies/mg for infected tissue.*
[3]*Viral load in fetal brain quantified.*
[4]*Amniotic fluid.*

infection and higher viral loads in the amnion and yolk sac than infection at 21 dGA. However, neither the timing of maternal infection nor the experimental endpoint had a significant effect on placental viral load. Higher viral loads were noted in placentas from our strain 2X13 hybrid pregnancies when compared to Hartley guinea pigs, but there was no other evidence that indicated that infection was more severe in the inbred animals. Presuming that there would be minimal animal-to-animal variation in the placental response to infection in guinea pigs with a consistent maternal and fetal genetic background, we focused on the strain 2X13 animals in our subsequent analysis of the effect of infection on placental function.

GPCMV Infection After Mid-Gestation Significantly Alters Placental Gene Expression

Having found that the timing of maternal GPCMV infection did not affect placental viral loads, we next compared how infection at our earlier and later time point affected placental gene expression. For this analysis, placentas were randomly selected from inbred guinea pigs that had been GPCMV- or mock-infected either at 21 or 35 dGA and euthanized at 21 dpi. RNA was extracted from four placentas from four GPCMV-infected dams and four placentas from three control dams per group and sequenced (**Table S1**). A principal component analysis of RNA-Seq data revealed that the samples clustered based upon the gestational age of placenta (**Figure 3A**). GPCMV- infected and control placenta from the early infection groups clustered tightly, while there was clear separation between GPCMV- and mock-infected samples after maternal infection at 35 dGA. Pairwise gene expression comparisons between age-matched groups of GPCMV and mock-infected tissues affirmed these findings. GPCMV infection at 21 dGA had a limited effect on placental gene expression at 21 dpi: only 8 transcripts were differentially regulated (≥2 fold, $p < 0.05$). In contrast, maternal infection at 35 dGA resulted in the differential regulation of 126 transcripts (≥2 fold, $p < 0.05$) at 21 dpi. A gene set enrichment analysis was performed on the transcripts that were differentially expressed after GPCMV infection late in pregnancy (58). This analysis found that several gene ontology terms related to the immune response (including GO:0002376, immune system process) were significantly enriched after GPCMV infection at 35 dGA (**Figure S3A**).

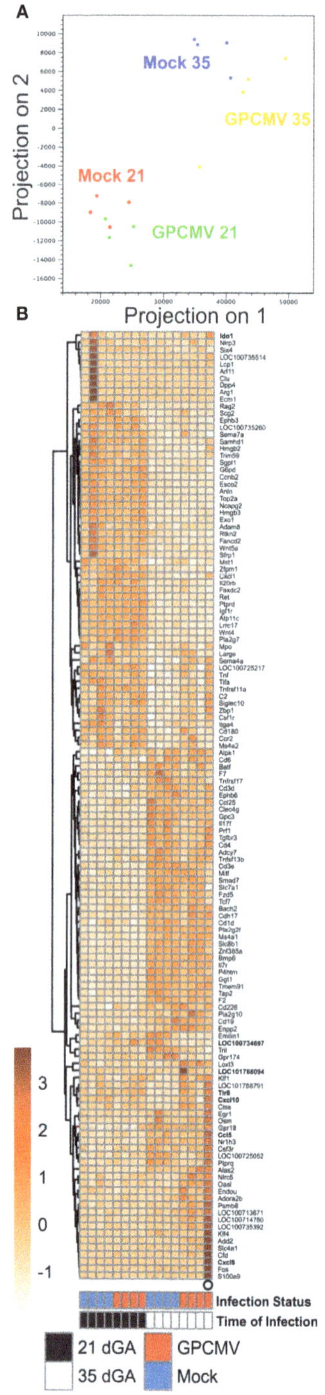

FIGURE 3 | Transcriptome profiling of GPCMV-infected placenta. Time mated guinea pigs were GPCMV- or mock-infected at 21 or 35 dGA and euthanized 21 days later. RNA was extracted from placentas (N=4/group) and gene expression was quantified by Illumina RNA-Seq. **(A)** Principal component analysis illustrating the similarity in gene expression between samples. **(B)** Heat map illustrating the relative expression of transcripts that function as part of an immune system processes (GO:0002376) that were differentially expressed in placenta either during normal development or after GPCMV infection. Transcripts that were also analyzed by RT-ddPCR are shown in bold.

In a pairwise gene expression analysis that compared the two groups of mock-infected placentas, the gestational age of placentas was found to have a much more significant effect on gene expression than GPCMV infection: 1438 transcripts were differentially regulated (≥2 fold, $p < 0.05$) between the two groups of control tissue. Gene ontogeny analysis found numerous terms related to the regulation of the mitotic cell, signaling receptor activity, and condensed chromosome regions were enriched in this pairwise comparison (**Figure S3B**). Many of the gene expression differences between normal placenta from 42 and 56 dGA appear to be related to the relatively higher expression of transcripts involved in cell division and the cell cycle by the younger tissue. While transcripts that function as part of an immune system process were not found to be significantly enriched in our comparison of normal placentas, 116 transcripts related to the immune response were differentially expressed between the two groups (**Figure 3B**, **Table S3**). We hypothesize that these normal changes in placental immunity may cause GPCMV infection after mid-gestation to significantly affect placental gene expression.

As only four samples of placenta per group were analyzed by RNA-seq, sample-to-sample variation in gene expression could be caused either by regional differences in transcription in the relatively large guinea pig placenta or represent the unique responses of individual fetuses to GPCMV infection. To better elucidate host factors that regulate the placenta's response to GPCMV, we used reverse transcriptase droplet digital PCR (RT-ddPCR) to measure the expression of select transcripts that function as part of the inflammatory response in additional placenta samples. For this experiment, RNA was extracted from two placentas per dam (including the samples that had been previously analyzed by RNA-Seq). RT-ddPCR confirmed that four genes– *Cxcl10*, *Ido1*, *Tgtp1*, and *Tlr8*–were significantly upregulated after maternal infection at 35 dGA when compared to age-matched control placentas (**Figure 4**). This analysis also found that *Cxcl10* and *Ido1* are normally downregulated as the guinea pig placenta matures and that GPCMV infection at 21 dGA leads to decreased *Ido1* expression relative to age-matched normal placenta. RT-ddPCR analysis did not support the RNA-Seq finding that several other inflammatory mediators—*Ccl5*, *Ccl15-l*, *Cxcl8*, *Il1b*, and *Il36b-l*—were differentially regulated by maternal GPCMV infection at 35 dGA (**Figure S4**). In the case of *Cxcl8* and *Il1b*, high levels of cytokine transcription were noted in the placenta of a dam that had been euthanized while delivering stillborn pups at 56 dGA (these placentas are represented as open circles in **Figures 3**, **4**, and **Figure S4**). The elevated transcription of these cytokines may not be specific to GPCMV infection and instead be inflammatory markers of preterm labor or *in utero* fetal demise (70, 71). Cumulatively, our gene expression analyses of GPCMV-infected placenta suggest that the immune response is dysregulated by GPCMV infection after mid-gestation but not after infection earlier in pregnancy.

The Junctional Zone Becomes Infected by GPCMV After Maternal Infection After Mid-Gestation

Finally, we compared the frequency and localization of GPCMV-infected cells in the placenta using *in situ* hybridization. For this

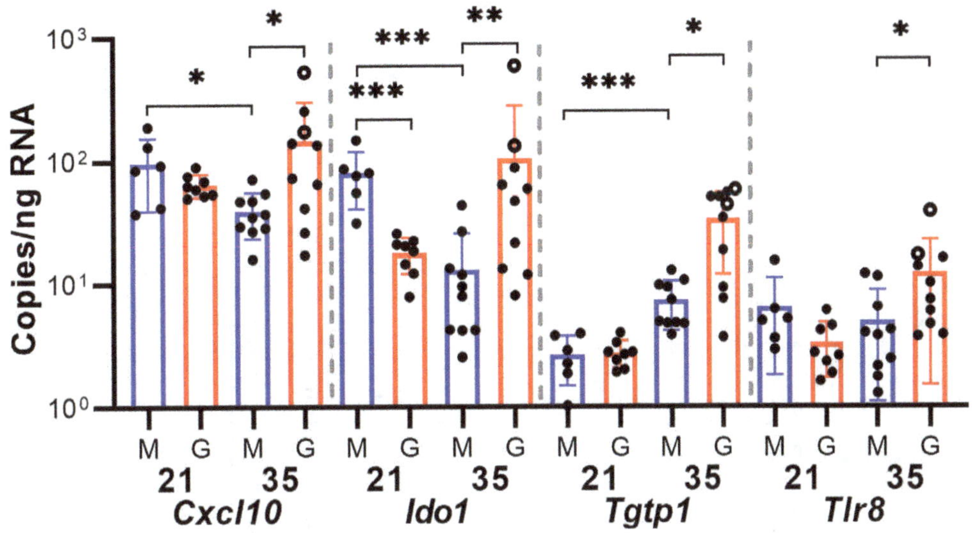

FIGURE 4 | GPCMV infection dysregulates immune gene transcription. A two-step RT-ddPCR protocol was used to quantify the expression of select transcripts in GPCMV- (G) and mock-infected (M) placentas after maternal infection at either 21 or 35 dGA. Data from two placentas per dam is shown. Statistically significant differences were calculated by Mann-Whitney test (*$p < 0.05$, **$p < 0.01$, ***$p < 0.001$).

study, we designed an RNAscope probe specific to the GPCMV transcript *gp3*. RNA-Seq analysis had revealed that *gp3* is highly expressed during all phases of GPCMV replication (**Figure S5**) (46). *gp3*+ foci, each representing either an individual infected cell or a group of infected cells, were manually counted in stained placenta sections (**Figure 5**). A small number of *gp3*+ foci were observed in the interlobium and labyrinth of all GPCMV-infected placenta (**Figure 5C**). When the placentas of dams infected at 21 and 35 dGA were compared, significantly more GPCMV infected cells were noted in the margin of placentas, including either the parietal yolk sac or marginal syncytium, after infection at the later time. Large areas of *gp3*+ cells were detected in the junctional zone in eight of ten of the placentas from the late infection group (**Figures 5A, B, D**). These large areas of GPCMV-infected cells were often adjacent to either the subplacenta or large blood vessels and were never detected after maternal infection at 21 dGA. Whether GPCMV infection of the junctional zone reflects the recruitment of infected cells to the placenta late in pregnancy or if there is a cell type in this region that becomes permissive to GPCMV infection as the placenta matures remains to be determined.

DISCUSSION

The timing of HCMV infection during pregnancy is a determinant of fetal outcomes, yet how placental development affects the course and severity of cCMV remains poorly understood (25, 72). Using the GPCMV model, we assessed how the placenta and fetal membranes are differentially affected by maternal infection at two times: 21 and 35 dGA. Prior research has found that GPCMV infection early in pregnancy can resolve prenatally while infection after mid-gestation often causes stillbirth and fetal growth restriction (42–44). Our study identified several possible explanations for these adverse pregnancy outcomes, including an increased rate of fetal membrane and junctional zone infection late in gestation and a transcriptional response to GPCMV that may indicate that placental immunopathology only occurs after maternal infection at later times in pregnancy.

This study found that GPCMV infects both the amnion and the yolk sack, that viral loads in the two membranes are correlated, and that the highest rates of infection and viral loads in the membranes occur after maternal infection late in pregnancy (46). While GPCMV joins HCMV on a short list of viruses that have been observed to infect the fetal membranes, it remains unclear whether or how viral infections of the fetal membrane affect the fetus (24, 73). In contrast, ascending bacterial infections, a significant cause of preterm labor, have a much better understood effect on fetal membrane physiology. Bacterial infection, treatment with inflammatory cytokines, or exposure to pathogen-associated molecular patterns can all trigger preterm labor in animal models and/or cause fetal membrane explants to biomechanically weaken *ex vivo* (71, 74–76). Several studies have suggested that viral infection may sensitize the fetal membranes to later damage from bacteria (77–79). It has also been hypothesized that fetal membrane infection may allow viruses to circumvent the potent antiviral defense of the placenta to infect the fetus (80). In this paraplacental route of infection, viruses that infect the chorioamnion may be shed into amniotic fluid and infect the fetus. Given that this study's primary focus was on the effect of infection on the placenta, future experiments that specifically analyze the effect of GPCMV on the fetal membranes are merited.

Developmentally programmed changes in maternal, placental, and fetal immunity are critical for healthy

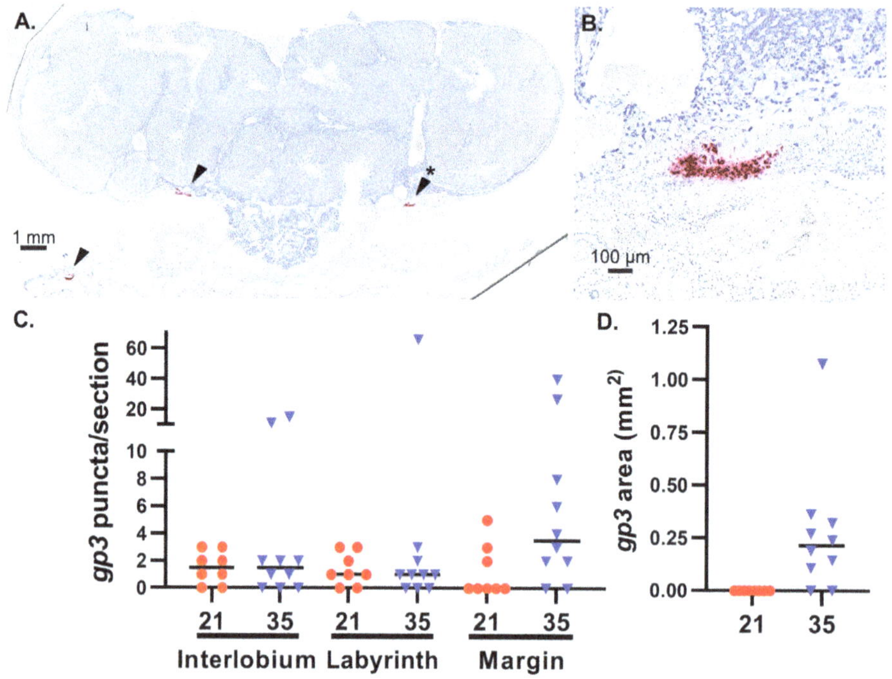

FIGURE 5 | GPCMV localization in infected placenta. An RNAscope probe specific to GPCMV *gp3* was used to detect infected cells in sections of placenta by *in situ* hybridization. **(A)** A representative section of a placenta from a dam infected at 35 dGA, illustrating large areas of GPCMV infected cells in the junctional zone and decidua (red, indicated by arrows). **(B)** High-magnification image of infected cells in the junctional zone (*). **(C)** *gp3*+ puncta, representing individual infected cells or small groups of infected cells, were counted based on their localization in the placenta after maternal infection at 21 or 35 dGA and collection at 21 dpi. **(D)** The measured area of *gp3*+ stained cells in the junctional zone of placentas is shown.

pregnancy, helping to establish and maintain maternal-fetal tolerance, remodel the uterus, and regulate parturition (30, 71). Alterations in maternal immunity can increase the severity of viral infections late in pregnancy (81). Severe, third-trimester infections caused by viruses such as influenza and hepatitis E can cause fetal injury or demise. High rates of maternal demise have been reported in some GPCMV infection studies (38, 82). However, HCMV infections are typically mild and there is no evidence that the virus causes more severe illness in pregnant individuals (83). We found that the timing of maternal GPCMV infection did not significantly affect maternal, placental, or fetal viral loads, and severe illness was not noted in dams that had been infected at the later time. Having eliminated severe maternal illnesses as a cause of adverse pregnancy outcomes in our experiments, the remainder of this study focused on the placental response to GPCMV infection.

Prior work in placental cells and explants has found that gestational age affects how permissive the cells or tissue are to viral infection and the nature of the inflammatory response that is triggered by infection (84, 85). Our study found that maternal infection at 35 dGA significantly altered placental gene expression while infection at 21 dGA had remarkably little effect on placental gene expression. Infection after mid-gestation upregulated numerous transcripts that function as part of an immune system process. Two transcripts that are dysregulated by placental GPCMV infection, *Cxcl10* and *Ido1*, are particularly relevant to the pathogenesis of cCMV. CXCL10, a biomarker of VUE, chronic chorioamnionitis, and late preterm birth, is found at elevated concentrations in amniotic fluid and maternal sera during cCMV (31, 86–89). Curiously, while the concentration of CXCL10 in amniotic fluid correlates with CMV genome abundance, the chemokine does not appear to accumulate in amniotic fluid when other viruses cause intrauterine infections (32). We and others have found that CXCL10 transcription is upregulated when placental cells or tissue are infected with HCMV or GPCMV *in vitro* (46, 84, 85). Indoleamine-2,3-dioxygenase (IDO) is an enzyme that is encoded by two genes, *IDO1* and *IDO2*, that catalyze the rate-limiting step in tryptophan catabolism. IDO production by the placenta and the subsequent metabolism of tryptophan prevents the rejection of the allogeneic fetus by suppressing T cell proliferation and activity (90). IDO is more highly expressed by the human placenta during the first-trimester than at term and HCMV infection suppressed IDO expression in early placenta (91). While our gene expression analysis was limited to a single time point post-infection, GPCMV may cause placental immunopathology but only after maternal infection relatively late in pregnancy.

In an analysis of placental pathology after GPCMV infection, pregnant Hartley guinea pigs were inoculated with GPCMV at 30 dGA. Infection caused ischemic injury and necrosis associated with acute or chronic inflammation beginning at 14 dpi and

GPCMV-specific antigens and viral particles were most frequently observed at 28 dpi in the marginal and interlobar transitional zones of the main placenta (39). We used *in situ* hybridization to compare the localization of GPCMV in the placenta 21 days after infection at 21 or 35 dGA. Like Griffith and colleagues, we detected occasional infected cells in the main placenta after infection at either time. However, the most consistent pattern of infection and largest lesions localized to the junctional zone, which is situated between the main placenta and the maternal decidua. These lesions were only found after infection at 35 dGA and may indicate that a ring of GPCMV-sensitive cells develop at the base of the placenta as term approaches. Given how frequently we detected this pattern of junctional zone infection, we were surprised it had not been previously reported. However, because our RNAscope assay targets a viral transcript (*gp3*) that is highly expressed during all phases of GPCMV's replication, *in situ* hybridization may be more sensitive than electron microscopy or immunohistochemistry for detecting GPCMV infected cells.

Cumulatively, our data suggests the placenta becomes more sensitized to GPCMV infection-associated injury late in gestation either due to a potentially pathogenic immune response or by the fetal membranes and junctional zone becoming more permissive to infection. Numerous questions remain. Because GPCMV-associated lesions had previously been reported exclusively in the main placenta, we extracted DNA and RNA for viral load quantification and gene expression analyses from this tissue (37, 39). A more nuanced analysis that compares the rate of GPCMV infection and the immune response in the decidua, junctional zone, and main placenta is justified. Our study did not investigate the effects of infection during the earliest stages of pregnancy. One report has noted that maternal GPCMV infection immediately prior to conception caused high rates of fetal demise, suggesting that the virus may perturb early placental development and function (40). Due to the limited availability of normal tissue between twenty weeks gestation and term, how viral infection effects the function of the human placenta after mid-gestation remains poorly characterized. Given similarities in the placental response of humans and guinea pigs to CMV infection and that comparative gene expression analyses suggest that murine placental development largely parallels the first half of human pregnancy, guinea pigs may be particularly well suited to model intrauterine infection after mid-gestation (92).

ETHICS STATEMENT

The animal study was reviewed and approved by Institutional Animal Care and Use Committee at the University of Minnesota.

AUTHOR CONTRIBUTIONS

CB conceived and designed the study. CB, ZB, and DP collected the data. All authors participated in data analysis and interpretation. CB drafted the manuscript. All authors contributed to the article and approved the submitted version.

FUNDING

This project was supported by grants from the Minnesota Masonic Charities (Masonic Early Investigator Award) and the National Institutes of Health (R21HD087496, R01HD098866, and UL1TR002494).

ACKNOWLEDGMENTS

Breeding pairs of strain 13 guinea pigs were generously shared by the U.S. Army Medical Research Institute of Infectious Diseases. Next-generation sequencing library generation and Illumina sequencing were completed by the University of Minnesota Genomics Center. Histopathologic studies were supported by Colleen Forster of the University of Minnesota Histology and Research Laboratory, which is supported by the National Institutes of Health's National Center for Advancing Translational Sciences, grant UL1TR002494, and the resources and staff of the University of Minnesota University Imaging Centers (UIC, SCR_020997). Grants from the National Institutes of Health (R21HD087496 to CB and R01HD098866 to MS) and the Minnesota Masons (Masonic Early Investigator Award to CB) supported this work. The funders had no role in study design, data collection, analysis, decision to publish, or preparation of the manuscript.

REFERENCES

1. Pereira L. Congenital Viral Infection: Traversing the Uterine-Placental Interface. *Annu Rev Virol* (2018) 5(1):273–99. doi: 10.1146/annurev-virology-092917-043236
2. Kenneson A, Cannon MJ. Review and Meta-Analysis of the Epidemiology of Congenital Cytomegalovirus (Cmv) Infection. *Rev Med Virol* (2007) 17 (4):253–76. doi: 10.1002/rmv.535
3. Mocarski ESJr., Shenk T, Griffiths PD, Pass RF. Cytomegaloviruses. In: Knipe DM, Howley PM, editors. *Fields Virology, 6th.* Philadelphia, PA: Wolters Kluwer/Lippincott Williams & Wilkins Health (2013). p. 1960–2014.
4. Iwasenko JM, Howard J, Arbuckle S, Graf N, Hall B, Craig ME, et al. Human Cytomegalovirus Infection Is Detected Frequently in Stillbirths and Is Associated With Fetal Thrombotic Vasculopathy. *J Infect Dis* (2011) 203 (11):1526–33. doi: 10.1093/infdis/jir121
5. Pereira L, Petitt M, Fong A, Tsuge M, Tabata T, Fang-Hoover J, et al. Intrauterine Growth Restriction Caused by Underlying Congenital Cytomegalovirus Infection. *J Infect Dis* (2014) 209(10):1573–84. doi: 10.1093/infdis/jiu019
6. Panhani S, Heinonen KM. Screening for Congenital Cytomegalovirus Infection Among Preterm Infants Born Before the 34th Gestational Week in Finland. *Scand J Infect Dis* (1994) 26(4):375–8. doi: 10.3109/00365549409008607

7. Gibson CS, Goldwater PN, MacLennan AH, Haan EA, Priest K, Dekker GA, et al. Fetal Exposure to Herpesviruses May Be Associated With Pregnancy-Induced Hypertensive Disorders and Preterm Birth in a Caucasian Population. *BJOG* (2008) 115(4):492–500. doi: 10.1111/j.1471-0528.2007.01653.x
8. Shi TL, Huang LJ, Xiong YQ, Zhong YY, Yang JJ, Fu T, et al. The Risk of Herpes Simplex Virus and Human Cytomegalovirus Infection During Pregnancy Upon Adverse Pregnancy Outcomes: A Meta-Analysis. *J Clin Virol* (2018) 104:48–55. doi: 10.1016/j.jcv.2018.04.016
9. Preece PM, Blount JM, Glover J, Fletcher GM, Peckham CS, Griffiths PD. The Consequences of Primary Cytomegalovirus Infection in Pregnancy. *Arch Dis Child* (1983) 58(12):970–5. doi: 10.1136/adc.58.12.970
10. Bodeus M, Hubinont C, Goubau P. Increased Risk of Cytomegalovirus Transmission In Utero During Late Gestation. *Obstet Gynecol* (1999) 93(5 Pt 1):658–60. doi: 10.1097/00006250-199905000-00005
11. Gindes L, Teperberg-Oikawa M, Sherman D, Pardo J, Rahav G. Congenital Cytomegalovirus Infection Following Primary Maternal Infection in the Third Trimester. *BJOG* (2008) 115(7):830–5. doi: 10.1111/j.1471-0528.2007.01651.x
12. Bodeus M, Kabamba-Mukadi B, Zech F, Hubinont C, Bernard P, Goubau P. Human Cytomegalovirus in Utero Transmission: Follow-Up of 524 Maternal Seroconversions. *J Clin Virol* (2010) 47(2):201–2. doi: 10.1016/j.jcv.2009.11.009
13. Picone O, Vauloup-Fellous C, Cordier AG, Guitton S, Senat MV, Fuchs F, et al. A Series of 238 Cytomegalovirus Primary Infections During Pregnancy: Description and Outcome. *Prenat Diagn* (2013) 33(8):751–8. doi: 10.1002/pd.4118
14. Pass RF, Fowler KB, Boppana SB, Britt WJ, Stagno S. Congenital Cytomegalovirus Infection Following First Trimester Maternal Infection: Symptoms at Birth and Outcome. *J Clin Virol* (2006) 35(2):216–20. doi: 10.1016/j.jcv.2005.09.015
15. Faure-Bardon V, Magny JF, Parodi M, Couderc S, Garcia P, Maillotte AM, et al. Sequelae of Congenital Cytomegalovirus Following Maternal Primary Infections Are Limited to Those Acquired in the First Trimester of Pregnancy. *Clin Infect Dis* (2019) 69(9):1526–32. doi: 10.1093/cid/ciy1128
16. Lipitz S, Yinon Y, Malinger G, Yagel S, Levit L, Hoffman C, et al. Risk of Cytomegalovirus-Associated Sequelae in Relation to Time of Infection and Findings on Prenatal Imaging. *Ultrasound Obstet Gynecol* (2013) 41(5):508–14. doi: 10.1002/uog.12377
17. Foulon I, Naessens A, Foulon W, Casteels A, Gordts F. A 10-Year Prospective Study of Sensorineural Hearing Loss in Children With Congenital Cytomegalovirus Infection. *J Pediatr* (2008) 153(1):84–8. doi: 10.1016/j.jpeds.2007.12.049
18. Elkan Miller T, Weisz B, Yinon Y, Weissbach T, De Castro H, Avnet H, et al. Congenital Cytomegalovirus Infection Following Second and Third Trimester Maternal Infection Is Associated With Mild Childhood Adverse Outcome Not Predicted by Prenatal Imaging. *J Pediatr Infect Dis Soc* (2021) 10(5):562–8. doi: 10.1093/jpids/piaa154
19. Garcia AG, Fonseca EF, Marques RL, Lobato YY. Placental Morphology in Cytomegalovirus Infection. *Placenta* (1989) 10(1):1–18. doi: 10.1016/0143-4004(89)90002-7
20. Muhlemann K, Miller RK, Metlay L, Menegus MA. Cytomegalovirus Infection of the Human Placenta: An Immunocytochemical Study. *Hum Pathol* (1992) 23(11):1234–7. doi: 10.1016/0046-8177(92)90290-j
21. Tsuge M, Hida AI, Minematsu T, Honda N, Oshiro Y, Yokoyama M, et al. Prospective Cohort Study of Congenital Cytomegalovirus Infection During Pregnancy With Fetal Growth Restriction: Serologic Analysis and Placental Pathology. *J Pediatr* (2019) 206:42–8 e2. doi: 10.1016/j.jpeds.2018.10.003
22. Maidji E, Nigro G, Tabata T, McDonagh S, Nozawa N, Shiboski S, et al. Antibody Treatment Promotes Compensation for Human Cytomegalovirus-Induced Pathogenesis and a Hypoxia-Like Condition in Placentas With Congenital Infection. *Am J Pathol* (2010) 177(3):1298–310. doi: 10.2353/ajpath.2010.091210
23. Sinzger C, Muntefering H, Loning T, Stoss H, Plachter B, Jahn G. Cell Types Infected in Human Cytomegalovirus Placentitis Identified by Immunohistochemical Double Staining. *Virchows Arch A Pathol Anat Histopathol* (1993) 423(4):249–56. doi: 10.1007/BF01606887
24. Uenaka M, Morizane M, Tanimura K, Deguchi M, Kanzawa M, Itoh T, et al. Histopathological Analysis of Placentas With Congenital Cytomegalovirus Infection. *Placenta* (2019) 75:62–7. doi: 10.1016/j.placenta.2019.01.003
25. Yockey LJ, Lucas C, Iwasaki A. Contributions of Maternal and Fetal Antiviral Immunity in Congenital Disease. *Science* (2020) 368(6491):608–12. doi: 10.1126/science.aaz1960
26. Tabata T, Petitt M, Zydek M, Fang-Hoover J, Larocque N, Tsuge M, et al. Human Cytomegalovirus Infection Interferes With the Maintenance and Differentiation of Trophoblast Progenitor Cells of the Human Placenta. *J Virol* (2015) 89(9):5134–47. doi: 10.1128/JVI.03674-14
27. Tabata T, Petitt M, Fang-Hoover J, Rivera J, Nozawa N, Shiboski S, et al. Cytomegalovirus Impairs Cytotrophoblast-Induced Lymphangiogenesis and Vascular Remodeling in an In Vivo Human Placentation Model. *Am J Pathol* (2012) 181(5):1540–59. doi: 10.1016/j.ajpath.2012.08.003
28. Zydek M, Petitt M, Fang-Hoover J, Adler B, Kauvar LM, Pereira L, et al. Hcmv Infection of Human Trophoblast Progenitor Cells of the Placenta is Neutralized by a Human Monoclonal Antibody to Glycoprotein B and Not by Antibodies to the Pentamer Complex. *Viruses* (2014) 6(3):1346–64. doi: 10.3390/v6031346
29. Mor G, Aldo P, Alvero AB. The Unique Immunological and Microbial Aspects of Pregnancy. *Nat Rev Immunol* (2017) 17(8):469–82. doi: 10.1038/nri.2017.64
30. Yockey LJ, Iwasaki A. Interferons and Proinflammatory Cytokines in Pregnancy and Fetal Development. *Immunity* (2018) 49(3):397–412. doi: 10.1016/j.immuni.2018.07.017
31. Scott GM, Chow SS, Craig ME, Pang CN, Hall B, Wilkins MR, et al. Cytomegalovirus Infection During Pregnancy With Maternofetal Transmission Induces a Proinflammatory Cytokine Bias in Placenta and Amniotic Fluid. *J Infect Dis* (2012) 205(8):1305–10. doi: 10.1093/infdis/jis186
32. Gervasi MT, Romero R, Bracalente G, Chaiworapongsa T, Erez O, Dong Z, et al. Viral Invasion of the Amniotic Cavity (VIAC) in the Midtrimester of Pregnancy. *J Matern Fetal Neonatal Med* (2012) 25(10):2002–13. doi: 10.3109/14767058.2012.683899
33. Hartley JW, Rowe WP, Huebner RJ. Serial Propagation of the Guinea Pig Salivary Gland Virus in Tissue Culture. *Proc Soc Exp Biol Med* (1957) 96 (2):281–5. doi: 10.3181/00379727-96-23455
34. Choi YC, Hsiung GD. Cytomegalovirus Infection in Guinea Pigs. II. Transplacental and Horizontal Transmission. *J Infect Dis* (1978) 138 (2):197–202. doi: 10.1093/infdis/138.2.197
35. Morrison JL, Botting KJ, Darby JRT, David AL, Dyson RM, Gatford KL, et al. Guinea Pig Models for Translation of the Developmental Origins of Health and Disease Hypothesis Into the Clinic. *J Physiol* (2018) 596(23):5535–69. doi: 10.1113/JP274948
36. Mess A, Zaki N, Kadyrov M, Korr H, Kaufmann P. Caviomorph Placentation as a Model for Trophoblast Invasion. *Placenta* (2007) 28(11-12):1234–8. doi: 10.1016/j.placenta.2007.08.003
37. Kaufmann P, Davidoff M. The Guinea-Pig Placenta. *Adv Anat Embryol Cell Biol* (1977) 53(2):5–91. doi: 10.1007/978-3-642-66618-6
38. Auerbach MR, Yan D, Vij R, Hongo JA, Nakamura G, Vernes JM, et al. A Neutralizing Anti-Gh/Gl Monoclonal Antibody is Protective in the Guinea Pig Model of Congenital Cmv Infection. *PloS Pathog* (2014) 10(4):e1004060. doi. 10.1371/journal.ppat.1004060
39. Griffith BP, McCormick SR, Fong CK, Lavallee JT, Lucia HL, Goff E. The Placenta as a Site of Cytomegalovirus Infection in Guinea Pigs. *J Virol* (1985) 55(2):402–9. doi: 10.1128/JVI.55.2.402-409.1985
40. Harrison CJ, Myers MG. Relation of Maternal Cmv Viremia and Antibody Response to the Rate of Congenital Infection and Intrauterine Growth Retardation. *J Med Virol* (1990) 31(3):222–8. doi: 10.1002/jmv.1890310309
41. Kumar ML, Prokay SL. Experimental Primary Cytomegalovirus Infection in Pregnancy: Timing and Fetal Outcome. *Am J Obstet Gynecol* (1983) 145 (1):56–60. doi: 10.1016/0002-9378(83)90339-3
42. Griffith BP, Lucia HL, Hsiung GD. Brain and Visceral Involvement During Congenital Cytomegalovirus Infection of Guinea Pigs. *Pediatr Res* (1982) 16 (6):455–9. doi: 10.1203/00006450-198206000-00010
43. Griffith BP, Hsiung GD. Cytomegalovirus Infection in Guinea Pigs. IV. Maternal Infection at Different Stages of Gestation. *J Infect Dis* (1980) 141 (6):787–93. doi: 10.1093/infdis/141.6.787
44. Harrison CJ, Britt WJ, Chapman NM, Mullican J, Tracy S. Reduced Congenital Cytomegalovirus (Cmv) Infection After Maternal Immunization With a Guinea Pig CMV Glycoprotein Before Gestational Primary Cmv Infection in the Guinea Pig Model. *J Infect Dis* (1995) 172(5):1212–20. doi: 10.1093/infdis/172.5.1212

45. Yang D, Tamburro K, Dittmer D, Cui X, McVoy MA, Hernandez-Alvarado N, et al. Complete Genome Sequence of Pathogenic Guinea Pig Cytomegalovirus From Salivary Gland Homogenates of Infected Animals. *Genome Announc* (2013) 1(2):e0005413. doi: 10.1128/genomeA.00054-13
46. Putri DS, Berkebile ZW, Mustafa HJ, Fernandez-Alarcon C, Abrahante JE, Schleiss MR, et al. Cytomegalovirus Infection Elicits a Conserved Chemokine Response From Human and Guinea Pig Amnion Cells. *Virology* (2020) 548:93–100. doi: 10.1016/j.virol.2020.06.005
47. Hoying JJ. *Selection and Histochemical Identification of Epithelial-Like Cells From Guinea Pig Lung. [M.s.].* Dayton, Ohio: W.S.U. Printing Service: Wright State University (1975).
48. Britt WJ. Human Cytomegalovirus: Propagation, Quantification, and Storage. *Curr Protoc Microbiol* (2010) 18:14E.3.1–3.17. doi: 10.1002/97804717 29259.mc14e03s18
49. Schleiss MR, Bourne N, Stroup G, Bravo FJ, Jensen NJ, Bernstein DI. Protection Against Congenital Cytomegalovirus Infection and Disease in Guinea Pigs, Conferred by a Purified Recombinant Glycoprotein B Vaccine. *J Infect Dis* (2004) 189(8):1374–81. doi: 10.1086/382751
50. Bierle CJ, Fernandez-Alarcon C, Hernandez-Alvarado N, Zabeli JC, Janus BC, Putri DS, et al. Assessing Zika Virus Replication and the Development of Zika-Specific Antibodies After a Mid-Gestation Viral Challenge in Guinea Pigs. *PloS One* (2017) 12(11):e0187720. doi: 10.1371/journal.pone.0187720
51. Bolger AM, Lohse M, Usadel B. Trimmomatic: A Flexible Trimmer for Illumina Sequence Data. *Bioinformatics* (2014) 30(15):2114–20. doi: 10.1093/bioinformatics/btu170
52. Siren J, Valimaki N, Makinen V. Indexing Graphs for Path Queries With Applications in Genome Research. *IEEE/ACM Trans Comput Biol Bioinform* (2014) 11(2):375–88. doi: 10.1109/TCBB.2013.2297101
53. Trapnell C, Roberts A, Goff L, Pertea G, Kim D, Kelley DR, et al. Differential Gene and Transcript Expression Analysis of RNA-seq Experiments With TopHat and Cufflinks. *Nat Protoc* (2012) 7(3):562–78. doi: 10.1038/nprot.2012.016
54. Liao Y, Smyth GK, Shi W. The Subread Aligner: Fast, Accurate and Scalable Read Mapping by Seed-and-Vote. *Nucleic Acids Res* (2013) 41(10):e108. doi: 10.1093/nar/gkt214
55. Robinson MD, McCarthy DJ, Smyth GK. Edger: A Bioconductor Package for Differential Expression Analysis of Digital Gene Expression Data. *Bioinformatics* (2010) 26(1):139–40. doi: 10.1093/bioinformatics/btp616
56. Edgar R, Domrachev M, Lash AE. Gene Expression Omnibus: NCBI Gene Expression and Hybridization Array Data Repository. *Nucleic Acids Res* (2002) 30(1):207–10. doi: 10.1093/nar/30.1.207
57. Metsalu T, Vilo J. ClustVis: a web tool for visualizing clustering of multivariate data using Principal Component Analysis and heatmap. *Nucleic Acids Res* (2015) 43(W1):W566–70. doi: 10.1093/nar/gkv468
58. Raudvere U, Kolberg L, Kuzmin I, Arak T, Adler P, Peterson H, et al. G: Profiler: A Web Server for Functional Enrichment Analysis and Conversions of Gene Lists (2019 Update). *Nucleic Acids Res* (2019) 47(W1):W191–W8. doi: 10.1093/nar/gkz369
59. Shannon P, Markiel A, Ozier O, Baliga NS, Wang JT, Ramage D, et al. Cytoscape: A Software Environment for Integrated Models of Biomolecular Interaction Networks. *Genome Res* (2003) 13(11):2498–504. doi: 10.1101/gr.1239303
60. Merico D, Isserlin R, Stueker O, Emili A, Bader GD. Enrichment Map: A Network-Based Method for Gene-Set Enrichment Visualization and Interpretation. *PloS One* (2010) 5(11):e13984. doi: 10.1371/journal.pone.0013984
61. Oesper L, Merico D, Isserlin R, Bader GD. Wordcloud: A Cytoscape Plugin to Create a Visual Semantic Summary of Networks. *Source Code Biol Med* (2011) 6:7. doi: 10.1186/1751-0473-6-7
62. Morris JH, Apeltsin L, Newman AM, Baumbach J, Wittkop T, Su G, et al. Clustermaker: A Multi-Algorithm Clustering Plugin for Cytoscape. *BMC Bioinf* (2011) 12:436. doi: 10.1186/1471-2105-12-436
63. Reimand J, Isserlin R, Voisin V, Kucera M, Tannus-Lopes C, Rostamianfar A, et al. Pathway Enrichment Analysis and Visualization of Omics Data Using G: Profiler, GSEA, Cytoscape and Enrichmentmap. *Nat Protoc* (2019) 14(2):482–517. doi: 10.1038/s41596-018-0103-9
64. Butler H. *An Atlas for Staging Mammalian and Chick Embryos.* In: Juurlink BHJ, editor. Boca Raton, Fla: CRC Press (1987).
65. Harman MT, Dobrovolny MP. The Development of the External Form of the Guinea-Pig (Cavia Cobaya) Between the Ages of 21 Days and 35 Days of Gestation. *J Morphol* (1933) 54(3):493–519. doi: 10.1002/jmor.1050540306
66. Wright S. *The Effects of Inbreeding and Crossbreeding on Guinea Pigs: I. Decline in Vigor : II. Differentiation Among Inbred Families.* Washington, D.C: U.S. Dept. of Agriculture (1922).
67. Fong CK, Lucia H, Bia FJ, Hsiung GD. Histopathologic and Ultrastructural Studies of Disseminated Cytomegalovirus Infection in Strain 2 Guinea Pigs. *Lab Invest* (1983) 49(2):183–94.
68. Nozawa N, Yamamoto Y, Fukui Y, Katano H, Tsutsui Y, Sato Y, et al. Identification of a 1.6 Kb Genome Locus of Guinea Pig Cytomegalovirus Required for Efficient Viral Growth in Animals But Not in Cell Culture. *Virology* (2008) 379(1):45–54. doi: 10.1016/j.virol.2008.06.018
69. Griffith BP, McCormick SR, Booss J, Hsiung GD. Inbred Guinea Pig Model of Intrauterine Infection With Cytomegalovirus. *Am J Pathol* (1986) 122(1):112–9.
70. Goldstein JA, Gallagher K, Beck C, Kumar R, Gernand AD. Maternal-Fetal Inflammation in the Placenta and the Developmental Origins of Health and Disease. *Front Immunol* (2020) 11:531543. doi: 10.3389/fimmu.2020.531543
71. Romero R, Espinoza J, Goncalves LF, Kusanovic JP, Friel L, Hassan S. The Role of Inflammation and Infection in Preterm Birth. *Semin Reprod Med* (2007) 25(1):21–39. doi: 10.1055/s-2006-956773
72. Chatzakis C, Ville Y, Makrydimas G, Dinas K, Zavlanos A, Sotiriadis A. Timing of Primary Maternal Cytomegalovirus Infection and Rates of Vertical Transmission and Fetal Consequences. *Am J Obstet Gynecol* (2020) 223 (6):870–83.e11. doi: 10.1016/j.ajog.2020.05.038
73. Tabata T, Petitt M, Fang-Hoover J, Zydek M, Pereira L. Persistent Cytomegalovirus Infection in Amniotic Membranes of the Human Placenta. *Am J Pathol* (2016) 186(11):2970–86. doi: 10.1016/j.ajpath.2016.07.016
74. Kumar D, Moore RM, Mercer BM, Mansour JM, Redline RW, Moore JJ. The Physiology of Fetal Membrane Weakening and Rupture: Insights Gained From the Determination of Physical Properties Revisited. *Placenta* (2016) 42:59 73. doi: 10.1016/j.placenta.2016.03.015
75. Yoshimura K, Hirsch E. Effect of Stimulation and Antagonism of Interleukin-1 Signaling on Preterm Delivery in Mice. *J Soc Gynecol Investig* (2005) 12 (7):533–8. doi: 10.1016/j.jsgi.2005.06.006
76. McCarthy R, Martin-Fairey C, Sojka DK, Herzog ED, Jungheim ES, Stout MJ, et al. Mouse Models of Preterm Birth: Suggested Assessment and Reporting Guidelines. *Biol Reprod* (2018) 99(5):922–37. doi: 10.1093/biolre/ioy109
77. Potter JA, Tong M, Aldo P, Kwon JY, Pitruzzello M, Mor G, et al. Viral Infection Dampens Human Fetal Membrane Type I Interferon Responses Triggered by Bacterial Lps. *J Reprod Immunol* (2020) 140:103126. doi: 10.1016/j.jri.2020.103126
78. Cross SN, Potter JA, Aldo P, Kwon JY, Pitruzzello M, Tong M, et al. Viral Infection Sensitizes Human Fetal Membranes to Bacterial Lipopolysaccharide by MERTK Inhibition and Inflammasome Activation. *J Immunol* (2017) 199 (8):2885–95. doi: 10.4049/jimmunol.1700870
79. Bakaysa SL, Potter JA, Hoang M, Han CS, Guller S, Norwitz ER, et al. Single and Double-Stranded Viral RNA Generate Distinct Cytokine and Antiviral Responses in Human Fetal Membranes. *Mol Hum Reprod* (2014) 20(7):701–8. doi: 10.1093/molehr/gau028
80. Tabata T, Petitt M, Puerta-Guardo H, Michlmayr D, Wang C, Fang-Hoover J, et al. Zika Virus Targets Different Primary Human Placental Cells, Suggesting Two Routes for Vertical Transmission. *Cell Host Microbe* (2016) 20(2):155–66. doi: 10.1016/j.chom.2016.07.002
81. Kourtis AP, Read JS, Jamieson DJ. Pregnancy and Infection. *N Engl J Med* (2014) 370(23):2211–8. doi: 10.1056/NEJMra1213566
82. Griffith BP, Lucia HL, Tillbrook JL, Hsiung GD. Enhancement of Cytomegalovirus Infection During Pregnancy in Guinea Pig. *J Infect Dis* (1983) 147(6):990 8. doi: 10.1093/infdis/147.6.990
83. Davis NL, King CC, Kourtis AP. Cytomegalovirus Infection in Pregnancy. *Birth Defects Res* (2017) 109(5):336–46. doi: 10.1002/bdra.23601

84. Weisblum Y, Panet A, Zakay-Rones Z, Vitenshtein A, Haimov-Kochman R, Goldman-Wohl D, et al. Human Cytomegalovirus Induces a Distinct Innate Immune Response in the Maternal-Fetal Interface. *Virology* (2015) 485:289–96. doi: 10.1016/j.virol.2015.06.023
85. Weisblum Y, Oiknine-Djian E, Vorontsov OM, Haimov-Kochman R, Zakay-Rones Z, Meir K, et al. Zika Virus Infects Early- and Midgestation Human Maternal Decidual Tissues, Inducing Distinct Innate Tissue Responses in the Maternal-Fetal Interface. *J Virol* (2017) 91(4):e01905–16. doi: 10.1128/JVI.01905-16
86. Lee J, Romero R, Chaiworapongsa T, Dong Z, Tarca AL, Xu Y, et al. Characterization of the Fetal Blood Transcriptome and Proteome in Maternal Anti-Fetal Rejection: Evidence of a Distinct and Novel Type of Human Fetal Systemic Inflammatory Response. *Am J Reprod Immunol* (2013) 70(4):265–84. doi: 10.1111/aji.12142
87. Romero R, Chaemsaithong P, Chaiyasit N, Docheva N, Dong Z, Kim CJ, et al. CXCL10 and IL-6: Markers of Two Different Forms of Intra-Amniotic Inflammation in Preterm Labor. *Am J Reprod Immunol* (2017) 78(1): e12685. doi: 10.1111/aji.12685
88. Gervasi MT, Romero R, Bracalente G, Erez O, Dong Z, Hassan SS, et al. Midtrimester Amniotic Fluid Concentrations of Interleukin-6 and Interferon-Gamma-Inducible Protein-10: Evidence for Heterogeneity of Intra-Amniotic Inflammation and Associations With Spontaneous Early (<32 Weeks) and Late (>32 Weeks) Preterm Delivery. *J Perinat Med* (2012) 40(4):329–43. doi: 10.1515/jpm-2012-0034
89. Lee J, Kim JS, Park JW, Park CW, Park JS, Jun JK, et al. Chronic Chorioamnionitis is the Most Common Placental Lesion in Late Preterm Birth. *Placenta* (2013) 34(8):681–9. doi: 10.1016/j.placenta.2013.04.014
90. Munn DH, Zhou M, Attwood JT, Bondarev I, Conway SJ, Marshall B, et al. Prevention of Allogeneic Fetal Rejection by Tryptophan Catabolism. *Science* (1998) 281(5380):1191–3. doi: 10.1126/science.281.5380.1191
91. Lopez H, Benard M, Saint-Aubert E, Baron M, Martin H, Al Saati T, et al. Novel Model of Placental Tissue Explants Infected by Cytomegalovirus Reveals Different Permissiveness in Early and Term Placentae and Inhibition of Indoleamine 2,3-Dioxygenase Activity. *Placenta* (2011) 32 (7):522–30. doi: 10.1016/j.placenta.2011.04.016
92. Soncin F, Khater M, To C, Pizzo D, Farah O, Wakeland A, et al. Comparative Analysis of Mouse and Human Placentae Across Gestation Reveals Species-Specific Regulators of Placental Development. *Development* (2018) 145(2): dev156273. doi: 10.1242/dev.156273
93. Kearse M, Moir R, Wilson A, Stones-Havas S, Cheung M, Sturrock S, et al. Geneious Basic: An Integrated and Extendable Desktop Software Platform for the Organization and Analysis of Sequence Data. *Bioinformatics* (2012) 28 (12):1647–9. doi: 10.1093/bioinformatics/bts199

10

HIF-1α-Deficiency in Myeloid Cells Leads to a Disturbed Accumulation of Myeloid Derived Suppressor Cells (MDSC) During Pregnancy and to an Increased Abortion Rate in Mice

Natascha Köstlin-Gille[1], Stefanie Dietz[1], Julian Schwarz[1], Bärbel Spring[1], Jan Pauluschke-Fröhlich[2], Christian F. Poets[1] and Christian Gille[1]*

[1] *Department of Neonatology, Tuebingen University Children's Hospital, Tuebingen, Germany,* [2] *Department of Obstetrics and Gynecology, Tuebingen, Germany*

***Correspondence:**
Natascha Köstlin-Gille
natascha.koestlin@med.uni-tuebingen.de

Abortions are the most important reason for unintentional childlessness. During pregnancy, maternal immune cells are in close contact to cells of the semi-allogeneic fetus. Dysregulation of the maternal immune system leading to defective adaptation to pregnancy often plays a role in pathogenesis of abortions. Myeloid-derived suppressor cells (MDSC) are myeloid cells that suppress functions of other immune cells, especially T-cells, thereby negatively affecting diseases such as cancer, sepsis or trauma. They seem, however, also necessary for maintenance of maternal-fetal tolerance. Mechanisms regulating MDSC expansion and function during pregnancy are only incompletely understood. In tumor environment, hypoxia is crucial for MDSC accumulation and activation. Hypoxia is also important for early placenta and embryo development. Effects of hypoxia are mediated through hypoxia-inducible factor 1α (HIF-1α). In the present study we aimed to examine the role of HIF-1α in myeloid cells for MDSC accumulation and MDSC function during pregnancy and for pregnancy outcome. We therefore used a mouse model with targeted deletion of HIF-1α in myeloid cells (myeloid HIF-KO) and analyzed blood, spleens and uteri of pregnant mice at gestational day E 10.5 in comparison to non-pregnant animals and wildtype (WT) animals. Further we analyzed pregnancy success by determining rates of failed implantation and abortion in WT and myeloid HIF-KO animals. We found that myeloid HIF-KO in mice led to an abrogated MDSC accumulation in the pregnant uterus and to impaired suppressive activity of MDSC. While expression of chemokine receptors and integrins on MDSC was not affected by HIF-1α, myeloid HIF-KO led to increased apoptosis rates of MDSC in the uterus. Myeloid-HIF-KO resulted in increased proportions of non-pregnant animals after positive vaginal plug and increased abortion rates, suggesting that activation of HIF-1α dependent pathways in MDSC are important for maintenance of pregnancy.

Keywords: HIF, pregnancy, MDSC, abortion, apoptosis

INTRODUCTION

Abortions are one of the most important pregnancy complication; at least 25%, probably up to 50% of women are affected (1). Recurrent Abortions (RA) are defined as three or more consecutive abortions and affect about 1-3% of couples of childbearing age (2). Besides chromosomal abnormalities, anatomic anomalies and infections, a dysregulation of the immune system seems to play an important role (1, 2). During pregnancy, maternal immune cells and cells of the semi-allogeneic fetus are in close contact. To avoid rejection of the fetus, the maternal immune system has tightly to be regulated (3). Mechanisms inducing maternal-fetal tolerance during pregnancy and those leading to complications like recurrent abortions are incompletely understood.

Myeloid derived suppressor cells (MDSC) are myeloid cells with suppressive activity on other immune cells, especially on T-cells (4). Depending on their phenotype, they can be sub-grouped in two populations - monocytic MDSC (MO-MDSC) and granulocytic MDSC (GR-MDSC). In mice, MDSC can be identified by co-expression of the myeloid lineage differentiation antigen Gr-1 and CD11b. MO-MDSC and GR-MDSC can further be differentiated by the expression of the two epitopes of Gr-1, i.e., Ly6G and Ly6C; MO-MDSC are defined as $CD11b^+/Ly6G^-/Ly6C^{high}$ and GR-MDSC as $CD11b^+/Ly6G^+/Ly6C^{low}$ (5, 6). Primarily, accumulation of MDSC has been described in cancer patients (7, 8) and tumor bearing mice (5), where they inhibit T-cell response against the tumor leading to disease progression. Later, we and others could show that MDSC and especially GR-MDSC also accumulate during pregnancy in the fetal and maternal organism and that their immune-modulatory properties may be crucial for maternal-fetal tolerance (9–13) and immune adaptation of the newborn (14–17). However, only little is known about mechanisms leading to MDSC-accumulation during pregnancy.

Hypoxia plays an important role in normal placental development as well as in pathogenesis of placental pathologies (18, 19). Hypoxia-inducible factor 1 (HIF-1) is a key regulator of the response to hypoxia, initiating transcription of various genes. HIF-1 is a heterodimer consisting of the subunits HIF-1α and HIF-1β; HIF-1β is constitutively expressed, while expression of HIF-1α is induced under hypoxic conditions (20). During early gestation, HIF-1α is highly expressed in the placenta, which is characterized by low oxygen pressure (21). In the context of malignancies HIF-1α may be critical for MDSC-activation in the hypoxic environment of tumors (22–24). Until now, nothing is known about the role of HIF-1α for MDSC accumulation and activation during pregnancy.

In the present study, we evaluated the impact of HIF-1α on MDSC accumulation and activation during pregnancy in a mouse model of HIF-1α deficiency in myeloid cells. We found that HIF-1α deficiency in myeloid cells (myeloid HIF-KO) (1) led to a diminished accumulation of MDSC during pregnancy, especially in the uterus of pregnant mice, (2) MDSC from myeloid HIF-KO mice had lower suppressive activity than wildtype (WT) MDSC, (3) MDSC from myeloid HIF-KO mice exhibited higher apoptosis rates and (4) myeloid HIF-KO mice had increased abortion rates compared to WT animals.

Taken together, we describe a role of HIF-1α for MDSC accumulation and function during pregnancy and for pregnancy maintenance. Disturbed activation of HIF-1α and resulting alterations in MDSC homeostasis during pregnancy may be a yet unknown mechanism for immunological pregnancy complications.

Abbreviations: BM, bone marrow; GR-MDSC, granulocytic MDSC; HIF-1α, hypoxia inducible factor 1 α; HIF-KO, HIF-1α knockout; MDSC, myeloid derived suppressor cells; MO-MDSC, monocytic MDSC; NK, natural killer; WT, wildtype.

METHODS

Mice

HIF-$1\alpha^{flox}$ (B6.129-Hif1a^{tm3Rsjo}/J) mice and LysMcre (B6.129P2-*Lyzs*$^{tm1(cre)Ifo}$/J) mice were obtained from The Jackson Laboratory (Bar Harbor, Maine, USA). HIF-$1\alpha^{flox}$ mice and LysMcre mice were crossed to get animals double homozygous for HIF-$1\alpha^{flox}$ and LysMcre, carrying a deletion of HIF-1α in myeloid cells (HIF-$1\alpha^{flox}$/LysMre, myeloid HIF-KO). C57BL/6J (WT) mice were also obtained from The Jackson Laboratory. All animals were maintained under pathogen-free conditions in the research animal facility of Tuebingen University, Tuebingen, Germany. All experimental animal procedures were conducted according to German federal and state regulations.

Syngeneic matings of myeloid HIF-KO and WT mice were set up at 8-12 weeks of age. Gestational ages were determined by visualizing the presence of a vaginal plug (E0.5 = vaginal plug day).

Abortion rates were determined by visual inspection of fetal-placental units and defined as ratio between resorbing units and total implantation sites. Resorbing units were either dark, small and necrotic or pale, small and with no visible fetus inside the amniotic cavity.

Tissue Collection and Single Cell Preparations

Non-pregnant and pregnant mice at gestational age E10.5 were euthanized by CO_2 inhalation. Blood (0.5–1 ml) was collected by intracardial puncture immediately after death and placed into EDTA-tubes. Red blood cells were removed from whole blood by Ammonium chloride lysis. Spleens were removed and tissue was pushed through a 100 μm filter (Greiner bio-one, Frickenhausen, Germany) using a syringe plunger. Red blood cells were removed by Ammonium chloride lysis and the resulting cell suspension was then passed again through a 40 μm filter (Greiner bio-one, Frickenhausen, Germany) Uterine horns were removed in toto. The fetuses and the fetal part of placenta were dissected from the uteri and blood vessels were removed. Uteri were then placed into PBS, minced into ~1 mm^3 pieces and pushed through a 40 μm filter. All cell suspensions were then adjusted to 1–4 × 10^6 cells/ml in PBS.

In-vitro Generation of MDSC

in-vitro generation of MDSC was performed according to previously established protocols (25, 26). For *in-vitro* generation of MDSC non-pregnant WT and myeloid HIF-KO mice were euthanized and femora removed. Bone marrow was collected by rinsing the bones with PBS with a syringe and a 25G needle. Bone marrow cells were then washed, adjusted to $3x10^5$ cells/ml and cultured for 72 h at 37°C in culture medium [Dulbecco's modified eagle medium, DMEM (Thermo Fisher Scientific, Darmstadt, Germany), supplemented with 10% fetal calf serum (FCS, Biochrom, Berlin, Germany) and 1% Penicilline/Streptomycin (Biochrom, Berlin, Germany)] supplemented with 100 ng/ml recombinant murine G-CSF (Peprotech, Hamburg, Germany) and 12.5 ng/ml recombinant murine GM-CSF (Peprotech, Hamburg, Germany). After 72 h of culture non-adherent cells were removed and adherent MDSC detached with trypsin (Biochrom GmbH, Berlin, Germany). >90% of cells were Gr-1^+/CD11b$^+$ as determined by flow cytometry, thereby exhibiting surface characteristics of MDSC.

Cell Isolation and Flow Cytometry

For isolation of CD4$^+$ from splenocytes, cells were labeled with T-cell Biotin-Antibody Cocktail followed by two sequential Anti-Biotin magnetic bead separation steps (Miltenyi Biotec, Bergisch-Gladbach, Germany) according to the manufacturer's instructions. Purity of CD4$^+$ T-cells after separation was >90%, as assessed by flow cytometry.

For extracellular staining, freshly isolated cells were washed in washing buffer [PBS with 0.1% bovine serum albumin (BSA)] and FcRs were blocked with purified anti-CD16/32 (clone 2.4G2) for 10 min. Then, fluorescent-conjugated extracellular antibodies were added. Antibodies were purchased from BD biosciences [CD3 (145-2C11), CD4 (RM4-5), CD8a (53-6.7), CD11b (M1/79), CD19 (1D3), CD45 (30-F11), NK1.1 (PK136), Gr-1 (RB6-8C5), Ly-6C (AL-21), Ly-6G (1A8), CXCR5 (2G8), annexin V] and R&D systems [CXCR1 (FAB8628P), CXCR2 (FAB2164C), CXCR4 (FAB21651C), CXC3CR1 (FAB5825P), IL4-Rα (FAB530P), Integrin-α4 (FAB2450P) Integrin-β2 (FAB2618P), L-Selectin (FAB5761P)]. For immune cell quantification, cells were pre-gated to CD45. Among CD45$^+$ cells, cell types were identified as follows: T-cells CD3$^+$, T-Helper cells CD3$^+$/CD4+, cytotoxic T-cells CD3$^+$/CD8$^+$ B-cells CD3$^-$/CD19$^+$, NK-cells CD3$^-$/NK1.1$^+$, MDSC CD11b$^+$/Gr-1$^+$, MO-MDSC CD11b$^+$/Ly6C$^+$/Ly6G$^-$, GR-MDSC CD11b$^+$/Ly6C^{low}/Ly6G$^+$, monocytes CD11b$^+$/Gr-1$^-$.

Data acquisition was performed with a FACScalibur flow cytometer (BD Bioscience) and analyzed via CellQuest (BD Biosciences).

T-Cell Suppression Assay

Freshly isolated CD4$^+$ splenocytes were stained with carboxyfluorescein-succinimidyl ester (CFSE, Invitrogen, Heidelberg, Germany) according to the manufacturer's instructions. Cells were suspended in RPMI 1640 media containing 1% penicillin/streptomycin and 10% FCS. CFSE-labeled CD4$^+$ T-cells (2×10^5) suspended in 100 μl media were stimulated with 2×10^5 mouse T-Activator CD3/CD28 Dynabeads (Thermo Fisher Scientific, Dreieich, Germany) and 50 ng recombinant murine Interleukin-2 (rmIL-2, R&D Systems, Wiesbaden-Nordenstadt, Germany). *In-vitro* generated MDSC also suspended in RPMI 1640 containing 1% penicillin/streptomycin and 10% FCS were added in different ratios (1:1, 1:2 and 1:4). After 5 days of culture, CD4$^+$ T-cell proliferation was determined by CFSE dye dilution by flow cytometry. Proliferation index, defined as the ratio of CD4$^+$ T-cell proliferation after addition of MDSC and CD4$^+$ T-cell proliferation without MDSC, was determined. CD4$^+$ T-cell proliferation without MDSC was set to a fixed value of 1.

Statistical Analysis

Statistical analysis was done using GraphPad Prism 5.0 (GraphPad Software, La Jolla, CA). Data were analyzed for Gaussian distribution using D'Agostino and Pearson omnibus normality test. Immune cell quantification experiments were analyzed using the Kruskal Wallis test and Dunn's multiple comparison test. T-cell suppression was analyzed using the Wilcoxon matched pairs signed rank test. Expression of surface receptors and apoptosis rates were analyzed using the Mann-Whitney test. Data analyzing pregnancy success (rate of pregnant animals after positive vaginal plug and rate of animals with at least one abortion) were analyzed by Fishers exact test. Abortion rate was analyzed by Mann-Whitney test. Normally distributed data were analyzed using paired *t*-test, not normally distributed data were evaluated using the Wilcoxon matched pairs signed rank test. A p-value < 0.05 was considered as statistically significant.

RESULTS

HIF-1α Deficiency in Myeloid Cells Leads to a Diminished Accumulation of MDSC in the Pregnant Uterus

HIF-1α has been shown to be essential for MDSC function in the tumor environment (22). Therefore, we first asked whether HIF-1α plays a role for MDSC accumulation also during pregnancy. We analyzed expression of MDSC in blood, spleens and uteri of non-pregnant and pregnant WT mice at embryonic day 10.5 (E10.5) in comparison to myeloid HIF-KO mice. Pregnant WT mice had significantly higher proportions of CD11b$^+$/Gr-1$^+$ MDSC in blood, spleen and uteri than non-pregnant WT mice (**Figures 1A–C**). In myeloid HIF-KO mice, MDSC counts in non-pregnant animals tended to be higher in blood, spleen and uterus compared to WT mice. Pregnancy induced further MDSC accumulation only in blood, not in spleens or uteri. In the latter, we even found a tendency toward lower MDSC numbers in pregnant than in non-pregnant myeloid HIF-KO mice (**Figures 1A–I**). MDSC-accumulation in WT animals was mainly attributed to the CD11b$^+$/Ly6G$^+$/Ly6C^{low} GR-MDSC subpopulation (**Figures 1D–F**), not the CD11b$^+$/Ly6G$^-$/Ly6C^{high} MO-MDSC subpopulation (**Figures 1G–I**). Gating strategy for MDSC, GR-MDSC and MO-MDSC in spleens and uteri are depicted in **Figures 1J–K**.

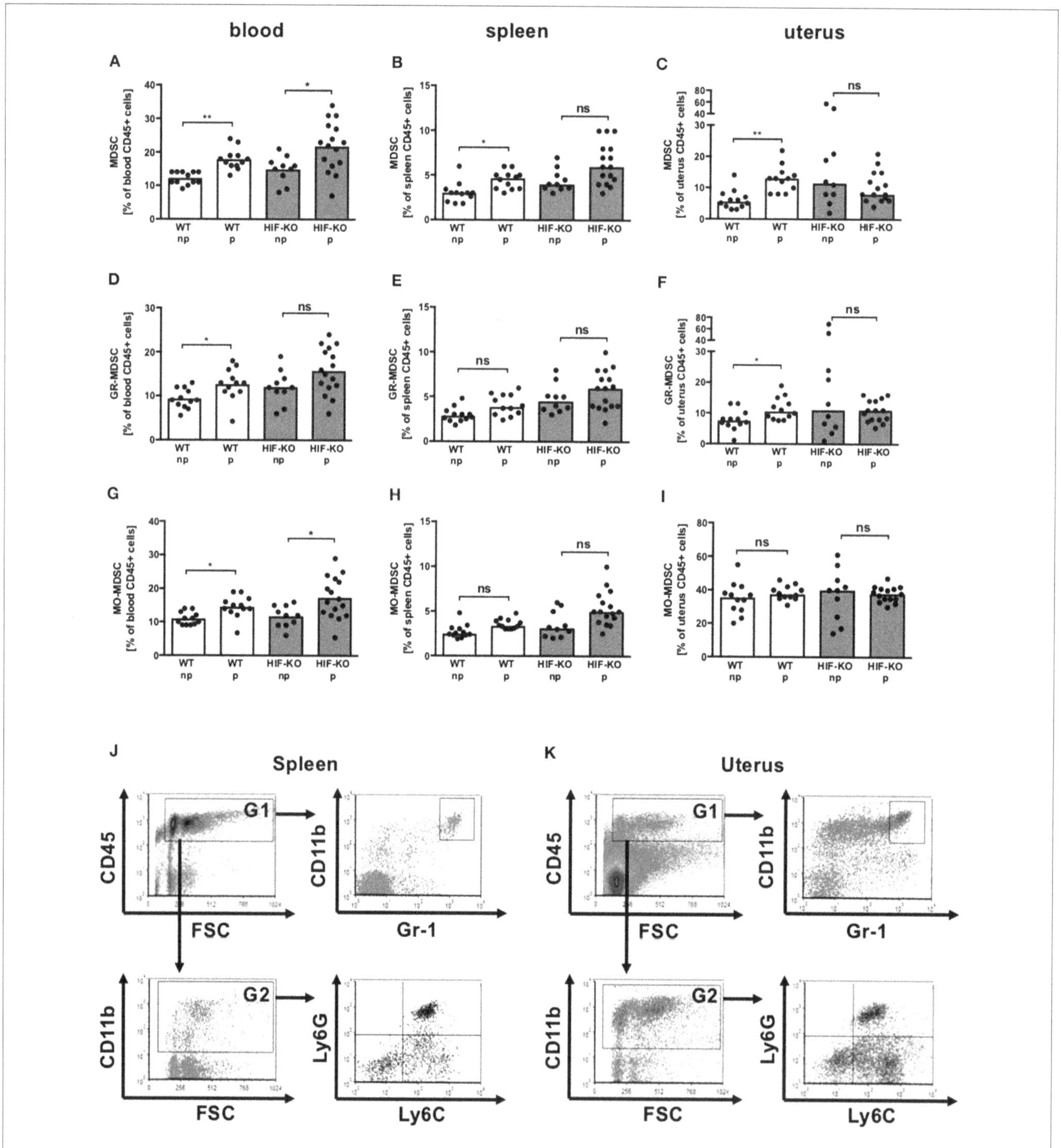

FIGURE 1 | Quantification of MDSC in blood, spleens and uteri of wildtype and myeloid HIF-KO mice. Non-pregnant (np) and E10.5 pregnant (p) wildtype (WT) and myeloid HIF-KO (HIF-KO) mice were euthanized and blood, spleens and uteri were collected. Tissues were homogenized and filtered to obtain single cell suspensions. Cells were then analyzed by flow cytometry. **(A–I)** Scatter diagrams with bars showing percentages of total MDSC **(A–C)** GR-MDSC **(D–F)**, and MO-MDSC **(G-I)** from total CD45$^+$ leucocytes in peripheral blood **(A,D,G)**, spleens **(B,E,H)** and uteri **(C,E,I)**. Each symbol represents an individual sample and the median is indicated. $n = 10$–16, $^*p < 0.05$; $^{**}p < 0.01$; ns not significant; Kruskal-Wallis test and Dunn's multiple comparison test. **(J,K)** Representative density plots showing the gating strategy for total MDSC (CD11b$^+$/Gr-1$^+$), GR-MDSC (CD11b$^+$/Ly6C^{low}/Ly6G$^+$) and MO-MDSC (CD11b$^+$/Ly6C^{high}/Ly6G$^-$) in spleens **(J)** and uteri **(K)**.

Regarding other leucocyte subpopulations, we found a decrease in percentages of B-cells in blood and NK-cells in spleens of both WT-mice and myeloid HIF-KO-mice during pregnancy (**Supplementary Figures 1D,H**). Percentages of T-cells decreased in uteri of myeloid HIF-KO mice during pregnancy, but remained unchanged in WT-mice

(**Supplementary Figure 1C**). Percentages of monocytes increased in blood and spleens of pregnant myeloid HIF-KO but not WT-mice (**Supplementary Figures 1J,K**), while they decreased in uteri of pregnant WT-mice and remained unchanged in uteri of myeloid HIF-KO mice (**Supplementary Figure 1L**).

HIF-1α Deficiency Leads to Diminished Suppressive Activity of MDSC

Next, we asked whether HIF-1α deficiency also has effects on suppressive activity of MDSC. To test this hypothesis, we generated MDSC from bone marrow (BM) of WT mice and myeloid HIF-KO mice and tested their suppressive activity on $CD4^+$ T-cell proliferation. MDSC generated from BM of WT mice efficiently suppressed $CD4^+$ T-cell proliferation in a concentration dependent manner to 48.0 ± 14.2 % (1:4), 24.6% ± 12.5% (1:2) and 14.3% ± 3.4% (1:1). In contrast, MDSC generated from BM of myeloid HIF-KO mice displayed substantially lower suppressive activity on $CD4^+$ T-cell (103.2% ± 25.2% (4:1) $p < 0.01$ vs. WT mice, 71.6% ± 26.5% (2:1) $p < 0.01$ vs. WT mice and 47.5% ± 15.4% (1:1) $p < 0.05$ vs. WT mice, $n = 5$, **Figures 2A,B**).

Diminished Accumulation of MDSC in the Pregnant Uterus Is Not Due to an Altered Expression of Chemokine Receptors or Integrins

As the most impressive difference between WT mice and myeloid HIF-KO mice was a diminished influx of MDSC into the pregnant uterus in myeloid HIF-KO mice, we asked whether deficiency for HIF-1α might lead to a diminished expression of chemokine receptors or integrins on MDSC leading to defects in their migratory capacity. Therefore, we analyzed expression of chemokine receptors CXCR1 (CD181), CXCR2 (CD182), CXCR4 (CD84), CXCR5 (CD185), CX3CR1 and IL4Rα (CD124), as well as ITGA4 (CD49d), ITGB2 (CD18) and L-selectin (CD62L) in MDSC from spleens and uteri of WT and myeloid HIF-KO mice. We found no differences in the expression of CXCR1, CXCR2, CXCR4, CXCR5, and CX3CR1 between WT and myeloid HIF-KO mice, neither in splenic MDSC nor in uterine MDSC. Interestingly, we even found higher expression of IL4Rα, ITGA4, ITGB2, and L-Selectin on myeloid HIF-KO MDSC (**Supplementary Figure 2** and **Figure 3**), not explaining the diminished accumulation in pregnant uteri.

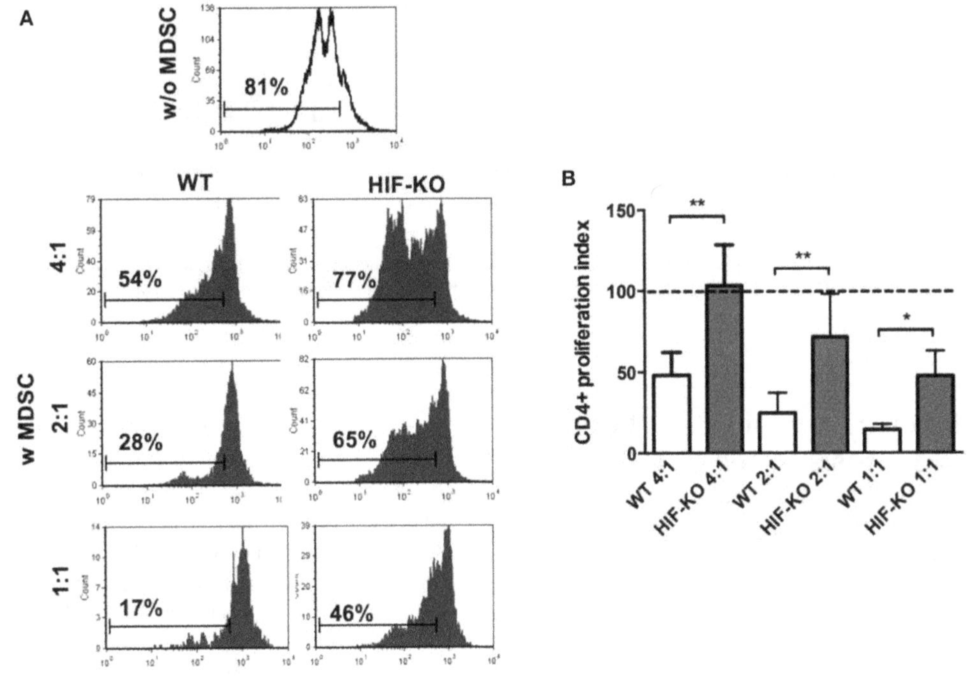

FIGURE 2 | Inhibition of $CD4^+$ T-cell proliferation by MDSC generated from wildtype and myeloid HIF-KO mice. Non-pregnant wildtype (WT) mice and myeloid HIF-KO mice (HIF-KO) were euthanized and bone marrow cells were collected. Cells were cultured for 4 days with G-CSF and GM-CSF. After 4 days non-adherent cells were removed and adherent MDSC were detached with Trypsin/EDTA. MDSC were then added to $CD4^+$ T-cells, freshly isolated from spleens of non-pregnant wildtype mice by MACS, stained with CFSE and stimulated with anti-CD3/CD28 microbeads. After 4 days, proliferation of $CD4^+$ T-cells was assessed by CFSE dye dilution. Proliferation index was determined as ratio of T-cell proliferation with and without addition of MDSC. **(A)** Representative histogram plots showing proliferation of $CD4^+$ T-cells without (white histogram, w/o MDSC) addition of MDSC and with (gray histograms, w MDSC) addition of MDSC generated from WT mice (left side) and from HIF-KO mice (right side) in T-cell:MDSC ratios of 4:1, 2:1 and 1:1. **(B)** Inhibitory effect of MDSC from WT mice (white bars) and HIF-KO mice (gray bars) on proliferation of $CD4^+$ T-cells. Dashed line shows proliferation of target $CD4^+$ T-cells without addition of MDSC. Inhibition of T-cell proliferation by MDSC was measured at the indicated ratios by CFSE dye dilution. Bars show mean and standard deviation of 5 samples pooled from 5 independent experiments. $^*p < 0.05$; $^{**}p < 0.01$ compared with target cells alone; Wilcoxon matched-pairs signed-rank test.

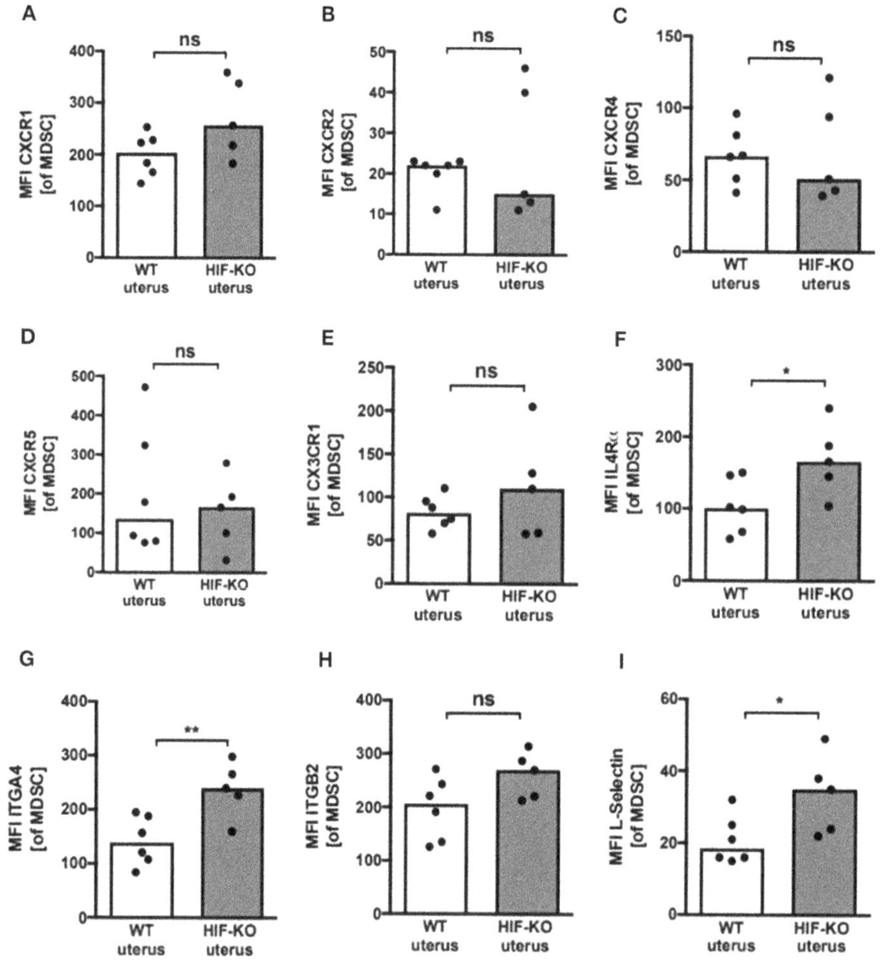

FIGURE 3 | Expression of chemokine receptors and integrins on uterine MDSC from wildtype and myeloid HIF-KO mice. **(A–I)** E10.5 pregnant wildtype (WT) and myeloid HIF-KO (HIF-KO) mice were euthanized and uteri were collected. Tissues were homogenized and filtered to obtain single cell suspensions. Cells were then analyzed by flow cytometry. Scatter diagrams with bars showing MFI for indicated chemokine receptor and integrin expression on $CD11b^+/Gr\text{-}1^+$ MDSC from wildtype (white bars) and myeloid HIF-KO (HIF-KO) mice. Each symbol represents an individual sample and the median is indicated. $n = 5–6$, $^*p < 0.05$; $^{**}p < 0.01$; ns, not significant; Mann-Whitney test.

HIF-1α Deficiency in Myeloid Cells Leads to Increased Apoptosis Rates of MDSC

To further figure out the mechanism(s) underlying the diminished accumulation of MDSC in uteri of pregnant myeloid HIF-KO mice, we analyzed apoptosis rates of MDSC in spleens and uteri of pregnant WT and myeloid HIF-KO mice by annexin V staining. We found that apoptosis rates of MDSC from spleens and uteri of myeloid HIF-KO mice were about twice as high as those of WT-MDSC (median 20.6 vs. 8.1% for spleens and 39.5 vs. 25.6% for uteri, $n = 5–6$, $p < 0.05$, **Figures 4A–C**).

HIF-1α Deficiency in Myeloid Cells Leads to an Increased Abortion Rate in Mice

To evaluate the clinical significance of myeloid HIF-KO during pregnancy, we analyzed pregnancy outcomes in myeloid HIF-KO mice and WT mice at E10.5. Placentae were prepared and numbers of resorbing units quantified. Resorbing units were either dark, small and necrotic, pale or small and with no visible fetus inside the amniotic cavity. We found that the rate of non-pregnant animals after positive vaginal plug was significantly higher in myeloid HIF-KO animals (16 vs. 7%, $n = 13–20$, $p < 0.05$, Fishers exact test, **Figure 5A**). Furthermore, we found a higher rate of animals with at least one abortion in myeloid HIF-KO animals than in WT mice (87 vs. 58%, $n = 12–16$, $p < 0.0001$, Fishers exact test, **Figure 5B**). At day E10.5, we found no differences in the number of implantation sites between myeloid HIF-KO mice and WT mice (**Supplementary Figure 3**), however, myeloid HIF-KO mice had significant higher abortion rates than WT mice (median 19.5% vs. 9.5%, $n = 12–16$, $p < 0.05$, **Figures 5C,D**).

Discussion

The role of MDSC in maintaining pregnancy is increasingly recognized. Molecular mechanisms leading to MDSC-accumulation during pregnancy, however, are still incompletely understood. In the present study, we investigated

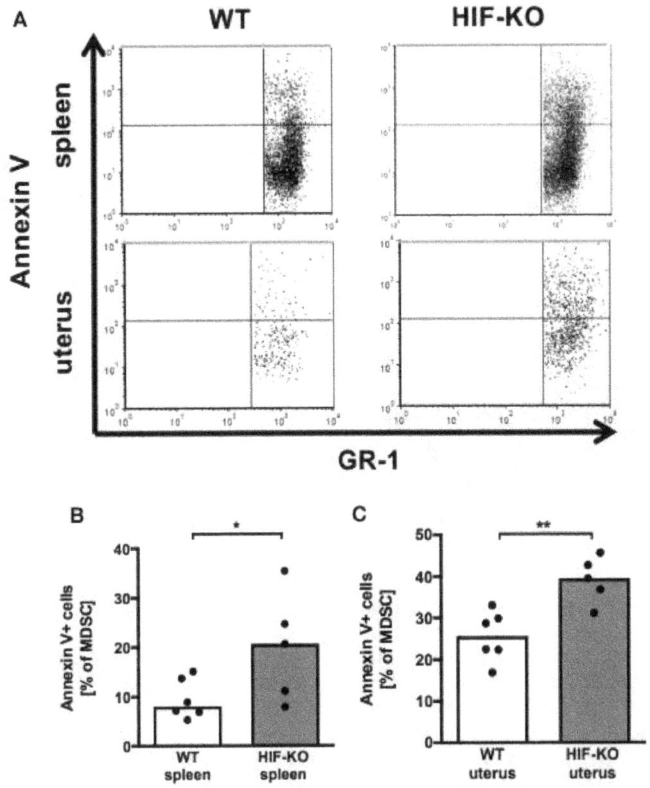

FIGURE 4 | Apoptosis of MDSC from spleens and uteri from wildtype and myeloid HIF-KO mice. E10.5 pregnant wildtype (WT) and myeloid HIF-KO (HIF-KO) mice were euthanized and spleens and uteri were collected. Tissues were homogenized and filtered to obtain single cell suspensions. Cells were then analyzed for apoptosis annexin V staining and flow cytometry. **(A)** Representative density plots from spleens (upper plots) and uteri (lower plots) of Wildtype (WT) and myeloid HIF-KO (HIF-KO) mice for GR-1 vs. annexin V. **(B,C)** Scatter diagrams with bars showing percentages of annexin V^+ MDSC from total MDSC in spleens **(B)** and uteri **(C)** from wildtype (white bars) and myeloid HIF-KO (HIF-KO) mice. Each symbol represents an individual sample and the median is indicated. $n = 5–6$, $^*p < 0.05$; $^{**}p < 0.01$; Mann-Whitney test.

the role of the hypoxia-regulated transcription factor HIF-1α for MDSC-accumulation during pregnancy and for pregnancy outcome.

First, we found that knockout of HIF-1α in myeloid cells led to a diminished accumulation of MDSC in the pregnant uterus, illustrating a relationship between myeloid HIF-1α expression and MDSC accumulation during pregnancy. One other study recently described a HIF-1α dependent accumulation of MDSC under tumor conditions; in a mouse model of hepatocellular carcinoma, HIF-1α activation in tumor cells led to an overexpression of the ectonucleotidase CD39 mediating a differentiation arrest of MDSC thereby leading to their accumulation (27). Other studies investigating the interplay between HIF-1α-activation and MDSC focused on MDSC function and not on MDSC accumulation (22–24). Interestingly, besides the uterine milieu, where hypoxia is known to play a role during different stages of pregnancy (18, 19), we also found a diminished MDSC-accumulation in spleens of myeloid HIF-KO mice. This suggests that, in addition to hypoxia, other factors may activate HIF-1α during pregnancy. Besides inflammatory pathways such as NF-κB that has been described to activate HIF-1α (28), one study reported an activation of HIF-1α by the sex hormone estrogen (29). Furthermore it has been shown that *in vitro* estrogen activates MDSC during pregnancy (30). The impact of estrogen on HIF-1α activation in MDSC and their functional activation during pregnancy is content of ongoing studies.

Interestingly, MDSC-accumulation in the pregnant uterus of wildtype mice was accompanied by a reduction of uterine monocytes. This reduction was not observed in uteri of myeloid HIF-KO mice. Since MDSC can differentiate to mature myeloid cells and hypoxia has been described to prevent MDSC differentiation via HIF-1α (27), the decreased monocyte numbers in pregnant uteri of WT mice might be a result of a HIF-1α-driven maturational arrest.

Second, we found that MDSC generated from myeloid HIF-KO mice had substantially reduced suppressive activity compared to MDSC generated from WT mice. This is in line with other studies describing an increased suppressive activity of MDSC under hypoxic tumor conditions mediated by HIF-1α (22). We now show that lack of HIF-1α leads to impaired suppressive activity of MDSC also in normoxia. The underlying mechanism for reduced suppressive activity of HIF-KO MDSC remains unclear. One of the main effector mechanisms used

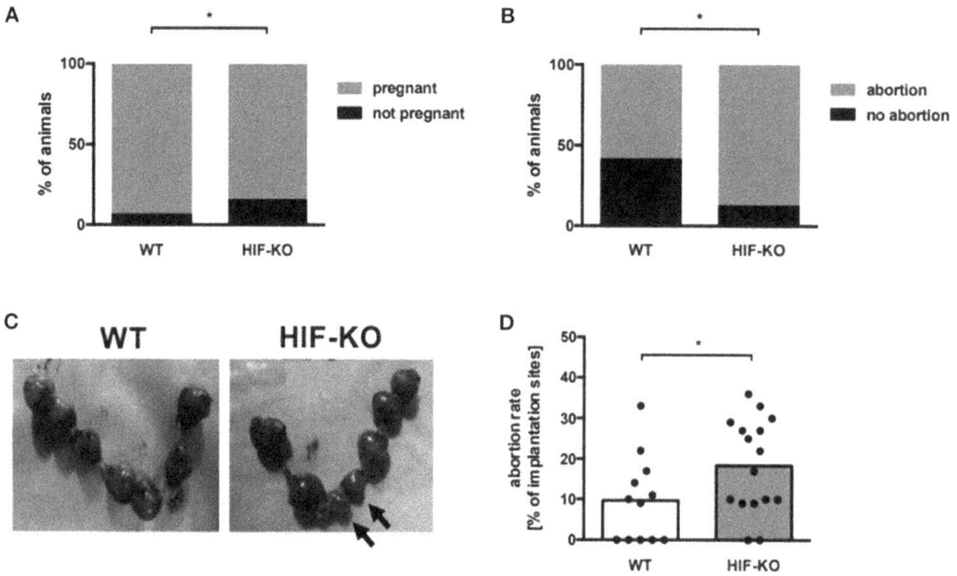

FIGURE 5 | Pregnancy success in wildtype and myeloid HIF-KO mice. Wildtype and myeloid HIF-KO mice were term-bred and the day when a vaginal plug was detected was defined as day E0.5. At day E10.5 mice were euthanized and the abdominal cavity was opened. Uteri containing foeto-placental units were removed and inspected. Total implantation sides and resorbing units were counted. **(A)** Bar graph showing the percentages of non-pregnant (black part) and pregnant (gray part) animals among wildtype (WT) and myeloid HIF-KO (HIF-KO) mice after positive evaluation for vaginal plug. $n = 13–20$, $^*p < 0.05$, Fishers exact test. **(B)** Bar graph shows the percentages of individuals without (black part) and with (gray part) at least one abortion among wildtype (WT) and myeloid HIF-KO (HIF-KO) mice. $n = 12–16$, $^*p < 0.05$, Fishers exact test. **(C)** Representative pictures of uteri from a pregnant wildtype (WT) and a pregnant myeloid HIF-KO mouse (HIF-KO). Arrows indicate resorbing units. **(D)** Scatter diagram with bars showing abortion rates of pregnant wildtype (white bar) and pregnant myeloid HIF-KO mice (gray bar). Abortion rates were defined as ratio between resorbing units and total implantation sites. Each symbol represents an individual animal and the median is indicated. $n = 12–16$, $^*p < 0.05$; Mann-Whitney test.

by MDSC to suppress T-cells is the production of iNOS (6). It has been shown that the Th1-cytokine IFN-γ activates HIF-1α leading to increased iNOS expression (31) and that myeloid cells acquire suppressive activity under hypoxic tumor conditions that can be abrogated by inhibiton of iNOS (23) so that it could be speculated that decreased generation of NO in HIF-KO MDSC leads to their decreased suppressive activity. Another mechanism linking HIF-1α activation and MDSC-function is the expression of the immune checkpoint molecule PD-L1. Noman et al. showed that expression of PD-L1 on myeloid cells can be stimulated by Hypoxia via HIF-1α and that blockade of PD-L1 decreases MDSC-mediated T-cell suppression by down-regulating MDSC IL-6 and IL-10 (24). Our group showed that expression of PD-L1 on human MDSC can be stimulated by E.coli (32). Thus, stimulation of PD-L1 expression via HIF-1α could also be a mechanism for MDSC activation during pregnancy.

To figure out mechanisms leading to the disturbed accumulation of MDSC in the pregnant uterus of myeloid HIF-KO mice we analyzed expression of chemokine receptors and integrins on MDSC. Although upregulation via HIF-1α signaling pathways has been described for many surface receptors including CXCR1 and CXCR2 (33), CXCR4 (34), and IL-4Rα (35), we found no differences in their expression on MDSC from WT and myeloid HIF-KO mice. ITGB2 and ITGA4 were found to be upregulated in HIF-KO MDSC confirming other studies that showed negative regulation of ITGA4 by HIF-1α (36) but not explaining the reduced MDSC-accumulation in the uterus. Taken together, our results suggest that HIF-1α knockout in myeloid cells does not alter MDSC migration to the uterus.

We found increased apoptosis rates of MDSC isolated from spleens and uteri of myeloid HIF-KO mice compared to WT mice. This is in line with most previous studies indicating that HIF-1α promotes survival in cancer and endothelial cells (37–41). In contrast, there are also studies describing a proapoptotic role for HIF-1α (42, 43). During pregnancy, data on the role of HIF-1α for apoptosis are conflicting (44, 45). However, previous studies focused on placental cells and not immune cells in the uterus. Regarding our results, the increased apoptosis rates in HIF-KO MDSC may explain their reduced accumulation in the pregnant uterus. Correspondingly, in peripheral organs, myeloid HIF-KO MDSC still expanded, albeit to a lesser extent than WT-MDSC.

Last, we show that myeloid HIF-KO mice had higher rates of non-pregnant animals after positive vaginal plug and higher abortion rates than WT-mice pointing to the potential clinical relevance of reduced MDSC accumulation in the uterus. General loss of HIF-1α causes severe failure in placental formation, resulting in embryo lethality by E10.5. In these animals, placental defects are mainly caused by disturbed development of vascularization and disruption of trophoblast differentiation (46–48). In the embryo, HIF-1α is required for heart development, chondrogenesis and bone formation (49–51). Clinical studies showed upregulation of HIF-1α in trophoblasts of patients with missed abortions (52, 53), and increased HIF-1α activity in placental tissues has been associated with preeclampsia (54–56). However, reports on HIF-1α-regulation in myeloid cells during pregnancy are lacking. The role of hypoxia and HIF-1α in myeloid cells during other inflammatory processes is inconclusive. In a mouse model of LPS-induced Sepsis, HIF-1α induced a proinflammatory phenotype in monocytes and deletion of HIF-1α led to improved survival (57). In dendritic cells, hypoxia and HIFs are described to mediate both, proinflammatory and anti-inflammatory properties (58, 59). Under tumor conditions however, hypoxia and HIF-1α seem to drive the development and function of immunosuppressive myeloid cells like TAMs and MDSCs (23, 60, 61). Correspondingly, a recent study showed that overexpression of HIF-1α in myeloid cells leads to diminished transplant rejection and induction of a regulatory phenotype in myeloid cells in a model of heart transplantation (62). To our knowledge, our study is the first describing an impact of myeloid HIF-1α-expression on pregnancy outcome. Several previous studies in humans (11, 63, 64) and mice (10, 64–66) have shown that reduced MDSC accumulation is associated with abortions. Adoptive transfer experiments with abortion-prone mice furthermore showed that abortion rates were reduced by MDSC-transfer (65, 66). Absence of MDSC also led to failed implantation (13). These results together with our finding of a reduced MDSC-accumulation in myeloid HIF-KO mice make it tempting to speculate that diminished MDSC accumulation is responsible for the disturbed course of pregnancy in these animals.

In conclusion, we show here that HIF-1α expression in myeloid cells is required for a successful pregnancy and that loss of HIF-1α in myeloid cells leads to diminished accumulation, increased apoptosis and impaired MDSC function in the pregnant uterus. These results not only enlarge our knowledge about regulation of MDSC-accumulation and function during pregnancy, but may also help to better understand MDSC biology in other hypoxic conditions such as in solide tumors and inflamed tissues. Targeting HIF-1α may be a promising strategy to modulate MDSC-function.

ETHICS STATEMENT

This study was carried out in accordance with the recommendations of the Einrichtung für Tierschutz, Tierärztlichen Dienst und Versuchtierkunde Tübingen. The protocol was approved by the Einrichtung für Tierschutz, Tierärztlichen Dienst und Versuchtierkunde Tübingen and the Regierungspräsidium Tübingen.

AUTHOR CONTRIBUTIONS

NK and CG conceptualized and designed the study. NK, SD, JS, and BS performed experiments. NK, SD, and CG analyzed data. NK drafted the initial manuscript. NK, JP-F, CP, and CG reviewed and revised the manuscript. All authors approved the final manuscript as submitted and agreed to be accountable for all aspects of the work.

ACKNOWLEDGMENTS

Thanks to Prof. Bernhard Brüne, Institute for Biochemistry, Pathobiochemistry, Frankfurt, Germany for his kind help with HIF-1α KO mice. This work was supported by research grants of the Ministerium für Wissenschaft, Forschung und Kunst Baden-Württemberg and the European Social Fund, the German Center for Infection Research (DZIF), the Deutsche Forschungsgemeinschaft (DFG) and by a research grant of the Medical Faculty of Tuebingen University, grant no. F 1275151.

REFERENCES

1. Rai R, Regan L. Recurrent miscarriage. *Lancet* (2006) 368:601–11. doi: 10.1016/S0140-6736(06)69204-0
2. (AGIM), D.G.f.G.u.G.D.u.d.A.I.i.d.G.u.G. (2013). Diagnostik und therapie beim wiederholten Spontanabort. *AWMF-Register* 015/050.
3. Warning JC, McCracken SA, Morris JM. A balancing act: mechanisms by which the fetus avoids rejection by the maternal immune system. *Reproduction* (2011) 141:715–24. doi: 10.1530/REP-10-0360
4. Budhwar S, Verma P, Verma R, Rai S, Singh K. The Yin and Yang of myeloid derived suppressor cells. *Front Immunol.* (2018) 9:2776. doi: 10.3389/fimmu.2018.02776
5. Youn JI, Nagaraj S, Collazo M, Gabrilovich DI. Subsets of myeloid-derived suppressor cells in tumor-bearing mice. *J Immunol.* (2008) 181:5791–802. doi: 10.4049/jimmunol.181.8.5791
6. Gabrilovich DI, Nagaraj S. Myeloid-derived suppressor cells as regulators of the immune system. *Nat Rev Immunol* (2009) 9:162–74. doi: 10.1038/nri2506
7. Rodriguez PC, Ochoa AC. Arginine regulation by myeloid derived suppressor cells and tolerance in cancer: mechanisms and therapeutic perspectives. *Immunol Rev.* (2008) 222:180–91. doi: 10.1111/j.1600-065X.2008.00608.x
8. Brandau S, Trellakis S, Bruderek K, Schmaltz D, Steller G, Elian M, et al. Myeloid-derived suppressor cells in the peripheral blood of cancer patients contain a subset of immature neutrophils with impaired migratory properties. *J Leukoc Biol.* (2011) 89:311–7. doi: 10.1189/jlb.0310162
9. Kostlin N, Kugel H, Spring B, Leiber A, Marme A, Henes M, et al. Granulocytic myeloid derived suppressor cells expand in human pregnancy and modulate T-cell responses. *Eur J Immunol.* (2014) 44:2582–91. doi: 10.1002/eji.201344200
10. Zhao H, Kalish F, Schulz S, Yang Y, Wong RJ, Stevenson DK. Unique roles of infiltrating myeloid cells in the murine uterus during early to midpregnancy. *J Immunol.* (2015) 194:3713–22. doi: 10.4049/jimmunol.1401930
11. Kostlin N, Hofstadter K, Ostermeir AL, Spring B, Leiber A, Haen S, et al. Granulocytic myeloid-derived suppressor cells accumulate in human placenta and polarize toward a Th2 phenotype. *J Immunol.* (2016) 196:1132–45. doi: 10.4049/jimmunol.1500340

12. Kostlin N, Ostermeir AL, Spring B, Schwarz J, Marme A, Walter CB, et al. HLA-G promotes myeloid-derived suppressor cell accumulation and suppressive activity during human pregnancy through engagement of the receptor ILT4. *Eur J Immunol.* (2017a) 47:374–84. doi: 10.1002/eji.201646564
13. Ostrand-Rosenberg S, Sinha P, Figley C, Long R, Park D, Carter D, et al. Frontline Science: Myeloid-derived suppressor cells (MDSCs) facilitate maternal-fetal tolerance in mice. *J Leukoc Biol.* (2017) 101:1091–101. doi: 10.1189/jlb.1HI1016-306RR
14. Rieber N, Gille C, Kostlin N, Schafer I, Spring B, Ost M, et al. Neutrophilic myeloid-derived suppressor cells in cord blood modulate innate and adaptive immune responses. *Clin Exp Immunol.* (2013) 174:45–52. doi: 10.1111/cei.12143
15. Kostlin N, Vogelmann M, Spring B, Schwarz J, Feucht J, Hartel C, et al. Granulocytic myeloid derived suppressor cells from human cord blood modulate T-helper-cell response towards an anti-inflammatory phenotype. *Immunology* (2017b) 152:89–101. doi: 10.1111/imm.12751
16. Schwarz J, Scheckenbach V, Kugel H, Spring B, Pagel J, Hartel C, et al. Granulocytic myeloid-derived suppressor cells (GR-MDSC) accumulate in cord blood of preterm infants and remain elevated during the neonatal period. *Clin Exp Immunol* (2017) 91:328–37. doi: 10.1111/cei.13059
17. He YM, Li X, Perego M, Nefedova Y, Kossenkov AV, Jensen EA, et al. Transitory presence of myeloid-derived suppressor cells in neonates is critical for control of inflammation. *Nat Med.* (2018) 24, 224–31. doi: 10.1038/nm.4467
18. Caniggia I, Mostachfi H, Winter J, Gassmann M, Lye SJ, Kuliszewski M, et al. Hypoxia-inducible factor-1 mediates the biological effects of oxygen on human trophoblast differentiation through TGFbeta(3). *J Clin Invest.* (2000) 105:577–87. doi: 10.1172/JCI8316
19. Rajakumar A, Conrad KP. Expression, ontogeny, and regulation of hypoxia-inducible transcription factors in the human placenta. *Biol Reprod.* (2000) 63:559–69. doi: 10.1095/biolreprod63.2.559
20. Semenza GL. HIF-1 and mechanisms of hypoxia sensing. *Curr Opin Cell Biol.* (2001) 13:167–71. doi: 10.1016/S0955-0674(00)00194-0
21. Tal R, Shaish A, Barshack I, Polak-Charcon S, Afek A, Volkov A, et al. Effects of hypoxia-inducible factor-1alpha overexpression in pregnant mice: possible implications for preeclampsia and intrauterine growth restriction. *Am J Pathol.* (2010) 177:2950–62. doi: 10.2353/ajpath.2010.090800
22. Corzo CA, Condamine T, Lu L, Cotter MJ, Youn JI, Cheng P, et al. HIF-1alpha regulates function and differentiation of myeloid-derived suppressor cells in the tumor microenvironment. *J Exp Med.* (2010) 207:2439–53. doi: 10.1084/jem.20100587
23. Doedens AL, Stockmann C, Rubinstein MP, Liao D, Zhang N, DeNardo DG, et al. Macrophage expression of hypoxia-inducible factor-1 alpha suppresses T-cell function and promotes tumor progression. *Cancer Res.* (2010) 70:7465–75. doi: 10.1158/0008-5472.CAN-10-1439
24. Noman MZ, Desantis G, Janji B, Hasmim M, Karray S, Dessen P, et al. PD L1 is a novel direct target of HIF-1alpha, and its blockade under hypoxia enhanced MDSC-mediated T cell activation. *J Exp Med.* (2014) 211:781–90. doi: 10.1084/jem.20131916
25. Koehn BH, Apostolova P, Haverkamp JM, Miller JS, McCullar V, Tolar J, et al. GVHD-associated, inflammasome-mediated loss of function in adoptively transferred myeloid-derived suppressor cells. *Blood* (2015) 126:1621–8. doi: 10.1182/blood-2015-03-634691
26. Messmann JJ, Reisser T, Leithauser F, Lutz MB, Debatin KM, Strauss G. *In vitro*-generated MDSCs prevent murine GVHD by inducing type 2 T cells without disabling antitumor cytotoxicity. *Blood* (2015) 126:1138–48. doi: 10.1182/blood-2015-01-624163
27. Chiu DK, Tse AP, Xu IM, Di Cui J, Lai RK, Li LL, et al. Hypoxia inducible factor HIF-1 promotes myeloid-derived suppressor cells accumulation through ENTPD2/CD39L1 in hepatocellular carcinoma. *Nat Commun.* (2017) 8:517. doi: 10.1038/s41467-017-00530-7
28. van Uden P, Kenneth NS, Rocha S. Regulation of hypoxia-inducible factor-1alpha by NF-kappaB. *Biochem J.* (2008) 412:477–84. doi: 10.1042/BJ20080476
29. Yang J, AlTahan A, Jones DT, Buffa FM, Bridges E, Interiano RB, et al. Estrogen receptor-alpha directly regulates the hypoxia-inducible factor 1 pathway associated with antiestrogen response in breast cancer. *Proc Natl Acad Sci USA.* (2015) 112:15172–7. doi: 10.1073/pnas.1422015112
30. Pan T, Zhong L, Wu S, Cao Y, Yang Q, Cai Z, et al. 17beta-estradiol enhances the expansion and activation of myeloid-derived suppressor cells via STAT3 signaling in human pregnancy. *Clin Exp Immunol.* (2016b) 185:86–97. doi: 10.1111/cei.12790
31. Takeda N, O'Dea EL, Doedens A, Kim JW, Weidemann A, Stockmann C, et al. Differential activation and antagonistic function of HIF-{alpha} isoforms in macrophages are essential for NO homeostasis. *Genes Dev.* (2010) 24:491–501. doi: 10.1101/gad.1881410
32. Leiber A, Schwarz J, Kostlin N, Spring B, Fehrenbach B, Katava N, et al. Neonatal myeloid derived suppressor cells show reduced apoptosis and immunosuppressive activity upon infection with *Escherichia coli*. *Eur J Immunol.* (2017) 47:1009–21. doi: 10.1002/eji.201646621
33. Maxwell PJ, Gallagher R, Seaton A, Wilson C, Scullin P, Pettigrew J, et al. HIF-1 and NF-kappaB-mediated upregulation of CXCR1 and CXCR2 expression promotes cell survival in hypoxic prostate cancer cells. *Oncogene* (2007) 26:7333–45. doi: 10.1038/sj.onc.1210536
34. Zhang T, Kawaguchi N, Hayama E, Furutani Y, Nakanishi T. High expression of CXCR4 and stem cell markers in a monocrotaline and chronic hypoxia-induced rat model of pulmonary arterial hypertension. *Exp Ther Med.* (2018) 15:4615–22. doi: 10.3892/etm.2018.6027
35. Yamaji-Kegan K, Su Q, Angelini DJ, Johns RA. IL-4 is proangiogenic in the lung under hypoxic conditions. *J Immunol.* (2009) 182:5469–76. doi: 10.4049/jimmunol.0713347
36. Choi JH, Lee YB, Jung J, Hwang SG, Oh IH, Kim GJ. Hypoxia inducible factor-1alpha regulates the migration of bone marrow mesenchymal stem cells via integrin alpha 4. *Stem Cells Int.* (2016) 2016:7932185. doi: 10.1155/2016/7932185
37. Alvarez-Tejado M, Naranjo-Suarez S, Jimenez C, Carrera AC, Landazuri MO, del Peso L. Hypoxia induces the activation of the phosphatidylinositol 3-kinase/Akt cell survival pathway in PC12 cells: protective role in apoptosis. *J Biol Chem.* (2001). 276:22368–74. doi: 10.1074/jbc.M011688200
38. Piret JP, Lecocq C, Toffoli S, Ninane N, Raes M, Michiels C. Hypoxia and CoCl2 protect HepG2 cells against serum deprivation- and t-BHP-induced apoptosis: a possible anti-apoptotic role for HIF-1. *Exp Cell Res.* (2004) 295:340–9. doi: 10.1016/j.yexcr.2004.01.024
39. Yu EZ, Li YY, Liu XH, Kagan E, McCarron RM. Antiapoptotic action of hypoxia-inducible factor-1 alpha in human endothelial cells. *Lab Invest.* (2004) 84:553–61. doi: 10.1038/labinvest.3700071
40. Zhang Q, Zhang ZF, Rao JY, Sato JD, Brown J, Messadi DV, et al. Treatment with siRNA and antisense oligonucleotides targeted to HIF-1alpha induced apoptosis in human tongue squamous cell carcinomas. *Int J Cancer* (2004) 111:849–57. doi: 10.1002/ijc.20334
41. Sasabe E, Tatemoto Y, Li D, Yamamoto T, Osaki T. Mechanism of HIF-1alpha-dependent suppression of hypoxia-induced apoptosis in squamous cell carcinoma cells. *Cancer Sci.* (2005) 96:394–402. doi: 10.1111/j.1349-7006.2005.00065.x
42. Carmeliet P, Dor Y, Herbert JM, Fukumura D, Brusselmans K, Dewerchin M, et al. Role of HIF-1alpha in hypoxia-mediated apoptosis, cell proliferation and tumour angiogenesis. *Nature* (1998) 394:485–90. doi: 10.1038/28867
43. Guo K, Searfoss G, Krolikowski D, Pagnoni M, Franks C, Clark K, et al. Hypoxia induces the expression of the pro-apoptotic gene BNIP3. *Cell Death Differ.* (2001) 8:367–76. doi: 10.1038/sj.cdd.4400810
44. Aban C, Martinez N, Carou C, Albamonte I, Toro A, Seyahian A, et al. Endocannabinoids participate in placental apoptosis induced by hypoxia inducible factor-1. *Apoptosis* (2016) 21:1094–105. doi: 10.1007/s10495-016-1274-x
45. Kenchegowda D, Natale B, Lemus MA, Natale DR, Fisher SA. Inactivation of maternal Hif-1alpha at mid-pregnancy causes placental defects and deficits in oxygen delivery to the fetal organs under hypoxic stress. *Dev Biol.* (2017) 422:171–85. doi: 10.1016/j.ydbio.2016.12.013
46. Adelman DM, Gertsenstein M, Nagy A, Simon MC, Maltepe E. Placental cell fates are regulated *in vivo* by HIF-mediated hypoxia responses. *Genes Dev.* (2000) 14:3191–203. doi: 10.1101/gad.853700
47. Cowden Dahl KD, Fryer BH, Mack FA, Compernolle V, Maltepe E, Adelman DM, et al. Hypoxia-inducible factors 1alpha and 2alpha regulate trophoblast differentiation. *Mol Cell Biol.* (2005) 25:10479–91. doi: 10.1128/MCB.25.23.10479-10491.2005

48. Dunwoodie SL. The role of hypoxia in development of the Mammalian embryo. *Dev Cell* (2009) 17:755–73. doi: 10.1016/j.devcel.2009.11.008
49. Ryan HE, Lo J, Johnson RS. HIF-1 alpha is required for solid tumor formation and embryonic vascularization. *EMBO J.* (1998) 17:3005–15. doi: 10.1093/emboj/17.11.3005
50. Amarilio R, Viukov SV, Sharir A, Eshkar-Oren I, Johnson RS, Zelzer E. HIF1alpha regulation of Sox9 is necessary to maintain differentiation of hypoxic prechondrogenic cells during early skeletogenesis. *Development* (2007) 134:3917–28. doi: 10.1242/dev.008441
51. Krishnan J, Ahuja P, Bodenmann S, Knapik D, Perriard E, Krek W, et al. Essential role of developmentally activated hypoxia-inducible factor 1alpha for cardiac morphogenesis and function. *Circ Res.* (2008) 103:1139–46. doi: 10.1161/01.RES.0000338613.89841.c1
52. Fang Y, Yu S, Ma Y, Sun P, Ma D, Ji C, et al. Association of Dll4/notch and HIF-1a -VEGF signaling in the angiogenesis of missed abortion. *PLoS ONE* (2013) 8:e70667. doi: 10.1371/journal.pone.0070667
53. Zhu LJ, Chen YP, Chen BJ, Mei XH. Changes in reactive oxygen species, superoxide dismutase, and hypoxia-inducible factor-1alpha levels in missed abortion. *Int J Clin Exp Med.* (2014) 7:2179–84.
54. Rajakumar A, Brandon HM, Daftary A, Ness R, Conrad KP. Evidence for the functional activity of hypoxia-inducible transcription factors overexpressed in preeclamptic placentae. *Placenta* (2004) 25:763–9. doi: 10.1016/j.placenta.2004.02.011
55. Nevo O, Soleymanlou N, Wu Y, Xu J, Kingdom J, Many A, et al. Increased expression of sFlt-1 in in vivo and in vitro models of human placental hypoxia is mediated by HIF-1. *Am J Physiol Regul Integr Comp Physiol.* (2006) 291:R1085–93. doi: 10.1152/ajpregu.00794.2005
56. Robb KP, Cotechini T, Allaire C, Sperou A, Graham CH. Inflammation-induced fetal growth restriction in rats is associated with increased placental HIF-1alpha accumulation. *PLoS ONE* (2017) 12:e0175805. doi: 10.1371/journal.pone.0175805
57. Peyssonnaux C, Cejudo-Martin P, Doedens A, Zinkernagel AS, Johnson RS, Nizet V. Cutting edge: essential role of hypoxia inducible factor-1alpha in development of lipopolysaccharide-induced sepsis. *J Immunol.* (2007) 178:7516–9. doi: 10.4049/jimmunol.178.12.7516
58. Jantsch J, Chakravortty D, Turza N, Prechtel AT, Buchholz B, Gerlach RG, et al. Hypoxia and hypoxia-inducible factor-1 alpha modulate lipopolysaccharide-induced dendritic cell activation and function. *J Immunol.* (2008) 180:4697–705. doi: 10.4049/jimmunol.180.7.4697
59. Mancino A, Schioppa T, Larghi P, Pasqualini F, Nebuloni M, Chen IH, et al. Divergent effects of hypoxia on dendritic cell functions. *Blood* (2008) 112:3723–34. doi: 10.1182/blood-2008-02-142091
60. Talks KL, Turley H, Gatter KC, Maxwell PH, Pugh CW, Ratcliffe PJ, et al. The expression and distribution of the hypoxia-inducible factors HIF-1alpha and HIF-2alpha in normal human tissues, cancers, and tumor-associated macrophages. *Am J Pathol.* (2000) 157:411–21. doi: 10.1016/S0002-9440(10)64554-3
61. Corzo CA, Cotter MJ, Cheng P, Cheng F, Kusmartsev S, Sotomayor E, et al. Mechanism regulating reactive oxygen species in tumor-induced myeloid-derived suppressor cells. *J Immunol.* (2009) 182:5693–701. doi: 10.4049/jimmunol.0900092
62. Keranen MAI, Raissadati A, Nykanen AI, Dashkevich A, Tuuminen R, Krebs R, et al. Hypoxia-inducible factor controls immunoregulatory properties of myeloid cells in mouse cardiac allografts - an experimental study. *Transpl Int.* (2019) 32:95–106. doi: 10.1111/tri.13310
63. Nair RR, Sinha P, Khanna A, Singh K. Reduced myeloid-derived suppressor cells in the blood and endometrium is associated with early miscarriage *Am J Reprod Immunol.* 73:479–86. doi: 10.1111/aji.12351
64. Kang X, Zhang X, Liu Z, Xu H, Wang T, He L, et al. Granulocytic myeloid-derived suppressor cells maintain feto-maternal tolerance by inducing Foxp3 expression in CD4+CD25-T cells by activation of the TGF-beta/beta-catenin pathway. *Mol Hum Reprod.* (2016b) 22:499–511. doi: 10.1093/molehr/gaw026
65. Kang X, Zhang X, Liu Z, Xu H, Wang T, He L, et al. CXCR2-mediated granulocytic myeloid-derived suppressor cells' functional characterization and their role in maternal fetal interface. *DNA Cell Biol.* (2016a) 35:358–65. doi: 10.1089/dna.2015.2962
66. Pan T, Liu Y, Zhong LM, Shi MH, Duan XB, Wu K, et al. Myeloid-derived suppressor cells are essential for maintaining feto-maternal immunotolerance via STAT3 signaling in mice. *J Leukoc Biol.* (2016a) 100:499–511. doi: 10.1189/jlb.1A1015-481RR

11

ZIKV Disrupts Placental Ultrastructure and Drug Transporter Expression in Mice

Cherley Borba Vieira Andrade[1], *Victoria Regina de Siqueira Monteiro*[1], *Sharton Vinicius Antunes Coelho*[2], *Hanailly Ribeiro Gomes*[1], *Ronny Paiva Campos Sousa*[1], *Veronica Muller de Oliveira Nascimento*[1], *Flavia Fonseca Bloise*[1], *Stephen Giles Matthews*[3,4,5,6], *Enrrico Bloise*[7], *Luciana Barros Arruda*[2] *and Tania Maria Ortiga-Carvalho*[1*]

[1] *Institute of Biophysics Carlos Chagas Filho, Federal University of Rio de Janeiro, Rio de Janeiro, Brazil,* [2] *Institute of Microbiology Paulo de Góes, Federal University of Rio de Janeiro, Rio de Janeiro, Brazil,* [3] *Department of Physiology, Faculty of Medicine, University of Toronto, Toronto, ON, Canada,* [4] *Department of Obstetrics & Gynecology, Faculty of Medicine, University of Toronto, Toronto, ON, Canada,* [5] *Department of Medicine, Faculty of Medicine, University of Toronto, Toronto, ON, Canada,* [6] *Lunenfeld-Tanenbaum Research Institute, Mount Sinai Hospital, Toronto, ON, Canada,* [7] *Department of Morphology, Federal University of Minas Gerais, Belo Horizonte, Brazil*

***Correspondence:**
Tania Maria Ortiga-Carvalho
taniaort@biof.ufrj.br

Congenital Zika virus (ZIKV) infection can induce fetal brain abnormalities. Here, we investigated whether maternal ZIKV infection affects placental physiology and metabolic transport potential and impacts the fetal outcome, regardless of viral presence in the fetus at term. Low (10^3 PFU-ZIKV$_{PE243}$; low ZIKV) and high ($5x10^7$ PFU-ZIKV$_{PE243}$; high ZIKV) virus titers were injected into immunocompetent (ICompetent C57BL/6) and immunocompromised (ICompromised A129) mice at gestational day (GD) 12.5 for tissue collection at GD18.5 (term). High ZIKV elicited fetal death rates of 66% and 100%, whereas low ZIKV induced fetal death rates of 0% and 60% in C57BL/6 and A129 dams, respectively. All surviving fetuses exhibited intrauterine growth restriction (IUGR) and decreased placental efficiency. High-ZIKV infection in C57BL/6 and A129 mice resulted in virus detection in maternal spleens and placenta, but only A129 fetuses presented virus RNA in the brain. Nevertheless, pregnancies in both strains produced fetuses with decreased head sizes ($p<0.05$). Low-ZIKV-A129 dams had higher IL-6 and CXCL1 levels ($p<0.05$), and their placentas showed increased CCL-2 and CXCL-1 contents ($p<0.05$). In contrast, low-ZIKV-C57BL/6 dams had an elevated CCL2 serum level and increased type I and II IFN expression in the placenta. Notably, less abundant microvilli and mitochondrial degeneration were evidenced in the placental labyrinth zone (Lz) of ICompromised and high-ZIKV-ICompetent mice but not in low-ZIKV-C57BL/6 mice. In addition, decreased placental expression of the drug transporters P-glycoprotein (P-gp) and breast cancer resistance protein (Bcrp) and the lipid transporter Abca1 was detected in all ZIKV-infected groups, but Bcrp and Abca1 were only reduced in ICompromised and high-ZIKV ICompetent mice. Our data indicate that gestational ZIKV infection triggers specific proinflammatory responses and affects placental turnover and transporter expression in a manner dependent on virus concentration and maternal immune status. Placental damage may impair proper fetal-maternal exchange function and fetal growth/survival, likely contributing to congenital Zika syndrome.

Keywords: ZIKV, placenta, P-glycoprotein (P-gp) breast cancer resistance protein (BCRP), ABCA1, ABCG1, ultrastructure, cytokine, chemokine 2

INTRODUCTION

Congenital Zika virus (ZIKV) infection can be associated with adverse pregnancy outcomes. Neonates born from ZIKV-positive pregnancies may develop severe neurological abnormalities, placental pathologies and intrauterine growth restriction (IUGR), among other complications (1). ZIKV vertical transmission has become a major public health issue worldwide, especially in Brazil, where more than 200,000 ZIKV-positive cases have been confirmed and over 2,000 congenital microcephaly births have been reported (2–6). These numbers represent a 20-fold rise in the incidence of congenital microcephaly in Brazil during the years of the ZIKV pandemic, with similar increases reported elsewhere in Latin America (2, 3, 7). Importantly, while the ZIKV pandemic is currently thought to be controlled, evidence points to a possible silent ZIKV spread across the Americas (8, 9), highlighting the need for improved knowledge of the possible routes of vertical ZIKV transmission and its association with disruptive inflammatory and developmental phenotypes and the need for new avenues of prevention and treatment.

Previous studies have investigated the possible pathways involved in vertical ZIKV transmission. Miranda and colleagues (10) showed that in humans, ZIKV infection changed the pattern of tight junction proteins, such as claudin-4, in syncytiotrophoblasts. Jurado et al. (2016) suggested that the migratory activities of Hofbauer cells (feto-placental macrophages) could help disseminate ZIKV to the fetal brain (11). Other recent studies have shown that placental villous fibroblasts, cytotrophoblasts, endothelial cells and Hofbauer cells are permissive to ZIKV, and placentae from ZIKV-infected women had chorionic villi with a high mean diameter (11–14). Furthermore, in 2019, Rathore et al. demonstrated that pregnant mice carrying high levels of antibodies against dengue virus (DENV) exhibited increased ZIKV vertical transmission associated with severe microcephaly-like syndrome, demonstrating another possible mechanism of antibody-dependent vertical ZIKV transmission (15). However, at present, further studies are required to identify the precise mechanism of maternal-fetal ZIKV transmission.

Many mouse models have been developed to identify how ZIKV overcomes placental defenses. Initially, limited information was obtained due to the apparent inability of the virus to infect wild-type (WT) mice (16). ZIKV NS5 targets the interferon signaling pathway in humans but not in mice (17). Thus, WT mice show no clear evidence of clinical disease (17, 18) and are of limited use in modeling the disease. However, mice lacking an interferon signaling response show evidence of disease and have been widely used to investigate ZIKV infection during pregnancy (8, 17, 19).

The interferon system, especially type III interferon, is a key mechanism of host defense and a viral target for immune evasion (20). Type III interferons have a role in protection against ZIKV infection in human syncytiotrophoblasts from term placenta (21). Luo et al. have shown that inhibition of Toll-like receptors 3 and 8 inhibits the cytokine output of ZIKV-infected trophoblasts (22). In addition, viral replication coincides with the induction of proinflammatory cytokines, such as interleukin [IL]-6. This cytokine has a crucial role in inflammation and affects the homeostatic processes related to tissue injury and activation of stress-related responses (23, 24). ZIKV infection can trigger an inflammatory response with IL-6 release (11, 25).

Maternal infection has profound effects on placental permeability to drugs and environmental toxins. Changes in the expression and function of specific ABC transporters in the placenta and yolk sac following infective and inflammatory stimuli have been demonstrated (26–30). ABC transporters are efflux transporters that control the biodistribution of several endogenous and exogenous substrates, including xenobiotics (antiretrovirals and synthetic glucocorticoids), steroid hormones (estrogens and androgens), nutrients (folate and cholesterol) and immunological factors (chemokines and cytokines) within the maternal-fetal interface (31). The best described ABC transporters in the placenta are P-glycoprotein (P-gp; also known as multidrug resistance protein 1, MDR1), breast cancer resistance protein (Bcrp) and the lipid Abca1 and Abcg1 transporters. P-gp and Bcrp transporters are responsible for preventing fetal accumulation of xenobiotics and environmental toxins that may be present in the maternal circulation, whereas Abca1 and Abcg1 control the placental exchange of cytotoxic oxysterol and lipid permeability throughout pregnancy; therefore, they play an important role in fetal protection and placental lipid homeostasis (26).

Despite the limited number of studies showing ZIKV infection in immunocompetent mice, intrauterine inoculation with a high virus titer was previously demonstrated to result in decreased fetal viability, with worse outcomes following infection in early gestation (32). In another report, intravenous infection on a very early embryonic day resulted in fetal demise even though the virus was not found in the fetal compartment in most of the treated animals (33). In the present study, we hypothesize that maternal exposure to ZIKV affects placental function, including placental ultrastructure and ABC transporter (P-gp, Bcrp, Abca1 and Abcg1) protein expression, even in the absence of vertical transmission and that these effects are dependent on viral infective titers and maternal immune status.

MATERIALS AND METHODS

Virus Preparation and Storage

The Brazilian $ZIKV_{PE243}$ (GenBank ref. number KX197192) strain was isolated from a febrile case during the ZIKV outbreak in the state of Pernambuco, Brazil and was kindly provided by Dr Ernesto T. Marques Jr. (Centro de Pesquisa Aggeu Magalhães, FIOCRUZ, PE). Viruses were propagated in C6/36 cells, and viral titers were determined by plaque assays in Vero cells, as previously described (34). Supernatants of noninfected C6/36 cells cultured under the same conditions were used as mock controls.

Animal Experimentation and Study Design

Two mouse strains were used in the study: immunocompetent (ICompetent) C57BL/6 and immunocompromised (ICompromised) (type 1 *Ifnr*-deficient) A129 strains. Since we were unable to consistently produce viable pregnancies by mating A129 males and females in our experimental settings, we mated A129 females (n=15) with C57BL/6 males (n=4) to produce ICompromised C57BL6/A129 pregnancies, whereas ICompetent C57BL/6 pregnancies were obtained by mating male (n=6) and female (n=35) C57BL/6 mice (8-10 weeks old). Animals were kept in a controlled temperature room (23°C) with a light/dark cycle of 12 hours and *ad libitum* access to water and food. After detection of the proestrous/estrous phase *via* vaginal cytology, copulation was confirmed by visualization of the vaginal plug and considered gestational day 0.5 (GD0.5). Maternal weight was monitored for confirmation of pregnancy; thus, females were weighed on GD0.5 and GD12.5, and females with a weight gain greater than 3 g were considered pregnant and entered randomly in the experimental groups. Experimental protocols were approved by the Animal Care Committee of the Health Sciences Center, Federal University of Rio de Janeiro (CEUA-036/16 and 104/16) and registered with the Brazilian National Council for Animal Experimentation Control.

On GD12.5, pregnant mice (ICompetent and ICompromised pregnancies) were injected with a single intravenous (i.v.) titer of ZIKV or mock control. ICompetent and ICompromised pregnant mice were randomly subdivided into three experimental groups: the mock (control) group, which received an injection of supernatant from noninfected C6/36 cells (ICompetent mock and ICompromised mock); the high-ZIKV-titer group, inoculated with $5x10^7$ plaque-forming units (PFU) of $ZIKV_{PE243}$ (ICompetent high and ICompromised high); and the ZIKV low-titer group, injected with 10^3 PFU of $ZIKV_{PE243}$ (ICompetent low and ICompromised low).

On the morning of GD18.5, all animals were euthanized with a sodium phenobarbital overdose of 300 mg/kg. Maternal blood was collected *via* cardiac puncture, centrifuged (10 min, 4000 g) and stored at -20°C. The maternal brain and spleen and all placentae and all fetuses were dissected, collected and weighed, followed by fetal head isolation and measurement. The three placentae closest to the mean weight in a litter were selected for further analysis and cut in half using umbilical cord insertion as a reference (35–37). One-half of the placental disk was frozen in liquid nitrogen for qPCR, and the other half was fixed overnight in buffered paraformaldehyde (4%, Sigma-Aldrich, Brazil) for ultrastructural and protein expression/localization analysis. Matched fetal heads, maternal brains and spleens were frozen in liquid nitrogen for qPCR. Of important note, all fetuses obtained from ICompromised pregnancies were heterozygous.

ZIKV RNA Quantification *via* RT-qPCR

ZIKV load was evaluated in maternal blood, brains and spleens and in the placentae and fetal heads. Brains, spleens, placentae and fetal heads were macerated in RPMI medium (Gibco™ RPMI 1640 Medium) normalized by the ratio of 0.2 mg of tissue to every 1 µl of medium and plotted per gram of tissue. The macerated volume was centrifuged at 4500 g for 5 min to remove tissue residues, and then, 500 µl of the centrifuged volume was used for RNA extraction using 1 mL of TRIzol reagent (Life Technologies, Thermo Fischer, USA). Treatment with DNase I (Ambion, Thermo Fischer, USA) was performed to prevent contamination by genomic DNA. cDNA was synthesized using a cDNA High Capacity Kit (Applied Biosystems, Thermo Fischer, USA) according to the manufacturer's instructions by subjecting the samples to the following cycle: 25°C for 10 min, 37°C for 120 min and 85°C for 5 min. qPCR was performed using a StepOnePlus Real-Time qPCR system, TaqMan Master Mix Reagents (Applied Biosystems, Thermo Fischer, USA) and primers and probes specific for the protein E sequence (38). Samples were then subjected to the following cycle: 50°C for 2 min, followed by 40 cycles of 95°C for 10 min, 95°C for 15 sec, and 60°C for 1 min.

RT-qPCR

The placenta was macerated in 1.5 mL of TRIzol reagent (Life Technologies, Thermo Fischer, USA). RNA extraction was performed following the manufacturer's protocol. cDNA was prepared using High Capacity cDNA Reverse Transcription Kit (Applied Biosystems, CA, USA). The reaction was carried out for selected genes using intron-spanning primers (**Table 1**) and the StepOnePlus Real-Time PCR system (Life Technologies, Thermo Fischer, USA). Samples were subjected to the following cycle: 95° C for 10 min, followed by 40 amplification cycles consisting of DNA denaturation for 30 sec at 95°C and annealing of primers for 30 sec at 60°C. The threshold cycle (Ct) was determined for each gene of interest and for the reference genes glycerol 3-phosphate dehydrogenase (*Gapdh*) and RNA Polymerase II Subunit A (*Polr2a*). The relative expression of each gene was calculated using $2^{-\Delta\Delta CT}$ (39) and graphically expressed as the fold-increase. The efficiency was calculated using the standard curve method. The melting curves were analyzed for each sample.

Detection of Cytokines and Chemokines In Maternal Serum and the Placenta

Initially, placental tissue was homogenized in extraction buffer (50 mM Tris, 150 mM NaCl, 1X Triton, 0.1% SDS, 5 mM EDTA, 5 mM NaF, 50 mM sodium pyrophosphate, 1 mM sodium

TABLE 1 | Primer sequences for the real-time PCR assay.

Gene	Primer sequences	GenBank accession no.
ZIKV	5'CCGCTGCCCAACACAAG3' 5'CCACTAACGTTCTTTTGCAGACAT3'	
Il6	5'TCATATCTTCAACCAAGAGGTA3' 5'CAGTGAGGAATGTCCACAAACTG3'	NM_031168.2
Il1b	5'GTAATGAAAGACGGCACACC3' 5'ATTAGAAACAGTCCAGCCCA3'	XM_006498795.4
Il10	5'TAAGGGTTACTTGGGTTGCCAAG3' 5'CAAATGCTCCTTGATTTCTGGGC3'	NM_010548.2
Ifng	5'AGCAACAGCAAGGCGAAAA3' 5'CTGGACCTGTGGGTTGTTGA3'	NM_008337.4
Ifn1	5'CTGGAGCAGCTGAATGGAAAG3' 5'CTTGAAGTCCGCCCTGTAGGT3'	NM_010510.1
Gapdh	5'CTTTGTCAAGCTCATTTCCTGG3' 5'TCTTGCTCAGTGTCCTTGC3'	XM_017321385.2
Tnf	5'CCTCACACTCAGATCATCTTCTCA3' 5'TGGTTCTCTTTGAGATCCATGC3'	NM_013693.3
Polr2a	5'TCTGCCAAGAATGTGACGCT3' 5'CCAAGCGGCAAAGAATGTCC3'	NM_001291068.1

orthovanadate, pH 7.4) containing complete protease inhibitor cocktail (Roche Applied Science, Germany) with TissueLyser LT (Qiagen, Germany). The protein concentration of each sample was analyzed using a Pierce™ BCA Protein Assay Kit (Thermo Scientific, USA) according to the manufacturer's instructions. Analysis of the cytokines IL-6 and IL-1β and the chemokines monocyte chemoattractant protein-1 (MCP-1/CCL2) and chemokine (C-X-C motif) ligand 1 (CXCL1) in maternal serum and placenta was performed with MILLIPLEX MAP Mouse Cytokine/Chemokine Magnetic Bead Panel – Immunology Multiplex Assays (MCYTOMAG-70K, Merck Millipore, Germany) following the manufacturer's recommendations. The plate with samples and magnetic beads was analyzed on a MAGPIX® System (Merck Millipore, Germany). The analyses were performed using Luminex xPonent® for MAGPIX® v software. 4.2 (Luminex Corp., USA). For each reaction well, the MAGPIX Luminex® platform reports the median fluorescence intensity (MFI) for each of the analytes in the sample. The levels of each analyte were then calculated against the standard curve. The ratio between the value obtained and the protein quantification for each sample was determined and plotted.

Virus Titration by Plaque Assay

Blood from mock- and $ZIKV_{PE243}$-infected mice was collected from the base of the tail at 4 hours, 48 hours and 144 hours following the appropriate treatments and subsequently centrifuged at 400 g for 30 min for plasma separation. Samples obtained at different periods post infection were titrated using a plaque assay. Vero cells (obtained from ATCC® CCL81™) (African green monkey kidney epithelial cell line) were plated in 24-well plates at $4x10^4$ cells per well in Dulbecco's modified Eagle's medium (DMEM) (GIBCO, Thermo Fisher, USA) supplemented with 5% fetal bovine serum (FBS) (GIBCO, Thermo Fisher, USA) and 1% gentamicin (10 µg/ml) (GIBCO, Thermo Fisher, USA) and cultured overnight for complete adhesion at 37°C with 5% CO_2. Then, the medium was removed, and the cells were washed with 1x PBS and incubated with serial (base 10) dilutions of virus in FBS-free medium. After 90 min of incubation under gentle shaking, the medium was removed, and the cells were washed with 1x PBS and cultured with 1.5% carboxymethylcellulose (CMC) supplemented with 1% FBS (GIBCO, Thermo Fisher, USA). After 5 days, the cells were fixed overnight with 4% formaldehyde and stained with 1% crystal violet in 20% methanol (ISOFAR, Brazil) for 1 hour. Plaques were counted, and the virus yield was calculated and expressed as plaque-forming units per milliliter (PFU/ml).

Histological, Immunohistochemistry, and TUNEL Analyses of the Placenta

Placental fragments were fixed overnight and subjected to dehydration (increasing ethanol series; ISOFAR, Brazil), diaphanization with xylol (ISOFAR, Brazil) and paraffin (Histopar, Easypath, Brazil). Sections (5 µm) were prepared using a Rotatory Microtome CUT 5062 (Slee Medical GmbH, Germany) and subjected to immunohistochemistry and TUNEL analyses.

For immunohistochemistry, blocking of endogenous peroxidase was performed with 3% hydrogen peroxide diluted in PBS, followed by microwave antigenic recovery in Tris-EDTA (pH=9) and sodium citrate (pH=6) buffers (15 min for Tris-EDTA buffer and 8 min for citrate buffer). Sections were washed in PBS + 0.2% Tween and exposed to 3% PBS/BSA for 1 hour. Sections were then incubated overnight at 4°C with the following primary antibodies: anti-Ki-67 (1:100 – [M3064]; Spring Bioscience, USA), anti-P-gp (1:500 – Mdr1[sc-55510]; Santa Cruz Biotechnology, USA), anti-Bcrp (1:100 – Bcrp [MAB4146]; Merck Millipore, USA), anti-Abcg1 (1:100 – [PA5-13462]; Thermo Fisher Scientific, USA) or anti-Abca1 (1:100 – [ab18180]; Abcam Plc, UK). The next day, sections were incubated with the biotin-conjugated secondary antibody SPD-060 (Spring Bioscience, USA) for 1 hour at room temperature. Three washes were performed with PBS + 0.2% Tween followed by incubation with streptavidin (SPD-060 - Spring Bioscience, USA) for 30 min. Sections were stained with 3,3-diamino-benzidine (DAB) (SPD-060 - Spring Bioscience, USA), counterstained with hematoxylin (Proquímios, Brazil), dehydrated, diaphanized and mounted with a coverslip and Entellan (Merck, Germany).

For analysis of apoptotic nuclei, terminal deoxynucleotidyl transferase dUTP nick-end labeling (TUNEL) staining was performed using an ApopTag® In Situ Peroxidase Detection Kit (S7100, Merck Millipore, USA) according to the manufacturer's recommendations and as previously described (36). All negative controls were prepared with omission of the primary antibody.

Image acquisition was performed using a high-resolution Olympus DP72 (Olympus Corporation, Japan) camera coupled to an Olympus BX53 light microscope (Olympus Corporation, Japan). For nuclear quantification of Ki-67 and TUNEL immunolabeling, Stepanizer software (40) was used. For this analysis, we evaluated 15 images from different random fields of the Lz (labyrinth zone) and Jz (junctional zone) for each animal, in a total of five animals from each ICompetent group and three animals from each ICompromised group. A total of 360 digital images (40X) randomly captured per placental region (180 Lz imagens and 180 Jz images) were evaluated in each experimental group. The total number of immunolabeled Ki-67 or TUNEL nuclei in each digital image was normalized by the total image area to obtain an index of the estimated number of proliferative and apoptotic nuclei in the entire histological section analyzed. Analysis was undertaken by two investigators blinded to the treatment.

Quantification of P-gp, Bcrp, Abca1 and Abcg1 staining was performed using the Image-Pro Plus, version 5.0 software (Media Cybernetics, USA) mask tool. The percentage of viable tissue area was considered upon exclusion of negative spaces. A total of 360 digital images (40X) randomly captured per placental region (180 Lz imagens and 180 Jz images) were evaluated in each experimental group. Analysis was undertaken by two investigators blinded to the treatment.

Transmission Electron Microscopy (TEM)

Sections of the placental Lz and Jz were fixed in paraformaldehyde 4% (Sigma-Aldrich, Brazil) for 48 hours, postfixed with osmium tetroxide (Electron Microscopy Sciences, USA) and potassium ferrocyanide (Electron Microscopy Sciences, USA) for 60 min and dehydrated with an increasing series of acetone (30%, 50%, 70%, 90% and two of 100%) (ISOFAR, Brazil). Sections were subsequently embedded with EPOXI resin (Electron Microscopy Sciences, USA) in acetone (1:2, 1:1 and 2:1, respectively) followed by EPOXI pure resin. After polymerization, ultrafine sections (70 nm) were prepared (Leica Microsystems, USA) and collected into 300 mesh copper grids (Electron Microscopy Sciences, USA). Tissue was contrasted with uranyl acetate and lead citrate and visualized using a JEOL JEM-1011 transmission electron microscope (JEOL, Ltd., Akishima, Tokyo, Japan). Digital micrographs were captured using an ORIUS CCD digital camera (Gatan, Inc., Pleasanton, California, EUA) at 6000× magnification. An overall qualitative analysis of the Lz and Jz in different groups was performed by investigating the ultrastructural characteristics of the mitochondria and the ER cisterns. The qualitative evaluation consisted of analyzing disruption of the mitochondrial membranes, mitochondrial morphology, preservation of mitochondrial cristae and matrix intensity (41). Ultrastructural analysis of nuclear morphology and the presence of microvilli in trophoblast sinusoidal giant cells was also undertaken. Analysis of ER cisterns was performed by evaluating the dilation of their lumen (42).

Statistical Analysis

GraphPad Prism 8 software (GraphPad Software, Inc., USA) was used for statistical analysis. A D'Agostino & Pearson normality test was used to evaluate normal distribution, and outliers were identified using a Grubbs test. The data are expressed as the mean ± SEM or individual values. One-way ANOVA followed by Tukey's posttest was used for comparisons between different inbred groups, whereas Student's t-test or a nonparametric Mann-Whitney test was performed to compare the outbred groups. Differences were considered significant when $p<0.05$. Pregnancy parameters were evaluated using the mean value of all fetuses and placentae in a litter per dam and not the individual conceptus, i.e., the mean value. In **Figures 1**, **2**, "n" represents the number of dams. For MET and immunostaining data, placentae closest to the mean weight of all placentae were selected from each litter; "n" represents the number of litters (35–37).

RESULTS

Weight Gain During Pregnancy Is Dependent on Maternal Immune Status in ZIKV-Infected Mice

To determine the effect of ZIKV infection on fetal and placental phenotypes at term (GD18.5), we infected Immunocompetent (ICompetent) C57BL/6 and immunocompromised (ICompromised) A129 mice with ZIKV at GD12.5 (**Figure 1A**). Given the very distinct susceptibility of C57BL/6 and A129 mice to ZIKV, systemic infection models were established by injecting high ($5x10^7$ PFU) and low (10^3 PFU) virus inoculum titers. As shown in **Figure 1B**, ICompetent C57BL/6 mice in all groups and ICompromised A129 dams inoculated with mock and low ZIKV titers exhibited higher maternal weight at GD18.5 than at GD12.5 and GD0.5 ($p<0.05$). On the other hand, ICompromised A129 mice presented significant weight loss at GD18.5, despite showing an increase at GD12.5 in relation to GD0.5 (**Figure 1B**).

Immunocompetent and Immunocompromised Mice Have Distinct Term Placental and Fetal Phenotypes in Response to High and Low ZIKV Titer Challenges in Mid-Pregnancy

The fetuses from C57BL/6 dams and sires were called ICompetent. The fetuses from the mating of A129 dams and C57BL/6 sires were called ICompromised. High-ZIKV ICompetent mice exhibited 34% fetal loss, whereas high-ZIKV-A129 mice had 100% fetal loss (**Figure 1C**). In the low-ZIKV groups, C57BL/6 mice had no (0%) fetal death, while A129 mice exhibited a 42% fetal death rate (**Figure 1C**). Fetal and fetal head sizes were decreased in A129 mice compared to those in C57BL/6 dams infected with the high ZIKV titer ($p=0.05$; **Figures 1D–G**). However, no changes in fetal weight or fetal head size were observed when the mice were infected with the low ZIKV titer (**Figures 1D–G**).

ZIKV Is Detected in the Fetal Brain of ICompromised, but Not ICompetent Mice

ZIKV RNA was detected in the spleens of pregnant ICompetent C57BL/6 mice inoculated with the highest ZIKV titer, confirming acute systemic infection. Viral RNA was also detected in the majority of the placentae of those mice (**Figures 2A, B**) but not in the maternal and fetal C57BL/6 brains (**Figures 2A, B**), suggesting

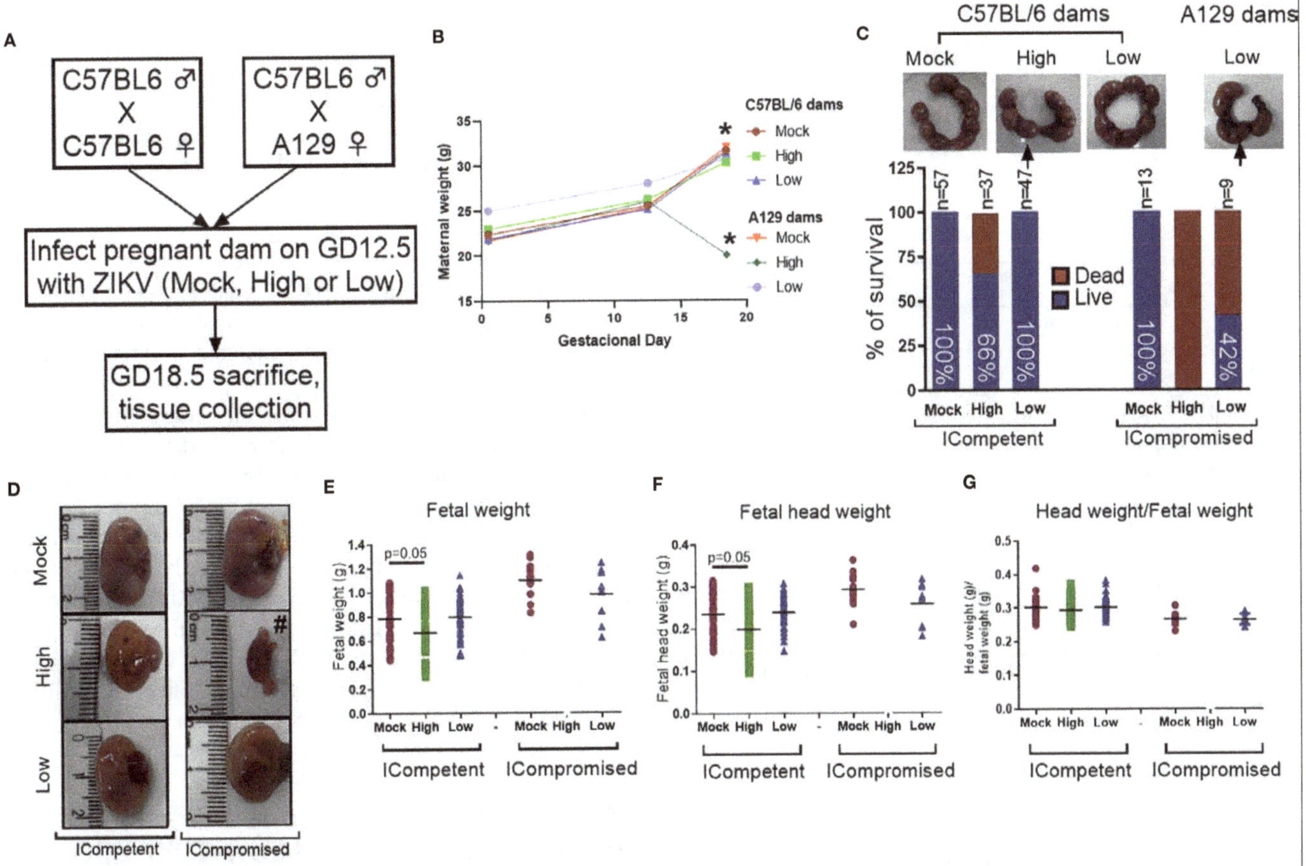

FIGURE 1 | ZIKV infection induced fetal changes during pregnancy. **(A)** Experimental design: matings of C57BL/6 dams x C57BL/6 sires (mock n=11 dams; high ZIKV n=15 dams; low ZIKV n=9 dams) and A129 dams x C57BL/6 sires (n=3 dams/group). The mock control consisted of noninfected C6/36 cell supernatants; high ZIKV titers consisted of 5×10^7 plaque-forming units (PFU) of $ZIKV_{PE243}$, and low ZIKV titers consisted of 10^3 PFU of $ZIKV_{PE243}$. Fetuses from C57BL/6 dams and sires were termed ICompetent, whereas fetuses from A129 dams and C57BL/6 sires were termed ICompromised. **(B)** Maternal weight gain throughout pregnancy. **(C)** Uterine horn and survival rates following ZIKV exposure (arrows show resorption sites). **(D)** Fetal/reabsorption images (#=example of fetal reabsorption). **(E)** Fetal weight, **(F)** fetal head weight and **(G)** fetal head weight/fetal weight ratio. One-way ANOVA followed by Tukey's posttest was used to assess changes among ICompetent groups, whereas an unpaired Student's t-test or nonparametric Mann-Whitney test was used to assess differences between ICompromised groups. Values are the mean of individual plotted values. $^*p < 0.05$, one-way ANOVA.

that the virus was not transmitted to the fetuses. In contrast, ZIKV RNA was detected in all analyzed organs from ICompromised A129 dams, including the maternal brain and spleen and the placenta and fetal brain (**Figures 2A, B**). Viremia in maternal plasma was evaluated at 4, 48 and 144 hours after infection. Within 4 hours, the presence of the virus was verified in the serum (high ICompetent=637.5 PFU/mL, low ICompetent=740 PFU/mL and low ICompromised=325 PFU/mL), indicating that the virus was correctly inoculated. Afterwards, ZIKV RNA was detected in ICompromised dams at 48 and 144 hours post inoculation but not in ICompetent dams (**Figure 2C**).

ZIKV Infection Induces Distinct Systemic and Placental Inflammatory Responses in ICompetent and ICompromised Mice

The maternal serum and placental protein levels of specific cytokines and chemokines related to fetal death and preterm delivery (43–45) were evaluated to probe whether midgestation ZIKV infection would induce a maternal inflammatory response at term in our two distinct models. Since A129 infected with 5×10^7 ZIKV-PFU showed 100% fetal loss, we proceeded using 5×10^7 PFU inoculation in C57BL/6 mice and 10^3 PFU inoculation in both C57BL/6 and A129 mice.

CCL2 was elevated in the serum of low-ZIKV ICompetent mice, but no other alteration was systemically detected in any ICompetent mice at this time point (**Figures 3A, B**). On the other hand, ICompromised dams showed significantly increased CXCL1 and IL-6 levels in the serum and a strong trend for an enhancement in CCL2 (**Figure 3C**). Analysis of cytokine and chemokine expression in the placenta demonstrated that the CXCL1 and CCL2 chemokines were also upregulated in ICompromised but not ICompetent mice (**Figures 3D–F**). Surprisingly, IL-6 protein expression was augmented in the placenta of some of the low-ZIKV ICompetent mice (58%;

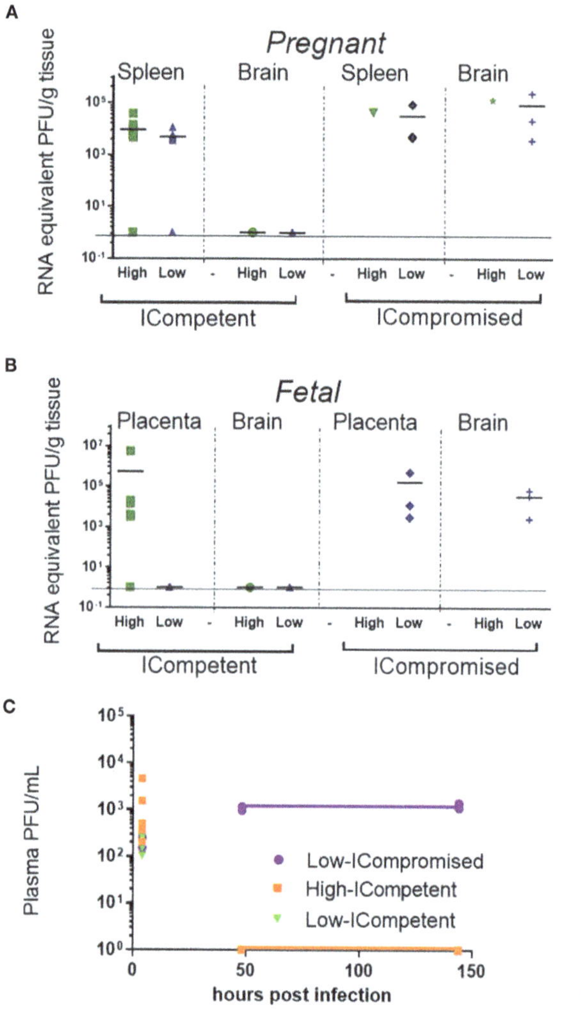

FIGURE 2 | Viral load detection in maternal and fetal tissues after ZIKV infection. Pregnant ICompetent and ICompromised mice were inoculated i.v. with low and high doses of ZIKV. **(A, B)** ZIKV RNA was measured *via* RT-qPCR in tissue samples obtained from maternal spleen and brain **(A)** and from placenta and fetal brain **(B)**. **(C)** The presence of ZIKV infectious particles in the plasma of infected dams was evaluated with a plaque assay 4, 48, and 144 hours post infection in ICompetent (mock n=11 dams; high ZIKV n=15 dams; low ZIKV n=9 dams) and ICompromised (mock n=3 dams; high ZIKV n=3 dams; low ZIKV n=3 dams) mice.

p<0.05) but not in high-ZIKV mice or ICompromised mice (**Figures 3D–F**).

We also assessed the placental mRNA expression of a range of cytokines related to placental infective responses: *Ifng, Il6, Ifn1, Tnf, Il1b* and *Il10.* All the infected mice showed a significant increase in *Tnf* mRNA expression, with higher levels detected in ICompetent mice (**Figures 3G-I**). The low-ZIKV ICompetent mice presented modest but significant *Ifn1* expression, which was not detected in the high-ZIKV group (**Figure 3G**). Additionally, both low-ZIKV-infected groups (ICompetent and ICompromised) presented increased *Ifng* mRNA expression (**Figures 3G, I**, p< 0.05). Interestingly, placental *Il6* mRNA levels were only elevated in ICompromised pregnancies compared to mock pregnancies (p=0.05) (**Figure 3I**). *Il1b* and *Il10* remained unchanged in all groups analyzed (**Figures 3G–I**).

ZIKV Affects Placental Proliferation and Apoptosis in a Viral Load- and Maternal Immune Status-Dependent Manner

We did not observe changes in placental weight or in the fetal: placental weight ratio in any of the groups investigated (data not shown). However, since we detected the presence of ZIKV RNA in the placentas, we investigated the cellular proliferation (Ki-67$^+$ cells) and apoptotic ratio in the Lz and Jz of the mouse placenta. Increased Ki-67 staining was observed in the Lz of high- and low-ZIKV-treated ICompetent animals compared to mock animals (**Figures 4A–D**, p=0.005 and p=0.015), whereas the apoptotic ratio in the Lz was increased in high-ZIKV dams and decreased in low-ZIKV dams (p=0.01, **Figures 4E–H**). Although no differences were observed in Ki67 staining (**Figures 5A-D**), a similar apoptotic pattern was detected in the Jz of ICompetent pregnancies (p=0.008 and p=0.004, respectively; **Figures 5E–H**). In contrast, in ICompromised dams, Lz Ki-67 staining was decreased (p=0.001; **Figures 4I–L**), while the apoptotic reaction was increased in ZIKV-infected animals (p=0.05; **Figures 4M–P**). Jz from ICompromised offspring exhibited increased Ki-67 labeling and no differences in the apoptotic reaction (p=0.001; **Figures 5I–P**).

Placental Ultrastructure Is Differently Impacted by High- and Low-Titer ZIKV Infection in ICompetent and ICompromised Trocaria Strains of Mice

Lz ultrastructural analyses of ICompetent and ICompromised-mock animals detected sinusoidal trophoblastic giant cells exhibiting regular microvilli, euchromatic nuclei, preserved mitochondrial ultrastructure and regular narrow ER cisternae (**Figures 6A, B**). In sharp contrast, high-ZIKV ICompetent (**Figure 6C**) infected placentae showed fewer villi in the sinusoidal giant trophoblastic cells, degenerated mitochondria, granular ER with dilated cisterns and euchromatic nuclei. The sinusoidal giant trophoblastic cells in the low-ZIKV ICompetent mice (**Figure 6D**) also had fewer villi and degenerated mitochondria than those in the mock placentae, but no effect on the ER or euchromatic nuclei observed. Low-ZIKV ICompromised infected placentae (**Figure 6E**) showed fewer villi in the sinusoidal giant trophoblastic cells, degenerated mitochondria, granular ER with dilated cisterns and euchromatic nuclei.

The Jz of mock ICompetent and ICompromised placentae (**Figures 7A, B**) exhibited euchromatic nuclei, with evident heterochromatin, preserved mitochondria and narrow cisternae in a granular ER. High-ZIKV ICompetent Jz had degenerated mitochondria, granular ER with dilated cisterns and euchromatic nuclei (**Figure 7C**). Low-ZIKV ICompetent (**Figure 7D**) placentae exhibited euchromatic nuclei with evident heterochromatin, preserved mitochondria and narrow cisternae in a granular ER, whereas low-ZIKV ICompromised placentae

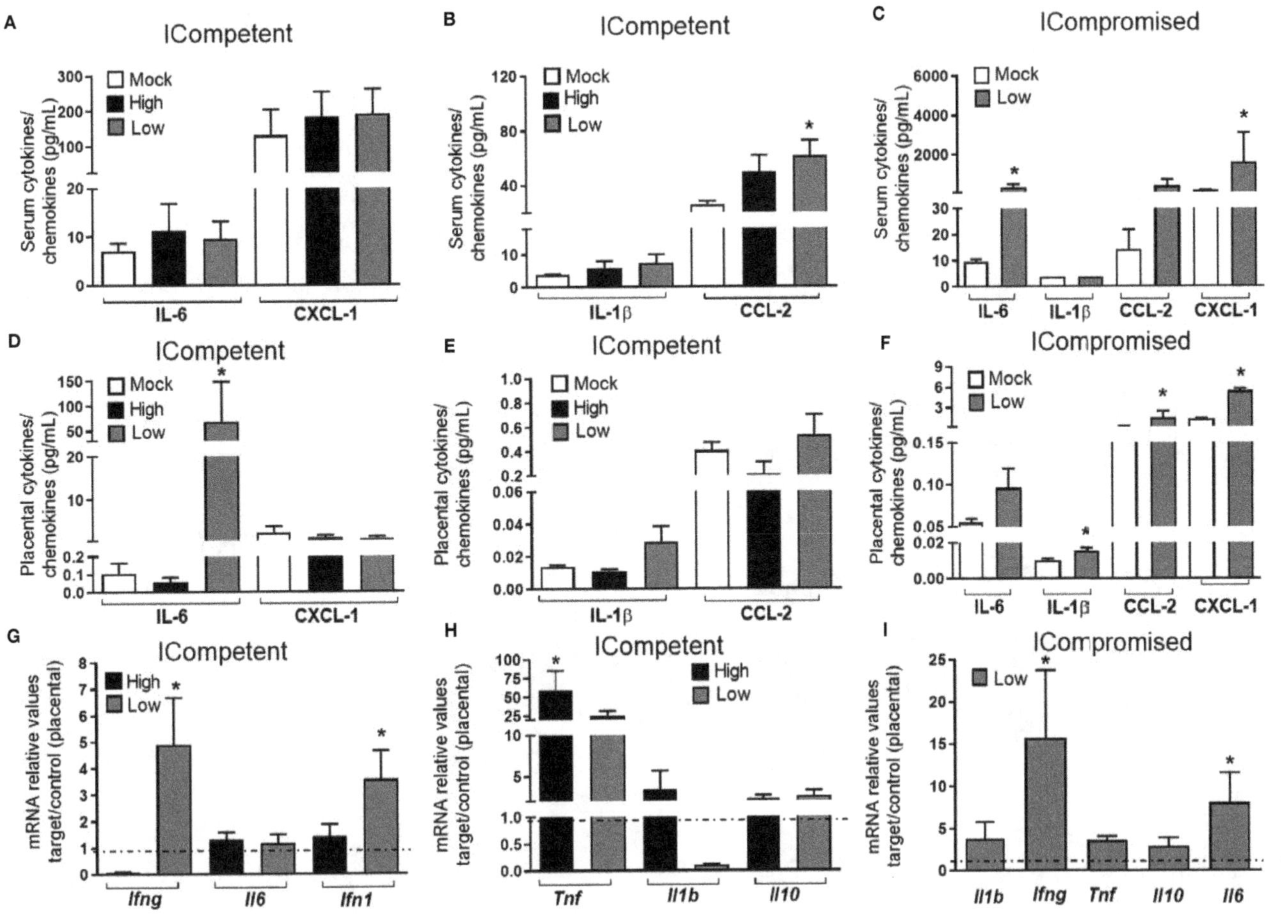

FIGURE 3 | ZIKV during pregnancy promotes an inflammatory response in the maternal serum and in the placenta. Levels of IL-1β, IL-6, CCL-2 and CXCL-1 in the maternal serum **(A–C)** and placenta **(D–F)** at GD18.5 in matings of C57BL/6 dams x C57BL/6 sires (ICompetent fetuses - mock n=11 dams; high ZIKV n=15 dams; low ZIKV n=9 dams) and A129 dams x C57BL/6 sires (ICompromised fetuses n=3 dams/group). Placental mRNA expression **(G–I)** of *Ifng*, *Ifn1*, *Il1b*, *Il6*, *Il10* and *Tnf*. Broken lines show the expression levels in both lineages in the mock group. One-way ANOVA followed by Tukey's posttest was used to assess changes among ICompetent groups, whereas an unpaired Student's t-test or nonparametric Mann-Whitney test was used to assess differences between ICompromised groups. The values are expressed as the mean ± SEM. *P < 0.05.

had degenerated mitochondria, granular ER with dilated cisterns and euchromatic nuclei (**Figure 7E**).

ZIKV Differentially Affects Placental Expression of Drug and Lipid ABC Transporter Systems

Evaluation of key ABC transporters in the Lz of mock and ZIKV-infected ICompetent and ICompromised placentae revealed that immunolabeling of the drug P-gp and Bcrp efflux transporter systems was primarily present at the cellular membranes of the sinusoidal trophoblastic giant cells, with diffuse cytoplasmic Bcrp staining. Labeling of the Abca1 and Abcg1 lipid efflux transporters was moderately and heterogeneously distributed within the Lz. Less Lz-P-gp was observed in ICompetent mice infected with both high- and low-ZIKV infective regimens than in mock-treated animals (p=0.001 and p=0.002, respectively; **Figures 8A–E**), whereas reduced Bcrp and Abca1 staining was observed in high-ZIKV-infected mice (p=0.003 and p=0.004, **Figures 8F–J** and **8K–O**, respectively). No changes in Abcg1 were observed in any of the ICompetent experimental groups (**Figures 8P–T**). P-gp, Bcrp and Abca1 transporter immunostaining was downregulated in ICompromised low ZIKV-treated animals (p=0.001, p=0.05 and p=0.05, **Figures 9A–D**, **9E–H** and **9I–L**, respectively). No changes in Abcg1 were observed in any of the ICompromised experimental groups (**Figures 9M–P**).

Next, the impact of ZIKV on ABC transporters in the Jz layer (structural and endocrine layers of the mouse placenta) was assessed. P-gp and Bcrp were predominantly localized at the cellular membranes of spongiotrophoblast cells, whereas Abca1 and Abcg1 exhibited membrane and cytoplasmic staining. P-gp staining was decreased in Jz cells from the low-ZIKV ICompromised placentae (p=0.006), with no other alterations observed (**Figures 10A–T**, **11A–P**).

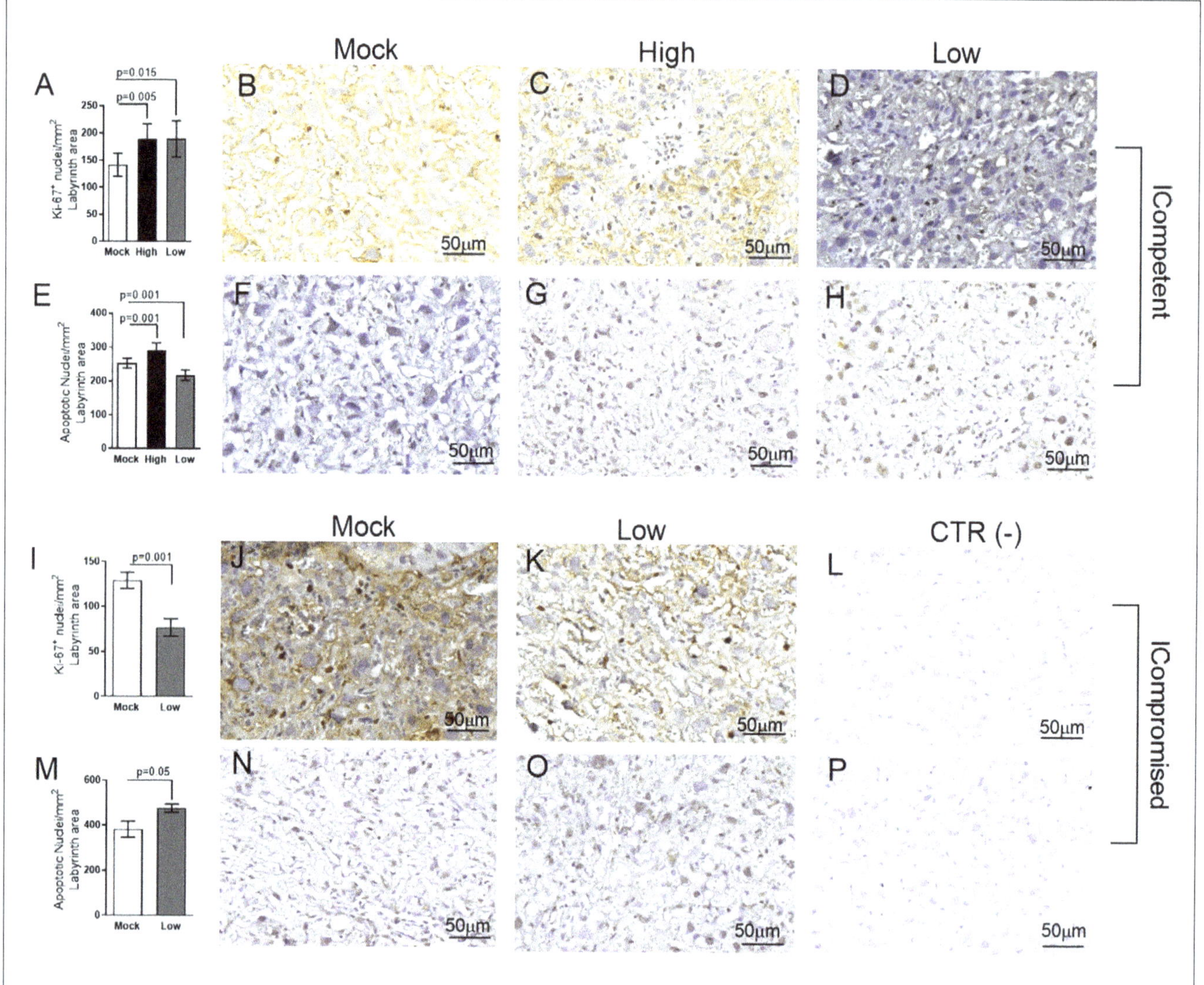

FIGURE 4 | Labyrinthine remodeling in ICompetent and ICompromised placentae is affected by gestational ZIKV infection. A total of 180 digital images (40X) randomly captured from the whole labyrinth zone (Lz) of each placenta per dam were evaluated. Immunolabeled nuclei from each digital image were quantified and normalized by the total digital image area to obtain an index of the estimated number of proliferative and apoptotic nuclei in the entire histological section. **(A, I)** Quantification and **(B–D, J, K)** representative photomicrographs of Ki-67$^+$ stained nuclei in the Lz of ICompetent (n=6 placentae from 6 independent dams/group) and ICompromised (n=3 placentae from 3 independent dams/group) placentae, respectively. **(E, M)** Quantification and **(F–H, N, O)** representative photomicrographs of apoptotic nuclei (TUNEL) in the Lz of ICompetent (n=5 placentae from 5 independent dams/group) and ICompromised (n=3 placentae from 3 independent dams/group) placentae, respectively. **(L, P)** Negative controls. One-way ANOVA followed by Tukey's posttest was used to assess changes among ICompetent groups, whereas an unpaired Student's t-test or nonparametric Mann-Whitney test was used to assess differences between ICompromised groups. The values are expressed as the mean ± SEM. Images were captured at 40X. Scale bar=50 μm.

DISCUSSION

In this study, we investigated several fetal and placental features at term (GD18.5) in ICompetent (C57BL/6) and ICompromised (A129) females exposed to ZIKV at mid-pregnancy (GD12.5). Fetal survival rates, systemic and placental inflammatory responses, placental ultrastructure and cell turnover, as well as the expression of key drug (P-gp and Bcrp) and lipid (Abca1) efflux transporter systems in the placenta, were consistently impacted by ZIKV in both strains. The magnitude of the effects was clearly related to the infective titer (high and low) of ZIKV and maternal immune status (ICompetent-C57BL/6 x and ICompromised-A129), and fetal alterations were not exclusively dependent on virus detection in the fetuses.

Infection of ICompetent mice with ZIKV did not result in viremia in the initial postinoculation phase, although viral RNA was detected in the maternal spleen in both the high- and low-ZIKV groups, confirming systemic infection. This is consistent with a previous report (46). Our data demonstrate that pregnant ICompetent C57BL/6 mice were more susceptible to high ZIKV titers than to low ZIKV infective. Since viral RNA was only detected in the placentae of high ZIKV-infected mice, fetal survival rates and weights were impacted to a greater extent in those mice. Strikingly, even though the virus was not present in

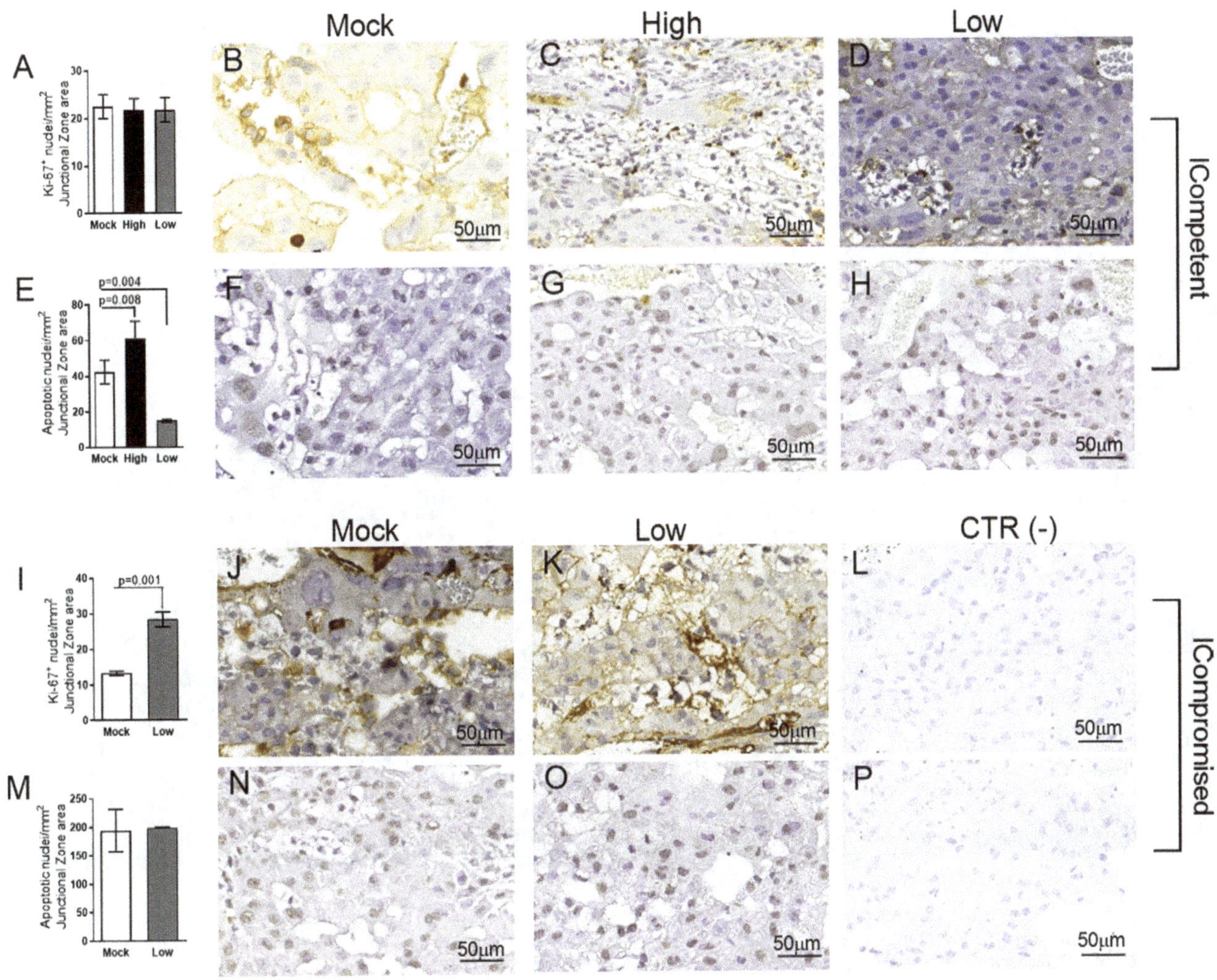

FIGURE 5 | Junctional zone remodeling in ICompetent and ICompromised placentae is affected by gestational ZIKV infection. A total of 180 digital images (40X) randomly captured from the whole junctional zone (Jz) of each placenta per dam were evaluated. Immunolabeled nuclei from each digital image were quantified and normalized by the total digital image area to obtain an index of the estimated number of proliferative and apoptotic nuclei in the entire histological section. **(A, I)** Quantification and **(B–D, J, K)** representative photomicrographs of Ki-67$^+$ stained nuclei in the Jz of ICompetent (n=6 placentae from 6 independent dams/group) and ICompromised (n=3 placentae from 3 independent dams/group) placentae, respectively. **(E, M)** Quantification and **(F–H, N, O)** representative photomicrographs of apoptotic nuclei (TUNEL) in the Jz of ICompetent (n=5 placentae from 5 independent dams/group) and ICompromised (n=3 placentae from 3 independent dams/group) placentae, respectively. **(L, P)** Negative controls. One-way ANOVA followed by Tukey's posttest was used to assess changes among ICompetent groups, whereas an unpaired Student's t-test or nonparametric Mann-Whitney test was used to assess differences between ICompromised groups. The values are expressed as the mean ± SEM. Images were captured at 40X. Scale bar = 50 μm.

the fetal brain (at least at term), fetal and fetal head weights were lower in mice subjected to the high-ZIKV titer regimen, suggesting that high infective viral load in mid-pregnancy, even in ICompetent individuals, can induce IUGR and lower fetal head weight despite a lack of transmission to the fetal brain (47). On the other hand, ICompromised placentae and fetal brains had detectable viral transcripts, with no changes in weight, which is consistent with previous data (19). In fact, in our models, the presence (ICompromised) or absence (ICompetent) of the virus in the fetal brain did not correspond to fetal head size (decreased in only high ICompetent). The data from ICompetent and ICompromised placentae demonstrate how important the maternal immunological status is to control viremia, fetal survival and accessibility of the virus to the fetal brain. The reason for the reduction in fetal brain size in C57BL/6 mice in the absence of fetal brain infection requires further investigation. It is possible that fetal brains in the ICompetent mice may have been exposed to ZIKV earlier in pregnancy, when viremia was present in the maternal blood, and this may have severely compromised brain development. Of note, one limitation of our study is that we measured fetal head weight instead of cortical thickness. Future studies should investigate whether high- and low-ZIKV exposure alters cortical thickness in ICompetent and ICompromised offspring.

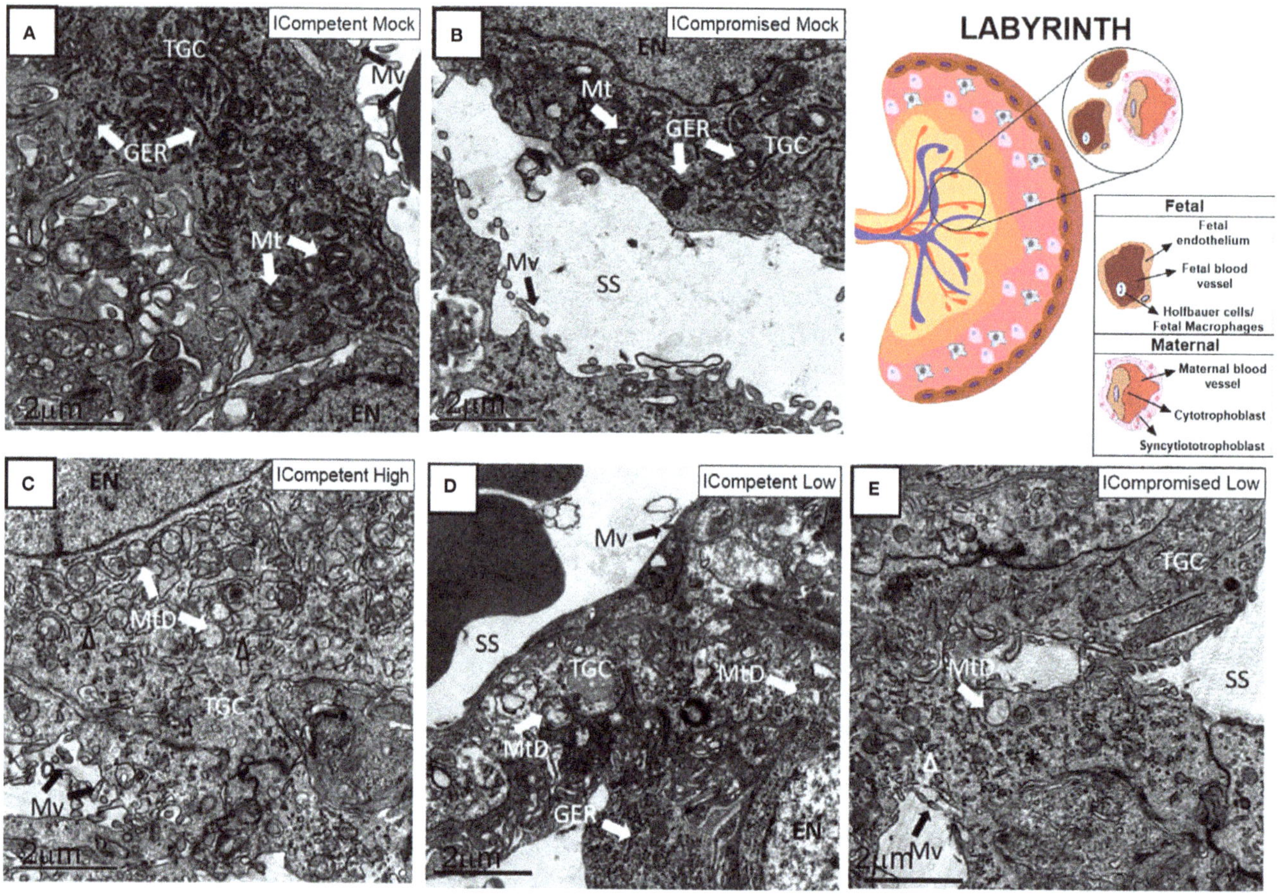

FIGURE 6 | Associated ultrastructural changes in the placental Lz after ZIKV infection. Transmission electron photomicrographs of ICompetent mock **(A)**, ICompromised mock **(B)**, ICompetent high **(C)**, ICompetent low **(D)** and ICompromised low **(E)** groups (n=5/group). We observed dilatation in the ER cisterns of ICompetent high placentas. Additionally, there was a reduction in the microvilli in both the ICompetent high and ICompetent low placentas. In the ICompromised low group, we found fragmented ER and microvillus reduction. All infected groups showed degenerate mitochondria. GER = granular endoplasmic reticulum; Δ = dilated granular endoplasmic reticulum; * = fragmented granular endoplasmic reticulum; Mt, mitochondria; MtD, degenerate mitochondria; Mv, microvilli; EN, euchromatic nuclei; SS, sinusoidal space; TGC, trophoblastic giant cell. Scale bar = 2 µm.

A distinct inflammatory profile was also detected in the three analyzed groups. At the protein level, low-ZIKV-ICompromised dams exhibited increased maternal IL-6 and CXCL-1 and placental CCL-2 and CXCL-1, whereas low-ZIKV-ICompetent dams had increased maternal CCL2 and placental IL-6 levels. CCCL-2 and CXCL-1 are related to fetal death and preterm delivery (43–45) and could be associated with pronounced fetal injury detected upon ICompromised pregnancy. In addition, IL-6 was previously demonstrated (48) to be related to fetal response syndrome, characterized by activation of the fetal immune system. This syndrome is known to increase fetal morbidity and affect several organs, such as the adrenal gland, brain and heart (32, 48–51). At the mRNA level, *Il6* expression was only detected in ICompromised placentae at term and may indicate a sustained harmful response in these mice until term. The IFN signaling pathway may be triggered by ZIKV (17) and is one of the key mechanisms of host defense and a viral target for immune evasion (20), but we only detected a slight increase in *Ifn1* in low-ZIKV ICompetent mice at term. However, we cannot rule out the possibility that these cytokines might have been produced earlier. Our findings showed that *Ifng* expression was significantly enhanced in both ICompetent and ICompromised low-ZIKV-derived placentae but not in high-ZIKV-infected mice. Although we could not assess cytokine expression in high-ZIKV ICompromised placentas, one may extrapolate that low-ZIKV infection could result in stimulation of *Ifng* producing cells, which has been previously shown to be protective for ZIKV-infected mice (52).

Both ICompromised and ICompetent mice showed increased expression of placental *Tnf* mRNA, which has been demonstrated to be directly related to placental damage, abortion and premature birth (53–56). In addition, an increased *Tnf* response is related to impaired placental hormone production and trophoblastic invasion and increased apoptosis in pregnancy (57, 58). Although we did not assess TNF-α protein levels in the placenta and maternal blood, this response could be implicated in the overall damage detected.

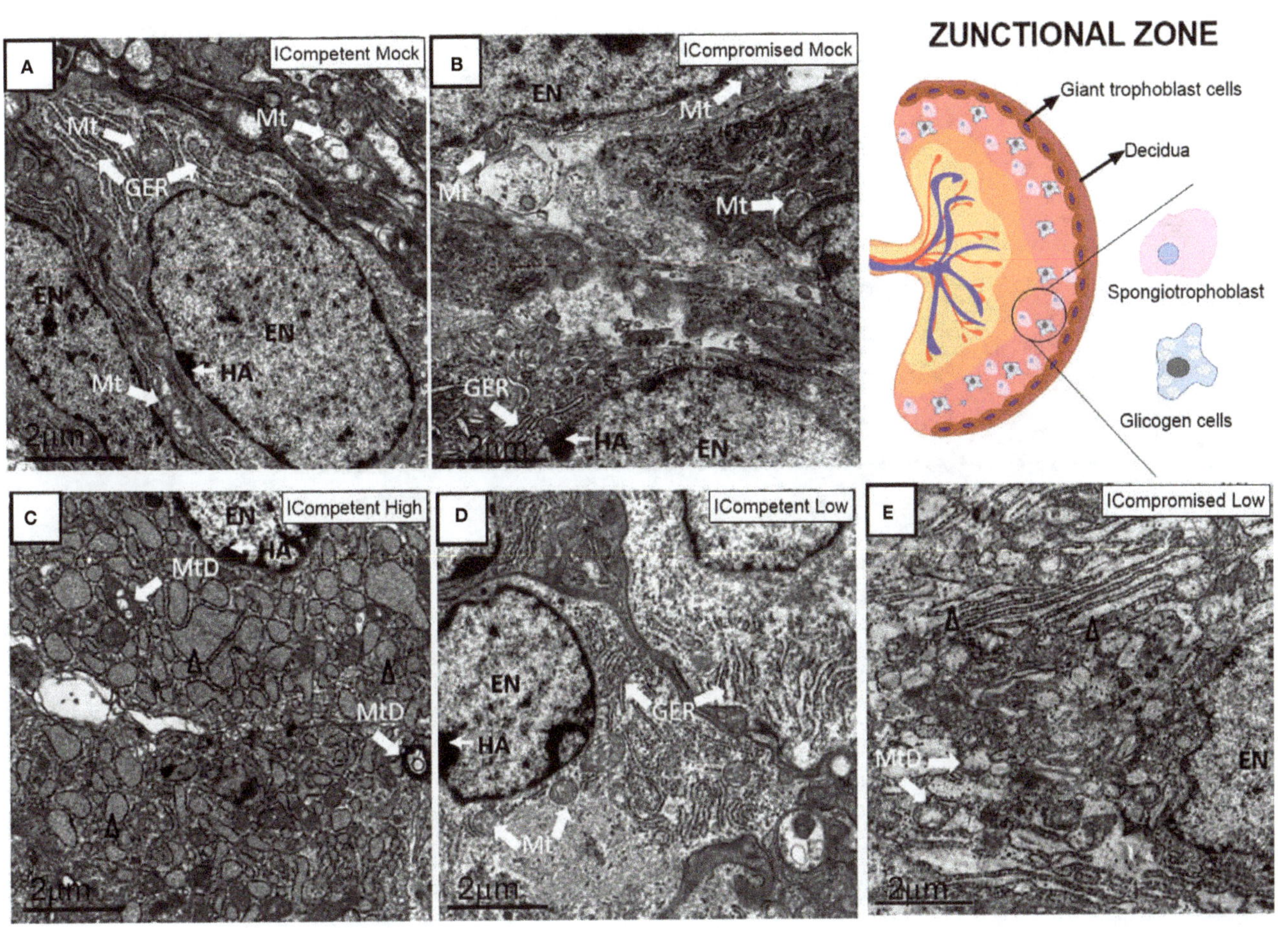

FIGURE 7 | Associated ultrastructural changes in the placental Jz after ZIKV infection. Transmission electron photomicrographs of ICompetent mock **(A)**, ICompromised mock **(B)**, ICompetent high **(C)**, ICompetent low **(D)** and ICompromised low **(E)** groups (n=5/group). We found deteriorating mitochondria and dilated reticulum endoplasmic cisterns in both the high ICompetent and low ICompromised groups. GER, granular endoplasmic reticulum; Δ, dilated granular endoplasmic reticulum; Mt, mitochondria; MtD, degenerate mitochondria; Mv, microvilli; EN, euchromatic nuclei; SS, sinusoidal space; TGC, trophoblastic giant cell; HA, heterochromatin area. Scale bar = 2 μm.

Although differences in placental weight were not observed, ZIKV infection mid-pregnancy had a profound effect on placental cellular turnover, dependent on virus titer, strain and/or placental compartment. The Lz is responsible for fetal and maternal nutrient, gas and waste exchange, while the Jz provides structural support, nutrient storage and hormone synthesis (35). ZIKV induced a consistent increase in Lz proliferation in all groups. However, the Lz apoptotic rate was increased only in the high-ZIKV-ICompetent and ICompromised groups and decreased in low-ZIKV-ICompetent mice. The mechanisms underlying these differences are unknown but may be related to the distinct maternal and placental proinflammatory responses and/or to the direct effect of the virus on the placenta (59). Increased Lz apoptosis in the high-ICompetent-ZIKV group may be one of the mechanisms driving the lower fetal and fetal head weight detected in this group. In this context, changes in placental turnover can determine placental maturation and function and lead to fetal distress and developmental abnormalities (60). An increase in the Lz apoptotic ratio may signify damage to this placental layer, which is consistent with the fact that diverse pathological lesions associated with congenital disorders were described in placentae from women infected by ZIKV at different stages of pregnancy (61). Conversely, no proliferative changes were observed in the Jz in high-ZIKV and low-ZIKV ICompetent mice, while increased and decreased apoptotic rates were detected. It follows that the lack of Jz-Ki-67 induction may suggest that this layer is less capable of restoring proliferation in response to high-ZIKV challenge, and this may be related to decreased fetal growth.

Our placental ultrastructural analysis detected consistent differences across ZIKV-exposed groups. The Lz and Jz layers from both strains exhibited signs of ER stress, i.e., dilated ER cisterns or fragmented ER granular structures. These alterations may result from the accumulation of folded or poorly folded viral proteins in the ER lumen (42, 62, 63). The *Flaviridae* family uses the ER to replicate (64), and according to Offerdahl et al. (63), there is evidence of ZIKV interacting with this organelle,

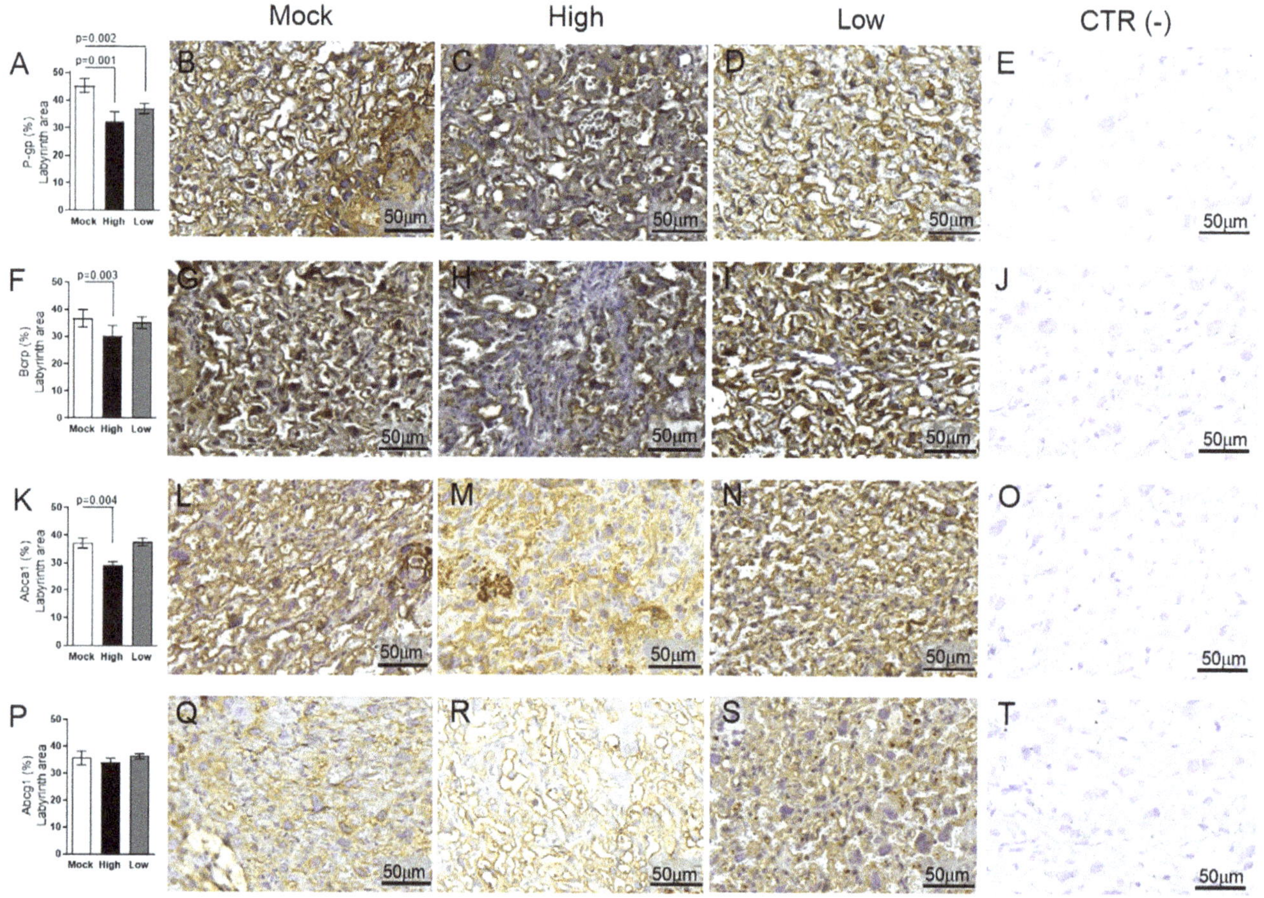

FIGURE 8 | ZIKV infection decreases P-gp, Bcrp and Abca1 expression in the placental Lz of infected mice in the ICompetent groups. A total of 180 digital images (40X) randomly captured from the whole labyrinth zone (Lz) of each placenta per dam were evaluated. Immunolabeling in each digital image was quantified by calculating the percentage area of the total stained labyrinthine tissue after exclusion of the total negative space. **(A)** Quantification and **(B–D)** representative photomicrographs of P-gp staining in the Lz of ICompetent (n=6 placentae from 6 independent dams/group) placenta. **(F)** Quantification and **(G–I)** representative photomicrographs of Bcrp staining in the Lz of ICompetent (n=6 placentae from 6 independent dams/group) placenta. **(K)** Quantification and **(L–N)** representative photomicrographs of Abca1 staining in the Lz of ICompetent (n=6 placentae from 6 independent dams/group) placenta. **(P)** Quantification and **(Q–S)** representative photomicrographs of Abcg1 staining in the Lz of ICompetent (n = 6 placentae from 6 independent dams/group) placenta. **(E, J, O, T)** Negative controls. One-way ANOVA followed by Tukey's post-test. The values are expressed as the mean ± SEM. Images were captured at 40X. Scale bar = 50 μm.

promoting an increased release of Ca^{+2} from the ER to the cell cytoplasm, thereby causing an increase in the production of reactive oxygen species (ROS) (65, 66).

The mitochondrial ultrastructure in the Lz and Jz layers was severely impacted by ZIKV exposure. We found evidence of mitochondrial degeneration, i.e., mitochondrial membrane rupture, absence of mitochondrial ridges and a less electron-dense mitochondrial matrix, in all the treated groups. Placental mitochondrial dysfunction is associated with IUGR (67, 68) and may be related, at least in part, to the lower fetal weight observed in high-ZIKV-ICompetent fetuses along with the altered placental apoptotic and proliferative patterns. Furthermore, mitochondrial dysfunction together with ER stress is likely to modify the placental ROS balance and generate local oxidative stress (69), which is associated with impaired fetal development (70). Of importance, associations between mitochondrial disruption, ER stress and placental cell senescence have been reported. Senescence is characterized as an irreversible interruption of the cell cycle and acquisition of a senescence-associated secretory phenotype (SASP) that promotes the release of cytokines, such as IL-1, IL-6, IL-8 and proinflammatory proteases (70). Therefore, the increased expression of IL-6 detected in the placentas of ICompromised mice suggests a SASP profile, which may be related to changes in the ER and mitochondrial ultrastructure, accompanied by important changes in apoptosis and cell proliferation. The interactions between mitochondria and the ER are critical for homeostasis and cell signaling (71). In conjunction with the ER, mitochondria can regulate cell death mediators in response to hypoxia and inflammation (72). The increase in apoptosis observed in the high-titer ICompetent groups and the low-titer ICompromised group may be related to the mitochondrial damage and ER stress observed. In fact, we observed an important decrease

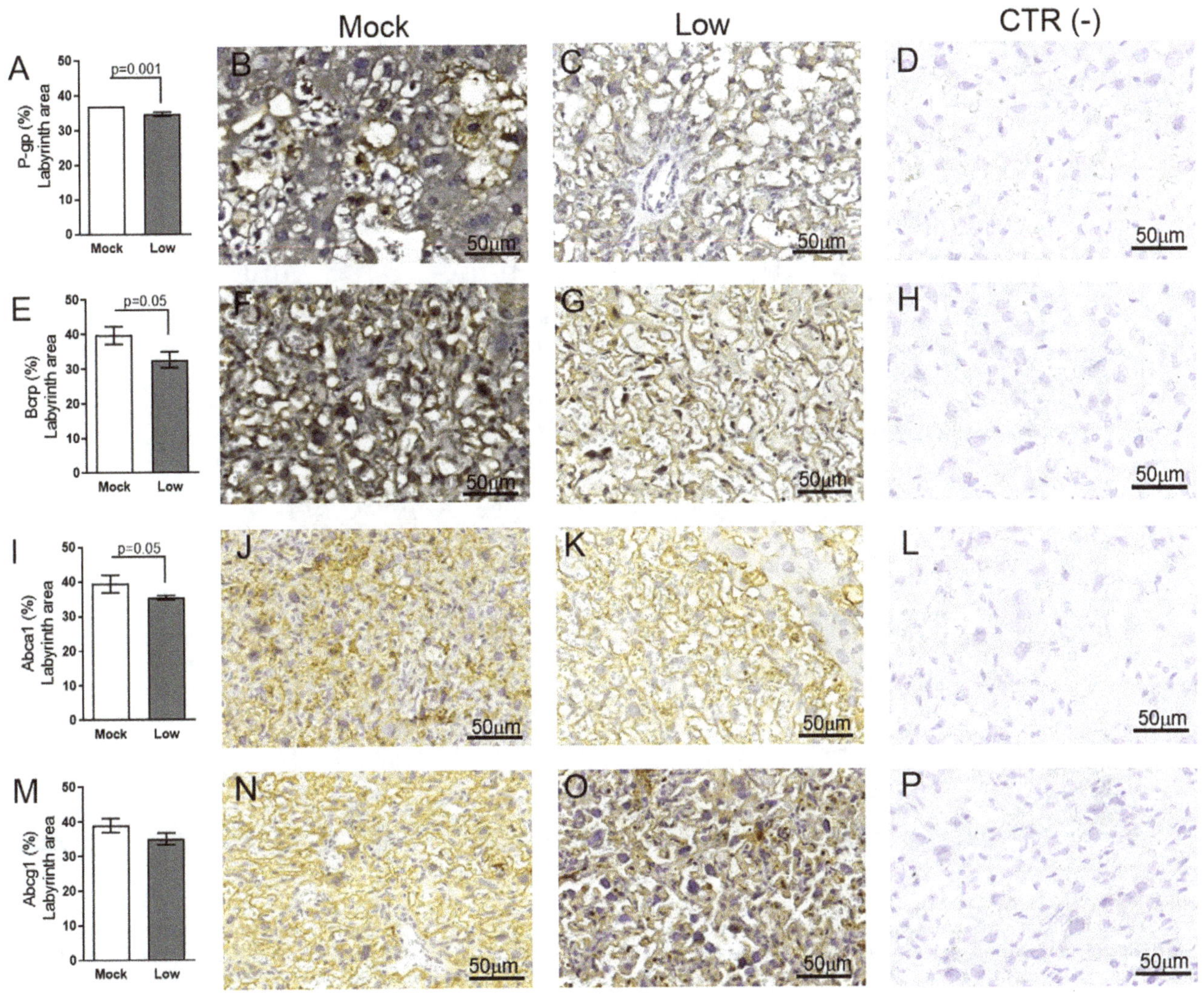

FIGURE 9 | ZIKV infection decreases P-gp, Bcrp and Abca1 protein expression in the placental Lz of infected mice in the ICompromised groups. A total of 180 digital images (40X) randomly captured from the whole labyrinth zone (Lz) of each placenta per dam were evaluated. Immunolabeling in each digital image was quantified by calculating the percentage area of the total stained labyrinth zone tissue after exclusion of the total negative space. **(A)** Quantification and **(B, C)** representative photomicrographs of P-gp staining in the Lz of ICompromised (n=3 placentae from 3 independent dams/group) placenta. **(E)** Quantification and **(F, G)** representative photomicrographs of Bcrp staining in the Lz of ICompromised (n=3 placentae from 3 independent dams/group) placenta. **(I)** Quantification and **(J, K)** representative photomicrographs of Abca1 staining in the Lz of ICompromised (n=3 placentae from 3 independent dams/group) placenta **(M)** quantification and **(N, O)** representative photomicrographs of Abcg1 staining in the Lz of ICompromised (n=3 placentae from 3 independent dams/group) placenta. **(D, H, L, P)** Negative controls. Unpaired Student's t-test or nonparametric Mann-Whitney test was used to assess differences between ICompromised groups. The values are expressed as the mean ± SEM. Images were captured at 40X. Scale ba r= 50 μm.

in microvillus abundance in sinusoidal giant trophoblast cells. Previously, we observed a decrease in microvillus density in the Lz of pregnancies exposed to malaria in pregnancy (MiP) (36). Together, our data show that different gestational infective stimuli (MiP and ZIKV) are capable of damaging placental microvillus abundance and impairing proper fetal-maternal exchange function and fetal growth/survival.

Next, to investigate whether maternal ZIKV exposure may influence fetal protection, we evaluated the placental localization and expression (semiquantitative) of the ABC efflux transporter systems P-gp, Bcrp, Abca1 and Abcg1, which are highly enriched in labyrinthine microvilli and in human syncytiotrophoblasts. These efflux transporters exchange drugs, environmental toxins, cytotoxic oxysterols and lipids within the maternal-fetal interface (26). We found a consistent decrease in labyrinthine P-gp expression in all ZIKV-exposed groups, demonstrating that ZIKV infection during pregnancy has the potential to increase fetal exposure to P-gp substrates, such as synthetic glucocorticoids, antibiotics, antiretrovirals, antifungals, stomach-protective drugs, and nonsteroidal anti-inflammatory drugs (26). Furthermore, Jz-P-gp was decreased in ICompromised placentae. Although little is known about the

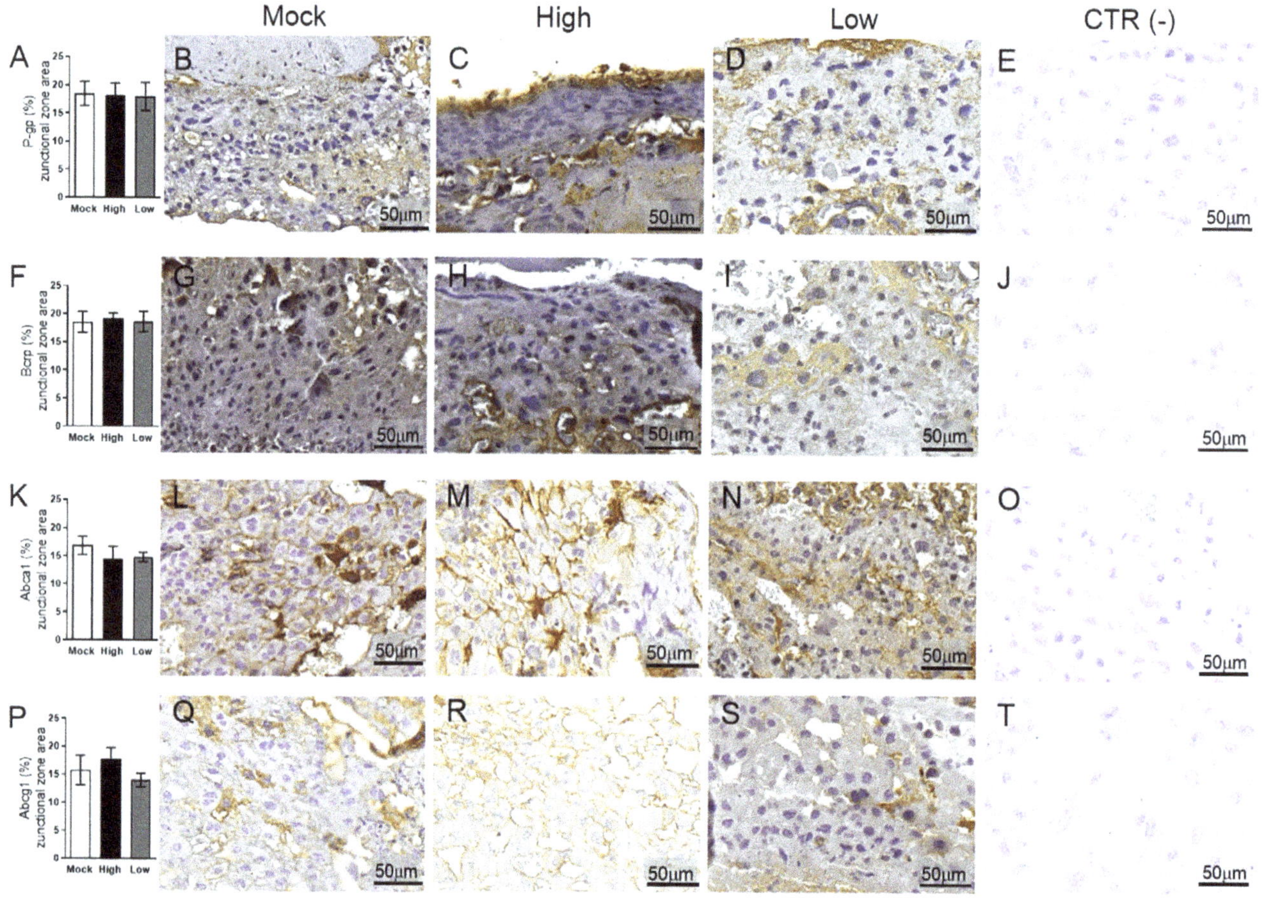

FIGURE 10 | ZIKV infection did not impact P-gp, Bcrp, Abca1 or Abcg1 protein expression in the placental Jz of infected mice in the ICompetent groups. A total of 180 digital images (40X) randomly captured from the whole junctional zone (Jz) of each placenta per dam were evaluated. Immunolabeling in each digital image was quantified by calculating the percentage area of the total stained junctional zone tissue after exclusion of the total negative space. **(A)** Quantification and **(B–D)** representative photomicrographs of P-gp staining in the Jz of ICompetent (n=6 placentae from 6 independent dams/group) placenta. **(F)** Quantification and **(G–I)** representative photomicrographs of Bcrp staining in the Jz of ICompetent (n=6 placentae from 6 independent dams/group) placenta. **(K)** Quantification and **(L–N)** representative photomicrographs of Abca1 staining in the Jz of ICompetent (n=6 placentae from 6 independent dams/group) placenta. **(P)** Quantification and **(Q–S)** representative photomicrographs of Abcg1 staining in the Jz of ICompetent (n=6 placentae from 6 independent dams/group) placenta. **(E, J, O, T)** Negative controls. One-way ANOVA followed by Tukey's post-test. The values are expressed as the mean ± SEM. Images were captured at 40X. Scale bar = 50 μm.

function of ABC transporters in the Jz, our data highlight the need for further studies investigating the biological importance of ABC transporters in the placental endocrine and structural zones of the rodent hemochorial placenta under normal and infective conditions.

ZIKV impaired Lz Bcrp and Abca1 expression in ICompetent (high) and ICompromised (low) mice. However, no effects were observed in ICompetent animals at a low ZIKV titer or in Abcg1 in any experimental setting. Thus, ZIKV also likely increases fetal accumulation of Bcrp substrates (antibiotics, antiretrovirals, sulfonylureas, folate, mercuric species, estrogenic mycotoxins, carcinogens and phototoxic compounds, among others) and disrupts placental lipid homeostasis (lipids, cholesterol, and cytotoxic oxysterols) by reducing placental Abca1 expression (26, 73–76). We can speculate that the increased fetal accumulation of the P-gp, Bcrp and Abca1 substrates during ZIKV infection may contribute to the establishment of congenital Zika syndrome, although additional studies are clearly required to answer this important question. The present data are in agreement with previous publications showing that bacterial, viral and protozoan inflammation alters the expression and/or function of P-gp, Bcrp and Abca1 in biological barriers, such as the placenta, yolk sac and blood-brain barriers (26, 27, 36, 64, 77–79).

CONCLUSION

Our data show that gestational ZIKV impacts the fetal phenotype independently of term fetal viremia. Abnormal placental cell turnover, ultrastructure and transporter expression may result from specific proinflammatory responses that depend on the ZIKV

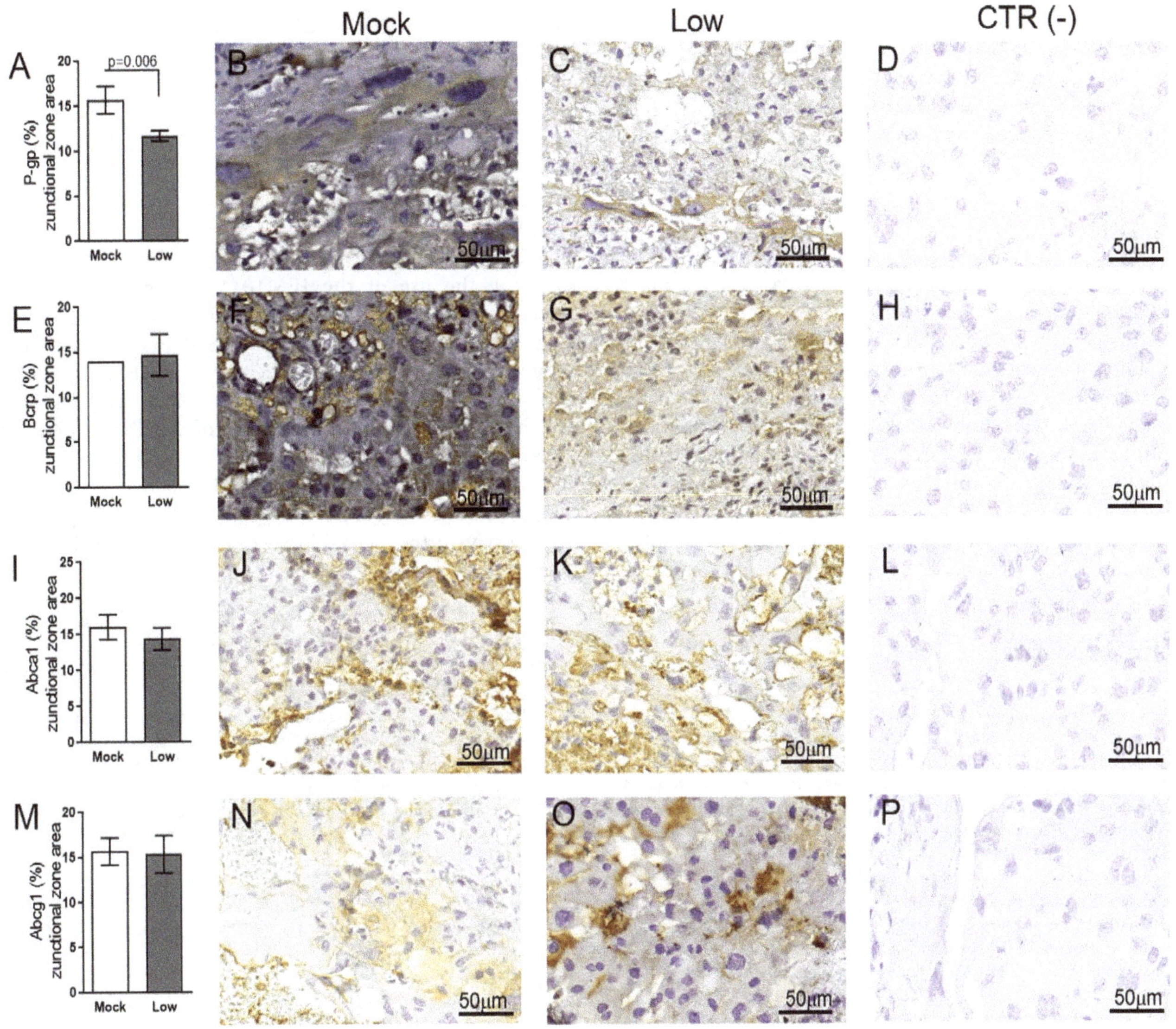

FIGURE 11 | ZIKV infection decreases Bcrp protein expression in the placental Jz of infected mice in the ICompromised group. A total of 180 digital images (40X) randomly captured from the whole junctional zone (Jz) of each placenta per dam were evaluated. Immunolabeling in each digital image was quantified by calculating the percentage area of the total stained junctional zone tissue after exclusion of the total negative space. **(A)** Quantification and **(B, C)** representative photomicrographs of P-gp staining in the Jz of ICompromised (n=3 placentae from 3 independent dams/group) placenta. **(E)** Quantification and **(F, G)** representative photomicrographs of Bcrp staining in the Jz of ICompromised (n=3 placentae from 3 independent dams/group) placenta. **(I)** Quantification and **(J, K)** representative photomicrographs of Abca1 staining in the Jz of ICompromised (n=3 placentae from 3 independent dams/group) placenta. **(M)** Quantification and **(N, O)** representative photomicrographs of Abcg1 staining in the Jz of ICompromised (n=3 placentae from 3 independent dams/group) placenta. **(D, H, L, P)** Negative controls. Unpaired Student's t-test or nonparametric Mann-Whitney test was used to assess differences between ICompromised groups. The values are expressed as the mean ± SEM. Images were captured at 40X. Scale bar = 50 μm.

infective load and maternal immune status. Fetal accumulation of drugs, environmental toxins and lipids within the fetal compartment may potentially be increased in ZIKV-infected pregnancies due to altered levels of key ABC transporters.

ETHICS STATEMENT

The animal study was reviewed and approved by Animal Care Committee of the Health Sciences Center, Federal University of Rio de Janeiro (CEUA-036/16 and 104/16).

AUTHOR CONTRIBUTIONS

CA, FB, EB, LA, and TO-C conceived and designed the experiments. CA, VM, SC, HG, RS, and VN performed the experiments. CA, SC, FB, EB, SM, LA, and TO-C analyzed the data. CA, VM, EB, LA, and TO-C wrote the paper and edited the manuscript. All authors contributed to the article and approved the submitted version.

FUNDING

This work was supported, in whole or in part, by the Bill & Melinda Gates Foundation [OPP1107597]. Under the grant conditions of the Foundation, a Creative Commons Attribution 4.0 Generic License has already been assigned to the Author Accepted Manuscript version that might arise from this submission. This study was also supported by the Canadian Institutes for Health Research (SGM: Foundation-148368), Conselho Nacional de Desenvolvimento Científico e Tecnológico (CNPq; TMO-C: 304667/2016-1, 422441/2016-3, 303734/2012-4, 422410/2016-0, EB:310578/2020-5, LBA: 310867/2018-5), Coordenação de Aperfeiçoamento Pessoal de Nível Superior(CAPES, finance Code 001), and Fundação de Amparo à Pesquisa do Estado do Rio de Janeiro (FAPERJ, CBVA 2002/010/2016, TMO-C: 201.341/2016, SVAC: 200.302/2020, LBA: 201.324/2016.

ACKNOWLEDGMENTS

We would like to thank Alan Moraes for supporting the acquisition of electron microscopy images and the electron microscopy laboratory at the UFF Biology Institute for allowing the use of the JEM1011 transmission electron microscope. We would also like to thank Mauro Jorge Castro Cabral for the use of the MAGPIX® System equipment at the Paulo de Góes Institute of Microbiology/UFRJ, Ernesto T. Marques Jr. (Centro de Pesquisa Aggeu Magalhães, FIOCRUZ, PE) for providing ZIKV to the Institute of Microbiology Paulo de Góes, Federal University of Rio de Janeiro, and the technicians, Juliana Gonçalves, Rakel Alves, and Ronaldo Rocha for their support during all the experiments. This study was preprinted in the Biorxiv (https://www.biorxiv.org/content/10.1101/2020.12.17.423218v6).

REFERENCES

1. Garcez PP, Loiola EC, Madeiro da Costa R, Higa LM, Trindade P, Delvecchio R, et al. Zika Virus Impairs Growth in Human Neurospheres and Brain Organoids. *Science* (2016) 352(6287):816–8. doi: 10.1126/science.aaf6116
2. Brasil P, Calvet GA, Siqueira AM, Wakimoto M, de Sequeira PC, Nobre A, et al. Zika Virus Outbreak in Rio De Janeiro, Brazil: Clinical Characterization, Epidemiological and Virological Aspects. Powers am, Editor. *PloS Negl Trop Dis* (2016) 10(4):e0004636. doi: 10.1371/journal.pntd.0004636
3. Brasil P, Nielsen-Saines K. More Pieces to the Microcephaly–Zika Virus Puzzle in Brazil. *Lancet Infect Dis* (2016) 16(12):1307–9. doi: 10.1016/S1473-3099(16)30372-3
4. Brasil P, Pereira JP, Moreira ME, Ribeiro Nogueira RM, Damasceno L, Wakimoto M, et al. Zika Virus Infection in Pregnant Women in Rio De Janeiro. *N Engl J Med* (2016) 375(24):2321–34. doi: 10.1056/NEJMoa1602412
5. Jaenisch T, Rosenberger KD, Brito C, Brady O, Brasil P, Marques ET. Risk of Microcephaly After Zika Virus Infection in Brazil, 2015 to 2016. *Bull World Health Organ* (2017) 95(3):191–8. doi: 10.2471/BLT.16.178608
6. Proenca-Modena JL, Milanez GP, Costa ML, Judice CC, Maranhão Costa FT. Zika Virus: Lessons Learned in Brazil. *Microbes Infect* (2018) 20: (11–12):661–9. doi: 10.1016/j.micinf.2018.02.008
7. Jouannic J-M, Friszer S, Leparc-Goffart I, Garel C, Eyrolle-Guignot D. Zika Virus Infection in French Polynesia. *Lancet* (2016) 387(10023):1051–2. doi: 10.1016/S0140-6736(16)00625-5
8. Musso D, Ko AI, Baud D. Zika Virus Infection — After the Pandemic. Longo DL, Editor. *N Engl J Med* (2019) 381(15):1444–57. doi: 10.1056/NEJMra1808246
9. Kasprzykowski JI, Fukutani KF, Fabio H, Fukutani ER, Costa LC, Andrade BB, et al. A Recursive Sub-Typing Screening Surveillance System Detects the Appearance of the ZIKV African Lineage in Brazil: Is There a Risk of a New Epidemic? *Int J Infect Dis* (2020) 96:579–81. doi: 10.1016/j.ijid.2020.05.090
10. Miranda J, Martín-Tapia D, Valdespino-Vázquez Y, Alarcón L, Espejel-Nuñez A, Guzmán-Huerta M, et al. Syncytiotrophoblast of Placentae From Women With Zika Virus Infection has Altered Tight Junction Protein Expression and Increased Paracellular Permeability. *Cells* (2019) 8(10):1174. doi: 10.3390/cells8101174
11. Jurado KA, Simoni MK, Tang Z, Uraki R, Hwang J, Householder S, et al. Zika Virus Productively Infects Primary Human Placenta-Specific Macrophages. *JCI Insight* (2016) 1(13):e88461. doi: 10.1172/jci.insight.88461
12. Quicke KM, Bowen JR, Johnson EL, McDonald CE, Ma H, O'Neal JT, et al. Zika Virus Infects Human Placental Macrophages. *Cell Host Microbe* (2016) 20(1):83–90. doi: 10.1016/j.chom.2016.05.015
13. Tabata T, Petitt M, Puerta-Guardo H, Michlmayr D, Wang C, Fang-Hoover J, et al. Zika Virus Targets Different Primary Human Placental Cells, Suggesting Two Routes for Vertical Transmission. *Cell Host Microbe* (2016) 20(2):155–66. doi: 10.1016/j.chom.2016.07.002
14. Simoni MK, Jurado KA, Abrahams VM, Fikrig E, Guller S. Zika Virus Infection of Hofbauer Cells. *Am J Reprod Immunol* (2017) 77(2):e12613. doi: 10.1111/aji.12613
15. Rathore APS, Saron WAA, Lim T, Jahan N, John ALS. Maternal Immunity and Antibodies to Dengue Virus Promote Infection and Zika Virus–Induced Microcephaly in Fetuses. *Sci Adv* (2019) 5(2):eaav3208. doi: 10.1126/sciadv.aav3208
16. Lazear HM, Govero J, Smith AM, Platt DJ, Fernandez E, Miner JJ, et al. A Mouse Model of Zika Virus Pathogenesis. *Cell Host Microbe* (2016) 19 (5):720–30. doi: 10.1016/j.chom.2016.03.010
17. Grant A, Ponia SS, Tripathi S, Balasubramaniam V, Miorin L, Sourisseau M, et al. Zika Virus Targets Human STAT2 to Inhibit Type I Interferon Signaling. *Cell Host Microbe* (2016) 19(6):882–90. doi: 10.1016/j.chom.2016.05.009
18. Yockey LJ, Varela L, Rakib T, Khoury-Hanold W, Fink SL, Stutz B, et al. Vaginal Exposure to Zika Virus During Pregnancy Leads to Fetal Brain Infection. *Cell* (2016) 166(5):1247–56. e4. doi: 10.1016/j.cell.2016.08.004
19. Garcez PP, Stolp HB, Sravanam S, Christoff RR, Ferreira JCCG, Dias AA, et al. Zika Virus Impairs the Development of Blood Vessels in a Mouse Model of Congenital Infection. *Sci Rep* (2018) 8(1):12774. doi: 10.1038/s41598-018-31149-3
20. Elong Ngono A, Shresta S. Immune Response to Dengue and Zika. *Annu Rev Immunol* (2018) 36(1):279–308. doi: 10.1146/annurev-immunol-042617-053142
21. Bayer A, Lennemann NJ, Ouyang Y, Bramley JC, Morosky S, Marques ETDAJ, et al. Type III Interferons Produced by Human Placental Trophoblasts Confer Protection Against Zika Virus Infection. *Cell Host Microbe* (2016) 19(5):705–12. doi: 10.1016/j.chom.2016.03.008
22. Luo H, Winkelmann ER, Fernandez-Salas I, Li L, Mayer SV, Danis-Lozano R, et al. Zika, Dengue and Yellow Fever Viruses Induce Differential Anti-Viral Immune Responses in Human Monocytic and First Trimester Trophoblast Cells. *Antiviral Res* (2018) 151:55–62. doi: 10.1016/j.antiviral.2018.01.003
23. Tanaka T, Narazaki M, Kishimoto T. IL-6 in Inflammation, Immunity, and Disease. *Cold Spring Harb Perspect Biol* (2014) 6(10):a016295. doi: 10.1101/cshperspect.a016295

24. Hunter CA, Jones SA. IL-6 as a Keystone Cytokine in Health and Disease. *Nat Immunol* (2015) 16(5):448–57. doi: 10.1038/ni.3153
25. Rabelo K, da Gonçalves AJS, de Souza LJ, Sales AP, de Lima SMB, Trindade GF, et al. Zika Virus Infects Human Placental Mast Cells and the HMC-1 Cell Line, and Triggers Degranulation, Cytokine Release and Ultrastructural Changes. *Cells* (2020) 9(4):975–90. doi: 10.3390/cells9040975
26. Bloise E, Ortiga-Carvalho TM, Reis FM, Lye SJ, Gibb W, Matthews SG. ATP-Binding Cassette Transporters in Reproduction: A New Frontier. *Hum Reprod Update* (2015) 22(2):164–81. doi: 10.1093/humupd/dmv049
27. do Imperio GE, Bloise E, Javam M, Lye P, Constantinof A, Dunk C, et al. Chorioamnionitis Induces a Specific Signature of Placental Abc Transporters Associated With an Increase of miR-331-5p in the Human Preterm Placenta. *Cell Physiol Biochem* (2018) 45(2):591–604. doi: 10.1159/000487100
28. Martinelli LM, Fontes KN, Reginatto MW, Andrade CBV, Monteiro VRS, Gomes HR, et al. Malaria in Pregnancy Regulates P-glycoprotein (P-Gp/Abcb1a) and ABCA1 Efflux Transporters in the Mouse Visceral Yolk Sac. *J Cell Mol Med* (2020) 00:1–12. doi: 10.1101/2020.06.27.175018
29. Reginatto MW, Fontes KN, Monteiro VRS, Silva NL, Andrade CBV, Gomes HR, et al. Effect of Sub-Lethal Prenatal Endotoxemia on Murine Placental Transport Systems and Lipid Homeostasis. *bioRxiv* (2020). doi: 10.1101/2020.08.04.236745
30. Martinelli LM, Reginatto MW, Fontes KN, Andrade CBV, Monteiro VRS, Gomes HR, et al. Breast Cancer Resistance Protein (Bcrp/Abcg2) is Selectively Modulated by Lipopolysaccharide (LPS) in the Mouse Yolk Sac. *Reprod Toxicol* (2020) 98:82–91. doi: 10.1016/j.reprotox.2020.09.001
31. Imperio GE, Javam M, Lye P, Constantinof A, Dunk CE, Reis FM, et al. Gestational Age-Dependent Gene Expression Profiling of ATP-binding Cassette Transporters in the Healthy Human Placenta. *J Cell Mol Med* (2019) 23(1):610–8. doi: 10.1111/jcmm.13966
32. Vermillion MS, Lei J, Shabi Y, Baxter VK, Crilly NP, McLane M, et al. Intrauterine Zika Virus Infection of Pregnant Immunocompetent Mice Models Transplacental Transmission and Adverse Perinatal Outcomes. *Nat Commun* (2017) 8(1):14575. doi: 10.1038/ncomms14575
33. Szaba FM, Tighe M, Kummer LW, Lanzer KG, Ward JM, Lanthier P, et al. Zika Virus Infection in Immunocompetent Pregnant Mice Causes Fetal Damage and Placental Pathology in the Absence of Fetal Infection. Coyne CB, Editor. *PloS Pathog* (2018) 14(4):e1006994. doi: 10.1371/journal.ppat.1006994
34. Coelho SVA, Neris RLS, Papa MP, Schnellrath LC, Meuren LM, Tschoeke DA, et al. Development of Standard Methods for Zika Virus Propagation, Titration, and Purification. *J Virol Methods* (2017) 246:65–74. doi: 10.1016/j.jviromet.2017.04.011
35. Connor KL, Kibschull M, Matysiak-Zablocki E, Nguyen TT-TN, Matthews SG, Lye SJ, et al. Maternal Malnutrition Impacts Placental Morphology and Transporter Expression: An Origin for Poor Offspring Growth. *J Nutr Biochem* (2020) 78:108329. doi: 10.1016/j.jnutbio.2019.108329
36. Fontes KN, Reginatto MW, Silva NL, Andrade CBV, Bloise FF, Monteiro VRS, et al. Dysregulation of Placental ABC Transporters in a Murine Model of Malaria-Induced Preterm Labor. *Sci Rep* (2019) 9(1):11488. doi: 10.1038/s41598-019-47865-3
37. Bloise E, Lin W, Liu X, Simbulan R, Kolahi KS, Petraglia F, et al. Impaired Placental Nutrient Transport in Mice Generated by *in Vitro* Fertilization. *Endocrinology* (2012) 153(7):3457–67. doi: 10.1210/en.2011-1921
38. Lanciotti RS, Kosoy OL, Laven JJ, Velez JO, Lambert AJ, Johnson AJ, et al. Genetic and Serologic Properties of Zika Virus Associated With an Epidemic, Yap State, Micronesia, 2007. *Emerg Infect Dis* (2008) 14(8):1232–9. doi: 10.3201/eid1408.080287
39. Livak KJ, Schmittgen TD. Analysis of Relative Gene Expression Data Using Real-Time Quantitative PCR and the 2-ΔΔct Method. *Methods* (2001) 25 (4):402–8. doi: 10.1006/meth.2001.1262
40. Tschanz SA, Burri PH, Weibel ER. A Simple Tool for Stereological Assessment of Digital Images: The STEPanizer: Tool FOR Stereological Assessment. *J Microscopy* (2011) 243(1):47–59. doi: 10.1111/j.1365-2818.2010.03481.x
41. Sesso A, Belizário JE, Marques MM, Higuchi ML, Schumacher RI, Colquhoun A, et al. Mitochondrial Swelling and Incipient Outer Membrane Rupture in Preapoptotic and Apoptotic Cells. *Anatomical Rec* (2012) 295(10):1647. doi: 10.1002/ar.22553
42. Montalbano R, Waldegger P, Quint K, Jabari S, Neureiter D, Illig R, et al. Endoplasmic Reticulum Stress Plays a Pivotal Role in Cell Death Mediated by the Pan-Deacetylase Inhibitor Panobinostat in Human Hepatocellular Cancer Cells. *Trans Oncol* (2013) 6(2):143–IN6. doi: 10.1593/tlo.12271
43. Hamilton SA, Tower CL, Jones RL. Identification of Chemokines Associated With the Recruitment of Decidual Leukocytes in Human Labour: Potential Novel Targets for Preterm Labour. *PloS One* (2013) 8(2):e56946. doi: 10.1371/journal.pone.0056946
44. Bloise E, Bhuiyan M, Audette MC, Petropoulos S, Javam M, Gibb W, et al. Prenatal Endotoxemia and Placental Drug Transport in The Mouse: Placental Size-Specific Effects. *PloS One* (2013) 8(6):e65728. doi: 10.1371/journal.pone.0065728
45. Romero R, Mazor M, Brandt F, Sepulveda W, Avila C, Cotton DB, et al. Interleukin-1α and Interleukin-1 β in Preterm and Term Human Parturition. *Am J Reprod Immunol* (1992) 27(3-4):117–23. doi: 10.1111/j.1600-0897.1992.tb00737.x
46. Larocca RA, Abbink P, Peron JPS, de A, Zanotto PM, Iampietro MJ, et al. Vaccine Protection Against Zika Virus From Brazil. *Nature* (2016) 536 (7617):474–8. doi: 10.1038/nature18952
47. Souza IN de O, Frost PS, França JV, Nascimento-Viana JB, Neris RLS, Freitas L, et al. Acute and Chronic Neurological Consequences of Early-Life Zika Virus Infection in Mice. *Sci Trans Med* (2018) 10(444):eaar2749. doi: 10.1126/scitranslmed.aar2749
48. Kalagiri RR, Carder T, Choudhury S, Vora N, Ballard AR, Govande V, et al. Inflammation in Complicated Pregnancy and Its Outcome. *Am J Perinatol* (2016) 33(14):1337–56. doi: 10.1055/s-0036-1582397
49. Barbeito-Andrés J, Pezzuto P, Higa LM, Dias AA, Vasconcelos JM, Santos TMP, et al. Congenital Zika Syndrome is Associated With Maternal Protein Malnutrition. *Sci Adv* (2020) 6(2):eaaw6284. doi: 10.1126/sciadv.aaw6284
50. Saito S, Nakashima A, Shima T, Ito M. Review ARTICLE: Th1/Th2/Th17 and Regulatory T-Cell Paradigm in Pregnancy. *Am J Reprod Immunol* (2010) 63 (6):601–10. doi: 10.1111/j.1600-0897.2010.00852.x
51. Gotsch F, Romero R, Kusanovic JP, Mazaki-Tovi S, Pineles BL, Erez O, et al. The Fetal Inflammatory Response Syndrome. *Clin Obstet Gynecol* (2007) 50 (3):652–83. doi: 10.1097/GRF.0b013e31811ebef6
52. Lucas CGO, Kitoko JZ, Ferreira FM, Suzart VG, Papa MP, Coelho SVA, et al. Critical Role of CD4 + T Cells and Ifnγ Signaling in Antibody-Mediated Resistance to Zika Virus Infection. *Nat Commun* (2018) 9(1):3136. doi: 10.1038/s41467-018-05519-4
53. Burdet J, Sacerdoti F, Cella M, Franchi AM, Ibarra C. Role of TNF-α in the Mechanisms Responsible for Preterm Delivery Induced by Stx2 in Rats. *Br J Pharmacol* (2013) 168(4):946. doi: 10.1111/j.1476-5381.2012.02239.x
54. Carpentier PA, Dingman AL, Palmer TD. Placental TNF-α Signaling in Illness-Induced Complications of Pregnancy. *Am J Pathol* (2011) 178 (6):2802–10. doi: 10.1016/j.ajpath.2011.02.042
55. Romanowska-Próchnicka K, Felis-Giemza A, Olesińska M, Wojdasiewicz P, Paradowska-Gorycka A, Szukiewicz D. The Role of TNF-α and Anti-TNF-α Agents During Preconception, Pregnancy, and Breastfeeding. *Int J Mol Sci* (2021) 22(6):2922. doi: 10.3390/ijms22062922
56. Sarr D, Bracken TC, Owino SO, Cooper CA, Smith GM, Nagy T, et al. Differential Roles of Inflammation and Apoptosis in Initiation of Mid-Gestational Abortion in Malaria-Infected C57BL/6 and A/J Mice. *Placenta* (2015) 36(7):738. doi: 10.1016/j.placenta.2015.04.007
57. Galinsky R, Polglase GR, Hooper SB, Black MJ, Moss TJM. The Consequences of Chorioamnionitis: Preterm Birth and Effects on Development. *J Pregnancy* (2013) 2013:412831. doi: 10.1155/2013/412831
58. Mor G, Cardenas I, Abrahams V, Guller S. Inflammation and Pregnancy: The Role of the Immune System at the Implantation Site. *Ann N Y Acad Sci* (2011) 1221(1):80–7. doi: 10.1111/j.1749-6632.2010.05938.x
59. Ribeiro MR, Moreli JB, Marques RE, Papa MP, Meuren LM, Rahal P, et al. Zika-Virus-Infected Human Full-Term Placental Explants Display Pro-Inflammatory Responses and Undergo Apoptosis. *Arch Virol* (2018) 163 (10):2687–99. doi: 10.1007/s00705-018-3911-x
60. Gown AM, Willingham MC. Improved Detection of Apoptotic Cells in Archival Paraffin Sections: Immunohistochemistry Using Antibodies to Cleaved Caspase 3. *J Histochem Cytochem* (2002) 50(4):449–54. doi: 10.1177/002215540205000401

61. de Noronha L, Zanluca C, Burger M, Suzukawa AA, Azevedo M, Rebutini PZ, et al. Zika Virus Infection at Different Pregnancy Stages: Anatomopathological Findings, Target Cells and Viral Persistence in Placental Tissues. *Front Microbiol* (2018) 9(2266):1–11. doi: 10.3389/fmicb.2018.02266
62. Lojpur T, Easton Z, Raez-Villanueva S, Laviolette S, Holloway AC, Hardy DB. Δ9-Tetrahydrocannabinol Leads to Endoplasmic Reticulum Stress and Mitochondrial Dysfunction in Human BeWo Trophoblasts. *Reprod Toxicol* (2019) 87:21–31. doi: 10.1016/j.reprotox.2019.04.008
63. Offerdahl DK, Dorward DW, Hansen BT, Bloom ME. Cytoarchitecture of Zika Virus Infection in Human Neuroblastoma and Aedes Albopictus Cell Lines. *Virology* (2017) 501:54–62. doi: 10.1016/j.virol.2016.11.002
64. Desuzinges-Mandon E, Arnaud O, Martinez L, Huché F, Di Pietro A, Falson P. Abcg2 Transports and Transfers Heme to Albumin Through Its Large Extracellular Loop. *J Biol Chem* (2010) 285(43):33123–33. doi: 10.1074/jbc.M110.139170
65. Ledur PF, Karmirian K, Pedrosa C da SG, Souza LRQ, Assis-de-Lemos G, Martins TM, et al. Zika Virus Infection Leads to Mitochondrial Failure, Oxidative Stress and DNA Damage in Human iPSC-derived Astrocytes. *Sci Rep* (2020) 10(1):1218. doi: 10.1038/s41598-020-57914-x
66. Reemst K, Noctor SC, Lucassen PJ, Hol EM. The Indispensable Roles of Microglia and Astrocytes During Brain Development. *Front Hum Neurosci* (2016) 10:566. doi: 10.3389/fnhum.2016.00566
67. Guitart-Mampel M, Gonzalez-Tendero A, Niñerola S, Morén C, Catalán-Garcia M, González-Casacuberta I, et al. Cardiac and Placental Mitochondrial Characterization in a Rabbit Model of Intrauterine Growth Restriction. *Biochim Biophys Acta (BBA) Gen Subj* (2018) 1862(5):1157–67. doi: 10.1016/j.bbagen.2018.02.006
68. Guitart-Mampel M, Juarez-Flores DL, Youssef L, Moren C, Garcia-Otero L, Roca-Agujetas V, et al. Mitochondrial Implications in Human Pregnancies With Intrauterine Growth Restriction and Associated Cardiac Remodelling. *J Cell Mol Med* (2019) 23(6):3962–73. doi: 10.1111/jcmm.14282
69. Zhang Z, Rong L, Li Y-P. Flaviviridae Viruses and Oxidative Stress: Implications for Viral Pathogenesis. *Oxid Med Cell Longev* (2019) 2019:1409582. doi: 10.1155/2019/1409582
70. Martínez F, Kiriakidou M, Strauss JF. Structural and Functional Changes in Mitochondria Associated With Trophoblast Differentiation: Methods to Isolate Enriched Preparations of Syncytiotrophoblast Mitochondria. *Endocrinology* (1997) 138(5):2172–83. doi: 10.1210/endo.138.5.5133
71. Burton GJ, Yung HW, Murray AJ. Mitochondrial – Endoplasmic Reticulum Interactions in the Trophoblast: Stress and Senescence. *Placenta* (2017) 52:146–55. doi: 10.1016/j.placenta.2016.04.001
72. Holland O, Dekker Nitert M, Gallo LA, Vejzovic M, Fisher JJ, Perkins AV. Review: Placental Mitochondrial Function and Structure in Gestational Disorders. *Placenta* (2017) 54:2–9. doi: 10.1016/j.placenta.2016.12.012
73. Bridges CC, Zalups RK, Joshee L. Toxicological Significance of Renal Bcrp: Another Potential Transporter in the Elimination of Mercuric Ions From Proximal Tubular Cells. *Toxicol Appl Pharmacol* (2015) 285(2):110–7. doi: 10.1016/j.taap.2015.03.027
74. Szilagyi JT, Gorczyca L, Brinker A, Buckley B, Laskin JD, Aleksunes LM. Placental BCRP/ABCG2 Transporter Prevents Fetal Exposure to the Estrogenic Mycotoxin Zearalenone. *Toxicol Sci* (2019) 168(2):394–404. doi: 10.1093/toxsci/kfy303
75. Scialis RJ, Aleksunes LM, Csanaky IL, Klaassen CD, Manautou JE. Identification and Characterization of Efflux Transporters That Modulate the Subtoxic Disposition of Diclofenac and Its Metabolites. *Drug Metab Dispos* (2019) 47(10):1080–92. doi: 10.1124/dmd.119.086603
76. Mao Q, Unadkat JD. Role of the Breast Cancer Resistance Protein (BCRP/ABCG2) in Drug Transport–an Update. *AAPS J* (2015) 17(1):65–82. doi: 10.1208/s12248-014-9668-6
77. Lye P, Bloise E, Javam M, Gibb W, Lye SJ, Matthews SG. Impact of Bacterial and Viral Challenge on Multidrug Resistance in First- and Third-Trimester Human Placenta. *Am J Pathol* (2015) 185(6):1666–75. doi: 10.1016/j.ajpath.2015.02.013
78. Girard S, Sebire G. Transplacental Transfer of Interleukin-1 Receptor Agonist and Antagonist Following Maternal Immune Activation. *Am J Reprod Immunol (N Y NY: 1989)* (2016) 75(1):8–12. doi: 10.1111/aji.12444
79. Bloise E, Petropoulos S, Iqbal M, Kostaki A, Ortiga-Carvalho TM, Gibb W, et al. Acute Effects of Viral Exposure on P-Glycoprotein Function in the Mouse Fetal Blood-Brain Barrier. *Cell Physiol Biochem: Int J Exp Cell Physiol Biochem Pharmacol* (2017) 41(3):1044–50. doi: 10.1159/000461569

12

Cross-Reactivity of Virus-Specific CD8+ T Cells Against Allogeneic HLA-C: Possible Implications for Pregnancy Outcome

*Anita van der Zwan, Ellen M. W. van der Meer-Prins, Paula P. M. C. van Miert, Heleen van den Heuvel, Jacqueline D. H. Anholts, Dave L. Roelen, Frans H. J. Claas and Sebastiaan Heidt**

Department of Immunohematology and Blood Transfusion, Leiden University Medical Center, Leiden, Netherlands

Correspondence:
Sebastiaan Heidt
s.heidt@lumc.nl

Heterologous immunity of virus-specific T cells poses a potential barrier to transplantation tolerance. Cross-reactivity to HLA-A and -B molecules has broadly been described, whereas responses to allo-HLA-C have remained ill defined. In contrast to the transplant setting, HLA-C is the only polymorphic HLA molecule expressed by extravillous trophoblasts at the maternal-fetal interface during pregnancy. Uncontrolled placental viral infections, accompanied by a pro-inflammatory milieu, can alter the activation status and stability of effector T cells. Potential cross-reactivity of maternal decidual virus-specific T cells to fetal allo-HLA-C may thereby have detrimental consequences for the success of pregnancy. To explore the presence of cross-reactivity to HLA-C and the other non-classical HLA antigens expressed by trophoblasts, HLA-A and -B-restricted CD8+ T cells specific for Epstein-Barr virus, Cytomegalovirus, Varicella-Zoster virus, and Influenza virus were tested against target cells expressing HLA-C, -E, and -G molecules. An HLA-B*08:01-restricted EBV-specific T cell clone displayed cross-reactivity against HLA-C*01:02. Furthermore, cross-reactivity of HLA-C-restricted virus-specific CD8+ T cells was observed for HCMV HLA-C*06:02/TRA CD8+ T cell lines and clones against HLA-C*03:02. Collectively, these results demonstrate that cross-reactivity against HLA-C can occur and thereby may affect pregnancy outcome.

Keywords: heterologous immunity, virus-specific T cells, allogeneic HLA, HLA-C, pregnancy

1. INTRODUCTION

High frequencies of memory T cells against several viruses such as Influenza virus (FLU), Epstein-Barr virus (EBV), Human Cytomegalovirus (HCMV), and Varicella-Zoster virus (VZV) have been described in healthy individuals (1–3). Primary infection or reactivation of these viruses can compromise graft survival after transplantation and during pregnancy result in fetal malformation and pregnancy complications such as preterm birth and intrauterine growth restriction (4–7). A significant proportion of virus-specific CD8+ T cells in healthy (non-HLA sensitized) individuals display alloreactivity against allogeneic human leukocyte antigens (allo-HLA) (8, 9). This phenomenon, referred to as heterologous immunity, enables the same T-cell receptor (TCR) to recognize its autologous virus-peptide presenting HLA allele as well as allo-HLA. The avidity of these cross-reactive T cells for their viral and allogeneic targets depends on the levels of peptide presentation (10). Within an individual, an HLA-restricted virus-specific T cell response can generate several clonotypes that have different patterns of allo-HLA cross-reactivity (11). Both naïve and memory T cells show alloreactive potential, though memory T cells pose a superior threat (12, 13). Their activation threshold is significantly lower as they have less need for co-stimulation while their cytotoxic function is enhanced (14, 15). To ensure a comprehensive immune response to foreign antigens, this high degree of cross-reactivity is an intrinsic and essential feature of antigen recognition by T cells, of which allo-HLA cross-reactivity is an inherent consequence (16).

In the pregnancy setting T cells have a dual role in mediating tolerance toward the allogeneic fetus and at the same time responding to infections. During gestation, fetal extravillous trophoblasts (EVT) deeply invade the maternal tissues (decidua) where they establish direct contact with the maternal immune cells. EVT do not express the highly polymorphic HLA-A and -B, but do express HLA-C, -E, and -G (17, 18). CD8+ T cells present in the decidua demonstrate a mixed transcriptional profile of T cell dysfunction, activation and effector function. They are not permanently suppressed, but maintain the capacity to respond to proinflammatory occurrences, such as infections (19). Significant numbers of HLA-A and -B-restricted virus-specific CD8+ T cells are found in decidual tissue of term pregnancy (20). Furthermore, in the maternal peripheral blood, cytotoxic T lymphocyte (CTL) responses to paternal allo-HLA (HLA-A/B) and minor histocompatibility antigens (mHag) have been detected during pregnancy (21–23). Thus, maternal CD8+ T cells can respond to viral, fetal and placental antigens during pregnancy but so far no evidence exists on the presence of HLA-C-restricted viral and mHag-specific CD8+ T cells and whether maternal HLA-A and -B-restricted virus-specific CD8+ T cells can cross-react with fetal HLA antigens, leading to possible pregnancy complications. Recognition of fetal HLA-C by both B cells and helper T cells is suggested by the presence of specific HLA-C IgG antibodies in women with recurrent miscarriages (24). Furthermore, HLA-C incompatibility is significantly increased in couples with unexplained recurrent miscarriages when compared to control subjects (25). In addition, certain combinations of maternal killer cell immunoglobulin-like receptor (KIR) genotypes, expressed by decidual NK cells, and fetal HLA-C are associated with pregnancy complications such as preeclampsia (26). These data indicate that fetal HLA-C could play a vital role in guiding the maternal immune response during pregnancy.

Studies on heterologous immunity in transplantation have focused on the cross-reactivity of HLA-A and -B-restricted virus-specific CD8+ T cells with allogeneic HLA-A and -B, with less attention for HLA-C considering its lower cell surface expression levels when compared to HLA-A and -B (27). In the context of pregnancy HLA-C is the only polymorphic antigen expressed on EVT and alloreactivity to HLA-C (and HLA-E and -G) is therefore unique and highly significant. The importance of HLA-C incompatibility in pregnancy complications coupled to the presence of virus-specific CD8+ T cells at the maternal-fetal interface, led us to investigate whether cross-reactivity of virus-specific CD8+ T cells against HLA-C, -E and -G is a common phenomenon in healthy individuals.

2. RESULTS

2.1. Alloreactivity of an EBV B8/FLR CD8+ T Cell Clone 4D5 Against HLA-C*01:02

To investigate the ability of virus-specific CD8+ T cells to cross-react with HLA-C, -E, and -G, 29 HLA-A and -B-restricted human CMV, FLU, VZV, and EBV-specific CD8+ T cell lines and clones (28) were tested against a panel of single antigen expressing lines (SALs) expressing HLA-C, -E, and -G alleles ($n = 11$) (29, 30). An HLA-A2-restricted EBV-specific CD8+ T cell clone isolated from placental decidua parietalis was also included (20). The specificities of the isolated virus-specific CD8+ T cell lines and clones are listed in **Table 1**. Lack of IFNγ production revealed that alloreactivity against HLA-C, -E, and -G is not common **Table 2**. Nonetheless, one HLA-B*08:01-restricted EBV-specific (EBV B8/FLR) T cell clone, 4D5, showed significant alloreactivity against HLA-C*01:02 **Figure 1A**. This T cell clone was isolated from an HLA-C*01:02 negative donor.

To corroborate alloreactivity against HLA-C*01:02, one EBV B8/FLR T cell line and four T cell clones were stimulated with a panel of SALs and EBV lymphoblastoid cell lines (EBV-LCLs) expressing HLA-C*01:02 and HLA-B*44:02 alleles for 24 h after which IFNγ production was measured. Alloreactivity of EBV B8/FLR T cells against HLA-B*44:02 is a commonly described occurrence (31). T cell clone 4D5 reacted against its virus-specific restriction allele HLA-B*08:01 loaded with FLR peptide as well as HLA-C*01:02 expressed by SALs and EBV-LCLs. Its lower alloreactivity against the second EBV-LCL donor expressing heterozygous HLA-C*01:02 may have been a result of low HLA-C expression. T cell clone 4D5 did not show alloreactivity against HLA-B*44:02 **Figure 1B**. T cell clone 4B8 (here shown as a representative example), comprising a different TCR Vα and Vβ usage than 4D5 **Table 3**, displayed no alloreactivity against HLA-C*01:02 and only cross-reacted with HLA-B*44:02 when loaded with the appropriate self-peptide (EEY). The other EBV B8/FLR CD8+ T cells tested also did not cross-react with HLA-C*01:02, but displayed cross-reactivity against HLA-B*44:02. No alloreactivity against HLA-E and -G was discerned **Figure S1**.

Alloreactivity of virus-specific CD8+ T cells can be cell type or tissue-specific (9, 32). Therefore, to further functionally

TABLE 1 | Specificities of isolated virus-specific CD8+ T cell lines and clones.

Virus	HLA	Antigen	Epitope
HCMV	HLA-A*02:01	pp65 (495-503)	NLVPMVATV
HCMV	HLA-B*35:01	pp65 (123-131)	IPSINVHHY
HCMV	HLA-C*06:02	pp65 (201-209)	TRATKMQVI
HCMV	HLA-C*07:02	IE-1 (309-317)	CRVLCCYVL
EBV	HLA-A*02:01	BMLF1 (280-288)	GLCTLVAML
EBV	HLA-B*08:01	EBNA-3A (325-333)	FLRGRAYGL
EBV	HLA-B*35:01	EBNA-3A (458-466)	YPLHEQHGM
FLU	HLA-A*02:01	IMP (58-66)	GILGFVFTL
VZV	HLA-A*02:01	IE-62 (593-601)	ALWALPHAA

HCMV, human Cytomegalovirus; EBV, Epstein-Barr virus; FLU, Influenza virus; VZV, Varicella-Zoster virus.

TABLE 2 | Alloreactivity of virus-specific CD8+ T cell lines and clones against HLA-C, -E, and -G.

Donor	Specificity	TCR Vβ	# T cell lines/clones tested	Allo-HLA-C	Allo-HLA-E, -G	Target cell (s)	Allo-HLA-C, -E, -G cross-reactivity
A	HCMV A2/NLV	2	2	2	2	SALs	No
	HCMV A2/NLV	8	3	2	3	SALs	No
	HCMV A2/NLV	13.1	1	0	1	SALs	No
	HCMV A2/NLV	5.2	1	0	1	SALs	No
	HCMV A2/NLV	#	9	0	9	SALs	No
A	HCMV B35/IPS	2	1	0	1	SALs	No
	HCMV B35/IPS	3	2	2	2	SALs	No
	HCMV B35/IPS	13.2	2	1	2	SALs	No
	HCMV B35/IPS	22	1	1	1	SALs	No
	HCMV B35/IPS	*	2	2	2	SALs	No
B	HCMV B35/IPS	3	3	2	3	SALs	No
C	HCMV B35/IPS	3	4	2	4	SALs	No
A	FLU A2/GIL	17	3	2	3	SALs	No
	FLU A2/GIL	17+18	1	0	1	SALs	No
D	FLU A2/GIL	17	4	1	4	SALs	No
B	FLU A2/GIL	#	3	2	3	SALs	No
E	FLU A2/GIL	#	2	1	2	SALs	No
F	FLU A2/GIL	#	1	0	1	SALs	No
F	VZV A2/ALW	#	1	1	1	SALs	No
G	VZV A2/ALW	#	1	1	1	SALs	No
H	EBV B35/YPL	14	1	1	1	SALs	No
	EBV B35/YPL	21.3	2	2	2	SALs	No
	EBV B35/YPL	*	1	1	1	SALs	No
I	EBV A2/GLC (decidua parietalis)	#	1	1	1	SALs	No
J	EBV B8/FLR	7	2	2	2	SALs, EBV-LCLs	No
K	EBV B8/FLR (4D5)	3	1	1	1	SALs, EBV-LCLs, PHA blasts	HLA-C*01:02
	EBV B8/FLR	4	2	2	2	SALs, EBV-LCLs	No
L	HCMV C*0702/CRV	6	1	1	1	721.221, EBV-LCLs	No
M	HCMV C*0602/TRA	13	2	2	2	SALs, EBV-LCLs	No
	HCMV C*0602/TRA (1A3, 7A12, 10C1)	28	2	2	2	SALs, EBV-LCLs, PHA blasts	HLA-C*03:02

Summary

Specificities	9
Donors	13
TCR tested	21
T cell lines/clones tested against HLA-C, -E, -G	34

* The TCR Vβ could not be determined with the TCR Vβ kit used.

Not tested.

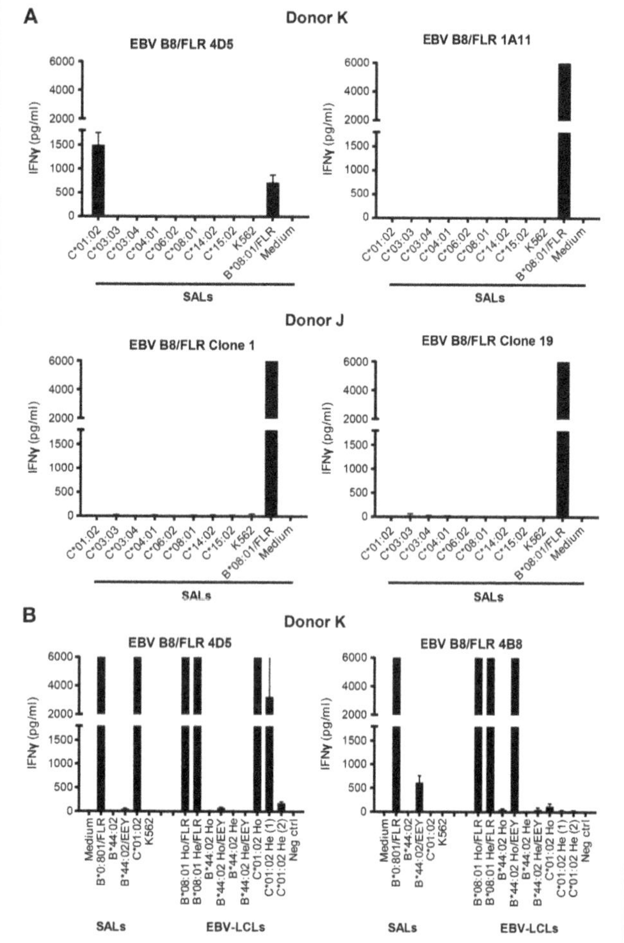

FIGURE 1 | Alloreactivity of EBV B8/FLR T cell clone 4D5 against HLA-C*01:02. **(A)** EBV B8/FLR T cell lines ($n = 9$; 1A11 shown) and T cell clones ($n = 6$; 4D5, clone 1, and clone 19 shown) were stimulated with a panel of HLA-C expressing SALs after which IFNγ production was measured. EBV B8/FLR T cell clone 4D5 showed alloreactivity against HLA-C*01:02. **(B)** One EBV B8/FLR T cell line and four EBV B8/FLR T cell clones (4B8 and 4D5 shown) were stimulated with a panel of SALs and EBV-LCLs expressing HLA B*08:01, HLA C*01:02, and HLA-B*44:02 alleles after which IFNγ production was measured. The range of the ELISA standard curve: 5–5120 pg/ml; Ho, homozygous; He, heterozygous. Bars represent duplicate values with standard deviation of the mean.

validate our results, cytotoxicity of the T cell clones 4D5 and 4B8 was investigated against ^{51}Chromium (^{51}Cr) -labeled human umbilical vein endothelial cells (HUVECs), SALs (myeloid origin), EBV-LCLs (B cells) and PHA blasts (T cells) expressing the recognized allo-HLA-C*01:02 allele and the virus-specific restriction allele HLA-B*08:01 loaded with viral peptide as a positive control. Target cells expressing no HLA-B*08:01 and HLA-C*01:02 were included as a negative control. The T cell clones were added to their targets in four effector: target ratios. Specific lysis of HLA-C*01:02 expressing SALs, EBV-LCLs and PHA blasts by T cell clone 4D5 was observed in a ratio-dependent manner. T cell clone 4D5 was however not lytic against HUVECs expressing HLA-C*01:02, presumably the result of the relevant self-peptide not being expressed by this cell type (33) **Figure 2A**. The robust cytolytic response of T cell clone 4D5 against EBV-LCLs expressing HLA-C*01:02 was substantially decreased by addition of an anti-CD8 blocking antibody, while lysis of target cells expressing the virus-specific restriction allele HLA-B*08:01 loaded with FLR peptide was not affected, indicating distinct TCR affinities **Figure 2B**. No specific lysis by T cell clone 4B8 was observed **Figure 2C**. Together, these results demonstrate that alloreactivity of HLA-A and -B-restricted virus-specific CD8+ T cells against HLA-C can occur and is dependent on CD8.

2.2. Characterization of HLA-C*06:02-Restricted HCMV-Specific T Cell Lines and Clones

HLA-C-restricted virus-specific CD8+ T cells have been described in the context of HIV infection where they recognize a highly conserved epitope and in HCMV infection where HLA-C*07:02-restricted CD8+ T cells dominate the T cell response to the immediate-early 1 (IE-1) viral antigen and their levels increase with age (34–36). Given their high allele frequency in the population, we set out to isolate HLA-C*06:02- and HLA-C*07:02-restricted HCMV-specific CD8+ T cells (37, 38) and explore their alloreactivity against HLA-C, -E, and -G. PBMC of HLA-C*06:02+HCMV+ donors ($n = 10$) were stained with an HLA-C*06:02 tetramer containing the HCMV TRA peptide (39) **Table 1**. From a donor with 15% positivity for the HLA-C*06:02/TRA tetramer, CD8+ T cell lines and clones were generated by sorting tetramer positive CD8+ T cells and expanding them *in vitro* **Figure 3A**; **Figure S2**. An established HLA-C*07:02-restricted HCMV-specific CD8+ T cell clone (LH) was included in the analysis (35). To examine the functionality of these HLA-C*06:02/TRA-restricted HCMV-specific T cell lines and clones, as well as the HLA-C*07:02/CRV-restricted HCMV-specific T cell clone LH, IFNγ production was measured after 24 h of co-culture with SALs and EBV-LCLs expressing HLA-C*06:02 or C*07:02 loaded with the appropriate viral peptide. All HLA-C*06:02-restricted T cell lines and clones, and the HLA-C*07:02-restricted clone LH responded against their virus-specific restriction HLA-allele loaded with viral peptide **Figure 3B**. In addition, specific lysis in a ratio-dependent manner of ^{51}Cr-labeled SALs, 721.221 cells expressing HLA-C*07:02, and EBV-LCLs was detected **Figure 3C**. These results confirmed functionality of the generated HLA-C*06:02-restricted T cell lines and clones (HCMV C*06:02/TRA), and the established HLA-C*07:02-restricted T cell clone LH (HCMV C*07:02/CRV).

2.3. Alloreactivity and Cytotoxicity of HCMV C*06:02/TRA T Cell Lines Against HLA-C*03:02

Next, the HCMV C*06:02/TRA CD8+ T lines and clones ($n = 4$), and HCMV C*07:02/CRV CD8+ T cell clone LH were tested against a panel of SALs expressing HLA-C, -E, and -G, in a co-culture system where IFNγ production was assessed. No alloreactivity was observed in this setting **Figures S3A,B**. Subsequently, in a similar manner, alloreactivity against a panel of EBV-LCLs covering the most common HLA alleles was

TABLE 3 | TCR Vα and Vβ usage of CD8+T cell lines and clones.

T cell line/clone	TRαV	TRαJ	CDR3α	TRβV	TRβJ	TRβD	CDR3β	Cross-reactivity
B8/FLR T cell clone 4B8	TRAV1-2*01 F	TRAJ36*01 F	C A V R D Q T G A N N L F F	TRBV4-3*02 (F)	TRBJ2-5*01 F	TRBD2*01 F	C A S S H G L A G I L E T Q Y F	No
B8/FLR T cell clone 4D5	TRAV40*01 F	TRAJ43*01 F	C L L G D N D M R F	TRBV3-1/2*01	TRBJ1-6*02 F	TRBD2*01 F	C A S S Q P P T G R S Y N S P L H F	HLA-C*01:02
C*0702/CRV T cell clone LH	TRAV27*03 (F)	TRAJ33*01 F	C A G G D M D S N Y Q L I W	TRBV6-2/3/6	TRBJ2-7*01 F	TRBD1*01 F	C A S G E V Y E Q Y F	No
C*0602/TRA T cell clone 1F12	TRAV19*01 F	TRAJ26*01 F	C A L S E G G S Y G Q N F V F	TRBV13*01/02 (F)	TRBJ2-1*01 F	TRBD2*01 F	C A S S L R D E Q F F	No
C*0602/TRA T cell line 1A3	TRAV12-2*02 (F)	TRAJ20*01 F (a)	C A V N N D Y K L S N	TRBV28*01 F	TRBJ2-1*01 F	TRBD2*01 F	C A S S S G G L E N E Q F F	HLA-C*03:02
C*0602/TRA T cell clone 10C1				TRBV28*01 F	TRBJ2-1*01 F	TRBD2*01 F	C A S S S G G L E N E Q F F	HLA-C*03:02

investigated **Table 4**. Interestingly, two HCMV C*06:02/TRA T cell lines cross-reacted with EBV-LCL donor 12 of which T cell line 1A3 is shown as a representative example **Figure 4A**. When comparing the HLA typing of all 20 EBV-LCL donors in the panel, HLA-C*03:02 expressed by donor 12 was the only non-overlapping HLA allele candidate. A SAL expressing HLA-C*03:02 is not present in the panel and therefore cross-reactivity against this allele was not picked up in the initial screening **Figures 3SA,B**. A role for HLA class II was ruled out. CD8+ T cell lines and clones cross-reacting against donor 12 disclosed a distinct TCR Vα and Vβ usage when compared to CD8+ T cells showing no alloreactivity **Table 3**. No alloreactivity of the HCMV C*07:02/CRV clone LH was observed **Figure 4A**.

To further gauge the alloreactivity against HLA-C*03:02, HCMV C*06:02/TRA T cell lines ($n = 2$) and clones ($n = 5$) with the same TCR Vβ usage as the two CD8+ T cell lines that cross-reacted with cells from donor 12 (and all isolated from an HLA-C*03:02 negative donor) were stimulated with EBV-LCLs and PHA blasts expressing the recognized allo-HLA-C*03:02 allele. Target cells expressing the virus-specific restriction allele HLA-C*06:02 loaded with viral peptide were included as a positive control. Alloreactivity against HLA-C*03:02 was detected for all HCMV C*06:02 T cells tested, with substantially more IFNγ production against EBV-LCLs than against PHA blasts 1 and 2, obtained from two different donors **Figure 4B**. Differential HLA expression levels on the cell surface may explain increased alloreactivity against PHA blast 3 expressing HLA-C*03:02, obtained from a third donor **Figure S4**.

Having identified IFNγ production against allo-HLA-C*03:02, HCMV C*06:02/TRA T cell lines and clones were tested for cytotoxicity against ^{51}Cr-labeled SALs, EBV-LCLs, and PHA blasts expressing HLA-C*03:02. Target cells expressing the virus-specific restriction allele HLA-C*06:02 loaded with viral peptide were included as a positive control. The CD8+ T cell lines and clone were added to their targets in four effector: target ratios. Specific lysis of HLA-C*03:02 expressing target cells was observed in a ratio-dependent manner **Figure 5A**. Subsequently, the T cell lines and clone were incubated with an anti-CD8 blocking antibody prior to co-culture with the ^{51}Cr-labeled target cells resulting in substantially decreased lysis of target cells expressing HLA-C*03:02. A decrease in lysis was not observed for target cells expressing the virus-specific restriction allele HLA-C*06:02 loaded with viral peptide, indicating distinct TCR affinities **Figure 5B**. These findings highlight the functionality of the isolated HCMV C*06:02/TRA T cell lines and clones and provide evidence that alloreactivity of HLA-C-restricted virus-specific CD8+ T cells against HLA-C is a phenomenon that occurs.

3. DISCUSSION

Alloreactivity of HLA-A and -B-restricted virus-specific CD8+ T cells against HLA-A and -B is common. Eighty percent of virus-specific T cell lines and 45% of virus-specific T cell clones disclosed cross-reactivity against allo-HLA molecules (9). Here, we have shown that alloreactivity of HLA-A and -B-restricted

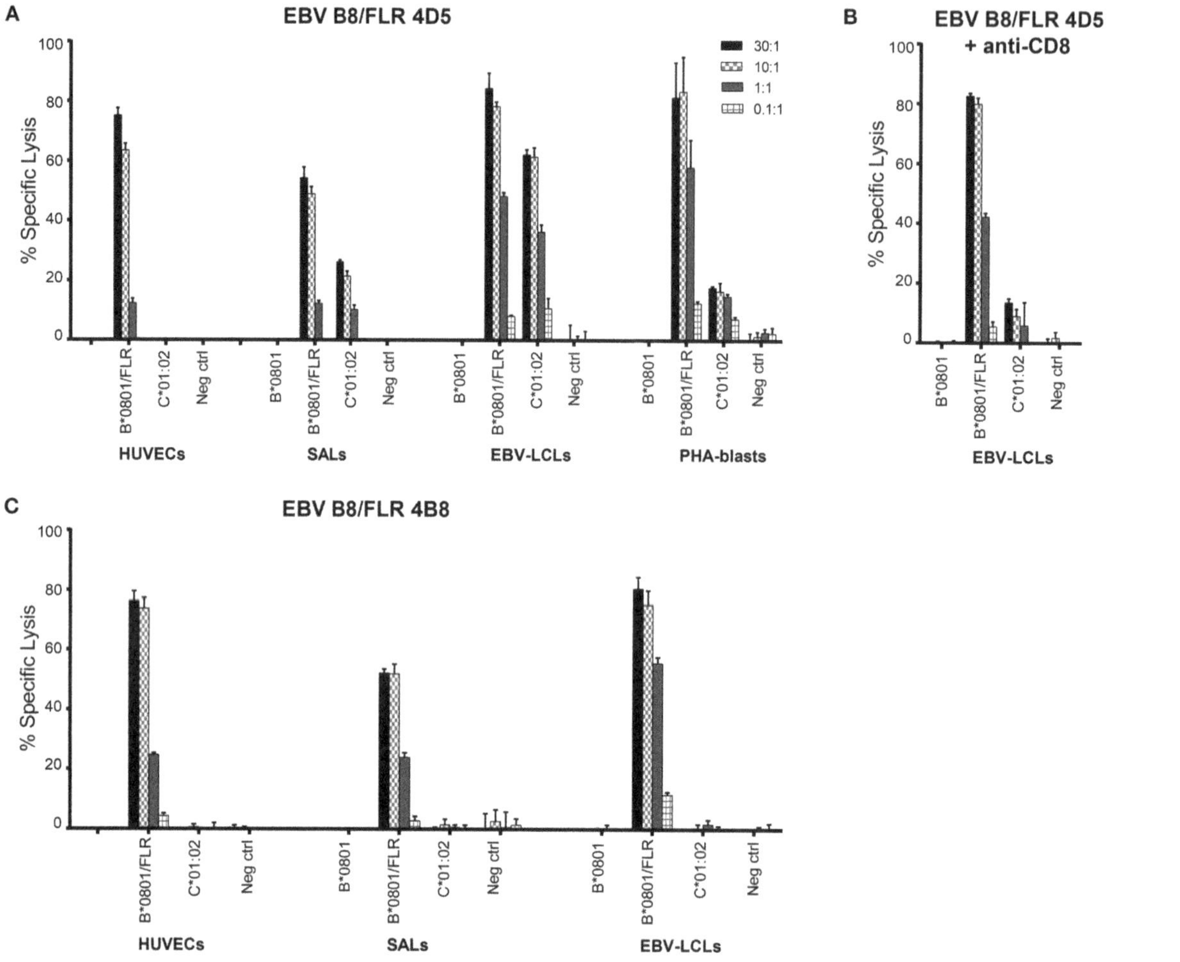

FIGURE 2 | EBV B8/FLR T cell clone 4D5 is cytotoxic against HLA-C*01:02. Cytotoxicity of T cell clones 4D5 **(A)** and 4B8 **(C)** was tested against ^{51}Cr-labeled HUVECs, SALs, EBV-LCLs, and PHA blasts expressing the recognized allo-HLA-C*01:02 allele and the virus-specific restriction HLA allele loaded with viral peptide as a positive control. As a negative control, target cells expressing no HLA-B*0801 and HLA-C*0102 were included. **(B)** T cell clone 4D5 was incubated with an anti-CD8 blocking antibody prior to co-culture with ^{51}Cr-labeled EBV-LCLs and specific lysis was measured. Bars represent triplicate values with standard deviation of the mean.

virus-specific CD8+ T cells against HLA-C can also occur. Amongst the 29 HLA-A and -B-restricted virus-specific T cells tested, one EBV B8/FLR CD8+ T cell clone 4D5 with distinct TCR Vα and Vβ usage displayed cross-reactivity and cytotoxicity against target cells expressing HLA-C*01:02, indicative of a more than 10 times lower frequency within the pool of HLA-A and -B-restricted virus-specific CD8+ T cells tested. This T cell clone did not reveal the classical described cross-reaction against HLA-B*44:02. Our preliminary data suggests that HLA-C cross-reactivity in HLA-C-restricted virus-specific T cells is more common. HLA-C*06:02-restricted HCMV-specific CD8+ T cells were successfully isolated from an HCMV+ donor by means of HLA-C tetramers and deemed fully functional *in vitro*. Alloreactivity of these HCMV C*06:02/CRV T cell lines and clones, with distinct TCR Vα and Vβ usage, was observed against HLA-C*03:02. This alloreactivity was mediated by IFNγ production and cytotoxicity. Viral specificity and alloreactivity are thought to be mediated by the same TCR (9), where in our setting anti-viral reactivity occurred independent of CD8, while allo-HLA-C reactivity was CD8 dependent. Differential recognition of HLA-C on SALs, EBV-LCLs, PHA blasts, and HUVECs, that did not provoke any alloreactivity, is an indication that cross-reactivity is determined by endogenous peptide (11) and supports the anticipation that tissue-specific peptides are presented and recognized. The nature of the endogenous peptide presented in HLA-C*01:02 and HLA-C*03:02, provoking the allo-response, is however unknown. Alternatively, expression of costimulatory and coinhibitory molecules by virus-specific T cells may have an influence on T cell signaling and thereby the extent of the allo-response (40). No alloreactivity against HLA-E and -G was observed. Our initial screening was against a panel of SALs expressing most, but not all HLA-C, -E, and -G molecules and we therefore may have underestimated the allo-response of virus-specific CD8+ T cells against these HLA alleles.

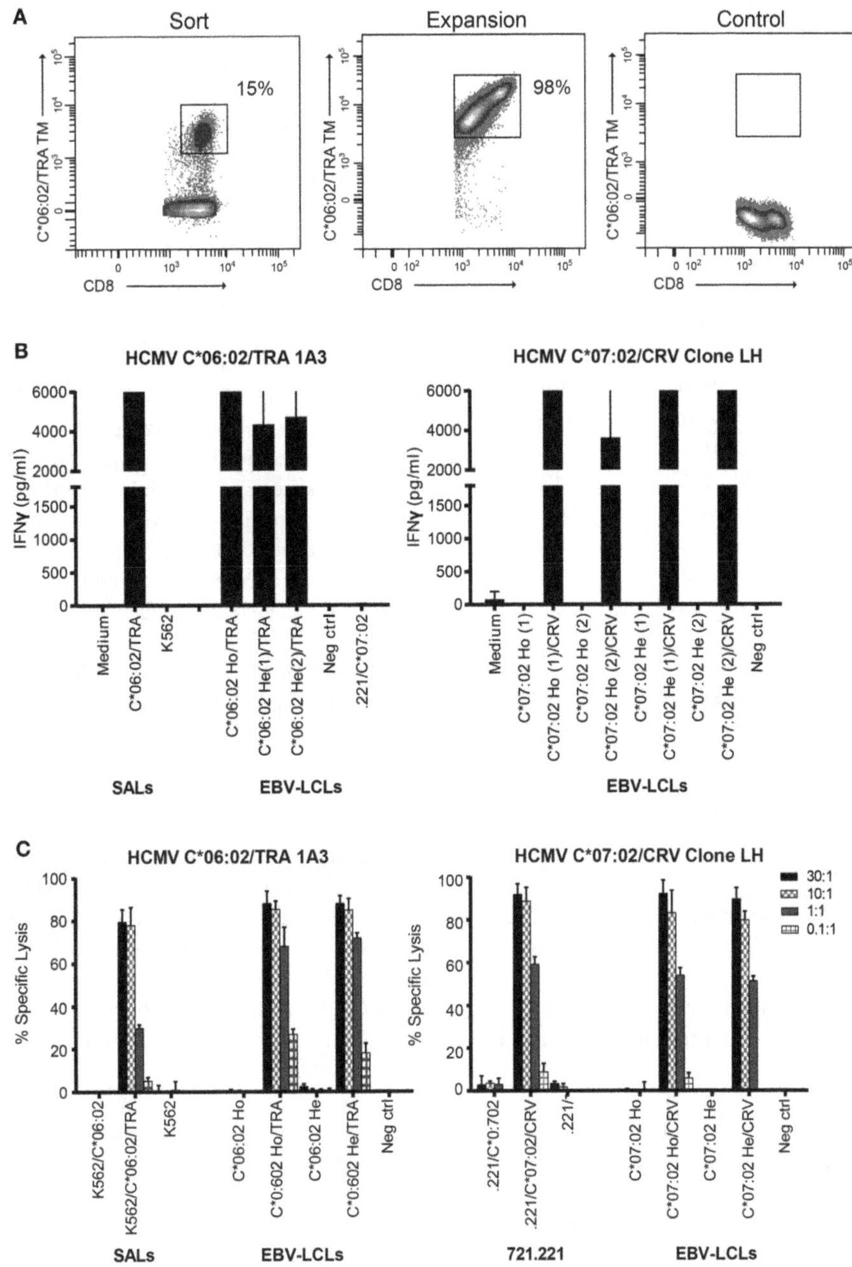

FIGURE 3 | Generated HCMV HLA-C*06:02/TRA T cell lines and clones, and the HCMV HLA-C*07:02/CRV T cell clone are cytolytic against their target cells. **(A)** FACS plots of HLA-C*06:02/TRA tetramer staining at time of sorting and 2 weeks after expansion of the tetramer-positive CD8+ T cells. **(B)** Two HCMV C*06:02/TRA T cell lines (1A3 shown) and two T cell clones, and HCMV C*07:02/CRV T cell clone LH were stimulated with SALs and EBV-LCLs expressing HLA-C*06:02 or C*07:02 loaded with viral peptide. **(C)** Cytotoxicity of one HCMV C*06:02/TRA T cell line (1A3 shown) and two T cell clones, and HCMV C*07:02/CRV T cell clone LH was tested against ^{51}Cr-labeled SALs, 721.221 cells and EBV-LCLs expressing the virus-specific restriction HLA allele alone or loaded with viral peptide. The range of the ELISA standard curve: 5–5120 pg/ml. Ho, homozygous; He, heterozygous. Bars represent triplicate values with standard deviation of the mean.

Variation of HLA-C expression at the cell surface can be a result of microRNA binding and discrepancies in exons that influence the structure of the peptide-binding cleft and the diversity of peptides bound by HLA-C molecules (27, 41). Differential expression of HLA-C has an influence on the ability of CD8+ T cells to mount an immune response. High expression of HLA-C has been associated with protection against infections, yet at the same time correlates with autoimmune disease (42). Nevertheless, when viral peptides are presented in the HLA-C locus, immune responses are still lower than to those presented in the HLA-A and -B loci (43). The lower expression of HLA-C at the cell surface and the differential

TABLE 4 | HLA class I typing of the EBV-LCL panel.

	HLA class I		
Panel ID	**A**	**B**	**C**
1	02:01, 32:01	08:01, 44:05	02:02, 07:01/06/18
2	24:02, 33:01	14:02	02:02/32, 08:02/29
3	03:01/22, 29:02/09	07:02/61/114, 44:03/105	07:02, 16:01
4	11:01/43, 33:03/51	18:01/17N, 52:01	07:02, 07:04
5	11:01/33, 30:01/54	13:02, 35:01/42	04:01, 06:02
6	01:01, 26:01	08:01, 49:01	07:01
7	11:01, 31:01	15:01, 57:01	03:03, 06:02/55
8	02:03, 24:02	38:02, 40:01	03:04, 07:02
9	29:02, 31:01	18:01/17N, 58:01	05:01, 07:18/01
10	24:03	51:01	15:02
11	26:01	38:01	12:03
12	24:02, 30:01	51:01, 58:01	01:02, 03:02
13	02:01, 03:01	15:01	03:03
14	68:01, 68:02	44:02/19N, 55:01	03:03, 07:04
15	24:02, 31:01	39:01, 55:01	03:03, 12:03
16	30:01, 68:02	42:01	17:01
17	01:01	41:01	17:01
18	02:01, 11:01	35:01, 44:03	04:01, 16:01
19	02:01, 25:01	18:01/17N/43, 44:02/19N/55	05:01, 12:03
20	24:02, 31:01/119	07:02/294/298, 07:05	07:02, 15:05

immune responses that it triggers when compared to HLA-A and -B (44) may be an explanation for less frequent alloreactivity against HLA-C.

We speculate that alloreactivity of virus-specific CD8+ T cells against HLA-C may play a role in pregnancy complications where HLA-C is the only polymorphic HLA allele expressed by EVT. Viral infections of the fetus or the placenta can lead to severe birth defects or pregnancy loss (5). Viruses are capable of downregulating surface HLA-A and -B expression upon infection, while HLA-C expression is spared (45). EVT also persistently express HLA-C when infected with HCMV (46). HLA-A and -B-restricted virus-specific CD8+ T cells are present at the maternal-fetal interface (20) and may be capable of cross-reacting with HLA-C under certain pro-inflammatory environmental circumstances and depending on (allo) peptide expression, thereby jeopardizing the success of pregnancy. It is yet to be established whether HLA-C-restricted virus-specific CD8+ T cells are present at the maternal-fetal interface and if so, whether they are capable of mounting an immune response. While the presence of anti-HLA-C IgG antibodies has been described in women with recurrent miscarriages, the competency of virus-specific CD8+ T cells to cross-react with HLA-C raises the question whether allo-HLA-C IgG antibodies are the only player in recurrent miscarriages or whether decidual virus-specific CD8+ T cells with cross-reactive potential also play their part in pregnancy complications.

Cross-reactivity of virus-specific CD8+ T cells against HLA-C can occur and consequently our results lay the foundation for further investigation into this cross-reactivity in the context of pregnancy. Future research will focus on isolating virus-specific CD8+ T cells from the peripheral blood of women with either a healthy pregnancy or recurrent miscarriage. Alloreactivity and differences thereof by these virus-specific CD8+ T cells, obtained after normal pregnancy and miscarriage cases, against target cells expressing allo-HLA-C, -E, and -G molecules can then be investigated. Isolating viable HLA-G+ EVT from first trimester and term placentas that express the correct HLA typing is challenging. Yet, it is important that allo-HLA reactive CD8+ T cells are tested against primary EVT expressing allo-HLA-C, as EVT may have protective mechanisms in place that prevent allo-HLA responses to ensure a successful pregnancy. A recent study described aberrant expression of HLA-DR in syncytiotrophoblasts and syncytiotrophoblast-derived extracellular vesicles (STEVs) in pre-eclampsia but not control placentae, addressing the importance of further examining heterologous immunity of not only decidual CD8+ T cells, but also decidual CD4+ T cells (47).

Not only in the pregnancy setting has HLA-C disparity been described as a possible cause of complication. In transplantation, HLA-C incompatibility has been associated with graft failure after bone marrow transplantation (48). Furthermore, HLA-C mismatches were significantly correlated with acute transplant rejection and increased chronic graft-vs.-host disease (GvHD) after hematopoietic stem cell transplantation (49, 50). Graft loss after solid organ transplantation and GvHD after hematopoietic stem cell transplantation (51) have been associated with heterologous immunity against allo-HLA-A and -B. The proven alloreactivity of virus-specific CD8+ T cells against HLA-C could lead to allo-immune responses and add an additional barrier to tolerance that requires further assessment in transplantation.

In conclusion, alloreactivity against HLA-C occurs and may have pronounced clinical implications in pregnancy, where the only polymorphic allo-HLA antigen expressed by EVT is HLA-C. It remains to be established how often this alloreactivity could lead to the development of pregnancy complications, such as recurrent miscarriages.

4. MATERIALS AND METHODS

4.1. Preparation of Responder and Target Cells

Peripheral blood leukocytes were isolated from buffy coats obtained from healthy blood donors after informed consent, at Sanquin Blood Supply, the Netherlands. PBMC were isolated by standard density gradient centrifugation and cryopreserved until use. Single HLA antigen–transfected K562 cells (SALs) were generated as described previously (52). HLA typing was performed by sequence-specific oligonucleotide or sequence-specific primer genotyping at the Department of Immunohematology and Blood Transfusion, LUMC, the

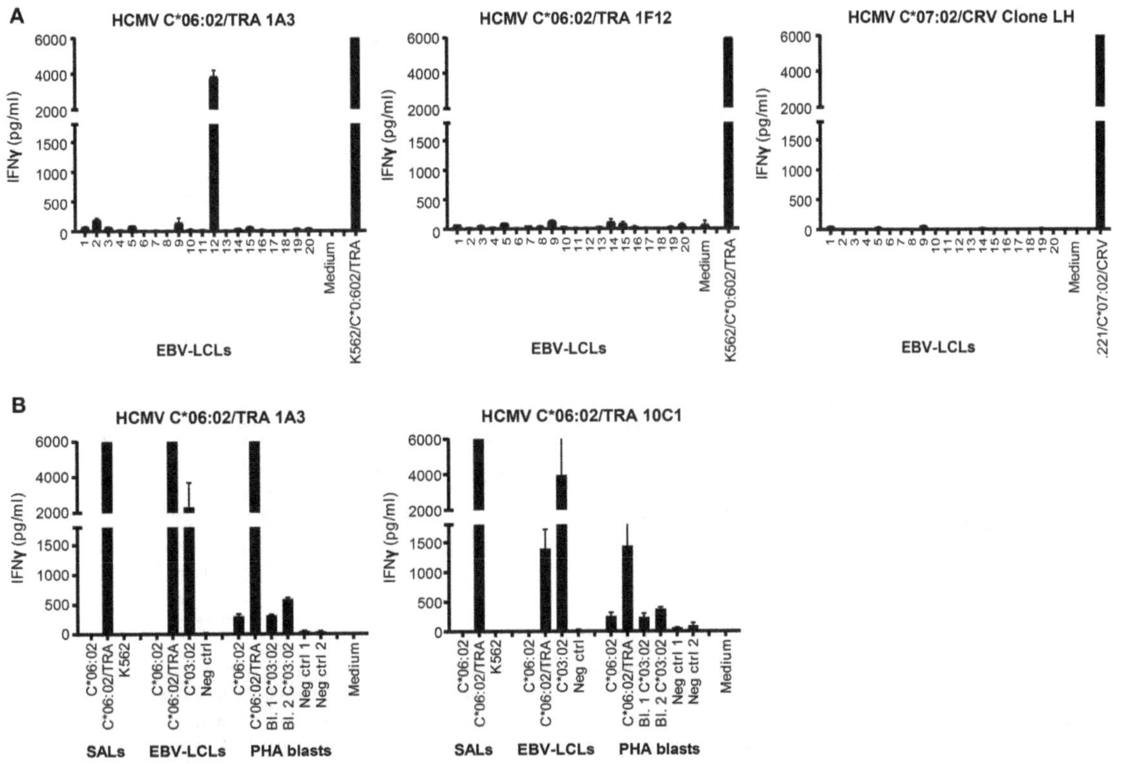

FIGURE 4 | Alloreactivity of HCMV C*06:02/TRA T cell lines against HLA-C*03:02. **(A)** Two HCMV C*06:02/TRA T cell lines (1A3 shown) and two T cell clones (1F12 shown), and HCMV C*07:02/CRV T cell clone LH were stimulated with a panel of EBV-LCLs after which IFNγ production was measured. **(B)** Three HCMV C*06:02/TRA T cell lines (1A3 shown) and five T cell clones (10C1 shown) were stimulated with EBV-LCLs and PHA blasts, obtained from two different donors, expressing the recognized allo-HLA-C*03:02 allele and the virus-specific restriction allele HLA-C*06:02 loaded with viral peptide as a positive control. SALs expressing HLA-C*06:02 loaded with viral peptide were also included as a positive control. The range of the ELISA standard curve: 5–5120 pg/ml. Bars represent duplicate values with standard deviation of the mean.

Netherlands. Epstein-Barr virus transformed lymphoblastoid cell lines (EBV-LCLs) were generated by incubating PBMC with the supernatant of the EBV-producing marmoset cell line B95.8 for 1.5 h at 37°C, and additional culture in RPMI 1640 Medium (Gibco Life Technologies, Carlsbad, CA) supplemented with 10% Fetal Calf Serum (FCS; Sigma Aldrich, St. Louis, Missouri), Penicillin/Streptavidin (Pen/Strep) and L-glutamine (all from Gibco). The 721.221 cell line expressing HLA-C*07:02 was kindly obtained from Professor Anthony W. Purcell (Monash University; cell line originally made by the laboratory of Prof. Andrew Brooks at the University of Melbourne).

Phytohaemagglutinin (PHA) blasts were generated by incubating PBMC for 8 days in RPMI 1640 Medium, Pen/Strep, L-glutamine, 15% human serum (HS, Sanquin, Amsterdam, the Netherlands), IL-2 (60 IU/ml; Novartis, Novartis, Horsham, UK) and PHA (4 μg/ml; Murex Biotech Ltd, Dartford, UK). Human umbilical vein endothelial cells (HUVECs) were cultured in M199 medium supplemented with 10% Newborn calf Serum (NCS), 1% sodium pyruvate, Pen/Strep (all from Gibco), 0,1% β-mercaptoethanol (0.05M, Sigma Aldrich), 1% sodium heparin (400 IE/ml; LUMC, Leiden, the Netherlands), and bovine purine extract (BPE; 100 μl in 20 ml; Invitrogen, Carlsbad, CA).

4.2. Generation of Virus-Specific CD8+ T Cell Lines and Clones

PBMC from EBV+, HCMV+, FLU+, and VZV+ blood donors were stained with phycoerythrin (PE)-labeled viral tetramers HCMV HLA-A*02:01/NLV, HCMV HLA-B*35:01/IPS, EBV HLA-A*02:01/GLC, EBV HLA-B*08:01/FLR, EBV HLA-B*35:01/YPL, FLU HLA-A*02:01/GIL, VZV HLA-A*02:01/ALW (Protein facility, Department of Immunohematology and Blood Transfusion, LUMC, Leiden, the Netherlands), and an Alexa-647-labeled viral tetramer HCMV pp65 HLA-C*06:02/TRA (NIH Tetramer Core Facility, Emory University, Atlanta, GA) **Table 1**. The HCMV HLA-C*07:02/CRV-specific CD8+ T cell clone was generated by CRV peptide stimulation of PBMC from an HCMV+ HLA-C*07:02+ donor. Additional staining with conjugated mouse anti-human monoclonal antibodies CD56, CD14, CD4, CD19 (FITC; BD Biosciences, San Jose, CA), CD45 (PE-Cy5; eBioscience, San Diego, CA), and CD8 (Pacific Orange; ThermoFisher, Waltham, MA) was performed. When staining with the HCMV pp65 HLA-C*06:02/TRA tetramer, CD158

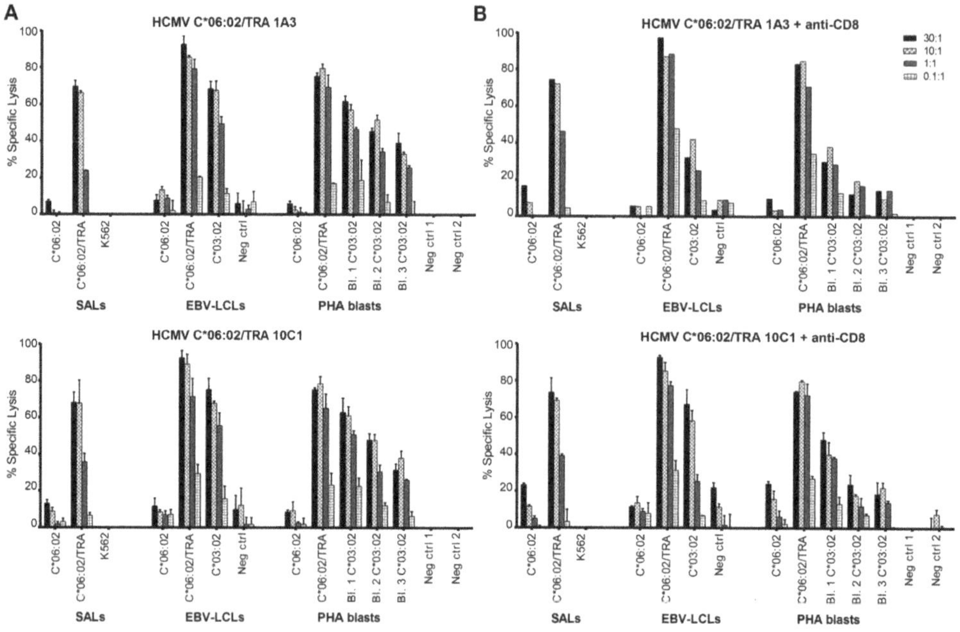

FIGURE 5 | HCMV C*06:02/TRA T cell lines and clones are cytotoxic against HLA-C*03:02. **(A)** Cytotoxicity of two HCMV C*06:02/TRA CD8+ T cell lines (1A3 shown) and one CD8+ T cell clone (10C1) was tested against ^{51}Cr-labeled EBV-LCLs and PHA blasts, obtained from three different donors, expressing the recognized allo-HLA-C*03:02 allele and the virus-specific restriction HLA allele loaded with viral peptide as a positive control. SALs expressing HLA-C*06:02 loaded with viral peptide were also included as a positive control. **(B)** The CD8+ T cell lines and clone were incubated with an anti-CD8 blocking antibody prior to co-culture with target cells and specific lysis was measured. Bars represent triplicate values with standard deviation of the mean.

(KIR2DL1/S1/S3/S5) and CD158b (KIR2DL2/L3) (PE-Cy7; Biolegend, San Diego, CA) were included in the panel to exclude binding of CD8+ T cells to the tetramer through KIR (38). Tetramer-positive CD8+ T cells were purified with FACS sort based on the expression of CD45+CD8+CD19-CD14-CD56-CD4-KIR- tetramer+ cells. CD8+ T cell lines were generated by sorting 10 tetramer-positive cells per round-bottom 96-well and CD8+ T cell clones by sorting 1 tetramer-positive cell per round-bottom 96-well, respectively. After sorting, tetramer-positive CD8+ T cells were expanded in 96-well plates with irradiated PBMC (4,000 Rad) isolated from buffy coats in Iscove's Modified Dulbecco's Medium (IMDM; Lonza, Basel, Switzerland) supplemented with Pen/Strep, L-Glutamine, 5% HS, 5% FCS, PHA (2 μl/ml; Remel, Lenexa, KS), and IL2 (60 IU/ml). TCR Vα and Vβ usage was determined by DNA sequencing using TCR-specific polymerase chain reaction primers (53) followed by use of the BigDye® Terminator V3.1 Cycle Sequencing Kit (Applied Biosystems, Foster City, CA).

4.3. Cytokine Production Assay

After 8 days of expansion with allogeneic irradiated PBMC, CD8+ T cell lines and clones (5 x 10^3) were incubated with EBV-LCLs and PHA blasts (5 x 10^4) expressing either self-HLA, self-HLA loaded with viral peptide (incubation 30 min at 37°C; washed thrice), or allo-HLA molecules (duplicate; 96-wells) in IMDM supplemented with Pen/Strep, L-Glutamine, 5% HS, 5% FCS, and IL-2 (60 IU /ml). PHA blasts were irradiated (5,000 Rad) before co-culture with T cells. After 24 h at 37°C, supernatants were collected and frozen until further use. IFNγ levels were measured in a standard enzyme-linked immunosorbent assay (ELISA), according to manufacturer's protocol (U-Cytech, Utrecht, the Netherlands). The range of the ELISA standard curve was 5–5120 pg/ml.

4.4. Cytotoxicity Assays

After 8 days of expansion with allogeneic irradiated PBMC, serial dilutions of responder CD8+ T cell lines and clones were incubated with ^{51}Chromium-labeled EBV-LCLs, SALs and/or 721.221 target cells, PHA blasts and HUVECs (responder/stimulator ratio 30:1; 10:1; 1:1; 0.1:1) in round-bottom 96-wells plates for 4 or 20 h at 37°C in IMDM supplemented with Pen/Strep, L-Glutamine, 5% HS, 5% FCS, and IL-2 (60 IU/ml). Where applicable, viral peptide was loaded onto the target cells for 60 min at 37°C, simultaneously with chromium incubation, and washed thrice. In addition, CD8+ T cell lines and clones were incubated with the anti-CD8 blocking antibody FK18 (4.3 μl/ml) for 60 min at 37°C, where after cells were washed twice. Supernatants were harvested for analysis on a gamma-counter (PerkinElmer 2470 Wizard2, Waltham, MA), counts from triplicate wells were averaged, and specific lysis was calculated as follows: (Condition of interest ^{51}Cr release − Spontaneous ^{51}Cr release)/(Maximum ^{51}Cr release

– Spontaneous ^{51}Cr release) x 100. Maximum ^{51}Cr release of the target cells was determined in PBS 1% Triton X-100 and spontaneous ^{51}Cr release in medium.

ETHICS STATEMENT

This study was carried out in accordance with the guidelines issued by the Medical Ethics Committee of the Leiden University Medical Center. All subjects gave written informed consent in accordance with the Declaration of Helsinki.

AUTHOR CONTRIBUTIONS

AvdZ, EvdM-P, FC, and SH designed the research and wrote the manuscript. AvdZ, EvdM-P and PvM performed the experiments. HvdH and EvdM-P generated the HLA-A and -B-restricted virus-specific T cell lines and clones. JA performed TCR sequencing analyses and DR provided extensive HLA typing.

FUNDING

This work was supported by the National Reference Center for Histocompatibility testing, the Netherlands.

ACKNOWLEDGMENTS

We thank professor Paul Moss and Louise Hosie from the University of Birmingham for providing us with the HCMV HLA-C*07:02/CRV CD8+ T cell clone, Professor Anthony Purcell from Monash University for providing us with the 721.221 cell line expressing HLA-C*07:02, the NIH tetramer core facility (Emory University) for providing the HCMV HLA-C*06:02/TRA tetramer, Jan-Wouter Drijfhout and Kees Franken for providing tetramers and giving technical advice, the LUMC HLA typing laboratory for performing HLA typing, professor Frits Koning for critical review of the manuscript and Tamara Tilburgs for helpful discussions on the topic.

REFERENCES

1. Benninger-Döring G, Pepperl S, Deml L, Modrow S, Wolf H, Jilg W. Frequency of CD8+ T lymphocytes specific for lytic and latent antigens of Epstein–Barr virus in healthy virus carriers. *Virology* (1999) 264:289–97. doi: 10.1006/viro.1999.9996
2. Asanuma H, Sharp M, Maecker HT, Maino VC, Arvin AM. Frequencies of memory T cells specific for varicella-zoster virus, herpes simplex virus, and cytomegalovirus by intracellular detection of cytokine expression. *J Infect Dis.* (2000) 181:859–66. doi: 10.1086/315347
3. Boon A, Fringuelli E, Graus Y, Fouchier R, Sintnicolaas K, Iorio A, et al. Influenza A virus specific T cell immunity in humans during aging. *Virology* (2002) 299:100–8. doi: 10.1006/viro.2002.1491
4. León-Juárez M, Martínez-Castillo M, González-García LD, Helguera-Repetto AC, Zaga-Clavellina V, García-Cordero J, et al. Cellular and molecular mechanisms of viral infection in the human placenta. *Pathog Dis.* (2017) 75:ftx093. doi: 10.1093/femspd/ftx093
5. Racicot K, Mor G. Risks associated with viral infections during pregnancy. *J Clin Invest.* (2017) 127:1591–9. doi: 10.1172/JCI87490
6. Fishman J. Infection in organ transplantation. *Am J Transplant.* (2017) 17:856–79. doi: 10.1111/ajt.14208
7. Lin R, Liu Q. Diagnosis and treatment of viral diseases in recipients of allogeneic hematopoietic stem cell transplantation. *J Hematol Oncol.* (2013) 6:94. doi: 10.1186/1756-8722-6-94
8. Gaston J, Rickinson A, Epstein M. Cross-reactivity of self-HLA-restricted Epstein-Barr virus-specific cytotoxic T lymphocytes for allo-HLA determinants. *J Exp Med.* (1983) 158:1804–21. doi: 10.1084/jem.158.6.1804
9. Amir AL, D'Orsogna LJ, Roelen DL, van Loenen MM, Hagedoorn RS, de Boer R, et al. Allo-HLA reactivity of virus-specific memory T-cells is common. *Blood* (2010) 115:3146–57. doi: 10.1182/blood-2009-07-234906
10. van den Heuvel H, Heutinck KM, van der Meer-Prins EM, Franke-van Dijk ME, van Miert PP, Zhang X, et al. The avidity of cross-reactive virus-specific T cells for their viral and allogeneic epitopes is variable and depends on epitope expression. *Hum Immunol.* (2018) 79:39–50. doi: 10.1016/j.humimm.2017.10.019
11. Felix NJ, Donermeyer DL, Horvath S, Walters JJ, Gross ML, Suri A, et al. Alloreactive T cells respond specifically to multiple distinct peptide-MHC complexes. *Nat. Immunol.* (2007) 8:388. doi: 10.1038/ni1446
12. Brook MO, Wood KJ, Jones ND. The impact of memory T cells on rejection and the induction of tolerance. *Transplantation* (2006) 82:1–9. doi: 10.1097/01.tp.0000226082.17507.da
13. D'Orsogna LJ, Roelen DL, Doxiadis II, Claas FH. Alloreactivity from human viral specific memory T-cells. *Transplant Immunol.* (2010) 23:149–55. doi: 10.1016/j.trim.2010.06.008
14. Byrne J, Butler J, Cooper M. Differential activation requirements for virgin and memory T cells. *J Immunol.* (1988) 141:3249–57.
15. Flynn K, Müllbacher A. Memory alloreactive cytotoxic T cells do not require costimulation for activation *in vitro*. *Immunol Cell Biol.* (1996) 74:413–20. doi: 10.1038/icb.1996.71
16. Mason D. A very high level of crossreactivity is an essential feature of the T-cell receptor. *Immunol Today* (1998) 19:395–404. doi: 10.1016/S0167-5699(98)01299-7
17. Apps R, Murphy SP, Fernando R, Gardner L, Ahad T, Moffett A. Human leucocyte antigen (HLA) expression of primary trophoblast cells and placental cell lines, determined using single antigen beads to characterize allotype specificities of anti-HLA antibodies. *Immunology* (2009) 127:26–39. doi: 10.1111/j.1365-2567.2008.03019.x
18. Hammer A, Hutter H, Dohr G. HLA class I expression on the materno-fetal interface. *Am J Reprod Immunol.* (1997) 38:150–7. doi: 10.1111/j.1600-0897.1997.tb00291.x
19. van der Zwan A, Bi K, Norwitz ER, Crespo ÂC, Claas FH, Strominger JL, et al. Mixed signature of activation and dysfunction allows human decidual CD8+ T cells to provide both tolerance and immunity. *Proc Natl Acad Sci USA.* (2018) 115:385–90. doi: 10.1073/pnas.1713957115
20. Van Egmond A, Van Der Keur C, Swings G, Scherjon S, Claas F. The possible role of virus-specific CD8+ memory T cells in decidual tissue. *J Reprod Immunol.* (2016) 113:1–8. doi: 10.1016/j.jri.2015.09.073
21. van Kampen CA, Versteeg-van der Voort MF, Langerak-Langerak J, van Beelen E, Roelen DL, Claas FH, et al. Pregnancy can induce long-persisting primed CTLs specific for inherited paternal HLA antigens. *Hum Immunol.* (2001) 62:201–7. doi: 10.1016/S0198-8859(01)00209-9
22. Verdijk RM, Kloosterman A, Pool J, van de Keur M, Naipal AM, van Halteren AG, et al. Pregnancy induces minor histocompatibility antigen-specific cytotoxic T cells: implications for stem cell transplantation and immunotherapy. *Blood* (2004) 103:1961–4. doi: 10.1182/blood-2003-05-1625
23. Lissauer D, Piper K, Goodyear O, Kilby MD, Moss PA. Fetal-specific CD8+ cytotoxic T cell responses develop during normal human pregnancy and exhibit broad functional capacity. *J Immunol.* (2012) 189:1072–80. doi: 10.4049/jimmunol.1200544
24. Meuleman T, van Beelen E, Kaaja R, van Lith J, Claas F, Bloemenkamp K. HLA-C antibodies in women with recurrent miscarriage suggests that antibody mediated rejection is one of the mechanisms leading to recurrent miscarriage. *J Reprod Immunol.* (2016) 116:28–34. doi: 10.1016/j.jri.2016.03.003

25. Meuleman T, Haasnoot GW, van Lith JM, Verduijn W, Bloemenkamp KW, Claas FH. Paternal HLA-C is a risk factor in unexplained recurrent miscarriage. *Am J Reprod Immunol.* (2018) 79:e12797. doi: 10.1111/aji.12797
26. Colucci F. The role of KIR and HLA interactions in pregnancy complications. *Immunogenetics* (2017) 69:557–65. doi: 10.1007/s00251-017-1003-9
27. Kaur G, Gras S, Mobbs JI, Vivian JP, Cortes A, Barber T, et al. Structural and regulatory diversity shape HLA-C protein expression levels. *Nat Commun.* (2017) 8:15924. doi: 10.1038/ncomms15924
28. Van den Heuvel H, Heutinck K, van der Meer-prins E, Yong S, van Miert P, Anholts J, et al. Allo-HLA cross-reactivities of cytomegalovirus-, influenza-, and varicella zoster virus-specific memory T cells are shared by different healthy individuals. *Am J Transplant.* (2017) 17:2033–44. doi: 10.1111/ajt.14279
29. D'orsogna L, Amir AL, Zoet YM, Van Der Meer-Prins P, Van Der Slik AR, Kester MG, et al. New tools to monitor the impact of viral infection on the alloreactive T-cell repertoire. *Tissue Antigens* (2009) 74:290–7. doi: 10.1111/j.1399-0039.2009.01311.x
30. Zoet YM, Eijsink C, Kardol MJ, Franke-van Dijk ME, Wilson GL, de Paus R, et al. The single antigen expressing lines (SALs) concept: an excellent tool for screening for HLA-specific antibodies. *Hum Immunol.* (2005) 66:519–25. doi: 10.1016/j.humimm.2005.01.007
31. Burrows S, Silins S, Moss D, Khanna R, Misko I, Argaet V. T cell receptor repertoire for a viral epitope in humans is diversified by tolerance to a background major histocompatibility complex antigen. *J Exp Med.* (1995) 182:1703–15. doi: 10.1084/jem.182.6.1703
32. van der Woude FJ, Daha MR, Andr'e M, Meyer-Paape ME, Bruyn JA, van Bockel HJ, et al. Renal allograft-infiltrated lymphocytes and proximal tubular cells: further analysis of donor specific lysis. *Hum Immunol.* (1990) 28:186–92. doi: 10.1016/0198-8859(90)90018-K
33. D'orsogna LJ, Roelen DL, van der Meer-Prins EM, van der Pol P, Franke-van Dijk ME, Eikmans M, et al. Tissue specificity of cross-reactive allogeneic responses by EBV EBNA3A-specific memory T cells. *Transplantation* (2011) 91:494–500. doi: 10.1097/TP.0b013e318207944c
34. Honeyborne I, Codoñer FM, Leslie A, Tudor-Williams G, Luzzi G, Ndung'u T, et al. HLA-Cw* 03-restricted CD8+ T-cell responses targeting the HIV-1 gag major homology region drive virus immune escape and fitness constraints compensated for by intracodon variation. *J Virol.* (2010) 84:11279–88. doi: 10.1128/JVI.01144-10
35. Hosie L, Pachnio A, Zuo J, Pearce H, Riddell S, Moss P. Cytomegalovirus-Specific T Cells Restricted by HLA-Cw* 0702 Increase Markedly with Age and Dominate the CD8+ T-Cell Repertoire in Older People. *Front Immunol.* (2017) 8:1776. doi: 10.3389/fimmu.2017.01776
36. Ameres S, Mautner J, Schlott F, Neuenhahn M, Busch DH, Plachter B, et al. Presentation of an immunodominant immediate-early CD8+ T cell epitope resists human cytomegalovirus immunoevasion. *PLoS Pathog.* (2013) 9:e1003383. doi: 10.1371/journal.ppat.1003383
37. Mack SJ, Tu B, Lazaro A, Yang R, Lancaster AK, Cao K, et al. HLA-A,-B,-C, and-DRB1 allele and haplotype frequencies distinguish Eastern European Americans from the general European American population. *Tissue Antigens* (2009) 73:17–32. doi: 10.1111/j.1399-0039.2008.01151.x
38. Schlott F, Steubl D, Ameres S, Moosmann A, Dreher S, Heemann U, et al. Characterization and clinical enrichment of HLA-C* 07: 02-restricted Cytomegalovirus-specific CD8+ T cells. *PLoS ONE* (2018) 13:e0193554. doi: 10.1371/journal.pone.0193554
39. Crough T, Beagley L, Smith C, Jones L, Walker DG, Khanna R. *Ex vivo* functional analysis, expansion and adoptive transfer of cytomegalovirus-specific T-cells in patients with glioblastoma multiforme. *Immunol Cell Biol.* (2012) 90:872–80. doi: 10.1038/icb.2012.19
40. Attanasio J, Wherry EJ. Costimulatory and coinhibitory receptor pathways in infectious disease. *Immunity* (2016) 44:1052–68. doi: 10.1016/j.immuni.2016.04.022
41. Kulkarni S, Savan R, Qi Y, Gao X, Yuki Y, Bass SE, et al. Differential microRNA regulation of HLA-C expression and its association with HIV control. *Nature* (2011) 472:495. doi: 10.1038/nature09914
42. Apps R, Qi Y, Carlson JM, Chen H, Gao X, Thomas R, et al. Influence of HLA-C expression level on HIV control. *Science* (2013) 340:87–91. doi: 10.1126/science.1232685
43. Hyun SJ, Sohn HJ, Lee HJ, Lee SD, Kim S, Sohn DH, et al. Comprehensive analysis of cytomegalovirus pp65 antigen-specific CD8+ T cell responses according to human leukocyte antigen class I allotypes and intraindividual dominance. *Front Immunol.* (2017) 8:1591. doi: 10.3389/fimmu.2017.01591
44. McCutcheon JA, Gumperz J, Smith KD, Lutz CT, Parham P. Low HLA-C expression at cell surfaces correlates with increased turnover of heavy chain mRNA. *J Exp Med.* (1995) 181:2085–95. doi: 10.1084/jem.181.6.2085
45. Keib A, Günther PS, Faist B, Halenius A, Busch DH, Neuenhahn M, et al. Presentation of a conserved adenoviral epitope on HLA-C* 0702 allows evasion of natural killer but not T cell responses. *Viral Immunol.* (2017) 30:149–56. doi: 10.1089/vim.2016.0145
46. Terauchi M, Koi H, Hayano C, Toyama-Sorimachi N, Karasuyama H, Yamanashi Y, et al. Placental extravillous cytotrophoblasts persistently express class I major histocompatibility complex molecules after human cytomegalovirus infection. *J Virol.* (2003) 77:8187–95. doi: 10.1128/JVI.77.15.8187-8195.2003
47. Tersigni C, Redman C, Dragovic R, Tannetta D, Scambia G, Di Simone N, et al. HLA-DR is aberrantly expressed at feto-maternal interface in pre-eclampsia. *J Reprod Immunol.* (2018) 129:48–52. doi: 10.1016/j.jri.2018.06.024
48. Petersdorf EW, Longton GM, Anasetti C, Mickelson EM, McKinney SK, Smith AG, et al. Association of HLA-C disparity with graft failure after marrow transplantation from unrelated donors. *Blood* (1997) 89:1818–23.
49. Frohn C, Fricke L, Puchta JC, Kirchner H. The effect of HLA-C matching on acute renal transplant rejection. *Nephrol Dial Transplant.* (2001) 16:355–60. doi: 10.1093/ndt/16.2.355
50. Morishima Y, Kashiwase K, Matsuo K, Azuma F, Morishima S, Onizuka M, et al. Biological significance of HLA locus matching in unrelated donor bone marrow transplantation. *Blood* (2014) 125:1189–97. doi: 10.1182/blood-2014-10-604785
51. Ingulli E. Mechanism of cellular rejection in transplantation. *Pediatr Nephrol.* (2010) 25:61. doi: 10.1007/s00467-008-1020-x
52. D'Orsogna LJ, van der Meer-Prins EM, Zoet YM, Roelen DL, Doxiadis II, Claas FH. Detection of allo-HLA cross-reactivity by virus-specific memory T-cell clones using single HLA-transfected K562 cells. In: Christiansen F, Tait B. Editors. *Immunogenetics. Methods in Molecular Biology (Methods and Protocols), vol 882.* Totowa, NJ: Humana Press (2012). p. 339–49.
53. Wei S, Charmley P, Robinson MA, Concannon P. The extent of the human germline T-cell receptor V beta gene segment repertoire. *Immunogenetics* (1994) 40:27–36. doi: 10.1007/BF00163961

13

Clonally Expanded Decidual Effector Regulatory T Cells Increase in Late Gestation of Normal Pregnancy, but Not in Preeclampsia, in Humans

Sayaka Tsuda[1], Xiaoxin Zhang[1], Hiroshi Hamana[2], Tomoko Shima[1], Akemi Ushijima[1], Kei Tsuda[1], Atsushi Muraguchi[3], Hiroyuki Kishi[3] and Shigeru Saito[1*]*

[1] Department of Obstetrics and Gynecology, University of Toyama, Toyama, Japan, [2] Department of Innovative Cancer Immunotherapy, Graduate School of Medicine and Pharmaceutical Sciences (Medicine), University of Toyama, Toyama, Japan, [3] Department of Immunology, Graduate School of Medicine and Pharmaceutical Sciences (Medicine), University of Toyama, Toyama, Japan

***Correspondence:**
Hiroyuki Kishi
immkishi@med.u-toyama.ac.jp
Shigeru Saito
s30saito@med.u-toyama.ac.jp

Background: Regulatory T (Treg) cells are necessary for the maintenance of allogenic pregnancy. However, the repertoire of effector Treg cells at the feto-maternal interface in human pregnancy remains unknown. Our objective was to study T cell receptor (TCR) repertoires of Treg cells during pregnancy compared to normal and complicated pregnancies.

Methods: Paired samples of peripheral blood and decidua in induced abortion and miscarriage cases were obtained from consenting patients. $CD4^+CD25^+CD127^{low/-}CD45RA^-$ effector Treg cells were single-cell sorted from mononuclear cells. cDNAs of complementarity determining region 3 (CDR3) in TCRβ were amplified from the single cells by RT-PCR and the sequences were analyzed. The TCRβ repertoires were determined by amino acid and nucleotide sequences. Treg cells were classified into clonally expanded and non-expanded populations by CDR3 sequences.

Results: We enrolled nine induced abortion cases in the 1st trimester, 12 cases delivered without complications in the 3rd trimester, 11 miscarriages with abnormal chromosomal karyotyped embryo, seven miscarriages with normal chromosomal karyotyped embryo, and seven cases of preeclampsia [median gestational week (interquartile range): 7 (7–9), 39 (38–40), 9 (8–10), 8 (8–10), and 34 (32–37), respectively]. The frequency of clonally expanded populations of effector Treg cells increased in decidua of 3rd trimester cases compared to 1st trimester cases [4.5% (1.4–10.8%) vs. 20.9% (15.4–28.1%), $p < 0.001$]. Clonally expanded Treg cells were rarely seen in peripheral blood. The ratio of clonally expanded populations of decidual effector Treg cells in miscarriages with abnormal and normal embryos was not significantly different compared with that in 1st trimester normal pregnancy. Interestingly, clonally expanded populations of effector Treg cells decreased in preeclampsia compared with that in 3rd trimester normal pregnancy [9.3% (4.4–14.5%) vs. 20.9% (15.4–28.1%), $p = 0.003$]. When repertoires in previous pregnancy and subsequent pregnancy were compared, some portions of the repertoire were shared.

Conclusion: TCR repertoires of decidual effector Treg cells are skewed in the 3rd trimester of normal pregnancy. Failure of clonal expansion of populations of decidual effector Treg cells might be related to the development of preeclampsia.

Keywords: effector regulatory T cell, human pregnancy, miscarriage, preeclampsia, regulatory T cell, T cell repertoire

INTRODUCTION

Regulatory T (Treg) cells are important in maintaining feto-maternal tolerance during pregnancy in humans and mice (1–6). Previous studies demonstrated the existence of fetal antigen specific Treg cells in a murine model of pregnancy (7–9). Rowe et al. (9) demonstrated that memory type-fetal antigen specific Treg cells induced fetal antigen specific tolerance in second pregnancy in mice. These results may explain why first pregnancy is a risk factor for preeclampsia. We have reported that fetal antigen specific Treg cells are recruited to uterine draining lymph nodes just before implantation in mice (10). Tilburgs et al. (11) suggested that human decidual Treg cells recognize self-fetal antigens by mixed lymphocyte reaction against umbilical cord blood. A suppressive reaction by decidual Treg cells, but not by systemic Treg cells, has been described (11). These findings suggest that fetal antigen specific memory type Treg cells induce feto-maternal tolerance at the feto-maternal interface in both mice and humans, although fetal antigen specific Treg cells have not yet been identified as a T cell receptor (TCR) repertoire in humans.

Human $CD4^+FoxP3^+$ cells contain a $CD4^+CD45RA^-FoxP3^{high}$ effector/activated Treg cell subset, $CD4^+CD45RA^+FoxP3^{low}$ naïve/resting Treg cell subset, and $CD45^+CD45RA^-FoxP3^{low}$ effector T cell subset (12, 13). $CD4^+CD45RA^-FoxP3^{high}$ effector Treg cells have the highest suppressive capability among these subsets. During human late gestation, $CD4^+CD45RA^-FoxP3^{high}$ effector Treg cells are the dominant Treg cell subset in peripheral blood and decidua (14). We have shown that $CD4^+CD45RA^-FoxP3^{high}$ effector Treg cells are significantly decreased in decidua of cases of miscarriage with normal chromosomal karyotyped embryo (15). Thus, the effector Treg cell subset might contain fetal antigen specific populations in human.

Previous reports suggested that systemic and local maldistribution and dysfunction of Treg cells could be one of the etiologies of miscarriage and preeclampsia (16–21). T cell receptor β variable (TRBV) repertoires of total Treg cells in peripheral blood and decidua were not significantly different between preeclampsia and normal pregnancy (22). Thus, how Treg cells relate to the development of preeclampsia remains unknown.

We hypothesized that decidual effector Treg cells that recognize fetal antigens are clonally expanded at the feto-maternal interface. To study the clonality of effector Treg cells, we used a single-cell based TCR repertoire analysis method that we previously described (23, 24). We also aimed to show whether altered TCR repertoires of effector Treg cells are present in miscarriage or preeclampsia.

MATERIALS AND METHODS

Subjects

The enrolled cases included nine cases of artificial abortion in the 1st trimester, 11 cases of 1st trimester miscarriage with abnormal embryo karyotype, seven cases of 1st trimester miscarriage with normal embryo karyotype, 12 cases delivered without pregnancy complications in the 3rd trimester, and seven cases delivered in the 3rd trimester with preeclampsia. Written informed consent was obtained from all the patients in accordance with a protocol approved by the Ethical Review Board of University of Toyama. Fetal heartbeat was confirmed before artificial abortion (induced abortion in the 1st trimester of normal pregnancy). Miscarriage was diagnosed when the fetal heart beat was lost, or when the fetal heartbeat was not detected inside the gestational sac for more than 2 weeks. All artificial abortion and miscarriage treatments were performed by dilation and curettage. Fetal chromosomal karyotype was determined by G-band staining in miscarriage cases. Preeclampsia was diagnosed when blood pressure exceeded 140/90 mmHg and urinary protein exceeded 0.3 g per day after the 20th week of gestation (25). Ten milliliters of venous blood and decidual sample were obtained simultaneously when induced abortion was performed or when subjects delivered a baby. The patients were recruited at Toyama University Hospital, Otogi no Mori Lady's Clinic and Yoshie Ladies Clinic.

Mononuclear Cell Isolation

Peripheral blood mononuclear cells (PBMC) were isolated by Ficoll Hypaque (Lymphoprep™; Alere Technologies, Norway) density gradient centrifugation. First trimester decidua was isolated from uterine content that was collected by induced abortion. Third trimester decidua was dissected from maternal surface of the delivered placenta. Decidua was rinsed with phosphate buffered saline (PBS) until the blood was removed, minced with a pair of scissors to produce 1–2 mm pieces, and filtered through 32-μm nylon mesh. All samples were cryopreserved.

Single-Cell Sorting

To sort the effector Treg cells, the following monoclonal antibodies were used: anti-CD3 (APC; BD Bioscience, USA), anti-CD4 (PerCP cy5.5; BD Bioscience), anti-CD45RA (APC cy7; BioLegend, USA), anti-CD25 (PE cy7; BioLegend), and anti-CD127 (PE; BD Bioscience). PBMC and decidual mononuclear cells were stained by these antibodies for 20 min on ice. After staining, the cells were washed with PBS and analyzed using a FACSAria II flow cytometer (BD Biosciences). $CD3^{+}CD4^{+}CD45RA^{-}CD25^{+}CD127^{low/-}$ effector Treg cells were single-cell sorted into wells of a 96-well PCR plate. The gating strategy used to sort the effector Treg cells is presented in **Figure 1**.

TCR Repertoire Analysis of Effector Treg Cells by Single-Cell RT-PCR and Sequencing

TCRs and FoxP3 cDNAs were amplified from single cells using one-step multiplex RT-PCR as described previously (24). All PCR primers are listed in **Supplementary Table 1**. Contents of the PCR reaction mixture are listed in **Supplementary Table 2**. Five microliters of the RT-PCR mixture was added to each well containing a single effector Treg cell. One-step RT-PCR was performed with the following program: 40 min at 45°C for the RT reaction, 98°C for 1 min and 30 cycles of 98°C for 10 s, 52°C for 5 s, and 72°C for 1 min. The products were diluted 10-fold and 2 μL of each was added to 18 μL of the second PCR mixture. In the second cycle, TCRβ and FoxP3 cDNAs were amplified. The program for the second PCR was as follows: 98°C for 1 min and 35 cycles of 98°C for 10 s, 52°C for 5 s, and 72°C for 30 s. The second PCR products were used for direct sequencing to determine CDR3 of TCRβ. The TCR repertoire was analyzed with the IMGT/VQuest tool (http://www.imgt.org/). We classified effector Treg cells with identical CDR3 as the clonal population and those with unique CDR3 as the non-clonal population. To compare the clonality of the effector Treg cells, frequencies of clonal populations among the analyzed TCRs were calculated. For the assessment of TCR repertoire distribution, we calculated the Gini-coefficient as previously described (26). This coefficient was originally used in economic studies to describe income distribution. However, it is also useful to describe TCR repertoire distribution (26, 27). The Gini coefficient (G) is calculated as:

$$G = \sum_{i=1}^{n} (2i - n - 1)\, xi/n \sum_{i=1}^{n} xi$$

where "xi" indicates the abundance of the ith sequence and "n" indicates the total number of TCR sequences. The score ranges from 0 to 1; $G = 1$ means that all the TCR clones are the same. When the variation of TCR repertoire is large, G approaches 0. The raw data supporting the conclusions of this manuscript, except the private information of the subjects, will be made available by the authors, without undue reservation, to any qualified researchers.

Statistical Analyses

Statistical analyses were performed with the JMP Pro 13.0.0 statistical analysis program (SAS Institute Inc., USA) and SPSS version 23 software (IBM, USA). The statistical tests used to determine statistical significance are indicated in the respective figure legends. Continuous variables are presented as median values with interquartile range, unless otherwise specified. A two-tailed $p < 0.05$ was considered significant.

RESULTS

Clinical Characteristics

Clinical characteristics of the subjects are shown in **Table 1**. Maternal ages of 1st trimester miscarriage and 3rd trimester normal pregnancy were higher than that of 1st trimester normal pregnancy. The frequency of cesarean section showed no significant difference between 3rd trimester normal pregnancy and preeclampsia.

TCR Repertoire Analysis of Effector Treg Cells in Normal Pregnancy

TCRβ and FoxP3 cDNAs were amplified from single cells and electrophoresed in agarose gel (**Figure 2A**). The number of analyzed TCRβ sequences of decidual effector Treg cells in 1st trimester normal pregnancy, 3rd trimester normal pregnancy, 1st trimester miscarriage with abnormal or normal embryo, and 3rd trimester pregnancy with preeclampsia for each subject was 49 (35.5–60), 46 (32.3–77.3), 36 (29–56), 43 (27–53), and 42 (31–45), respectively. The number of analyzed TCRβ sequences of effector Treg cells in PBMC in 1st trimester and 3rd trimester normal pregnancies was 70 (61.5–73.5) and 52 (43.5–60.8), respectively. Representative TCRβ repertoires in 1st trimester and 3rd trimester normal pregnancies are shown in **Figure 2B**. In the 3rd trimester, decidual effector Treg cells were clonally expanded and TCR repertoires were skewed (**Figure 2B**).

In normal pregnancy, the ratio of clonal populations of decidual effector Treg cells in the 3rd trimester was increased compared with the 1st trimester [4.5% (1.4–10.8%) vs. 20.9% (15.4–28.1%), $p < 0.001$]. In peripheral blood, the ratio for clonal populations of effector Treg cells was significantly smaller than that in paired decidual samples [0.0% (0.0–3.0%) vs. 4.5% (1.4–10.8%), $p = 0.039$ in the 1st trimester, 0.0% (0.0–3.3%) vs. 20.9% (15.4–28.1%), $p < 0.001$ in the 3rd trimester] and was not increased even in the 3rd trimester [0.0% (0.0–3.0%) vs. 0.0% (0.0–3.3%), $p = 0.935$; **Figure 3A**]. The Gini coefficient of the decidual TCRβ repertoire of effector Treg cells was higher in the 3rd trimester than in the 1st trimester [0.04 (0.02–0.09) vs. 0.22 (0.17–0.36), $p < 0.001$]. The Gini coefficient of the TCRβ repertoire of effector Treg cells in PBMC was lower than that in paired decidual samples in the 1st and 3rd trimesters [0.00 (0.00–0.03) vs. 0.04 (0.02–0.09), $p = 0.046$ in the 1st trimester, 0.00 (0.00–0.04) vs. 0.22 (0.17–0.36), $p < 0.001$ in the 3rd trimester; **Figure 3B**].

Frequencies of effector Treg cells among total Treg cells of 1st trimester decidua were significantly higher than that of peripheral blood [93.0% (82.4–94.6%) vs. 74.6% (58.0–91.4%), $p = 0.032$]. In the 3rd trimester, the p-value did not reach a significant level [87.0% (82.4–91.7%) vs. 79.6% (58.7–87.6%), $p = 0.094$; **Figure 3C**].

Next, we compared the TCR repertoires of peripheral blood and decidual effector Treg cells in each case. Common clonotype of effector Treg cells between PBMC and decidua appeared only

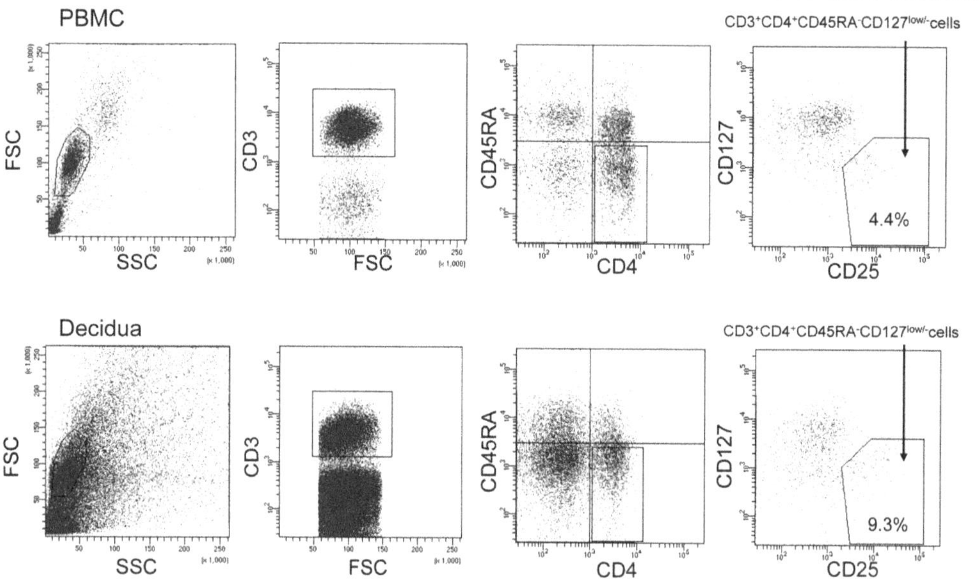

FIGURE 1 | Gating strategy to obtain CD4$^+$CD45RA$^-$CD25$^+$CD127$^{low/-}$ effector Treg cells. Lymphocyte in the peripheral blood (upper column) and decidua (lower column) were gated on forward and side scatter parameters. CD3$^+$CD4$^+$ T cells were classified into CD45RA$^+$ naïve T cells and CD45RA$^-$ effector T cells. Among CD45RA$^-$ effector T cells, CD25$^+$CD127$^{low/-}$ effector Treg cells were single-cell sorted.

TABLE 1 | Demographic and clinical characteristics.

	1st trimester normal pregnancy	3rd trimester normal pregnancy	1st trimester miscarriage with abnormal embryo	1st trimester miscarriage with normal embryo	3rd trimester preeclampsia
	(n = 9)	**(n = 12)**	**(n = 11)**	**(n = 7)**	**(n = 7)**
Maternal age (years), median (IQR)	28 (24–31)	36 (33–38)†	39 (38–41)†	38 (32–40)†	38 (31–41)
Gravidities, median (IQR)	3 (1–4)	5 (2–5)	3 (2–4)	3 (2–4)	2 (1–4)
No. of liveborn children, median (IQR)	0 (0–2)	0 (0–1)	0 (0–0)	0 (0–1)	0 (0–1)
No. of miscarriages, median (IQR)	0 (0–2)	2 (0–3)	1 (0–2)	1 (1–3)	(0–2)
Past history of stillbirth, n (%)	0 (0.0)	3 (25.0)	1 (9.1)	1 (14.3)	0 (0.0)
Nullipara, n (%)	5 (55.5)	5 (41.7)	8 (72.7)	3 (42.9)	4 (57.1)
Gestational weeks, median (IQR)	7 (7–9)	39 (38–40)	9 (8–10)	8 (8 10)	34 (32–37)
Cesarean section, n (%)		4 (33.3)			5 (71.4)

IQR, interquartile range. Steel–Dwass test for continuous variables and Fisher's exact test for categorical variables. †$p < 0.05$ vs. 1st trimester normal pregnancy.

in case #4 (two clones among 128 clones; 56 from decidua and 72 from PBMC) and case #16 (two clones among 82 clones; 40 from decidua and 42 from PBMC). The findings suggested marked differences in the characteristics of Treg cells between peripheral blood and decidua (**Figure 4**).

TCR Repertoire of Decidual Effector Treg Cells Between Previous and Subsequent Pregnancy

When repertoires of effector Treg cells were compared between past and subsequent pregnancies of the same subjects, sharing of some part of the repertoire of decidual effector Treg cells was evident. In case A, the TCR repertoires of cases #10 and #20, a pair of previous and subsequent 3rd trimester normal vaginal deliveries, shared three clones among 149 clones (**Figure 5A**; shared clones are underlined). In case B, the TCR repertoires of cases #13 and #17 revealed four shared clones among 129 clones (**Figure 5B**; underlined). In case C, case #25 was a previous pregnancy and resulted in miscarriage with normal embryo and case #47 was a subsequent pregnancy of the same subject and resulted in miscarriage with abnormal embryo. This pair shared one clone among 84 clones (**Figure 5C**; underlined). None of the TCR repertoires of effector Treg cells in PBMC were shared between previous and subsequent pregnancies (data not shown). Among the subjects who experienced pregnancies several times during the study period, no subject had their pregnancies ending up in preeclampsia.

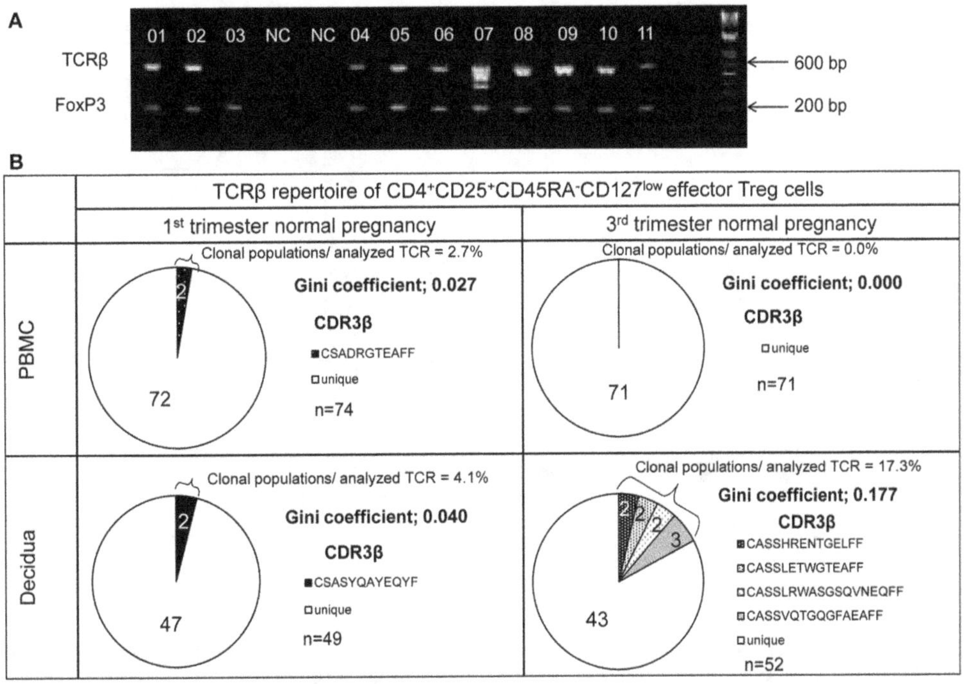

FIGURE 2 | TCRβ repertoire analysis of $CD4^+CD45RA^-CD25^+CD127^{low/-}$ effector Treg cells. **(A)** TCRβ and FoxP3 cDNAs amplified by multiplex one-step RT-PCR were resolved by agarose gel electrophoresis. Each single cell was numbered. NC denotes the cell-free negative control. FoxP3 and TCRβ mRNAs were expressed in 11/11 and 10/11, respectively. **(B)** Representative data of the TCRβ repertoire of $CD4^+CD45RA^-CD25^+CD127^{low/-}$ effector Treg cells in PBMC and decidua. The TCR repertoires were determined by amino acid and nucleotide sequences of complementarity determining region 3 (CDR3) of TCRβ chain. Each pie chart slice (shaded or closed) indicates clonal T cell population with the same clonotypic TCRβ. An open pie chart slice indicates T cells with unique TCRβ. Frequency of clonal populations among analyzed TCRβ and the Gini coefficients of the TCRβ repertoire were calculated.

TCR Repertoire of Decidual Effector Treg Cells of Normal Pregnancy and Miscarriage

In 1st trimester decidua, the frequencies of clonal populations of effector Treg cells and the Gini coefficients of TCR repertoires of miscarriage with abnormal embryo showed no significant differences between normal pregnancy, miscarriage with abnormal embryo, and miscarriage with normal embryo (**Figures 6A,B**). Proportions of $CD4^+CD45RA^-CD25^+CD127^{low/-}$ effector Treg cells among $CD4^+CD25^+CD127^{low/-}$ total Treg cells in decidua were significantly lower in miscarriage with normal embryo than normal pregnancy [80.0% (65.0–83.3%) vs. 90.6% (82.3–94.6%), $p = 0.049$; **Figure 6C**].

TCR Repertoire of Decidual Effector Treg Cells of Normal Pregnancy and Preeclampsia in 3rd Trimester

In 3rd trimester decidua, frequencies of clonal populations of effector Treg cells (**Figure 7A**) and Gini coefficients of TCR repertoires (**Figure 7B**) were significantly lower in preeclampsia than normal pregnancy [9.3% (4.4–14.5%) vs. 20.9% (15.4–28.1%), $p = 0.003$ and 0.09 (0.04–0.17) vs. 0.22 (0.17–0.36), $p = 0.005$, respectively]. The proportions of $CD4^+CD45RA^-CD25+CD127^{low/-}$ decidual effector Treg cells among $CD4^+CD25+CD127^{low/-}$ decidual total Treg cells did not differ significantly between the two groups [85.8% (71.1–88.4%) vs. 87.0% (82.4–91.7%), $p = 0.331$] (**Figure 7C**).

DISCUSSION

This study is the first report of the increase of clonally expanded decidual effector Treg cells in late gestation of normal pregnancy. In contrast, the repertoire of effector Treg cells of PBMC was not skewed in the 3rd trimester. A previous study showed that TRBV repertoires of total Treg cells differ in PBMC and decidua in the 3rd trimester (22). Our data support this finding. Neller et al. used 25 TRBV monoclonal antibodies in a TCR repertoire analysis. The analysis could not determine whether the skewed TCR repertoire occurred due to clonal expansion or not. We analyzed TCR repertoires more precisely based on CDR3 sequences that are a part of antigen binding site and provide high variety of TCR. Our results reveal that the skewed TCR repertoire in effector Treg cells in decidua, but not in peripheral blood during pregnancy, reflects clonal expansion of effector Treg cells in the decidua.

Concerning the relationship between the maldistribution or dysfunction of Treg cells and pregnancy complications, such as recurrent pregnancy loss or preeclampsia, the failure to maintain feto-maternal tolerance is thought to be one of the causes of these diseases (16–21). In the 1st trimester, miscarriage with normal embryo showed decreased population of decidual effector

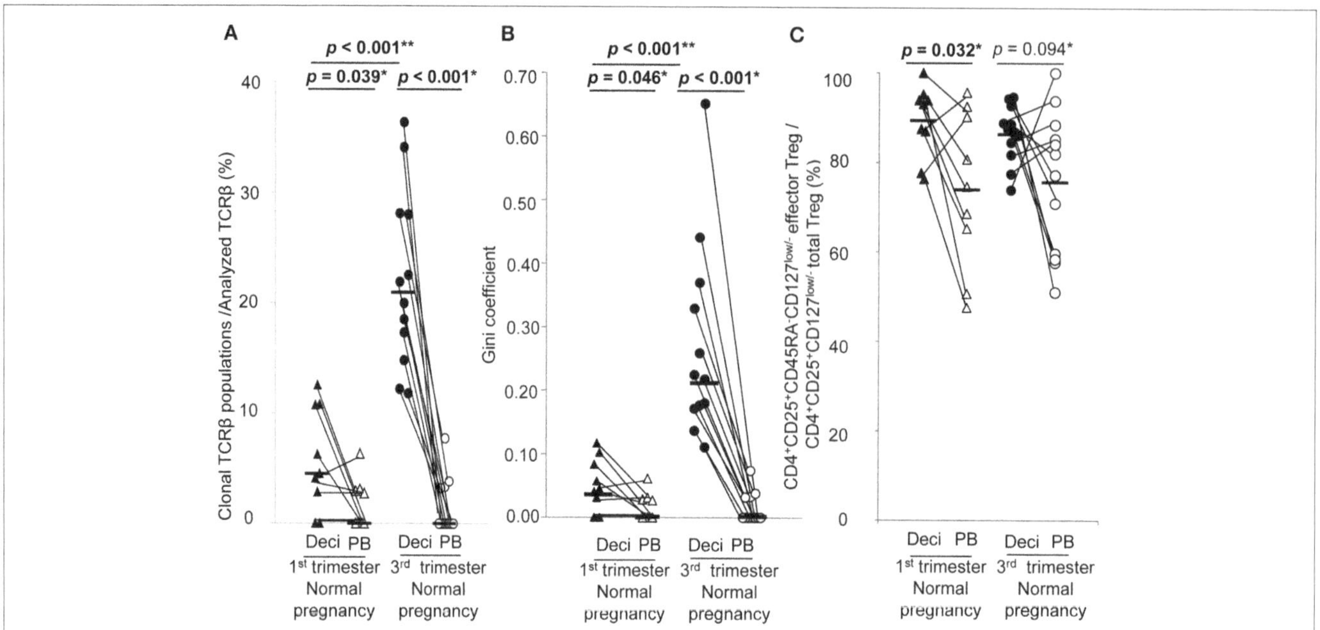

FIGURE 3 | TCRβ repertoire and flow cytometric analysis of effector Treg cells in 1st and 3rd trimester decidua and peripheral blood in normal pregnancy. **(A)** Frequencies of clonal populations among the analyzed TCRβ of effector Treg cells in 1st ($n = 9$) and 3rd trimester ($n = 12$) decidua and peripheral blood in normal pregnancies. **(B)** Gini coefficient of TCRβ repertoire of effector Treg cells. **(C)** Ratio of $CD4^+CD45RA^-CD25^+CD127^{low/-}$ effector Treg cells per $CD4^+CD25^+CD127^{low/-}$ total Treg cells. *p from Wilcoxon signed-rank test and **p from Mann–Whitney U-test. Each dot represents one donor, lines indicate median. Deci, decidua; PB, peripheral blood.

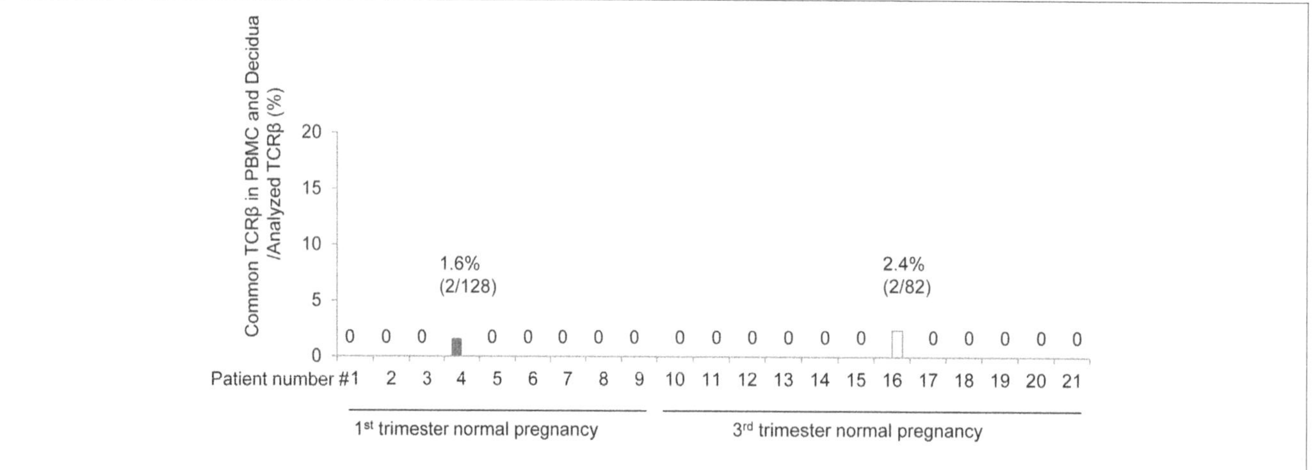

FIGURE 4 | Common clonotypic effector Treg cells between PBMC and decidua in 1st and 3rd trimester decidua and peripheral blood in normal pregnancy. Frequencies of common TCRβ in PBMC and decidua among analyzed TCRβ of effector Treg cells.

Treg cells compared with normal pregnancy. This result is consistent with our previous report of the decreased proportion of effector Treg cells in miscarriage with normal embryo than 1st trimester normal pregnancy (15). In contrast, the TCR repertoire in this study showed no significant skew between these populations (**Figure 6**). Taken together, our findings suggest that the decreased number of decidual effector Treg cells might be related to the pathogenesis of miscarriage with normal fetal karyotype, rather than an altered TCR repertoire. On the other hand, preeclampsia showed insufficient clonal expansion of decidual effector Treg cells compared with normal pregnancy in the 3rd trimester. In the 3rd trimester, effector Treg cells are the most dominant subset among Treg cells in PBMC and at the uteroplacental interface (14). The decrease in clonal populations of decidual effector Treg cells might be related to the pathogenesis of preeclampsia.

Concerning the TCR clonotypes of decidual effector Treg cells, we show for the first time that some TCR clonotypes in decidual effector Treg cells are shared between previous and subsequent pregnancies of the same subjects, but not those

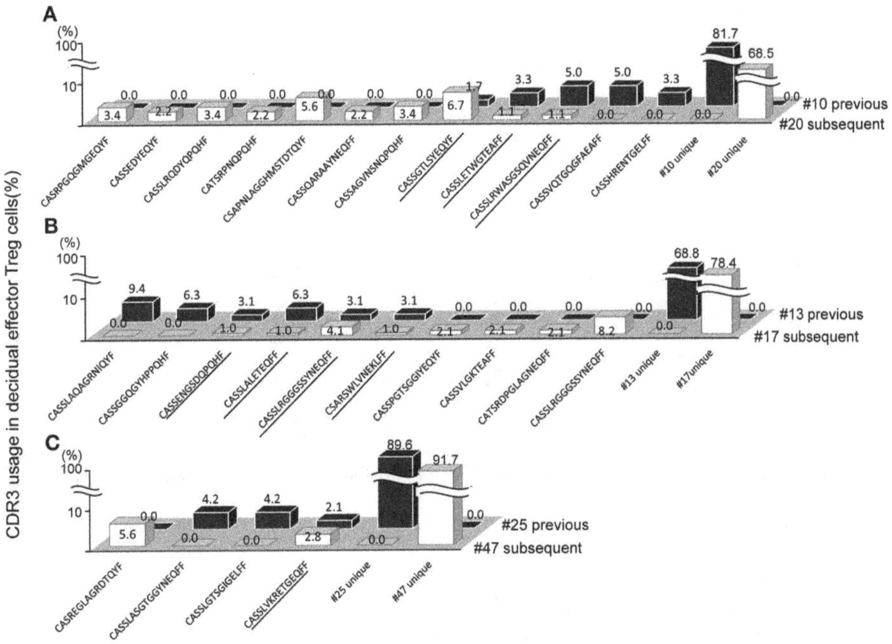

FIGURE 5 | Shared TCRβ repertoire of decidual effector Treg cells between previous and subsequent pregnancy. **(A–C)** Frequencies of decidual effector Treg cell clones expressing clonotypic TCRβ with the indicated CDR3 amino acid sequence. The underlined CDR3 sequences were shared in previous and subsequent pregnancies. **(A)** Case #10 previous pregnancy and case #20 subsequent pregnancy ending in the 3rd trimester with a normal vaginal delivery. **(B)** Case #13 previous pregnancy and case #17 subsequent pregnancy ending in the 3rd trimester with a normal vaginal delivery. **(C)** Case #25 previous pregnancy ending in miscarriage with a normal embryo and case #47 subsequent pregnancy ending in miscarriage with an abnormal embryo.

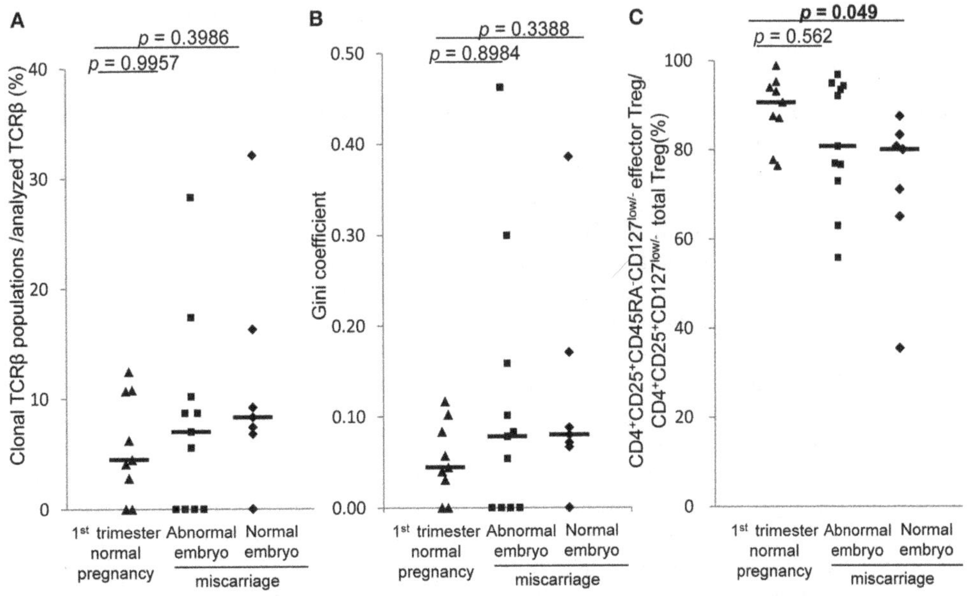

FIGURE 6 | TCRβ repertoire and flow cytometric analysis of decidual effector Treg cells in 1st trimester normal pregnancy and miscarriage. **(A)** Frequencies of clonal populations among analyzed TCRβ of effector Treg cells in 1st trimester normal pregnancy ($n = 9$) and miscarriage with abnormal embryo ($n = 11$) or normal embryo ($n = 7$). **(B)** Gini coefficient of TCRβ repertoire of effector Treg cells. **(C)** Ratio of $CD4^{+}CD45RA^{-}CD25^{+}CD127^{low/-}$ effector Treg cells per $CD4^{+}CD25^{+}CD127^{low/-}$ total Treg cells. *p from Steel's test. Each dot represents one donor; lines indicate median.

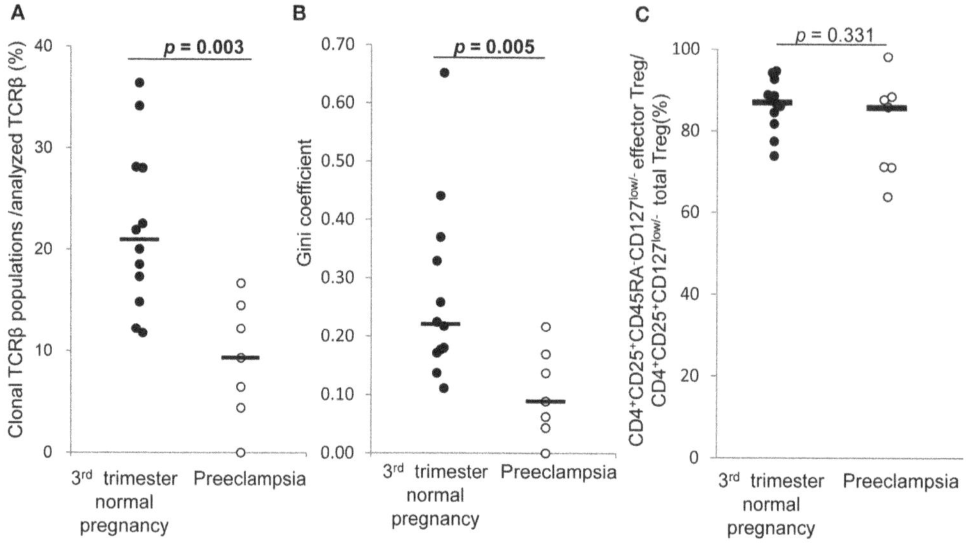

FIGURE 7 | TCRβ repertoire and flow cytometric analysis of decidual effector Treg cells in 3rd trimester normal pregnancy and preeclampsia. **(A)** Frequencies of clonal populations among analyzed TCRβ of effector Treg cells in 3rd trimester normal pregnancy ($n = 12$) and preeclampsia ($n = 7$). **(B)** Gini coefficient of TCRβ repertoire of effector Treg cells. **(C)** Ratio of $CD4^+CD45RA^-CD25^+CD127^{low/-}$ effector Treg cells per $CD4^+CD25^+CD127^{low/-}$ total Treg cells are shown. *p from Mann–Whitney *U*-test. Each dot represents one donor; lines indicate median.

in PBMC. The lower limit for the number of different CDR3 amino acid sequences in TCRβ is estimated to be $\sim 2 \times 10^7$ in young humans (28). This indicates that there is a very low probability of coincidence of the CDR3 amino acid sequence between two independent Treg cells if there is no force to skew the populations. Thus, effector Treg cell clones shared between previous and subsequent pregnancies might be recruited by reacting to the same antigens expressed in feto-maternal interface, suggesting that fetal antigen-specific Treg cells might accumulate at the feto-maternal interface.

The existence of fetal antigen-specific Treg cells and those recruited to the feto-maternal interface during pregnancy were reported in mice (8–10). An examination of functional differences of Treg cells from PBMC and decidua in humans led to the suggestion that decidual Treg cells contain fetal-antigen specific populations (11). However, fetal antigen-specific Treg cell clones have not been identified in humans. The present finding of common Treg cell clones in the decidua in previous and subsequent pregnancies raises the possibility that these clones might react to antigens expressed in feto-maternal interface and, thus, could be candidates of fetal antigen-specific Treg cells. Regarding the target antigen presenting cells for Treg cells in human decidua, it has been reported that HLA-C mismatched pregnancies feature an increased amount of Treg cells and higher activation of conventional T cells than non-mismatched pregnancies (29). HLA-C, E, F, and G are expressed in extravillous trophoblasts (30–33). These expressed HLAs might be potent antigens recognized by Treg cells.

Some limitations of our study have to be considered. Firstly, we could not amplify TCRα as efficiently as TCRβ. Thus, the TCR repertoire was analyzed based on TCRβ and not paired TCR. Secondly, our single cell TCR repertoire analysis covered only a limited number of Treg cell clones compared with the bulk TCR repertoire analysis by next-generation sequencing. Thirdly, the functionality of TCRs was not assessed. TCRs derived from antigen-specific Treg cells and their function were demonstrated by using TCR^{mini} mice, whose TCRβ is identical in all T cells (34, 35). In humans, a functional assay of target-specific polyclonal Treg cells has been developed (27). However, a direct functional assay of TCRs obtained from Treg cells is still not available, reflecting the limited knowledge about epitopes from physiological targets of Treg cells (27, 36). TCRs from tumor specific conventional $CD4^+$ T cells and $CD8^+$ T cells were identified using single-cell RT-PCR methods (23, 24, 37, 38). We also demonstrated a rapid and efficient functional assay for TCRs directly obtained from $CD8^+$ T cells using TCR-transduced lymphocytes in the absence of information on antigen or MHC haplotype (38). We tried to apply this technique to mixed lymphocyte reaction of paired αβ TCR-transduced maternal T cells or TCR-negative T cell lines against self-fetal umbilical cord blood but were unsuccessful. An assay method capable of identifying target-specific Treg or $CD4^+$ T cells using TCR-transduced responder cells in the absence of information concerning their antigen or MHC haplotype, to the best of our knowledge, has not been reported yet. It might be technically more difficult than analysis of TCRs obtained from $CD8^+$T cells, thus novel strategy might be needed to improve assay method of TCRs obtained from $CD4^+$ T cells. When the assay method is established, the function of obtained TCRs will be explored. Fourthly, we have not been able to demonstrate a relationship between the TCR clonotype and effector molecule expression. Zemmour et al. showed that Treg cells, which share the same

TCR clonotype, display similar transcriptional identities by single-cell analysis in mice (39). Combined single-cell TCR and gene expression analysis should be addressed, thereby providing further insight into features of heterogeneous decidual Treg cells.

In summary, we show for the first time that effector Treg cells are clonally expanded in 3rd trimester decidua, but not in peripheral blood in humans. In preeclampsia, the TCR repertoires of decidual effector Treg cells were not skewed. Clonally expanded effector Treg cell populations might be more important in the 3rd trimester than in the 1st trimester. Insufficient expansion of clonal effector Treg cells in decidua might be an etiological aspect in the development of preeclampsia. On the other hand, the frequency of effector Treg cells among the total Treg cells decreased in cases of miscarriage with normal fetal chromosomal content, but clonal effector Treg cells did not decrease. Our findings further the understanding of the mechanisms of feto-maternal tolerance and could provide clues for understanding the different aspects of the pathophysiology of preeclampsia and miscarriage.

ETHICS STATEMENT

This study was carried out in accordance with the recommendations of Ethical Guidelines for Medical and Health Research Involving Human Subjects, the Ministry of Health, Labor and Welfare, Japan. The protocol was approved by the ethics review committee of University of Toyama (Rin 28-144). All subjects gave written informed consent in accordance with the Declaration of Helsinki.

AUTHOR CONTRIBUTIONS

SS, HK, and AM: conception and design; ST, XZ, and AU: acquiring and processing samples; ST, XZ, HK, HH, AU, and KT: execution of experiment; ST and XZ: analysis of data; ST, XZ, HK, HH, TS, and SS: interpretation of data; ST, TS, and SS: drafting manuscript; XZ, HK, HH, TS, AU, KT, and AM: revision of the manuscript for important intellectual content.

FUNDING

This work was supported by grants from Ministry of Education, Culture, Sports, Science and Technology in Japan [KAKENHI Grant Number 15H04980 (SS), 17K11221 (TS), and 16H06499 (HK)] and AMED under Grant Number JP17gk0110018 (SS).

ACKNOWLEDGMENTS

The authors thank Hiroshi Furuya and Masanori Yoshie for providing samples.

SUPPLEMENTARY MATERIAL

Supplementary Table 1 | Primers for single-cell RT-PCR.

Supplementary Table 2 | Contents of single-cell RT-PCR reaction mix.

REFERENCES

1. Aluvihare VR, Kallikourdis M, Betz AG. Regulatory T cells mediate maternal tolerance to the fetus. *Nat Immunol.* (2004) 5:266–71. doi: 10.1038/ni1037
2. Sasaki Y, Sakai M, Miyazaki S, Higuma S, Shiozaki A, Saito S. Decidual and peripheral blood CD4+CD25+ regulatory T cells in early pregnancy subjects and spontaneous abortion cases. *Mol Hum Reprod.* (2004) 10:347–53. doi: 10.1093/molehr/gah044
3. Somerset DA, Zheng Y, Kilby MD, Sansom DM, Drayson MT. Normal human pregnancy is associated with an elevation in the immune suppressive CD25+ CD4+ regulatory T-cell subset. *Immunology* (2004) 112:38–43. doi: 10.1111/j.1365-2567.2004.01869.x
4. Zenclussen AC, Gerlof K, Zenclussen ML, Sollwedel A, Bertoja AZ, Ritter T, et al. Abnormal T-cell reactivity against paternal antigens in spontaneous abortion: adoptive transfer of pregnancy-induced CD4+CD25+ T regulatory cells prevents fetal rejection in a murine abortion model. *Am J Pathol.* (2005) 166:811–22. doi: 10.1016/S0002-9440(10)62302-4
5. Shima T, Sasaki Y, Itoh M, Nakashima A, Ishii N, Sugamura K, et al. Regulatory T cells are necessary for implantation and maintenance of early pregnancy but not late pregnancy in allogeneic mice. *J Reprod Immunol.* (2010) 85:121–9. doi: 10.1016/j.jri.2010.02.006
6. Samstein RM, Josefowicz SZ, Arvey A, Treuting PM, Rudensky AY. Extrathymic generation of regulatory T cells in placental mammals mitigates maternal-fetal conflict. *Cell* (2012) 150:29–38. doi: 10.1016/j.cell.2012.05.031
7. Moldenhauer LM, Diener KR, Thring DM, Brown MP, Hayball JD, Robertson SA. Cross-presentation of male seminal fluid antigens elicits T cell activation to initiate the female immune response to pregnancy. *J Immunol.* (2009) 182:8080–93. doi: 10.4049/jimmunol.0804018
8. Kahn DA, Baltimore D. Pregnancy induces a fetal antigen-specific maternal T regulatory cell response that contributes to tolerance. *Proc Natl Acad Sci USA.* (2010) 107:9299–304. doi: 10.1073/pnas.1003909107
9. Rowe JH, Ertelt JM, Xin L, Way SS. Pregnancy imprints regulatory memory that sustains anergy to fetal antigen. *Nature* (2012) 490:102–6. doi: 10.1038/nature11462
10. Shima T, Inada K, Nakashima A, Ushijima A, Ito M, Yoshino O, et al. Paternal antigen-specific proliferating regulatory T cells are increased in uterine-draining lymph nodes just before implantation and in pregnant uterus just after implantation by seminal plasma-priming in allogeneic mouse pregnancy. *J Reprod Immunol.* (2015) 108:72–82. doi: 10.1016/j.jri.2015.02.005
11. Tilburgs T, Roelen DL, van der Mast BJ, de Groot-Swings GM, Kleijburg C, Scherjon SA, et al. Evidence for a selective migration of fetus-specific CD4+CD25bright regulatory T cells from the peripheral blood to the decidua in human pregnancy. *J Immunol.* (2008) 180:5737–45. doi: 10.4049/jimmunol.180.8.5737
12. Miyara M, Yoshioka Y, Kitoh A, Shima T, Wing K, Niwa A, et al. Functional delineation and differentiation dynamics of human CD4+ T cells expressing the FoxP3 transcription factor. *Immunity* (2009) 30:899–911. doi: 10.1016/j.immuni.2009.03.019
13. Miyara M, Chader D, Sage E, Sugiyama D, Nishikawa H, Bouvry D, et al. Sialyl Lewis x (CD15s) identifies highly differentiated and most suppressive FOXP3high regulatory T cells in humans. *Proc Natl Acad Sci USA.* (2015) 112:7225–30. doi: 10.1073/pnas.1508224112
14. Loewendorf AI, Nguyen TA, Yesayan MN, Kahn DA. Normal human pregnancy results in maternal immune activation in the periphery and at the uteroplacental interface. *PLoS ONE* (2014) 9:e96723. doi: 10.1371/journal.pone.0096723

15. Inada K, Shima T, Ito M, Ushijima A, Saito S. Helios-positive functional regulatory T cells are decreased in decidua of miscarriage cases with normal fetal chromosomal content. *J Reprod Immunol.* (2015) 107:10–9. doi: 10.1016/j.jri.2014.09.053
16. Sasaki Y, Darmochwal-Kolarz D, Suzuki D, Sakai M, Ito M, Shima T, et al. Proportion of peripheral blood and decidual CD4(+) CD25(bright) regulatory T cells in pre-eclampsia. *Clin Exp Immunol.* (2007) 149:139–45. doi: 10.1111/j.1365-2249.2007.03397.x
17. Toldi G, Svec P, Vasarhelyi B, Meszaros G, Rigo J, Tulassay T, et al. Decreased number of FoxP3+ regulatory T cells in preeclampsia. *Acta Obstet Gynecol Scand.* (2008) 87:1229–33. doi: 10.1080/00016340802389470
18. Prins JR, Boelens HM, Heimweg J, Van der Heide S, Dubois AE, Van Oosterhout AJ, et al. Preeclampsia is associated with lower percentages of regulatory T cells in maternal blood. *Hypertens Pregnancy* (2009) 28:300–11. doi: 10.1080/10641950802601237
19. Hsu P, Santner-Nanan B, Dahlstrom JE, Fadia M, Chandra A, Peek M, et al. Altered decidual DC-SIGN+ antigen-presenting cells and impaired regulatory T-cell induction in preeclampsia. *Am J Pathol.* (2012) 181:2149–60. doi: 10.1016/j.ajpath.2012.08.032
20. Steinborn A, Schmitt E, Kisielewicz A, Rechenberg S, Seissler N, Mahnke K, et al. Pregnancy-associated diseases are characterized by the composition of the systemic regulatory T cell (Treg) pool with distinct subsets of Tregs. *Clin Exp Immunol.* (2012) 167:84–98. doi: 10.1111/j.1365-2249.2011.04493.x
21. Nguyen TA, Kahn DA, Loewendorf AI. Maternal-Fetal rejection reactions are unconstrained in preeclamptic women. *PLoS ONE* (2017) 12:e0188250. doi: 10.1371/journal.pone.0188250
22. Neller MA, Santner-Nanan B, Brennan RM, Hsu P, Joung S, Nanan R, et al. Multivariate analysis using high definition flow cytometry reveals distinct t cell repertoires between the fetal-maternal interface and the peripheral blood. *Front Immunol.* (2014) 5:33. doi: 10.3389/fimmu.2014.00033
23. Kobayashi E, Mizukoshi E, Kishi H, Ozawa T, Hamana H, Nagai T, et al. A new cloning and expression system yields and validates TCRs from blood lymphocytes of patients with cancer within 10 days. *Nat Med.* (2013) 19:1542–6. doi: 10.1038/nm.3358
24. Hamana H, Shitaoka K, Kishi H, Ozawa T, Muraguchi A. A novel, rapid and efficient method of cloning functional antigen-specific T-cell receptors from single human and mouse T-cells. *Biochem Biophys Res Commun.* (2016) 474:709–14. doi: 10.1016/j.bbrc.2016.05.015
25. Tranquilli AL, Dekker G, Magee L, Roberts J, Sibai BM, Steyn W, et al. The classification, diagnosis and management of the hypertensive disorders of pregnancy: a revised statement from the ISSHP. *Pregnancy Hypertens.* (2014) 4:97–104. doi: 10.1016/j.preghy.2014.02.001
26. van der Geest KS, Abdulahad WH, Horst G, Lorencetti PG, Bijzet J, Arends S, et al. Quantifying distribution of flow Cytometric TCR-Vbeta usage with economic statistics. *PLoS ONE* (2015) 10:e0125373. doi: 10.1371/journal.pone.0125373
27. Bacher P, Heinrich F, Stervbo U, Nienen M, Vahldieck M, Iwert C, et al. Regulatory T cell specificity directs tolerance versus allergy against Aeroantigens in humans. *Cell* (2016) 167:1067.e16–78.e16. doi: 10.1016/j.cell.2016.09.050
28. Qi Q, Liu Y, Cheng Y, Glanville J, Zhang D, Lee JY, et al. Diversity and clonal selection in the human T-cell repertoire. *Proc Natl Acad Sci USA.* (2014) 111:13139–44. doi: 10.1073/pnas.1409155111
29. Tilburgs T, Scherjon SA, van der Mast BJ, Haasnoot GW, Versteeg VDV-MM, Roelen DL, et al. Fetal-maternal HLA-C mismatch is associated with decidual T cell activation and induction of functional T regulatory cells. *J Reprod Immunol.* (2009) 82:148–57. doi: 10.1016/j.jri.2009.05.003
30. Kovats S, Main EK, Librach C, Stubblebine M, Fisher SJ, DeMars R. A class I antigen, HLA-G, expressed in human trophoblasts. *Science* (1990) 248:220–3. doi: 10.1126/science.2326636
31. Barakonyi A, Kovacs KT, Miko E, Szereday L, Varga P, Szekeres-Bartho J. Recognition of nonclassical HLA class I antigens by gamma delta T cells during pregnancy. *J Immunol.* (2002) 168:2683–8. doi: 10.4049/jimmunol.168.6.2683
32. Ishitani A, Sageshima N, Lee N, Dorofeeva N, Hatake K, Marquardt H, et al. Protein expression and peptide binding suggest unique and interacting functional roles for HLA-E, F, and G in maternal-placental immune recognition. *J Immunol.* (2003) 171:1376–84. doi: 10.4049/jimmunol.171.3.1376
33. Tilburgs T, Crespo AC, van der Zwan A, Rybalov B, Raj T, Stranger B, et al. Human HLA-G+ extravillous trophoblasts: immune-activating cells that interact with decidual leukocytes. *Proc Natl Acad Sci USA.* (2015) 112:7219–24. doi: 10.1073/pnas.1507977112
34. Lathrop SK, Bloom SM, Rao SM, Nutsch K, Lio CW, Santacruz N, et al. Peripheral education of the immune system by colonic commensal microbiota. *Nature* (2011) 478:250–4. doi: 10.1038/nature10434
35. Cebula A, Seweryn M, Rempala GA, Pabla SS, McIndoe RA, Denning TL, et al. Thymus-derived regulatory T cells contribute to tolerance to commensal microbiota. *Nature* (2013) 497:258–62. doi: 10.1038/nature12079
36. Bacher P, Scheffold, A. New technologies for monitoring human antigen-specific T cells and regulatory T cells by flow-cytometry. *Curr Opin Pharmacol.* (2015) 23:17–24. doi: 10.1016/j.coph.2015.04.005
37. Stevanovic S, Pasetto A, Helman SR, Gartner JJ, Prickett TD, Howie B, et al. Landscape of immunogenic tumor antigens in successful immunotherapy of virally induced epithelial cancer. *Science* (2017) 356:200–5. doi: 10.1126/science.aak9510
38. Shitaoka K, Hamana H, Kishi H, Hayakawa Y, Kobayashi E, Sukegawa K, et al. Identification of tumoricidal TCRs from tumor-infiltrating lymphocytes by single-cell analysis. *Cancer Immunol Res.* (2018) 6:378–88. doi: 10.1158/2326-6066.CIR-17-0489
39. Zemmour D, Zilionis R, Kiner E, Klein AM, Mathis D, Benoist C. Single-cell gene expression reveals a landscape of regulatory T cell phenotypes shaped by the TCR. *Nat Immunol.* (2018) 19:291–301. doi: 10.1038/s41590-018-0051-0

14

Human Innate Lymphoid Cells: Their Functional and Cellular Interactions in Decidua

Paola Vacca[1], Chiara Vitale[2,3], Enrico Munari[4,5], Marco Antonio Cassatella[6], Maria Cristina Mingari[2,3,7] and Lorenzo Moretta[1]*

[1] Department of Immunology, IRCCS Bambino Gesù Children's Hospital, Rome, Italy, [2] Department of Experimental Medicine (DIMES), University of Genoa, Genoa, Italy, [3] UOC Immunology, IRCCS Ospedale Policlinico San Martino Genova, Genoa, Italy, [4] Department of Pathology, Sacro Cuore Don Calabria Hospital, Negrar, Italy, [5] Department of Pathology AOUI, University of Verona, Verona, Italy, [6] Department of Medicine, Section of General Pathology, University of Verona, Verona, Italy, [7] Center of Excellence for Biomedical Research (CEBR), University of Genoa, Genoa, Italy

***Correspondence:**
Paola Vacca
paola.vacca@opbg.net

Innate lymphoid cells (ILC) are developmentally related cell subsets that play a major role in innate defenses against pathogens, in lymphoid organogenesis and in tissue remodeling. The best characterized ILC are natural killer (NK) cells. They are detectable in decidua in the early phases of pregnancy. During the first trimester, NK cells represent up to 50% of decidua lymphocytes. Differently from peripheral blood (PB) NK cells, decidual NK (dNK) cells are poorly cytolytic, and, instead of IFNγ, they release cytokines/chemokines that induce neo-angiogenesis, tissue remodeling, and placentation. dNK interact with resident myeloid cells and participate in the induction of regulatory T cells that play a pivotal role in maintaining an efficient fetal–maternal tolerance. dNK cells may originate from CD34$^+$ precursor cells present *in situ* and/or from immature NK cells already present in endometrial tissue and/or from PB NK cells migrated to decidua. In addition to NK cells, also ILC3 are present in human decidua during the first trimester. Decidual ILC3 include both natural cytotoxic receptor (NCR)$^+$ and NCR$^-$ cells, producing respectively IL-8/IL-22/GM-CSF and TNF/IL-17. NCR$^+$ILC3 have been shown to establish physical and functional interactions with neutrophils that, in turn, produce factors that are crucial for pregnancy induction/maintenance and for promoting the early inflammatory phase, a fundamental process for a successful pregnancy. While NCR$^+$ILC3 display a stable phenotype, most of NCR$^-$ILC3 may acquire phenotypic and functional features of NCR$^+$ILC3. In conclusion, both NK cells and ILC3 are present in human decidua and may establish functional interactions with immune and myeloid cells playing an important role both in innate defenses and in tissue building/remodeling/placentation during the early pregnancy. It is conceivable that altered numbers or function of these cells may play a role in pregnancy failure.

Keywords: innate lymphoid cell, innate immunity, natural killer cells, human pregnancy, neutrophils, stromal cells, inflammation, tolerance

INTRODUCTION

The fetus can be considered as a semi-allograft to the maternal host; therefore, pregnancy should include mechanisms to prevent allograft rejection (1–3). During the early phases of pregnancy, an appropriate balance between inflammation and tolerance is critical for a successful pregnancy (4, 5). Indeed, pro-inflammatory cytokines have been shown to contribute to tissue building/remodeling and neo-angiogenesis, thus favoring embryo implantation (6–8). The inflammatory phase is followed by a regulatory phase characterized by an increase in regulatory T cells (Tregs) that prevent an excessive inflammation and avoid fetal immuno-mediated rejection (9). Thus, relevant interactions among cells involved in immune response may occur at the fetal–maternal interface and play a fundamental role for a successful pregnancy.

GENERAL CHARACTERISTICS OF INNATE LYMPHOID CELLS (ILC) SUBSETS

Innate lymphoid cells are immune effector cells involved in host defenses against pathogens and tumors, in lymphoid organogenesis and in secondary lymphoid organ remodeling after birth. ILCs are tissue-resident cells mainly found at the mucosal surfaces of intestine (10), lungs (11), decidua (12), and skin (13, 14). Thanks to their strategic location, ILC are among the first immune cells to respond to pathogens. Recently, on the basis of their cytokine profile and transcription factors (TF), ILC have been classified into two main groups: cytotoxic- and helper-ILC (15–18). Natural killer (NK) cells, representing cytotoxic-ILC, are the first innate lymphoid cell population described, featuring the capacity of killing virus-infected or tumor cells and to release pro-inflammatory cytokines and chemokines. Human NK cell function is regulated by an array of inhibitory receptors, such as the HLA-I-specific killer immunoglobulin-like receptors and CD94/NKG2A, and by activating receptors, including natural cytotoxicity receptors (NCR, i.e., NKp46, NKp30, and NKp44), NKG2D, DNAM-1, and CD16 (19, 20). The other ILC are represented by "helper"-ILC that are further classified into three main subsets (ILC1/ILC2/ILC3) (21). ILC1 mainly produce IFNγ and provide defenses against intracellular bacteria and protozoa (22). In humans, two different subsets of ILC1 have been described in the intestine (23, 24). ILC2 mainly release type-2 cytokines, such as IL-5, IL-13, and IL-4 and contribute to type-2 immune responses. Finally, ILC3 are a heterogeneous subset, their signature cytokines are represented by IL-17 and IL-22 (25). ILC3 were first identified in the fetus and were originally defined lymphoid tissue inducer (LTi) cells because of their key role in driving lymphoid organogenesis. In particular, during embryogenesis, LTi cells interact with stromal cells and induce upregulation of adhesion molecules thus promoting the development of lymph node structure. After birth, ILC3 are mainly located in secondary lymphoid organs (SLO), tonsils, decidua, and intestinal lamina *propria* where they contribute to host defenses against extracellular pathogens and are defined as LTi-like cells. In humans, LTi/LTi-like cells are lineage (CD3/CD19/CD14/CD56)-negative and express CD127, CD117, retinoic acid receptor-related orphan receptor (ROR)-γt TF, and secrete primarily IL-17 and TNFα. A population of cells referred to as NCR + ILC3, sharing common features with both LTi-like cells and NK cells (type of cytokines production and NCR expression, respectively), has recently been identified in mucosal tissues and prevalently releases IL-22. ILC3-derived IL-22 acts on intestinal epithelial cells and induces not only production of antimicrobial peptides but also epithelial cell migration and wound healing. Moreover, ILC3 promote tissue repair and remodeling of SLO damaged by inflammatory processes. Conversely, ILC3 may also exert a pro-inflammatory role in intestinal inflammatory diseases.

All ILC subsets are developmentally related. Evidence in mice and humans indicates that NK cells and helper-ILC derive from a common ILC progenitor (CILP). As B and T lymphoid progenitors, the CILP derive from the common lymphoid progenitor. The acquisition of mature stages is dependent by different TF. Thus, NK cell differentiation involves Eomes, which regulates the expression of IFNγ and of the cytolytic machinery, while terminal differentiation of helper-ILC is regulated by other TF. In particular, ILC1 requires Tbet, ILC2 GATA3, and RORα, and ILC3 RORγt and AhR (26–29). Although, specific ILC3-committed precursors have been defined, a precise identification of a common ILC precursor in humans is still lacking. Moreover, it is still only partially understood which signals from the microenvironment are driving their differentiation. The low numbers of ILC3 that can be generated *in vitro* has so far hampered studies aimed to answer these questions. Moreover, limitations in cell numbers may be an obstacle for clinical application of ILC. Thus, the development of protocols allowing the generation of suitable numbers of given subsets of ILC for their use in adoptive cell therapy is required.

Along this line, it has become more evident that the fate of ILC determination and their stability is not set in stone, but that there is some plasticity between different ILC subsets, depending on various signaling, including cytokines and exposure to different tissue-specific microenvironments. This would indicate that microenvironmental conditions might drive this plasticity from an ILC subset to another (29). Accordingly, it is conceivable that also putative differentiated ILC may display intermediate phenotypic/functional characteristics (30, 31).

ILC IN HUMAN DECIDUA AND THEIR INTERACTIONS WITH DECIDUA MICROENVIRONMENT

Innate immune cells are important components of the decidual microenvironment. In this tissue, the best characterized and most abundant ILCs are NK cells (1, 2, 32). Remarkably, while the function of peripheral blood (PB) NK cells is to defend the host against infections and tumors, thanks to their cytolytic activity and production of cytokines, such as IFN-γ and TNF, decidual NK (dNK) cells are characterized by a regulatory function (33). It has been shown that the NK cell function is greatly influenced by the microenvironment, including cytokines (34), chemokines, and cell-to-cell interactions. A paradigmatic example of how NK cell function may be regulated in tissues is provided by human dNK cells. They represent as much as 50–70% of decidual infiltrating lymphocytes during the first trimester of pregnancy, and are characterized by $CD56^{bright}CD16^{-}KIR^{+}CD9^{+}$ phenotype (2, 35). In spite of their high content of cytolytic granules, dNK cells are poorly cytotoxic and release very low amounts of IFNγ as compared to PB-NK cells (2, 36–39). On the other hand, dNK cells release peculiar cytokines and chemokines, such as vascular endothelial growth factor (VEGF), stromal derived factor-1 (SDF-1 also identified as CXCL12), and IFN-γ-inducing protein 10 (IP10 also known as CXCL10), that mediate neo-angiogenesis, tissue remodeling, and placentation (3). Similarly, to humans, also murine dNK cells are abundant during the early phases of pregnancy and display unique phenotypic and functional features (40–44). Several reports revealed that NK cells are present also in non-pregnant endometrial tissue and that their proportions may vary during the menstrual cycle. It has been shown that, besides NK cells, other ILC populations are present in human decidua during the early phases of pregnancy (12, 41) This finding supports the notion that ILC participate to defensive/tissue building processes necessary for the maintenance/success of pregnancy (45, 46). Notably, decidual tissues contain different RORγt$^+$ ILC3 subsets displaying functional features similar to those previously described in other tissues. In particular, dILC3 not only express IL-22, but are also the main IL-8 producers, a functional activity previously assigned to dNK cells. Moreover, dILC3 have been shown to induce the expression of adhesion molecules (a functional activity referred to LTi-like cells) on decidual stromal cells (DSC), thus suggesting that, also dILC3, may play a role in tissue building/remodeling during the early phases of pregnancy.

ORIGIN OF DECIDUAL ILC

Given the relevant role of dNK cells in the maintenance of pregnancy, an important issue is to clarify their origin. NK cells are known to originate from CD34$^+$ hematopoietic stem cell, as revealed by a number of studies both *in vitro* and *in vivo*. These precursors are present mainly in the bone marrow, and also in PB and cord blood. Although, it is possible that dNK cells may derive from PB-NK cells migrated in decidua, where they acquire unique functional features upon exposure to the decidual microenvironment (47, 48), they may also derive from CD34$^+$ precursors detectable in decidua. In this context, previous studies described the presence of CD34$^+$VEGFR$^-$ precursors in decidual tissues and of immature NK cells in endometrial tissue (47–51). Both cell populations could undergo differentiation into dNK cells during pregnancy. Remarkably, dCD34$^+$ cells are committed toward the NK cell lineage as revealed by experiments showing that they undergo rapid *in vitro* differentiation toward mature NK cells both in the presence and in the absence of cytokines, provided they are co-cultured with DSC (3, 52).

The issue of the developmental relationship between different ILC is a matter of debate. In particular, the relationship between NK cells and ILC3 is unclear in humans, because the phenotypic features of immature NK cells and ILC3 are partially overlapping. It was originally proposed that NCR$^+$ILC3 represent an immature stage of NK cell development (53, 54). However, decidual ILC3, despite their extensive proliferative capacity, maintain their phenotypic and functional characteristic, while only a minor fraction could differentiate toward CD94$^+$ NK cells even in the presence of IL-15. Similarly, to NCR$^+$ILC3, also LTi-like cells virtually failed to generate NK cells. Thus, it is conceivable that the majority of NK cells present in decidual tissue may derive from PB-NK cells migrated to decidua, as well as from CD34$^+$ cell precursors detectable *in situ*. On the other hand, our recent studies support the notion that a developmental relationship exists between the two ILC3 subsets present in decidua. Indeed, NCR$^+$ILC3 (expressing CD56) could be derived from LTi-like CD56$^-$ cells. In these *in vitro* experiments, only a small percentage of LTi-like cells retained their phenotypic characteristics (Lin$^-$CD56$^-$CD117$^+$CD127$^+$), while they acquired the Lin$^-$CD56$^+$CD117$^+$CD127$^+$CD94$^-$NCR$^+$ phenotype (12). It cannot be excluded that, similarly to NK cells, also ILC3 may derive from precursors present in decidua. Indeed, ILC3 are not present in PB, implying that they should develop *in situ* from a precursor. Interestingly, dCD34$^+$ precursors are characterized by the expression of ID2 transcription factor, which is required for ILC development, suggesting that dCD34 cells may give rise not only to dNK cells but also to NCR$^+$ILC3 and LTi-like cells (12).

Although NK cells belong to the innate immune system, different reports suggested that they may display adaptive-like properties. These adaptive features include clonal expansion and the generation of long-lived memory cells (55–58). In humans, "trained/memory" NK cells are characterized by the expression of HLA-class I-specific activating receptor NKG2C (59). The NKG2C$^+$ NK cell subset undergo great expansion following human cytomegalovirus infection (55, 60). Several observations indicate that a major risk of a deficient placentation occurs in women that undergo first pregnancy (61, 62). These data suggest that, after the first pregnancy, the uterine microenvironment may acquire the ability to better sustain the early phase of placentation, including the inflammatory process. In this context, it has been shown recently that the dNK cell repertoire significantly differs in primigravidae as compared to multigravidae. Mulitgravid women display higher percentages of dNK cells expressing NKG2C and LILRB1, which also produce higher amounts of IFN-γ and VEGF as compared to dNK cells detectable in primigravid women. Precursors of these cells are present in the uterus between pregnancies and may become activated by the uterine microenvironment once a new pregnancy occurs. These cells could represent "trained" NK cells that would improve endometrial vascularization, angiogenesis, and maintenance of decidua through a more prompt and abundant secretion of functional VEGF and IFN-γ (63).

INVOLVEMENT OF ILC IN THE INFLAMMATORY AND TOLEROGENIC PHASES OF PREGNANCY

A successful pregnancy requires an early inflammatory phase that is necessary for successful implantation, while, subsequently, a regulatory/immunosuppressive phase should follow to prevent fetal rejection (5, 8, 64). Several studies highlighted the role of innate and adaptive immune cells in promoting either an inflammatory or an immunosuppressive environment. It is conceivable that functional activities thought to be exclusive of adaptive immunity, may actually be mediated also by ILC (65). Thus, not only uterine Th17 but also dILC releasing pro-angiogenetic factors are likely to play a role in the neo-angiogenesis and antimicrobial defenses during pregnancy.

The Inflammatory Phase

Different studies revealed the presence of neutrophils (N) with pro-angiogenetic capability in human decidua during the first and the second trimesters of pregnancy (66, 67). In particular, during the first trimester, N present in human decidual tissues are characterized by an "activated" phenotype, production of fibro/angiogenic factors and a prolonged survival. Previous studies reported that NCR$^+$ILC3 could mediate neutrophil activation in spleen *via* GM-CSF (68). It has been shown that dILC3 could functionally interact with N in decidual tissues (**Figure 1**). In particular, it is conceivable that dN recruitment to decidua, their activation, and expression of peculiar immunoregulatory factors (HB-EGF and IL1ra) may be related to interaction with dILC3 (69, 70). Indeed, thanks to their ability to release IL8 and GM-CSF, dILC3 could promote neutrophil recruitment and activation, respectively. These observations support the notion that both ILC3 and N may play an important role in early inflammatory phase and, subsequently, in the induction of tolerance.

Recent studies revealed that also cytokines released by NK cells might induce neutrophil activation, expression of activation markers, and production of cytokines and angiogenic factors (71–73). In addition, under suitable experimental conditions, NK cells have been shown to induce neutrophil apoptosis (74). Reciprocally, N may inhibit NK cell proliferation, cytolytic activity, cytokine production, and survival *via* contact-dependent or -independent mechanisms (73). In agreement with the concept of NK/N interactions in decidua, it has been observed that dN localize in close proximity of CD56$^+$ cells, suggesting a potential crosstalk with dNK cells. Thus, it is possible to speculate that also decidual N by interacting with dILC3 and/or dNK cells may contribute to the regulation of innate/adaptive immune responses occurring during pregnancy, by the release of soluble factors, or cell-to-cell contacts (67). These data shed new light on the cellular and molecular mechanisms involved in the initiation of an inflammatory response in the decidua.

The Tolerogenic Phase

Since fetus is a semi-allograft, successful pregnancy should also include mechanisms capable of preventing allograft rejection. Indeed, while effective immune responses must be maintained in order to protect the mother from harmful pathogens, immune reaction against fetal antigens should also be avoided. dNK cells express normal levels of HLA-class I-specific inhibitory receptors. Notably, certain HLA-class I molecules are expressed by trophoblast and are involved in the regulation of trophoblast growth, differentiation, and invasion (75). The fact that dNK cells are unable to kill different target cells has been tentatively explained with the poor ability to form appropriate immunological synapses and/or the expression of the inhibitory form of 2B4 co-receptor (39, 76). In addition, the fact that dNK cells do not kill trophoblastic

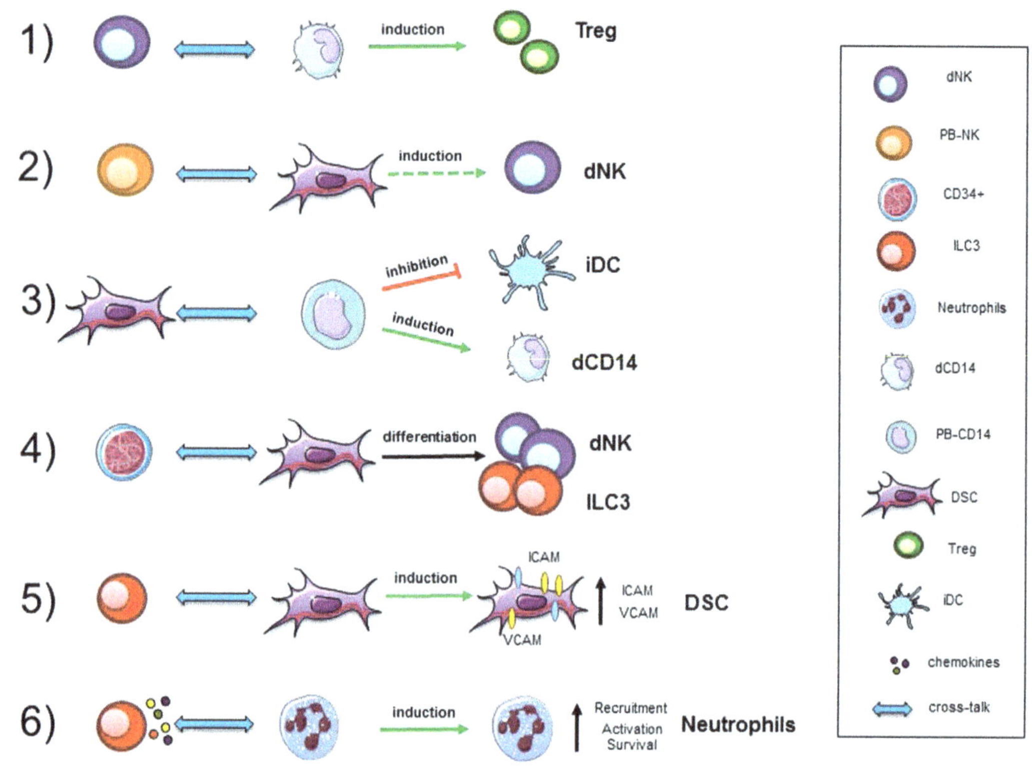

FIGURE 1 | Cellular interactions in human decidua. Representative interactions between immune cells, precursors, and stromal cells occurring in decidual tissues during the first trimester of pregnancy. Abbreviations: dNK, decidual natural killer cells; PB-NK, peripheral blood NK cells; ILC, innate lymphoid cells; dCD14, decidual myeloid cells; PB-CD14, peripheral blood myeloid cells; DSC, decidual stromal cells; Treg, regulatory T cells; iDC, immature dendritic cells.

cells has also been explained with the expression of inhibitory NK receptors, such as CD94/NKG2A specific for HLA-E, recognizing HLA-G KIR2DL4 and KIR2DL1/2/3 specific for HLA-C, i.e., the HLA-class I molecules expressed by human trophoblast. Therefore, both the poor ability to kill of dNK cells and a number of fail-safe mechanism may be responsible for the inability of dNK cells to kill the invading trophoblast (7). Notably, also Tregs have been detected during early pregnancy and are thought to exert an important protective role when the maternal immune cells come into contact with fetal antigens expressed by invading trophoblast cells. Accordingly, studies in humans revealed the presence of Tregs in the PB during the early phases of normal pregnancy, while a low Treg numbers have been reported in cases of recurrent pregnancy loss (77). In this context, it should be stressed that different Treg subpopulations occur, including naturally occurring Tregs, which derive from the thymus, and adaptive Tregs, which develop in the periphery, The development of Tregs requires the transcription factor Forkhead box P3 which currently represents their most specific marker. The secretion of inhibitory cytokines and contact-dependent inhibition are two identified mechanisms of Treg-mediated suppression. Tregs may contribute to prevent autoimmune diseases and play a role in transplantation tolerance. Previous studies indicated that the increase of Treg in decidual tissue may be due either to the local expansion or to their selective recruitment at the maternal–fetal interface (9, 78).

Another remarkable cell population present in the decidua is represented by CD14$^+$ cells, generally described as decidual myeloid cells (monocytes/macrophages) that did not express CD1a, a dendritic cell (DC) marker (79, 80). Histochemical analysis revealed that they may be in close association with dNK cells, and be involved in functional crosstalks with NK cells. *In vitro* experiments revealed that the interaction between dNK and dCD14$^+$ cells results in the production of IFN-γ which, in turn, induces indoleamine 2,3-dioxygenase (IDO) expression in dCD14$^+$ cells. Such "conditioned" dCD14$^+$ cells acquire the ability to induce Treg by a mechanism that involves TGF-β production. Our perception of the role of dNK cells has thus evolved indeed, not only they do not attack trophoblastic cells but also they can play a major role in immune regulation, by promoting the development of Tregs upon functional interaction with dCD14$^+$ cells (81) (**Figure 1**).

Decidual stromal cells represent other important component of decidual tissue. Indeed, decidual leukocytes are deeply influenced by these cells. On the other hand, also immune cells may modulate DSC function (82). Experimental evidences revealed that DSC, present in the early and late phases of pregnancy, may contribute to the induction of an anti-inflammatory and tolerogenic microenvironment crucial for the establishment/maintenance of successful pregnancy. In this context, DSC have been shown to induce downregulation of major activating NK receptors and to inhibit NK cell proliferation, cytotoxicity, and IFN-γ production. These inhibitory activities are related to the production of PGE2 and to the expression of IDO, resulting in kynurenine production. DSC display another important functional capability related to their ability to promote CD34$^+$ cell differentiation. In this context, it has been described that endometrium and decidua contain CD34$^+$ cell precursors (dCD34$^+$) capable of differentiating *in vitro* into NK cells. Interestingly, even in the absence of exogenous cytokines, dCD34$^+$ could give rise to dNK cells when co-cultured with DSC. Other leukocyte functional capabilities may be affected as a result of crosstalk with DSC (**Figure 1**). Thus, DSC, through IDO and PGE2, may affect the differentiation of PB-CD14$^+$ cells toward DCs (82). Moreover, previous studies showed that placenta-derived stromal cells can mediate T cell suppression and induce Treg expansion through a mechanism involving IDO, PGE2, and PD-L1 (83).

Interaction among different cell types may imply a bidirectional crosstalk. Accordingly, also immune cells may influence DSC properties. For example, decidual ILC3 (in particular LTi-like cells) can induce upregulation of ICAM1 and VCAM1 on DSC. This effect is one of the starting events necessary for the development of secondary and tertiary lymphoid organs. In decidua, this effect could be involved in tissue remodeling, placentation, and leukocyte recruitment. Moreover, engagement of RANK has been shown to promote production of CCL2, which, in turn, favors DSC survival and proliferation (84). Moreover, since decidual ILC3 express RANKL it would be of interest to explore whether they can interact with DSC *via* RANKL/RANK-mediated mechanisms.

CONCLUSION

As outlined in this contribution, during the first trimester of pregnancy, different cellular players deeply involved in the balance between inflammation and tolerance are present in decidual. In particular, decidual ILC, including NK cells, ILC3 and ILC1, upon interaction with stromal cells, neutrophils, myelomonocytic cells, and T lymphocytes may play a key role in the induction and maintenance of pregnancy. Notably, decidual ILC can originate from CD34$^+$ precursors or immature lymphoid cells present *in situ*. In view of the role of ILC in pregnancy, it is possible to speculate that defects in ILC generation or functional interactions in decidual tissues may be a possible cause of fetal losses. While a better knowledge on these cells is clearly required before planning any future clinical application, these concepts open new scenarios of investigation both in innate immunity and in reproductive immunology.

AUTHOR CONTRIBUTIONS

All authors discussed together the general outline of the article. PV, CV, and LM wrote the first draft that was subsequently reviewed by MAC, EM, and MCM. Thereafter, all authors contributed to the elaboration of the final version of the manuscript.

FUNDING

Supported by grants awarded by Associazione Italiana Ricerca per la Ricerca sul Cancro (AIRC)—Special Project "5 × 1000 Molecular Clinical Oncology Extension Program" no. 9962 (LM) and "5 × 1000 Immunity in Cancer Spreading and Metastasis (ISM) no. 21147 (LM); AIRC IG 2017 Id. 19920 (LM), AIRC 2014 Id. 15283 (LM), Ministero della Salute RF-2013, GR-2013-02356568 (PV).

REFERENCES

1. Erlebacher A. Immunology of the maternal-fetal interface. *Annu Rev Immunol* (2013) 31:387–411. doi:10.1146/annurev-immunol-032712-100003
2. Moffett-King A. Natural killer cells and pregnancy. *Nat Rev Immunol* (2002) 2(9):656–63. doi:10.1038/nri967
3. Vacca P, Moretta L, Moretta A, Mingari MC. Origin, phenotype and function of human natural killer cells in pregnancy. *Trends Immunol* (2011) 32(11):517–23. doi:10.1016/j.it.2011.06.013
4. Mortha A, Chudnovskiy A, Hashimoto D, Bogunovic M, Spencer SP, Belkaid Y, et al. Microbiota-dependent crosstalk between macrophages and ILC3 promotes intestinal homeostasis. *Science* (2014) 343(6178):1249288. doi:10.1126/science.1249288
5. Saito S, Nakashima A, Shima T, Ito M. Th1/Th2/Th17 and regulatory T-cell paradigm in pregnancy. *Am J Reprod Immunol* (2010) 63(6):601–10. doi:10.1111/j.1600-0897.2010.00852.x
6. Hanna J, Goldman-Wohl D, Hamani Y, Avraham I, Greenfield C, Natanson-Yaron S, et al. Decidual NK cells regulate key developmental processes at the human fetal-maternal interface. *Nat Med* (2006) 12(9):1065–74. doi:10.1038/nm1452
7. Vacca P, Cantoni C, Prato C, Fulcheri E, Moretta A, Moretta L, et al. Regulatory role of NKp44, NKp46, DNAM-1 and NKG2D receptors in the interaction between NK cells and trophoblast cells. Evidence for divergent functional profiles of decidual versus peripheral NK cells. *Int Immunol* (2008) 20(11):1395–405. doi:10.1093/intimm/dxn105
8. Mor G, Cardenas I, Abrahams V, Guller S. Inflammation and pregnancy: the role of the immune system at the implantation site. *Ann N Y Acad Sci* (2011) 1221:80–7. doi:10.1111/j.1749-6632.2010.05938.x
9. Aluvihare VR, Kallikourdis M, Betz AG. Regulatory T cells mediate maternal tolerance to the fetus. *Nat Immunol* (2004) 5(3):266–71. doi:10.1038/ni1037
10. Cherrier M, Ohnmacht C, Cording S, Eberl G. Development and function of intestinal innate lymphoid cells. *Curr Opin Immunol* (2012) 24(3):277–83. doi:10.1016/j.coi.2012.03.011
11. Monticelli LA, Sonnenberg GF, Abt MC, Alenghat T, Ziegler CG, Doering TA, et al. Innate lymphoid cells promote lung-tissue homeostasis after infection with influenza virus. *Nat Immunol* (2011) 12(11):1045–54. doi:10.1031/ni.2131
12. Vacca P, Montaldo E, Croxatto D, Loiacono F, Canegallo F, Venturini PL, et al. Identification of diverse innate lymphoid cells in human decidua. *Mucosal Immunol* (2015) 8(2):254–64. doi:10.1038/mi.2014.63
13. Klose CS, Artis D. Innate lymphoid cells as regulators of immunity, inflammation and tissue homeostasis. *Nat Immunol* (2016) 17(7):765–74. doi:10.1038/ni.3489
14. Villanova F, Flutter B, Tosi I, Grys K, Sreeneebus H, Perera GK, et al. Characterization of innate lymphoid cells in human skin and blood demonstrates increase of NKp44+ ILC3 in psoriasis. *J Invest Dermatol* (2014) 134(4):984–91. doi:10.1038/jid.2013.477
15. Diefenbach A, Colonna M, Romagnani C. The ILC world revisited. *Immunity* (2017) 46(3):327–32. doi:10.1016/j.immuni.2017.03.008
16. Colonna M. Innate lymphoid cells: diversity, plasticity, and unique functions in immunity. *Immunity* (2018) 48(6):1104–17. doi:10.1016/j.immuni.2018.05.013
17. Montaldo E, Vacca P, Moretta L, Mingari MC. Development of human natural killer cells and other innate lymphoid cells. *Semin Immunol* (2014) 26(2):107–13. doi:10.1016/j.smim.2014.01.006
18. Vacca P, Montaldo E, Croxatto D, Moretta F, Bertaina A, Vitale C, et al. NK cells and other innate lymphoid cells in hematopoietic stem cell transplantation. *Front Immunol* (2016) 7:188. doi:10.3389/fimmu.2016.00188
19. Moretta A, Bottino C, Vitale M, Pende D, Biassoni R, Mingari MC, et al. Receptors for HLA class-I molecules in human natural killer cells. *Annu Rev Immunol* (1996) 14:619–48. doi:10.1146/annurev.immunol.14.1.619
20. Moretta A, Bottino C, Vitale M, Pende D, Cantoni C, Mingari MC, et al. Activating receptors and coreceptors involved in human natural killer cell-mediated cytolysis. *Annu Rev Immunol* (2001) 19:197–223. doi:10.1146/annurev.immunol.19.1.197
21. Eberl G, Di Santo JP, Vivier E. The brave new world of innate lymphoid cells. *Nat Immunol* (2014) 16(1):1–5. doi:10.1038/ni.3059
22. McKenzie AN, Spits H, Eberl G. Innate lymphoid cells in inflammation and immunity. *Immunity* (2014) 41(3):366–74. doi:10.1016/j.immuni.2014.09.006
23. Bernink JH, Peters CP, Munneke M, te Velde AA, Meijer SL, Weijer K, et al. Human type 1 innate lymphoid cells accumulate in inflamed mucosal tissues. *Nat Immunol* (2013) 14(3):221–9. doi:10.1038/ni.2534
24. Fuchs A, Vermi W, Lee JS, Lonardi S, Gilfillan S, Newberry RD, et al. Intraepithelial type 1 innate lymphoid cells are a unique subset of IL-12- and IL-15-responsive IFN-gamma-producing cells. *Immunity* (2013) 38(4):769–81. doi:10.1016/j.immuni.2013.02.010
25. Diefenbach A, Colonna M, Koyasu S. Development, differentiation, and diversity of innate lymphoid cells. *Immunity* (2014) 41(3):354–65. doi:10.1016/j.immuni.2014.09.005
26. Lee JS, Cella M, McDonald KG, Garlanda C, Kennedy GD, Nukaya M, et al. AHR drives the development of gut ILC22 cells and postnatal lymphoid tissues via pathways dependent on and independent of Notch. *Nat Immunol* (2011) 13(2):144–51. doi:10.1038/ni.2187
27. Montaldo E, Juelke K, Romagnani C. Group 3 innate lymphoid cells (ILC3s): origin, differentiation, and plasticity in humans and mice. *Eur J Immunol* (2015) 45(8):2171–82. doi:10.1002/eji.201545598
28. Montaldo E, Teixeira-Alves LG, Glatzer T, Durek P, Stervbo U, Hamann W, et al. Human RORgammat(+)CD34(+) cells are lineage-specified progenitors of group 3 RORgammat(+) innate lymphoid cells. *Immunity* (2014) 41(6):988–1000. doi:10.1016/j.immuni.2014.11.010
29. Lim AI, Verrier T, Vosshenrich CA, Di Santo JP. Developmental options and functional plasticity of innate lymphoid cells. *Curr Opin Immunol* (2017) 44:61–8. doi:10.1016/j.coi.2017.03.010
30. Cella M, Otero K, Colonna M. Expansion of human NK-22 cells with IL-7, IL-2, and IL-1beta reveals intrinsic functional plasticity. *Proc Natl Acad Sci U S A* (2010) 107(24):10961–6. doi:10.1073/pnas.1005641107
31. Spits H, Cupedo T. Innate lymphoid cells: emerging insights in development, lineage relationships, and function. *Annu Rev Immunol* (2012) 30:647–75. doi:10.1146/annurev-immunol-020711-075053
32. Vacca P, Mingari MC, Moretta L. Natural killer cells in human pregnancy. *J Reprod Immunol* (2013) 97(1):14–9. doi:10.1016/j.jri.2012.10.008
33. Le Bouteiller P, Tabiasco J. Killers become builders during pregnancy. *Nat Med* (2006) 12(9):991–2. doi:10.1038/nm0906-991
34. Marcenaro E, Della Chiesa M, Bellora F, Parolini S, Millo R, Moretta L, et al. IL-12 or IL-4 prime human NK cells to mediate functionally divergent interactions with dendritic cells or tumors. *J Immunol* (2005) 174(7):3992–8. doi:10.4049/jimmunol.174.7.3992
35. Moffett-King A, Entrican G, Ellis S, Hutchinson J, Bainbridge D. Natural killer cells and reproduction. *Trends Immunol* (2002) 23(7):332–3. doi:10.1016/S1471-4906(02)02261-5
36. Verma S, King A, Loke YW. Expression of killer cell inhibitory receptors on human uterine natural killer cells. *Eur J Immunol* (1997) 27(4):979–83. doi:10.1002/eji.1830270426
37. Geiselhart A, Dietl J, Marzusch K, Ruck P, Ruck M, Horny HP, et al. Comparative analysis of the immunophenotypes of decidual and peripheral blood large granular lymphocytes and T cells during early human pregnancy. *Am J Reprod Immunol* (1995) 33(4):315–22. doi:10.1111/j.1600-0897.1995.tb00900.x
38. Sedlmayr P, Schallhammer L, Hammer A, Wilders-Truschnig M, Wintersteiger R, Dohr G. Differential phenotypic properties of human peripheral blood CD56dim+ and CD56bright+ natural killer cell subpopulations. *Int Arch Allergy Immunol* (1996) 110(4):308–13. doi:10.1159/000237321
39. Vacca P, Pietra G, Falco M, Romeo E, Bottino C, Bellora F, et al. Analysis of natural killer cells isolated from human decidua: Evidence that 2B4 (CD244) functions as an inhibitory receptor and blocks NK-cell function. *Blood* (2006) 108(13):4078–85. doi:10.1182/blood-2006-04-017343
40. Chiossone L, Vacca P, Orecchia P, Croxatto D, Damonte P, Astigiano S, et al. In vivo generation of decidual natural killer cells from resident hematopoietic progenitors. *Haematologica* (2014) 99(3):448–57. doi:10.3324/haematol.2013.091421
41. Montaldo E, Vacca P, Chiossone L, Croxatto D, Loiacono F, Martini S, et al. Unique eomes(+) NK cell subsets are present in uterus and decidua during early pregnancy. *Front Immunol* (2015) 6:646. doi:10.3389/fimmu.2015.00646

42. Gaynor LM, Colucci F. Uterine natural killer cells: functional distinctions and influence on pregnancy in humans and mice. *Front Immunol* (2017) 8:467. doi:10.3389/fimmu.2017.00467
43. Doisne JM, Balmas E, Boulenouar S, Gaynor LM, Kieckbusch J, Gardner L, et al. Composition, development, and function of uterine innate lymphoid cells. *J Immunol* (2015) 195(8):3937–45. doi:10.4049/jimmunol.1500689
44. Boulenouar S, Doisne JM, Sferruzzi-Perri A, Gaynor LM, Kieckbusch J, Balmas E, et al. The residual innate lymphoid cells in NFIL3-deficient mice support suboptimal maternal adaptations to pregnancy. *Front Immunol* (2016) 7:43. doi:10.3389/fimmu.2016.00043
45. Fu B, Zhou Y, Ni X, Tong X, Xu X, Dong Z, et al. Natural killer cells promote fetal development through the secretion of growth-promoting factors. *Immunity* (2017) 47(6):1100–13e6. doi:10.1016/j.immuni.2017.11.018
46. Xu Y, Romero R, Miller D, Silva P, Panaitescu B, Theis KR, et al. Innate lymphoid cells at the human maternal-fetal interface in spontaneous preterm labor. *Am J Reprod Immunol* (2018) 79(6):e12820. doi:10.1111/aji.12820
47. Carlino C, Stabile H, Morrone S, Bulla R, Soriani A, Agostinis C, et al. Recruitment of circulating NK cells through decidual tissues: a possible mechanism controlling NK cell accumulation in the uterus during early pregnancy. *Blood* (2008) 111(6):3108–15. doi:10.1182/blood-2007-08-105965
48. Santoni A, Carlino C, Stabile H, Gismondi A. Mechanisms underlying recruitment and accumulation of decidual NK cells in uterus during pregnancy. *Am J Reprod Immunol* (2008) 59(5):417–24. doi:10.1111/j.1600-0897.2008.00598.x
49. Male V, Hughes T, McClory S, Colucci F, Caligiuri MA, Moffett A. Immature NK cells, capable of producing IL-22, are present in human uterine mucosa. *J Immunol* (2010) 185(7):3913–8. doi:10.4049/jimmunol.1001637
50. Vacca P, Vitale C, Montaldo E, Conte R, Cantoni C, Fulcheri E, et al. CD34+ hematopoietic precursors are present in human decidua and differentiate into natural killer cells upon interaction with stromal cells. *Proc Natl Acad Sci U S A* (2011) 108(6):2402–7. doi:10.1073/pnas.1016257108
51. Keskin DB, Allan DS, Rybalov B, Andzelm MM, Stern JN, Kopcow HD, et al. TGFbeta promotes conversion of CD16+ peripheral blood NK cells into CD16- NK cells with similarities to decidual NK cells. *Proc Natl Acad Sci U S A* (2007) 104(9):3378–83. doi:10.1073/pnas.0611098104
52. Croxatto D, Vacca P, Canegallo F, Conte R, Venturini PL, Moretta L, et al. Stromal cells from human decidua exert a strong inhibitory effect on NK cell function and dendritic cell differentiation. *PLoS One* (2014) 9(2):e89006. doi:10.1371/journal.pone.0089006
53. Ahn YO, Blazar BR, Miller JS, Verneris MR. Lineage relationships of human interleukin-22-producing CD56+ RORgammat+ innate lymphoid cells and conventional natural killer cells. *Blood* (2013) 121(12):2234–43. doi:10.1182/blood-2012-07-440099
54. Montaldo E, Vitale C, Cottalasso F, Conte R, Glatzer T, Ambrosini P, et al. Human NK cells at early stages of differentiation produce CXCL8 and express CD161 molecule that functions as an activating receptor. *Blood* (2012) 119(17):3987–96. doi:10.1182/blood-2011-09-379693
55. Guma M, Angulo A, Vilches C, Gomez-Lozano N, Malats N, Lopez-Botet M. Imprint of human cytomegalovirus infection on the NK cell receptor repertoire. *Blood* (2004) 104(12):3664–71. doi:10.1182/blood-2004-05-2058
56. Guma M, Budt M, Saez A, Brckalo T, Hengel H, Angulo A, et al. Expansion of CD94/NKG2C+ NK cells in response to human cytomegalovirus-infected fibroblasts. *Blood* (2006) 107(9):3624–31. doi:10.1182/blood-2005-09-3682
57. Paust S, Gill HS, Wang BZ, Flynn MP, Moseman EA, Senman B, et al. Critical role for the chemokine receptor CXCR6 in NK cell-mediated antigen-specific memory of haptens and viruses. *Nat Immunol* (2010) 11(12):1127–35. doi:10.1038/ni.1953
58. Sun JC, Beilke JN, Lanier LL. Adaptive immune features of natural killer cells. *Nature* (2009) 457(7229):557–61. doi:10.1038/nature07665
59. Netea MG, Joosten LA, Latz E, Mills KH, Natoli G, Stunnenberg HG, et al. Trained immunity: a program of innate immune memory in health and disease. *Science* (2016) 352(6284):aaf1098. doi:10.1126/science.aaf1098
60. Della Chiesa M, Sivori S, Carlomagno S, Moretta L, Moretta A. Activating KIRs and NKG2C in viral infections: toward NK cell memory? *Front Immunol* (2015) 6:573. doi:10.3389/fimmu.2015.00573
61. Prefumo F, Canini S, Casagrande V, Pastorino D, Venturini PL, De Biasio P. Correlation between first-trimester uterine artery Doppler indices and maternal serum free beta-human chorionic gonadotropin and pregnancy-associated plasma protein A. *Fertil Steril* (2006) 86(4):977–80. doi:10.1016/j.fertnstert.2006.01.063
62. Kozuki N, Lee AC, Silveira MF, Sania A, Vogel JP, Adair L, et al. The associations of parity and maternal age with small-for-gestational-age, preterm, and neonatal and infant mortality: a meta-analysis. *BMC Public Health* (2013) 13(Suppl 3):S2. doi:10.1186/1471-2458-13-S3-S2
63. Gamliel M, Goldman-Wohl D, Isaacson B, Gur C, Stein N, Yamin R, et al. Trained memory of human uterine NK cells enhances their function in subsequent pregnancies. *Immunity* (2018) 48(5):951–62e5. doi:10.1016/j.immuni.2018.03.030
64. Robertson SA. Immune regulation of conception and embryo implantation-all about quality control? *J Reprod Immunol* (2010) 85(1):51–7. doi:10.1016/j.jri.2010.01.008
65. Sonnenberg GF, Artis D. Innate lymphoid cells in the initiation, regulation and resolution of inflammation. *Nat Med* (2015) 21(7):698–708. doi:10.1038/nm.3892
66. Amsalem H, Kwan M, Hazan A, Zhang J, Jones RL, Whittle W, et al. Identification of a novel neutrophil population: proangiogenic granulocytes in second-trimester human decidua. *J Immunol* (2014) 193(6):3070–9. doi:10.4049/jimmunol.1303117
67. Croxatto D, Micheletti A, Montaldo E, Orecchia P, Loiacono F, Canegallo F, et al. Group 3 innate lymphoid cells regulate neutrophil migration and function in human decidua. *Mucosal Immunol* (2016) 9(6):1372–83. doi:10.1038/mi.2016.10
68. Magri G, Miyajima M, Bascones S, Mortha A, Puga I, Cassis L, et al. Innate lymphoid cells integrate stromal and immunological signals to enhance antibody production by splenic marginal zone B cells. *Nat Immunol* (2014) 15(4):354–64. doi:10.1038/ni.2830
69. Jessmon P, Leach RE, Armant DR. Diverse functions of HBEGF during pregnancy. *Mol Reprod Dev* (2009) 76(12):1116–27. doi:10.1002/mrd.21066
70. Vinante F, Marchi M, Rigo A, Scapini P, Pizzolo G, Cassatella MA. Granulocyte-macrophage colony-stimulating factor induces expression of heparin-binding epidermal growth factor-like growth factor/diphtheria toxin receptor and sensitivity to diphtheria toxin in human neutrophils. *Blood* (1999) 94(9):3169–77.
71. Costantini C, Cassatella MA. The defensive alliance between neutrophils and NK cells as a novel arm of innate immunity. *J Leukoc Biol* (2011) 89(2):221–33. doi:10.1189/jlb.0510250
72. Costantini C, Micheletti A, Calzetti F, Perbellini O, Pizzolo G, Cassatella MA. Neutrophil activation and survival are modulated by interaction with NK cells. *Int Immunol* (2010) 22(10):827–38. doi:10.1093/intimm/dxq434
73. Scapini P, Cassatella MA. Social networking of human neutrophils within the immune system. *Blood* (2014) 124(5):710–9. doi:10.1182/blood-2014-03-453217
74. Thoren FB, Riise RE, Ousback J, Della Chiesa M, Alsterholm M, Marcenaro E, et al. Human NK Cells induce neutrophil apoptosis via an NKp46- and Fas-dependent mechanism. *J Immunol* (2012) 188(4):1668–74. doi:10.4049/jimmunol.1102002
75. Kieckbusch J, Gaynor LM, Moffett A, Colucci F. MHC-dependent inhibition of uterine NK cells impedes fetal growth and decidual vascular remodelling. *Nat Commun* (2014) 5:3359. doi:10.1038/ncomms4359
76. Kopcow HD, Allan DS, Chen X, Rybalov B, Andzelm MM, Ge B, et al. Human decidual NK cells form immature activating synapses and are not cytotoxic. *Proc Natl Acad Sci U S A* (2005) 102(43):15563–8. doi:10.1073/pnas.0507835102
77. Inada K, Shima T, Nakashima A, Aoki K, Ito M, Saito S. Characterization of regulatory T cells in decidua of miscarriage cases with abnormal or normal fetal chromosomal content. *J Reprod Immunol* (2013) 97(1):104–11. doi:10.1016/j.jri.2012.12.001
78. Tilburgs T, Roelen DL, van der Mast BJ, de Groot-Swings GM, Kleijburg C, Scherjon SA, et al. Evidence for a selective migration of fetus-specific CD4+CD25bright regulatory T cells from the peripheral blood to the decidua in human pregnancy. *J Immunol* (2008) 180(8):5737–45. doi:10.4049/jimmunol.180.8.5737
79. Kammerer U, Eggert AO, Kapp M, McLellan AD, Geijtenbeek TB, Dietl J, et al. Unique appearance of proliferating antigen-presenting cells expressing DC-SIGN (CD209) in the decidua of early human pregnancy. *Am J Pathol* (2003) 162(3):887–96. doi:10.1016/S0002-9440(10)63884-9
80. Gustafsson C, Mjosberg J, Matussek A, Geffers R, Matthiesen L, Berg G, et al. Gene expression profiling of human decidual macrophages: evidence for

immunosuppressive phenotype. *PLoS One* (2008) 3(4):e2078. doi:10.1371/journal.pone.0002078

81. Vacca P, Cantoni C, Vitale M, Prato C, Canegallo F, Fenoglio D, et al. Crosstalk between decidual NK and CD14+ myelomonocytic cells results in induction of Tregs and immunosuppression. *Proc Natl Acad Sci U S A* (2010) 107(26):11918–23. doi:10.1073/pnas.1001749107
82. Vacca P, Montaldo E, Vitale C, Croxatto D, Moretta L, Mingari MC. MSC and innate immune cell interactions: a lesson from human decidua. *Immunol Lett* (2015) 168(2):170–4. doi:10.1016/j.imlet.2015.05.006
83. Erkers T, Nava S, Yosef J, Ringden O, Kaipe H. Decidual stromal cells promote regulatory T cells and suppress alloreactivity in a cell contact-dependent manner. *Stem Cells Dev* (2013) 22(19):2596–605. doi:10.1089/scd.2013.0079
84. He YY, He XJ, Guo PF, Du MR, Shao J, Li MQ, et al. The decidual stromal cells-secreted CCL2 induces and maintains decidual leukocytes into Th2 bias in human early pregnancy. *Clin Immunol* (2012) 145(2):161–73. doi:10.1016/j.clim.2012.07.017

15

Progesterone Modulation of Pregnancy-Related Immune Responses

*Nishel M. Shah[1], Nesrina Imami[2] and Mark R. Johnson[1]**

[1] *Department of Surgery and Cancer, Imperial College London, Chelsea and Westminster Hospital, London, United Kingdom,*
[2] *Department of Medicine, Imperial College London, Chelsea and Westminster Hospital, London, United Kingdom*

Correspondence:
Mark R. Johnson
mark.johnson@imperial.ac.uk

Progesterone (P4) is an important steroid hormone for the establishment and maintenance of pregnancy and its functional withdrawal in reproductive tissue is linked with the onset of parturition. However, the effects of P4 on adaptive immune responses are poorly understood. In this study, we took a novel approach by comparing the effects of P4 supplementation longitudinally, with treatment using a P4 antagonist mifepristone (RU486) in mid-trimester pregnancies. Thus, we were able to demonstrate the immune-modulatory functions of P4. We show that, in pregnancy, the immune system is increasingly activated (CD38, CCR6) with greater antigen-specific cytotoxic T cell responses (granzyme B). Simultaneously, pregnancy promotes a tolerant immune environment (IL-10 and regulatory-T cells) that gradually reverses prior to the onset of labor. P4 suppresses and RU486 enhances antigen-specific CD4 and CD8 T cell inflammatory cytokine (IFN-γ) and cytotoxic molecule release (granzyme B). P4 and RU486 effectively modulate immune cell-mediated interactions, by regulating differentiated memory T cell subset sensitivity to antigen stimulation. Our results indicate that P4 and RU486, as immune modulators, share a reciprocal relationship. These data unveil key contributions of P4 to the modulation of the maternal immune system and suggests targets for future modulation of maternal immune function during pregnancy.

Keywords: pregnancy, progesterone, RU486, immune modulation, immune response

INTRODUCTION

Progesterone (P4) plays a key role in the establishment and maintenance of pregnancy and its withdrawal causes the onset of labor (1, 2). In humans, the production of P4 gradually rises throughout pregnancy; the corpus luteum is the major source in early pregnancy, but after 8 weeks, the placenta takes over (1). P4 and its metabolites work through a series of nuclear P4 (PR) and glucocorticoid (GR) receptors, as well as membrane-bound P4 receptors (mPR), to exert their effects (3–5). The majority of P4 actions on immune function are mediated by its interactions with GR (6–9). Human PBMCs are thought to express a number of endocrine receptors including: mPR, GR, and estrogen receptors (4, 6, 7, 10). In murine models, GR engagement increases regulatory T cell (Treg) immune-suppressive function, and P4 binding to GR is thought to be responsible for this finding in pregnancy (8, 9). In humans, GR agonists have been shown to increase apoptosis of $CD4^+$ T cells *via* the GR (7). In contrast to most animal models of pregnancy, where there is a systemic withdrawal of P4 prior to the onset of labor, in the human, the literature suggests that there is a functional withdrawal at the level of the PR at the end of pregnancy (11). In particular, there are differences seen in the level of expression of P4 receptor isoforms, P4 receptor gene polymorphisms in reproductive tissue, and a decline in secretion of a lymphocyte-derived immunomodulatory protein known as P4-induced blocking factor (PIBF) (1, 11). P4 acts, either directly, or indirectly through PIBF, to modulate the immune system to achieve a successful pregnancy. These include promoting a T_H2-dominant cytokine profile and upregulating HLA-G expression on trophoblast, which enables γδ T-cell activation and evasion of host defenses by acting as a ligand for inhibitory receptors on natural killer (NK) cells (1, 12–14). In fact, PIBF is a potent suppressor of cytotoxic immune cells and regulator of cytokine secretion (11, 15).

Pregnancy is associated with a series of immune adaptations that begin pre-implantation and span the length of the antenatal and postnatal period (16–18). As a result, maternal immune responses are different compared to non-pregnant women, and they fluctuate during the course of pregnancy (19, 20). In fact, some autoimmune conditions, such as rheumatoid arthritis, enter remission during pregnancy, but flare up in the postnatal period (21). Although clinical trials using HRT in women with rheumatoid arthritis have not shown the same effect as pregnancy, animal models using pregnancy-like levels of hormones have shown promising findings (22). In clinical practice, P4 supplementation is used in pregnancy as an effective treatment for the prevention of preterm birth (23). Its effects are likely to be a combination of immune modulation and a reversal of the functional withdrawal of P4 action in reproductive tissue. Spontaneous labor is associated with a loss of suppression of syngeneic and allogeneic T-cell responses (24). Interestingly, gestational changes are seen *ex vivo* where fetal-specific T effector memory (T_{EM}) cells and detectable fetal DNA are longitudinally increased in pregnancy (18). Peripheral blood IFN-γ, IL-4 spontaneous responses, and paternal antigen stimulated responses, measured using enzyme-linked immunospot (ELISpot), appear to peak at 35 weeks of pregnancy (19).

We investigated the hypothesis that in the peripheral circulation during pregnancy, P4 actively suppresses CD4 and CD8 T cell inflammatory cytokine and cytotoxic molecule production. In addition, we hypothesized that P4 alters T cell, NK cell, and dendritic cell (DC) phenotype to regulate immune responses. To determine the effects of P4, we began by determining the gestational changes in immune responses and leukocyte phenotype, longitudinally, in healthy uncomplicated pregnancies, which we expected may be affected by the use of P4. We then compared this cohort of patients to those supplemented with vaginal P4. Finally, to understand the potential effects of P4 antagonism in a clinical setting, we recruited patients receiving the most widely used P4 antagonist mifepristone (RU486) in second trimester pregnancies and analyzed its effects longitudinally. Our study takes a novel approach by comparing the effects of P4 supplementation and the use of RU486 in pregnancy. Importantly, this is the first study to investigate the immune-modulatory effects of RU486, *in vivo*, in the mid second trimester of pregnancy. We found that advancing pregnancy may be associated with an inherent loss of sensitivity to P4. More importantly, P4 reduces pro-inflammatory and cytotoxic T cell responses. It achieves this by a combination of effects to modulate immune cell-mediated interactions, including memory T cell antigen sensitivity and regulation of leukocyte migration.

MATERIALS AND METHODS

Ethics Statement

All subjects were recruited from Chelsea and Westminster Hospital, London, UK. This study was carried out in accordance with the recommendations of National Institute of Health Research (NIHR) Good Clinical Practice guidelines, and a NHS Research Ethics Committee. The protocol was approved by the National Research Ethics Service (NRES), London, UK committee as well as by Chelsea and Westminster NHS Trust, London, UK; Ref: 11/LO/0971. All subjects gave written informed consent in accordance with the Declaration of Helsinki.

Study Design

Based on the premise that maternal peripheral blood will provide a window to the systemic effects of P4 in pregnancy, a combination of ELISpot, 9-parameter flow cytometry, and multiplex assays were developed to assess functional cellular responses and leukocyte phenotype. A standardized protocol was used for all samples to ensure consistency and comparability. Blood samples were processed within 2 h of collection and all phenotypic and functional work was performed on fresh samples.

Study Participants

For the control group, healthy pregnant patients ($N = 42$) were recruited from the antenatal clinic from April 2013 to September 2014 at Chelsea and Westminster Hospital during their first visit before 20 weeks of gestation. These patients had no previous history of premature delivery defined as less than 37 weeks of gestation. Women with a history of previous vaginal deliveries were not excluded so that the sample population was comparable to the P4 supplemented cohort, which were often started on P4 due to a previous history. Once recruited, these patients were asked to provide peripheral blood samples longitudinally. The time points for sample collection were: at recruitment (range 11–20 weeks of gestation), 28, 34 weeks, in labor or at delivery, 24 h postnatal, and 6–8 weeks postnatal.

Pregnant patients receiving P4 supplementation ($N = 15$) (once a day Cyclogest® 400 mg per vaginum/rectum, Actavis UK) were recruited from the preterm antenatal clinic at Chelsea and Westminster Hospital between April 2013 and September 2014, ideally prior to 20 weeks of gestation (range 17–20 weeks of gestation). These patients were commenced on P4 due to: a previous history of preterm labor and delivery, second trimester loss, or ultrasonographic evidence of cervical shortening of <25 mm, which carries a significantly increased risk of preterm delivery at ≤32 weeks of gestation (23). These patients continued P4 treatment until 34 weeks of gestation. For these patients, the time points for longitudinal sample collection were: at recruitment, 28, 34, and 36 weeks of gestation. Since exogenous vaginal P4 (100 mg tablets) has a terminal half-life of approximately 14 h, the effect of P4 was thought to have substantially declined by the 36 weeks of gestation (25). The effects of supplementary P4 should disappear in the postnatal period. Since treatment stopped at 34 weeks of gestation, no differences were expected between the P4 treated and control subjects, and so these were not compared.

In order to understand the effects of P4 antagonism, pregnant patients ($N = 8$) undergoing medically indicated terminations of pregnancy due to fetal anomaly in an otherwise uncomplicated pregnancy were recruited from the fetal medicine unit at Chelsea and Westminster Hospital, from June 2013 to May 2015. As part of the termination process, these patients received RU486 (once only Mifegyne® 400 mg orally, Nordic Pharma UK) and then attended the hospital for prostaglandin-induced labor 2 days later. Once recruited, these patients were asked to provide peripheral blood samples prior to taking RU486, 48 and 72 h post RU486, which was 24 h post-delivery. The mean gestation at delivery was 19 weeks (SD ± 1.8).

Study inclusion criteria included: age at booking under 40 years as replicative senescence, immune exhaustion, and thymic output is age linked with the latter reduced beyond 40 years of age (26). Exclusion criteria included: failure to meet the inclusion criteria; the development of or past medical history of any pregnancy related or unrelated complications that affected the course of pregnancy, such as pre-eclampsia, gestational diabetes, or intrauterine growth restriction as well as any autoimmune, hypertensive, or renal conditions. Demographic data are summarized in Table S1 in Supplementary Material.

Non-pregnant female control samples were obtained from individuals working in the Centre for Immunology and Vaccinology, Imperial College London, UK and clinical staff working in the Maternity Department, Chelsea and Westminster Hospital.

Preparation of Cells

Approximately 35 ml of peripheral blood was obtained using a Vacutainer™ system and using 6 ml lithium heparin blood collection tubes (Becton Dickinson, Oxford, UK). PBMCs from adult peripheral blood were prepared by density gradient centrifuge on Histopaque (Sigma-Aldrich, Dorset, UK) as described previously (27). Viability was determined using a trypan blue exclusion test of cell viability and samples where this was greater than 80% were used. For functional work, the cells were suspended in TCM [RPMI-1640 with Penicillin and Streptomycin (Sigma-Aldrich), at final concentrations of 100 IU/ml and 100 µg/ml, and L-glutamine (Sigma-Aldrich) at a final concentration of 2 mM], and for phenotype the cells were suspended in Ca^{2+} and Mg^{2+} containing PBS (Sigma-Aldrich). All ELISpot and flow cytometry assays were performed on fresh samples. Processing was commenced within 2 h of obtaining peripheral blood. Plasma for multiplex immunoassay was collected, aliquoted, and stored at −80°C until use.

ELISpot Assay

IFN-γ, IL-10, IL-4, and Granzyme B ELISpot assays were performed in order to detect recall antigen/peptide specific T cell responses as previously described (28). Briefly, 1×10^5 PBMC/well were cultured in 10% (heat-inactivated) male AB plasma-RPMI (200 µl/well, Sigma-Aldrich) in 96-well polyvinylidene difluoride backed plates (Merck Millipore, Hertfordshire, UK), which were coated in antibodies for the cytokines and proteases of interest, namely IFN-γ, IL-10, Granzyme B, and IL-4 (MabTech, Nacka Strand, Sweden). PBMCs, in duplicate wells, were stimulated with 100 µl of an antigen/peptide pool obtained from NIBSC (NIBSC, Hertfordshire, UK) and Virion-Serion (Virion-Serion, Würzburg, Germany) at the manufacturer's recommended concentrations. These included: EBV, CMV, influenza A, measles, and HSV whole lysates; purified protein derivative (PPD) of *M. Tuberculosis* Tuberculin; purified tetanus toxoid (TTOX); and flu/EBV/influenza (FEC) peptide pool. Positive and negative controls were provided by phytohemagglutinin (5 µg/ml) and TCM. The plate was incubated at 37°C in 5% CO_2 for 48 h for anti IFN-γ, IL-10, and Granzyme B coated and 96 h for anti-IL-4 coated plates. Detection of spot forming cells (SFC) was carried out by the addition of biotinylated anti IFN-γ, IL-10, Granzyme B, or IL-4 (MabTech) and incubation, followed by the use of a concentrated streptavidin-alkaline phosphatase conjugate (MabTech). Finally, the development step required the use of a chromogen prepared from a premixed BCIP/NBT substrate kit (BioRad labouratories Ltd., Hertfordshire, UK). Spot reading and counting was performed using an AID ELISpot reader (Oxford Biosystems Cadama, Oxfordshire, UK).

Flow Cytometric Leukocyte Quantification

Multicolor color flow cytometry was used to phenotype CD4 and CD8 T-cell subsets, NK cells, and DC. In order to evaluate T cell subtypes, PBMCs were stained with the following murine, anti-human monoclonal antibodies according to the manufacturer's instructions: peridinin chlorophyll protein (PerCP) Cy5.5-labeled anti-CD3 (Biolegend, London, UK); allophyocyanin (APC)-H7-conjugated anti-CD8 (Biolegend); BD Horizon V450-labeled anti-CD38 (BD Biosciences, Oxford, UK), anti-CD127 (BD), and anti-CCR4 (BD); BD Horizon V500-labeled anti-HLA-DR (BD) and anti-CD4 (BD); fluorescein isothiocyanate (FITC)-labeled anti-CD31 (BD), anti-CD25 (BD), anti-CCR6 (R&D Systems, Abingdon, UK) and anti-PIBF (rabbit polyclonal; Biorbyt, Cambridge, UK); phycoerythrin (PE)-conjugated anti-CCR7 (R&D), anti-CCR5 (BD) and anti-CCR3 (BD); APC-labeled anti-CD28 (BD), anti-HLA-G (eBioscience, Cheshire, UK), anti-CXCR3 (BD); PECy7-labeled anti-CD45RA (BD), anti-CD45RO (BD) and anti-CXCR4 (BD). NK subsets were phenotyped with: BD Horizon V450-labeled anti-CD56 (BD); FITC-labeled anti-PIBF; PE-labeled anti-iNKT (BD); APC-labeled anti-TCR-γδ (BD); PE-Cy7-labeled anti-CD16 (BD); and PerCP-Cy 5.5-labeled anti-CD3. Approximately 2×10^6 cells were stained per tube, incubated in the dark at room temperature for 30 min, washed with PBS, and fixed with BD stabilizing fixative (BD Biosciences), before acquisition within 24 h. At least 100,000 events were acquired on a 3-laser flow cytometer (BD Biosciences LSR II) and subsequently gated according to respective isotype controls.

Dendritic cell of myeloid and plasmacytoid lineage, as well as HLA-G expressing tolerant variants were identified using the antibodies: Qdot® 605-labeled anti-CD3 and anti-CD19 (Invitrogen, Paisley, UK); BD Horizon V450-labeled anti-CD11c (BD); BD Horizon V500-labeled HLA-DR; FITC-labeled anti-CD16 (BD); PE-labeled anti-ILT4 (eBioscience); APC-labeled anti-HLA-G (eBioscience); PE-Cy7-labeled anti-CD83 (BD); PerCP-Cy 5.5-labeled CD123 (BD); and APC-H7-labeled anti-CD14 (BD). A minimum of 500,000 events were acquired according to the description detailed above. Analysis of flow cytometric data was performed using FlowJo version 7.65 (Tree Star Inc., Ashland, OR, USA).

Multiplex Immunoassay

A human 17-plex Bio-Plex Pro® Multiplex immunoassay kit (BioRad) was used to determine plasma cytokine and chemokine concentrations. The kit contained the following cytokines: G-CSF, GM-CSF, IFN-γ, IL-1β, IL-2, IL-4, IL-5, IL-6, IL-7, IL-8, IL-10, IL-12 (p70), IL-13, IL-17, MCP-1 (MCAF), MIP-1β, TNF-α. The multiplex immunoassay was performed according to the manufacturer's instructions and assays were read using a Bio-Plex© MAGPIX© reader (BioRad).

Statistics

Longitudinal analysis of un-supplemented pregnancies was undertaken using mixed-effects modeling to avoid a loss of statistical power by omitting patients with incomplete data. For normally distributed data, a linear mixed effects model was used, and pairwise multiple comparisons of estimated marginal means with sequential Bonferroni correction was performed where the main effect was significant. Where data did not follow a normal distribution, a generalized linear mixed effects model with gamma log-link was used. If the main effect was significant, pairwise multiple comparisons of estimated marginal means with sequential Bonferroni correction was performed. Data were analyzed following the methods outlined by Duricki et al. and using IBM© SPSS Version 21.0 (Armonk, New York, NY, USA) for mixed effects modeling (29). In addition, longitudinal ELISpot data presented as a heatmap was produced and the analysis and presentation of distributions was performed using SPICE version 5.1, downloaded from http://exon.niaid.nih.gov. Comparison of distributions was performed using a Student's t-test and a partial permutation test as described (30).

P4 supplemented and un-supplemented pregnancies were compared using a Students t-test where the data were continuous and parametric, and for non-parametric data, Mann–Whitney U test was used. For longitudinal analysis of P4 and RU486 treated pregnancies with repeated measures and parametric data, a one-way analysis of variance (ANOVA) with multiple group comparisons and a Tukey correction was used to compare group means. For non-parametric longitudinal repeated measures, data analysis was undertaken using a Friedman test with Dunn's correction. Statistical analysis was performed on GraphPad Prism version 6.0 (GraphPad Software, San Diego, CA, USA).

Data are presented as means ± SEM or medians ± interquartile range (IQR) as appropriate for the distribution normality. All P-values were two-tailed and significance was defined as $P < 0.05$.

RESULTS

Pregnancy Promotes a Tolerant Immune Environment in the Peripheral Circulation That Gradually Reverses Prior to the Onset of Delivery

Before investigating the effects of P4, leukocyte functional and phenotypic profiles were analyzed longitudinally in un-supplemented pregnancies. This established the effects of pregnancy and advancing gestation as well as providing a control group. Baseline results from pregnant participants were compared with non-pregnant volunteers. Where longitudinal analysis in pregnancy was significant, pairwise analysis comparing with baseline, 34 weeks and labor were reported. These co-responded to recruitment, prior to the onset of labor and labor/delivery.

T cell antigen-specific responses were determined using ELISpot and the results are summarized using the heat-map in **Figure 1A**. The majority of pregnant patients at baseline produced robust IFN-γ responses that were comparable to non-pregnant volunteers (**Figures 1A–C**; Figure S1 in Supplementary Material). Irrespective of the baseline response, labor and delivery was associated with a significant peak in cellular responses to CMV (**Figure 1C**) and HSV (**Figure 1A**). IL-10 cytokine responses behaved in a similar manner to IFN-γ. Our results showed that labor and delivery was characterized by a peak in responses to measles and CMV (**Figures 1B,C**) whole lysates, as well as TTOX (Figure S1 in Supplementary Material), PPD antigens, and FEC peptide pool (**Figure 1A**). Both IFN-γ and IL-10 responses returned to non-pregnant levels in the postnatal period. In contrast to IFN-γ, pregnancy was associated with improved IL-10 cellular responses throughout its course. The majority of IL-4 responses were below the positive threshold. When measurable, IL-4 response patterns were associated with an improved response to influenza A, PPD, TTOX, FEC peptide pool, and herpesvirus antigen (**Figure 1A**; Figure S1 in Supplementary Material). However, the peak response in pregnancy was at 34 weeks of gestation and the majority of these returned to non-pregnant levels in labor or 24 h post-delivery (**Figure 1A**). Most pregnant patients had positive cytotoxic granzyme B responses at baseline, but this was not true for all non-pregnant patients where some responses fell below the threshold of 20 per 10^6 SFC. When compared to baseline, 34 weeks of pregnancy showed a significant peak in SFC and a positive response to measles whole lysate and TTOX antigen (**Figure 1B**; Figure S1 in Supplementary Material).

The changes in functional responses were reflected in the leukocyte phenotype observed. CD38 is a surface glycoprotein and enzyme that is important for cell adhesion and regulation of T cell functions including proliferation (31). CD38 expression on CD4 and CD8 T cells was reduced at recruitment and then rose with advancing gestation (**Figures 2A,D**). This occurred without a similar increase in HLA-DR expression on CD4 or CD8 T cells (not shown). In addition, we observed longitudinal increases in CCR6 expression on CD4 T cells (**Figures 2B,D**), and increased CD83 expression on both mDC and pDC (**Figures 3A,D**). CCR6 is important for mucosal immunity. As well as being expressed on T_H17 cells, the expression of CCR6 on memory T cells enables their migration in response to CCL20 to sites of inflammation (32,33). Proportions of CD28 expressing effector memory subtypes fell longitudinally during pregnancy (**Figures 2C,D**). CD28 is an important co-stimulatory marker for T cell activation. However, on memory T cells, the loss of expression correlates with greater peripheral homing and effector function (34). Concurrently, T_H17 proportions, defined using chemokine markers CCR4 and CCR6 as previously described (35), were reduced in pregnancy compared to non-pregnant controls but saw a longitudinal increase

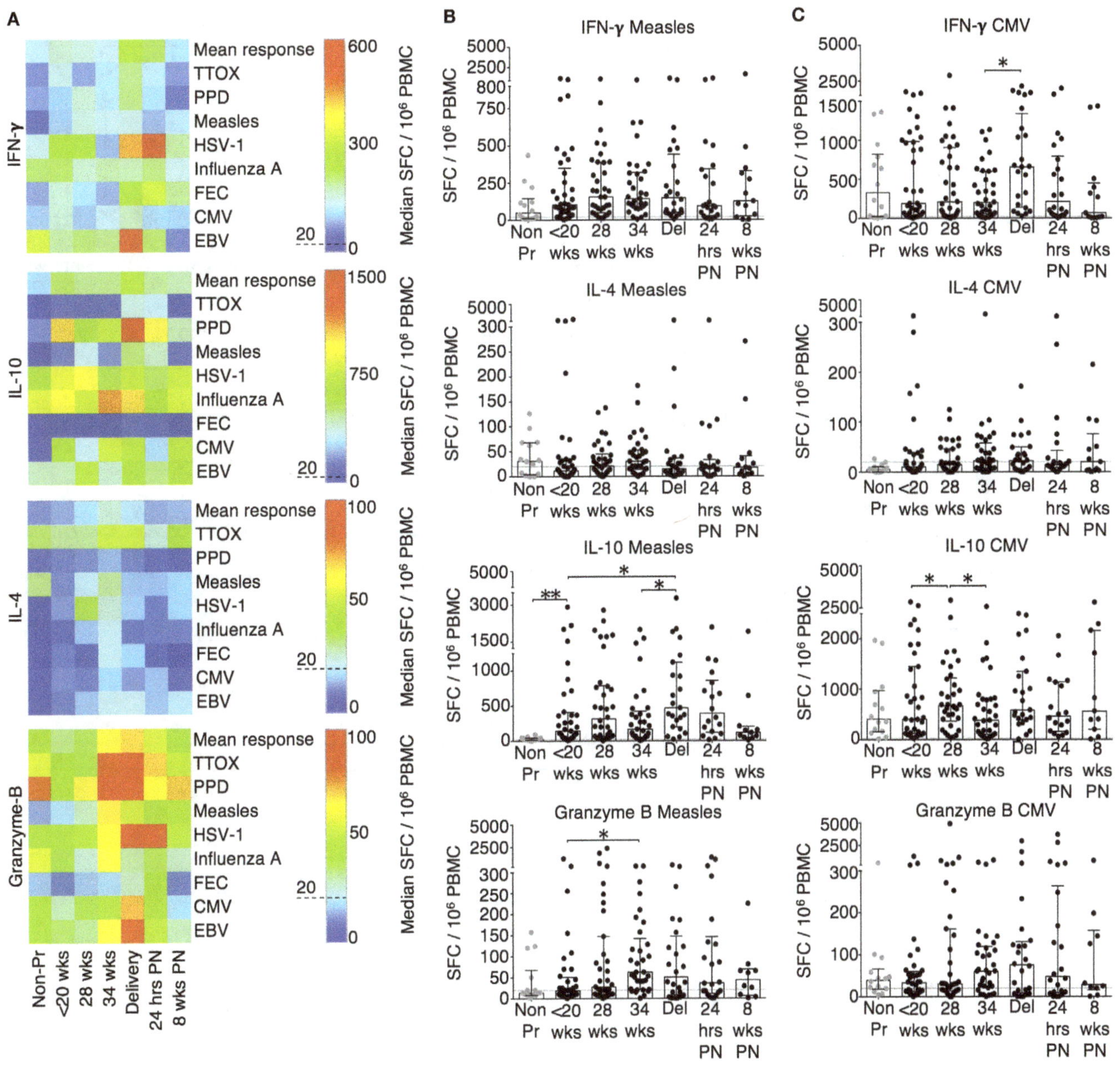

FIGURE 1 | Advancing pregnancy is associated with greater IFN-γ, IL-10, IL-4, and granzyme B ELISpot responses. **(A)** Summary heat-map of gestation specific median ELISpot responses to antigens/peptides as well as overall mean response for each analyte. The individual scales used for each cytokine is shown with the threshold of 20 spot forming cells (SFC)/10^6 PBMC indicated using a dashed line. The heat-map was generated and analyzed using SPICE (30). **(B)** ELISpot responses to measles and **(C)** CMV whole lysates. Columns indicate median and interquartile range. Gestation at sampling is indicated in pregnancy (●): < 20^{+0} weeks (*N* = *42*), 28 weeks (*N* = *35*), 34 weeks (*N* = *33*), at delivery (*N* = *24*), 24 h post-delivery (*N* = *22*), 6–8 weeks postnatal (*N* = *13*). Non-pregnant controls are depicted as ● (*N* = *14*). A dashed line represents <20 SFC/10^6. *P* values are two tailed and significance is defined as **P* < 0.05 and ***P* < 0.01. Non-pregnant and baseline pregnant data analyzed by Mann–Whitney *U* test. Longitudinal data analyzed by generalized linear mixed effects model with gamma log-link and pairwise multiple comparisons of estimated marginal means with sequential Bonferroni correction.

that peaked at 34 weeks (**Figures 3B,E**). In contrast, CD4 Treg proportions were increased in pregnancy at baseline compared to controls (**Figures 3C,F**). Collectively, these results were consistent with an initial immune suppression and its subsequent reversal during pregnancy. The perforin/granzyme pathway for target cell killing is used by both cytotoxic T lymphocytes and NK cells (36). Although CD38 expression on CD8 T cells showed a longitudinal increase in pregnancy (**Figure 2A**), the more cytotoxic NK cell subtype with the phenotype CD16$^+$CD56^{lo} (**Figure 4A**) were reduced and showed an increase in PIBF expression at 34 weeks (**Figure 4B**). Furthermore, the 9mer FEC peptide pool, which contains CD8 T cell epitopes, predominantly stimulated IL-4 and IL-10 responses (**Figure 1A**). This suggested that although we demonstrated functionally greater

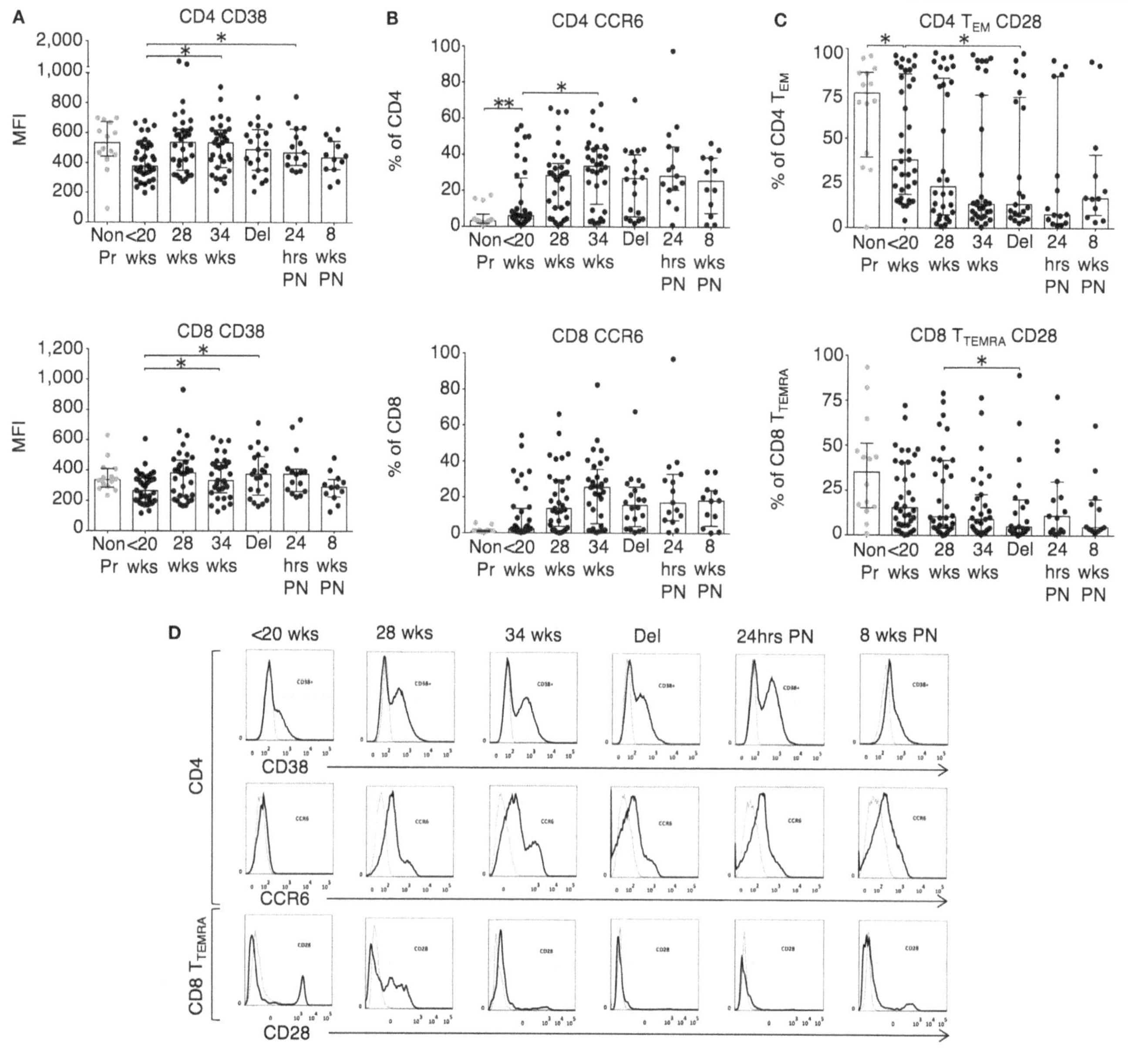

FIGURE 2 | Leukocyte phenotype during pregnancy shows increased activation and migratory potential. **(A)** CD38 mean fluorescence intensity and the proportion of expression of **(B)** CCR6 on CD4 and CD8 T cells; **(C)** CD28 expression on CD4 T_{EM} ($CCR7^{-}CD45RA^{-}$) and CD8 T_{TEMRA} ($CCR7^{-}CD45RA^{+}$) T cell subtypes analyzed longitudinally with gestation and compared to controls. Gestation at sampling is indicated in pregnancy (●): $<20^{+0}$ weeks (*N* = *42*), 28 weeks (*N* = 35), 34 weeks (*N* = *33*), at delivery (*N* = *24*), 24 h post-delivery (*N* = *22*), 6–8 weeks postnatal (*N* = *13*). Non-pregnant controls are depicted as ● (*N* = *14*). *P* values are two tailed and significance is defined as $^{*}P < 0.05$ and $^{**}P < 0.01$. Non-pregnant and baseline pregnant data analyzed by Mann–Whitney *U* test. Longitudinal data analyzed by generalized linear mixed effects model with gamma log-link and pairwise multiple comparisons of estimated marginal means with sequential Bonferroni correction. **(D)** Shows representative flow cytometry histograms across gestations with matched isotype controls for CD38 and CCR6 expression on CD4 T cells as well as CD28 expression on CD8 T_{TEMRA} and HLA-DR expression on CD8 T cells.

granzyme B responses with gestation, these were concurrently being modulated.

P4 Suppresses IFN-γ and Granzyme B Responses in Pregnancy

To determine the effects of P4, we recruited patients receiving either P4 supplementation or P4 antagonism with RU486 for clinically relevant indications as outlined in the Section "Materials and Methods." Longitudinal differences in IFN-g responses with P4 treatment were not significantly different (**Figure 5A**). However, when compared to untreated patients, P4 treatment significantly reduced pro-inflammatory IFN-γ responses to measles whole lysate at 34 weeks and TTOX antigen at 28 weeks of gestation (**Figure 5B**; Figure S2 in Supplementary Material). An opposite effect was seen in the RU486-treated group at 72 h where IFN-γ responses to EBV, influenza A, HSV, measles,

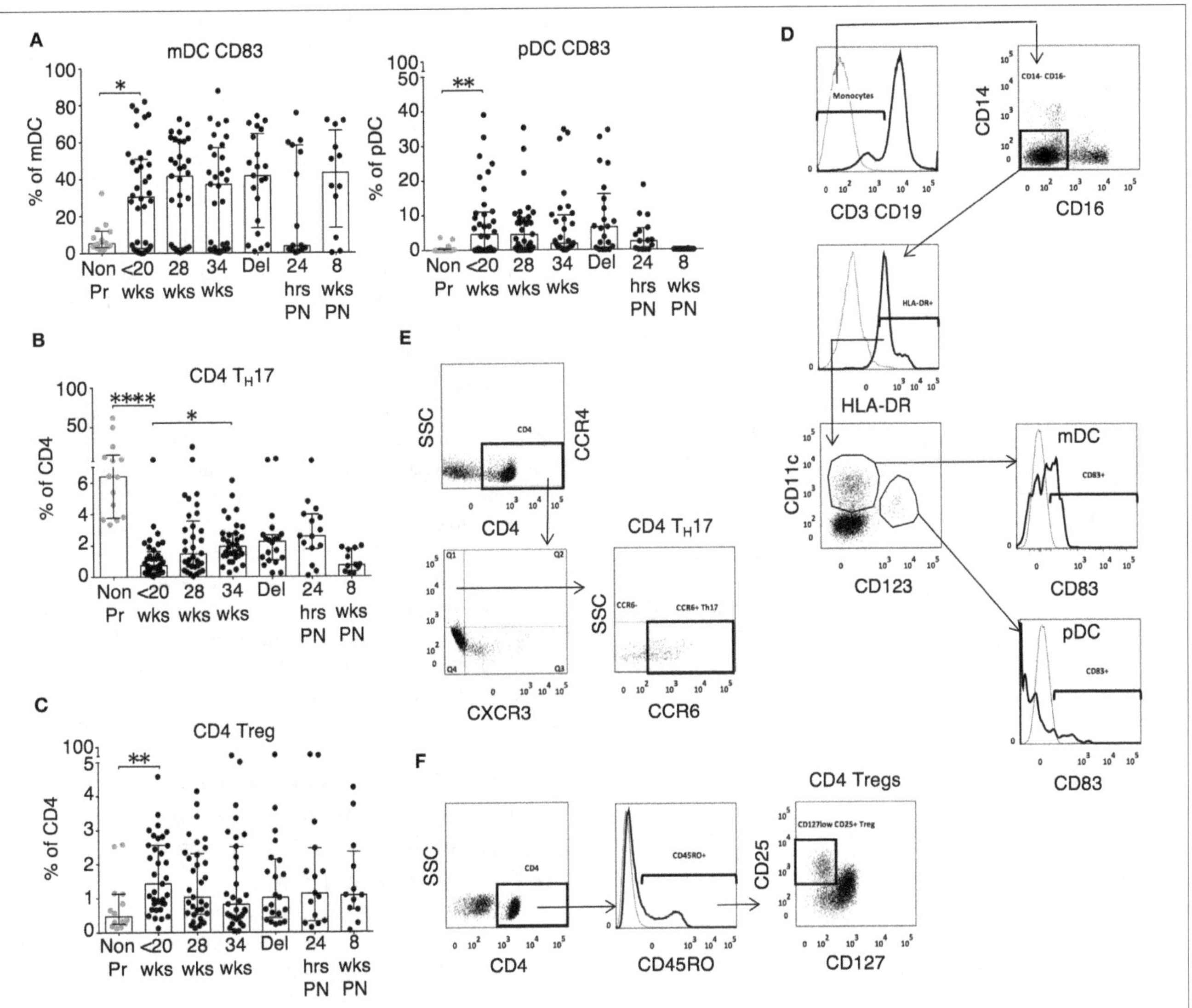

FIGURE 3 | Inflammatory, activated, and cytotoxic leukocyte subsets show gestational variation in pregnancy. **(A)** Proportions of activated mDC ($CD3^-CD19^-CD14^-CD16^-HLA\text{-}DR^+CD11c^+CD123^-CD83^+$) and pDC ($CD3^-CD19^-CD14^-CD16^-HLA\text{-}DR^+CD11c^+CD123^+CD83^+$) during pregnancy and compared with gestation matched controls. **(B)** Longitudinal analysis of T_H17 cells ($CCR4^+CXCR3^-CCR6^+$) and **(C)** regulatory T cell (Tregs) with phenotype $CD4^+CD45RO^+CD25^+CD127^{lo}$ in pregnancy and compared with gestation matched controls. Gestation at sampling is indicated in pregnancy (●): $<20^{+0}$ weeks ($N = 42$), 28 weeks ($N = 35$), 34 weeks ($N = 33$), at delivery ($N = 24$), 24 h post-delivery ($N = 22$), 6–8 weeks postnatal ($N = 13$). Non-pregnant controls are depicted as ● ($N = 14$). P values are two tailed and significance is defined as $^*P < 0.05$ and $^{**}P < 0.01$ $^{****}P < 0.0001$. Non-pregnant and baseline pregnant data analyzed by Mann–Whitney U test. Longitudinal data analyzed by generalized linear mixed effects model with gamma log-link and pairwise multiple comparisons of estimated marginal means with sequential Bonferroni correction. Representative flow cytometry plots of **(D)** dendritic cell subtypes mDC and pDC, **(E)** T_H17 CD4 T cells, and **(F)** $CD4^+$ Tregs and, and their respective gating strategies.

and PPD were significantly increased compared to baseline (**Figure 5C**; Figure S2 in Supplementary Material). Longitudinal and gestation matched analysis of P4 supplemented pregnancies did not show significant changes in antigen-specific IL-10 and IL-4 responses (**Figures 5D–F** and **6A–C**). However, longitudinal analysis of RU486 treated patients showed a significant increase in IL-10 response to measles whole lysate (**Figure 5F**). Cellular IL-4 production in response to measles whole lysate at 2 weeks post P4 treatment was reduced but remained largely unmeasurable (**Figure 6B**).

Granzyme B responses showed the same pattern as the IFN-γ responses (**Figures 6D,E**). P4 treatment was associated with a significantly reduced granzyme B response at 34 weeks of gestation to measles, influenza A and TTOX (**Figure 6E**; Figure S3 in Supplementary Material). An opposite effect was seen in the RU486 treated group. Although granzyme B production at baseline was below 20 per 10^6 SFCs, when measurable, PBMC from RU486 treated patients produced a greater number of granzyme B SFCs in response to measles and influenza A whole lysate, and FEC peptide pool measured 72 h post RU486 (**Figure 6F**; Figure S3 in Supplementary Material).

A representative sample of six patients, from the P4 and RU486 treated groups, with plasma samples taken longitudinally were analyzed to measure cytokine concentrations without cell

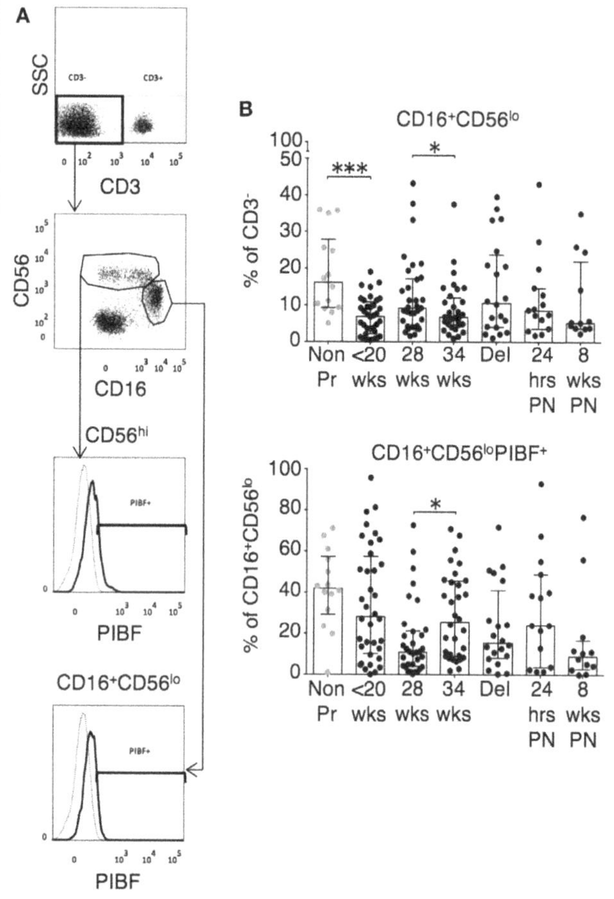

FIGURE 4 | Cytotoxic natural killer (NK) cell subtype with the phenotype $CD16^{+}CD56^{lo}$ are reduced and show an increase in P4-induced blocking factor (PIBF) expression in late pregnancy. **(A)** Representative flow cytometry plots are shown for NK cell subsets. **(B)** Longitudinal analysis of $CD16^{+}CD56^{lo}$ and their PIBF expression during pregnancy and compared with gestation matched controls. Gestation at sampling is indicated in pregnancy (●): $<20^{+0}$ weeks (*N* = *42*), 28 weeks (*N* = *35*), 34 weeks (*N* = *33*), at delivery (*N* = *24*), 24 h post-delivery (*N* = *22*), 6–8 weeks postnatal (*N* = *13*). Non-pregnant controls are depicted as ● (*N* = *14*). *P* values are two tailed and significance is defined as $^{*}P < 0.05$ and $^{***}P < 0.001$. Non-pregnant and baseline pregnant data analyzed by Mann—Whitney *U* test. Longitudinal data analyzed by generalized linear mixed effects model with gamma log-link and pairwise multiple comparisons of estimated marginal means with sequential Bonferroni correction.

culture or stimulation. Longitudinally, cytokine concentrations in P4 treated patients remained stable (**Figure 7A**). However, when compared to gestation-matched controls, baseline IFN-γ, IL-7, and IL-1β were significantly reduced in P4 treated patients (**Figure 7B** and not shown). This was sustained for IFN-γ and IL-7 at 28 weeks of gestation (**Figure 7B**). Despite these observations, longitudinal cytokine concentrations in the RU486-treated cohort remained stable (**Figure 7C**).

P4 Antagonism Results in Activation of CD4 and Memory T cell Subtypes

The longitudinal changes seen in the expression of CD38 and CCR6 on both CD4 and CD8 T cells in the un-supplemented group were reproduced in the P4 treated (**Figures 8A,D**). P4 had no impact on CD38 or CCR6 expression on CD4 T cells when compared to gestation-matched controls (**Figures 8B,E**). However, with P4 supplementation, CD38 expression on CD8 T cells at 34 weeks of gestation was increased (**Figure 8B**). Nonetheless, CD38 and CCR6 expression was unaffected by RU486 (**Figure 8C,F**). Supplemental P4 appeared to have no impact on CD4 and CD8 HLA-DR expression either longitudinally nor when compared to gestation-matched controls (**Figures 8G,H** and data not shown). However, antagonism with RU486 resulted in increased expression of HLA-DR on CD4 but not on CD8 T cells (**Figure 8I** and data not shown).

Memory T cells provide quantitatively enhanced responses to secondary or recall antigen challenge. In our study, these subsets were defined as previously described (37). Their activated and expansive potential was determined by their expression of HLA-DR and CD28 as these are associated with peptide presentation and co-stimulation (34). Proportions of CD4 terminally differentiated effector memory (T_{TEMRA}) T cells and CD8 T_{EM} and T_{TEMRA} were reduced 72 h post RU486 treatment (**Figures 9A–E**). CD4 T_{CM} expressing HLA-DR and CD28 (**Figures 10A,E** and not shown) showed an increase 72 h post RU486 and proportions of CD4 T_{EM} expressing HLA-DR increased 48 h following RU486 (**Figures 10B,E**). $HLA\text{-}DR^{+}$ CD8 T_{CM} proportions increased 72 h post RU486 but $HLA\text{-}DR^{+}$ CD8 T_{TEMRA} decreased 48 h post RU486 and returned to baseline 72 h post RU486 (**Figures 10C–E**).

P4 Was Associated With a Fall in Proportions of Tregs, but Had No Impact on T-Helper Subtypes or PIBF-Expressing T Cells

Although P4 has previously been shown to be able to generate induced Tregs *in vitro*, in our study, proportions of CD4 Tregs decreased longitudinally with P4 treatment (**Figure 11A**). However, when proportions of Tregs with P4 supplementation were compared to gestation matched controls, there were no differences (**Figure 11B**). In addition, the longitudinal P4 effects were not reciprocated with the use of RU486 (**Figure 11C**). This led us to assume *in vivo*, P4 supplementation has little effect on the induction of Tregs in the periphery. Similarly, proportions of T-helper subtypes $T_{H}1$, $T_{H}2$, and $T_{H}17$ were unaffected by the use of P4 or RU486 (not shown). There were no longitudinal effects of P4 supplementation on CD4 PIBF expression. However, when compared to controls (**Figure 11D**), PIBF expression on CD4 T cells was decreased at 34 weeks of gestation, but the reverse was not observed with RU486 treatment (**Figures 11E,F**). PIBF expression on CD3 γδ or CD8 T cells was unaffected by P4 or RU486 (not shown).

P4 Does Not Appear to Affect NK or DC Phenotype

Overall, P4 had no longitudinal effects on NK cell expression of PIBF (Figures S4A,D,E in Supplementary Material). $CD16^{+}CD56^{lo}$ NK cells expressing PIBF represented a smaller proportion when compared to un-supplemented pregnancies at 34 weeks (Figure S4B in Supplementary Material). However,

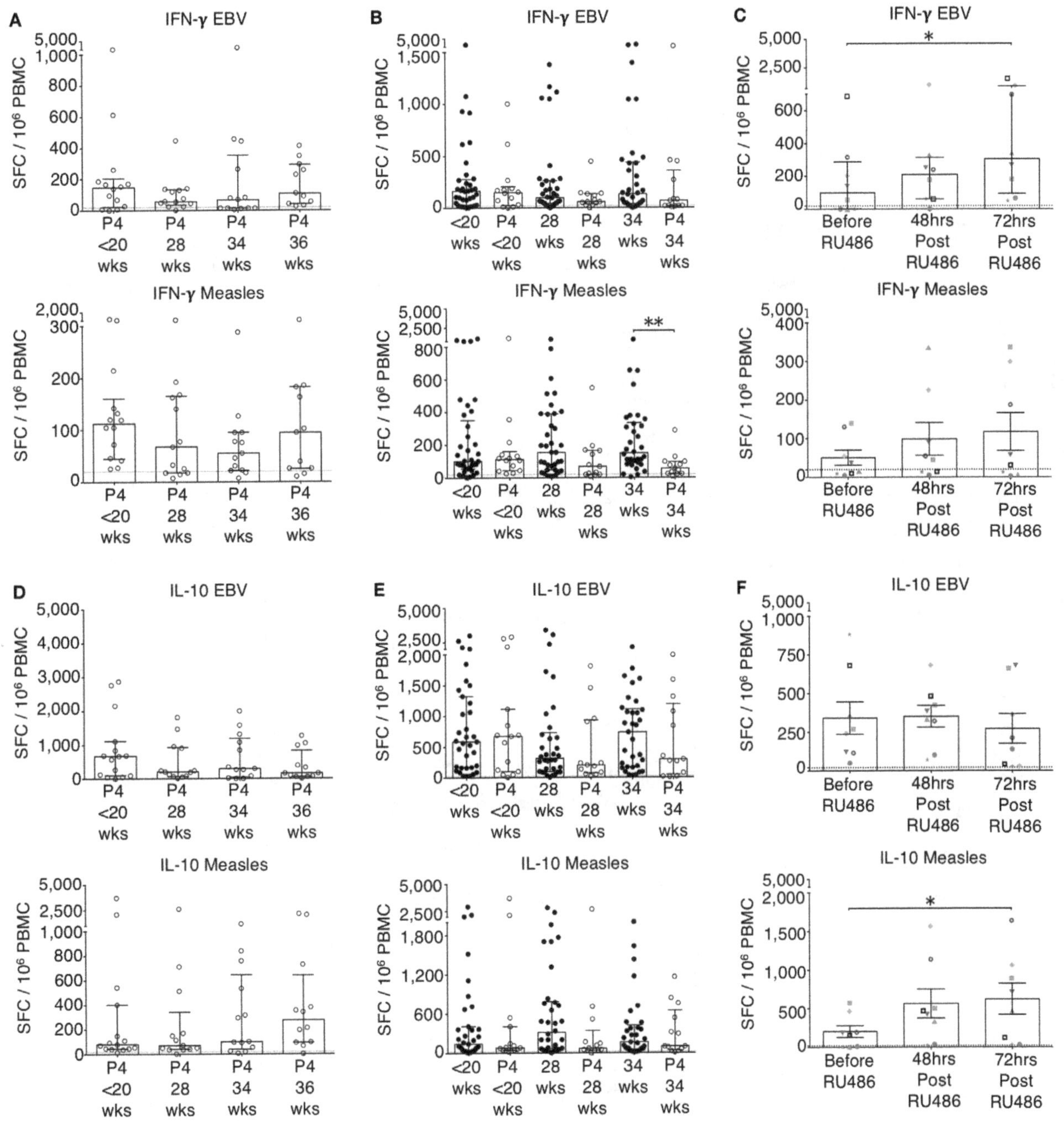

FIGURE 5 | P4 supresses IFN-γ and IL-10 enzyme-linked immunospot (ELISpot) responses. EBV and measles responses are shown. **(A)** Longitudinal analysis of IFN-γ responses in P4 treated. **(B)** IFN-γ responses in P4 treated compared to controls. Unpaired Mann–Whitney *U* test. **(C)** Longitudinal analysis of IFN-γ responses in RU486 treated. **(D)** Longitudinal analysis of IL-10 responses in P4 treated. **(E)** IL-10 responses in P4 treated compared to controls. Unpaired Mann–Whitney *U* test. **(F)** Longitudinal analysis of IL-10 responses in RU486 treated. Gestation at sampling is indicated: in pregnant controls (●) at $<20^{+0}$ weeks (*N* = 42), 28 weeks (*N* = 35), 34 weeks (*N* = 33); and P4 treated pregnancies (○) at $<20^{+0}$ weeks (*N* = 15), 28 weeks (*N* = 13), 34 weeks (*N* = 13), 36 weeks (*N* = 11). For RU486 treated (*N* = 8) symbols represent individual patients. A dashed line represents <20 spot forming cells/10^6. Longitudinal data were analyzed with either one-way analysis of variance with Tukey's *post hoc* correction or Freidman test with Dunn's *post hoc* correction depending on the data distribution. *P* values are two tailed and significance is defined as $^*P < 0.05$ and $^{**}P < 0.01$.

RU486 had no effect (Figure S4C in Supplementary Material). Likewise, proportions of CD56[hi] and iNKT did not change with P4 supplementation or RU486 treatment (Figures S4E,F,H,I in Supplementary Material).

Despite the previously mentioned changes seen on memory T cells, proportions of activated mDC and pDC expressing co-stimulatory markers, and HLA-G expressing CD14+ DC-10 (38) remained un-affected by P4 or RU486 (not shown).

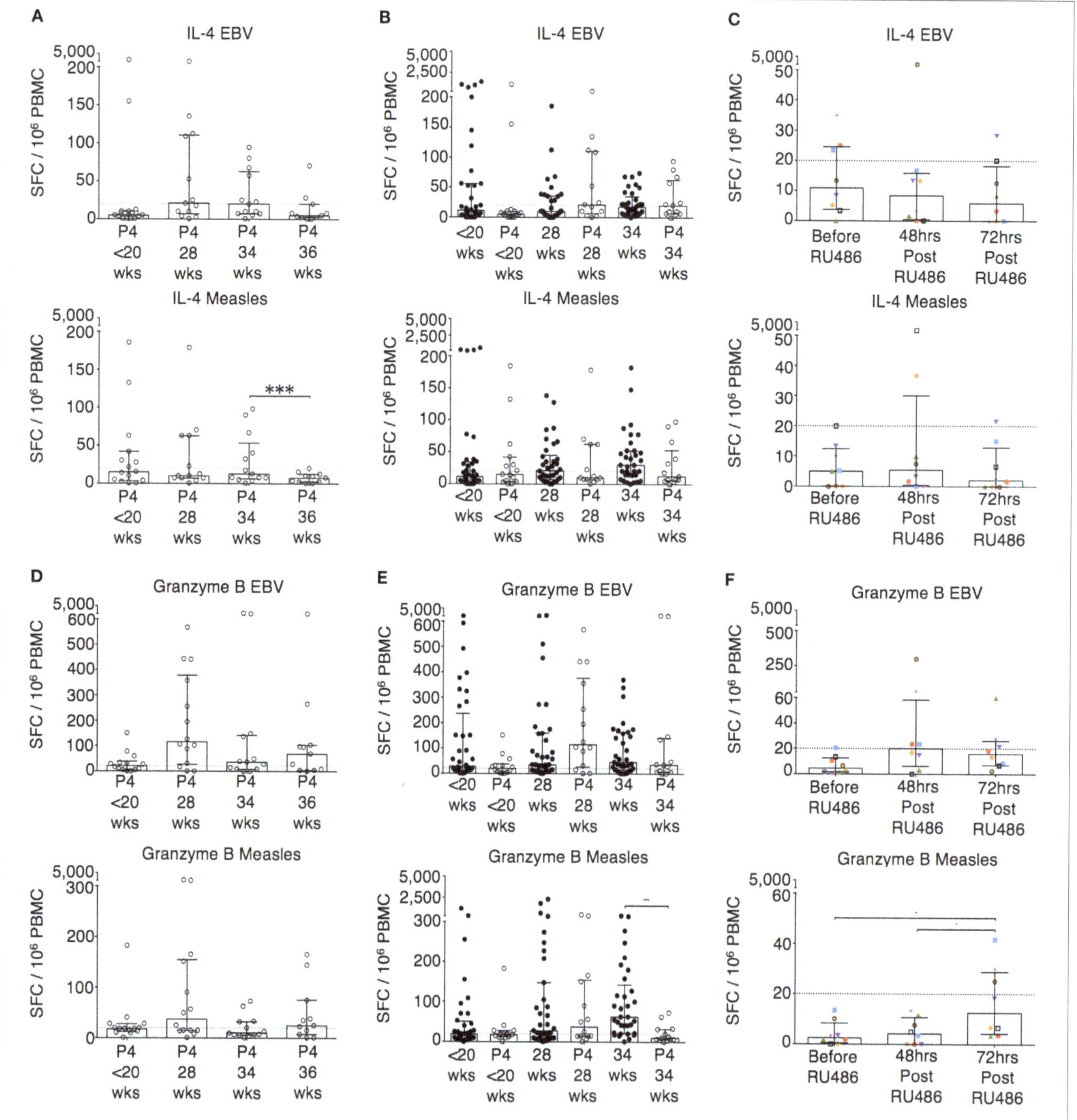

FIGURE 6 | P4 and RU486 have little impact on IL-4 B ELISpot responses but P4 suppresses and RU486 enhances Granzyme B ELISpot responses. EBV and measles responses are shown. **(A)** Longitudinal changes in IL-4 responses with P4 treatment. **(B)** Comparison of IL-4 responses in P4 treated and controls, and **(C)** longitudinal analysis in RU486 treated. **(D)** Longitudinal changes in granzyme B responses with P4 treatment. **(E)** Comparison of granzyme B responses in P4 treated and controls, and **(F)** longitudinal analysis in RU486 treated. Gestation at sampling is indicated: in pregnant controls (●) at $<20^{+0}$ weeks (*N* = *42*), 28 weeks (*N* = *35*), 34 weeks (*N* = *33*); and P4 treated pregnancies (○) at $<20^{+0}$ weeks (*N* = *15*), 28 weeks (*N* = *13*), 34 weeks (*N* = *13*), 36 weeks (*N* = *11*). For RU486 treated (*N* = *8*) symbols represent individual patients. A dashed line represents <20 spot forming cells/10^6. Longitudinal data were analyzed with either one-way analysis of variance with Tukey's *post hoc* correction or Freidman test with Dunn's *post hoc* correction depending on the data distribution. *P* values are two tailed and significance is defined as ***$P < 0.001$.

DISCUSSION

In this study, we investigated the effect of P4 on the peripheral maternal immune system. We used a novel approach by recruiting pregnant women taking P4 or RU486 using clinically effective regimens specifically designed to either reduce their risk of preterm labor or induce a functional P4 withdrawal with the aim of initiating labor. Furthermore, we are the first group to

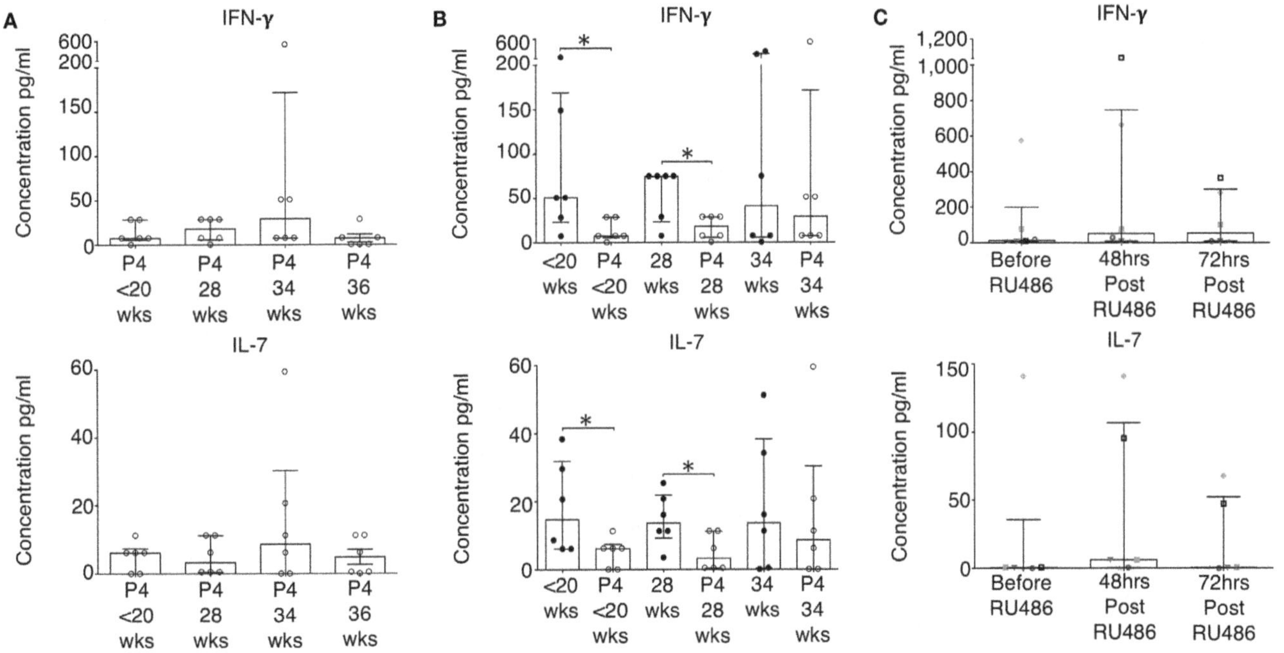

FIGURE 7 | Baseline concentrations of pro-inflammatory cytokines in the P4-treated group are reduced. Plasma concentrations of cytokines measured by 17-plex multiplex assay were determined. **(A)** Longitudinal analysis of IFN-γ and IL-7 concentrations of noted in the P4 treated group. **(B)** IFN-γ and IL-7 concentrations in P4 treated compared to gestation-matched controls. Unpaired Mann–Whitney *U* test. **(C)** Longitudinal analysis of RU486 effect on plasma cytokine concentrations. A representative sample of patients (*N* = *6*) were assessed. Gestation at sampling is indicated: in pregnant controls (●) at $<20^{+0}$ weeks (*N* = *42*), 28 weeks (*N* = *35*), 34 weeks (*N* = *33*); and P4 treated pregnancies (O) at $<20^{+0}$ weeks (*N* = *15*), 28 weeks (*N* = *11*), 34 weeks (*N* = *11*), 36 weeks (*N* = *10*). For RU486 treated (*N* = *6*) symbols represent individual patients. Longitudinal data were analyzed with Freidman test with Dunn's *post hoc* correction. *P* values are two tailed and significance is defined as **P* < 0.05.

examine the *in vivo* effects of RU486 on leukocyte function in the mid second trimester of pregnancy. Our data demonstrate that, in pregnancy, P4 reduces both pro-inflammatory and cytotoxic T cell responses, and that this suppressive effect is reversed with the use of RU486.

We have previously shown that, in normal pregnancy, IFN-γ and IL-10 responses to recall antigens are elevated in the third trimester (39). This occurs despite an increase in CD4 T_{EM} in the second trimester, suggesting that IL-10 may restrict the activation of the immune system by suppressing antigen specific T cell responses (39, 40). In the current study, our findings supported this concept. Both IFN-γ and IL-10 peripheral recall responses were largely elevated at delivery. Notably though, IL-10 responses showed marked increases in pregnancy across gestation despite a leukocyte phenotype that seemed to suggest a gradual decline of IL-10 antigen-induced immune tolerance with a longitudinal increase in T_H17 proportions, and the loss of any baseline pregnancy-related bias in CD4 Treg proportions. This occurred alongside an increasingly activated immune system, suggested by longitudinal increases in activated (CD38) and migratory (CCR6) T cells, mature memory T cells (CD28) with greater homing and effector function (34), and activated DCs (CD83). This gradual decline of immune-modulation was also evident in humoral and cytotoxic responses suggested by more frequent IL-4 SFCs in pregnancy, as well as increased granzyme B cytotoxic T cell activity, and IFN-γ and IL-10 responses to CD8 epitopes at delivery. In contrast, other studies have suggested that both humoral and cell-mediated immune responses are largely reduced in the third trimester, but innate responses to bacteria are increased (20, 41, 42). Our IL-4 findings likely reflect heightened humoral immune function in pregnancy, but the change in cytotoxic responses are suggestive of a loss of modulation of antigen specific memory CTL functions. We sought to determine how influential P4 may be as a driver of these changes.

Of note in our non-pregnant controls, we did not control for different phases in their menstrual cycle. In non-human primates, in peripheral blood, the luteal phase of the menstrual cycle, when P4 is at peak concentration, is associated with tolerant immune responses that favor successful pregnancy (43). It is assumed these changes transfer to humans. However, the majority of studies investigating the effects of menstruation show conflicting data. For example, although some researchers have shown Tregs initially expand during the follicular phase and then decrease mid-luteal, and that the luteal phase is associated with a decline in PBMC proliferation and IFN-γ production, T cell PHA responses are unchanged, and variations in Th1/Th2 cytokines have not been shown consistently in the literature (44–49). In contrast, NK cytotoxicity may be influenced by menstruation (44, 50). It is also important to appreciate that previous exposure to paternal antigens induces tolerance and so parity and sexual activity may enhance the effects of P4 (45, 51, 52). Furthermore, when compared to pregnant patients, the peak serum P4 concentration

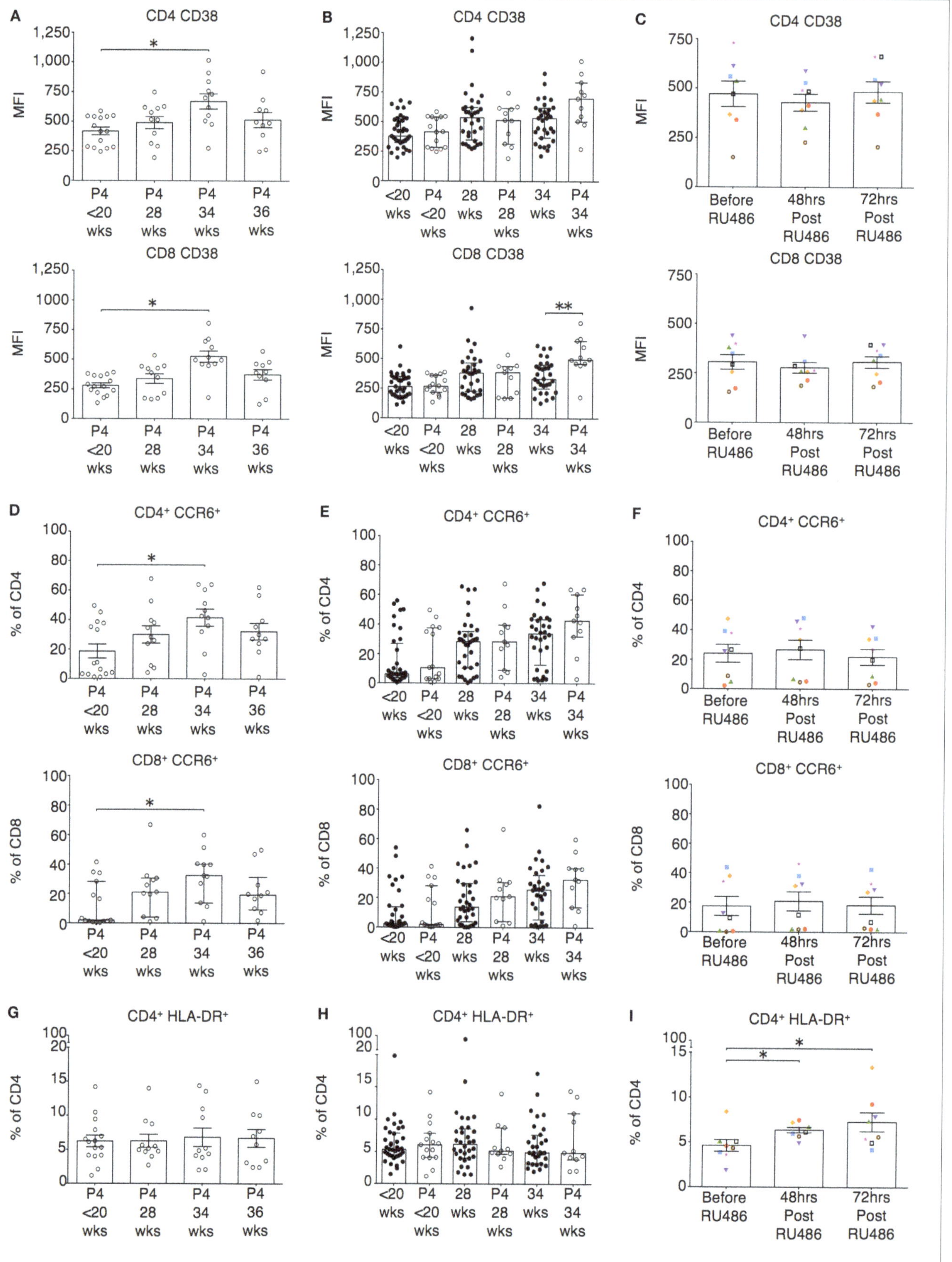

FIGURE 8 | Continued

FIGURE 8 | P4 does not suppress CD38 or CCR6 expression on T cells. However, RU486 increases HLA-DR expression on CD4 T cells. **(A)** Longitudinal analysis of CD38 expression measured by mean fluorescence intensity (MFI) on CD4 and CD8 T cells. **(B)** Comparing CD38 expression on CD4 and CD8 T cells in P4 treated with gestation matched controls. Unpaired Mann–Whitney *U* test. **(C)** Longitudinal analysis of the effect of RU486 on CD4 and CD8 T cell CD38 expression. **(D)** Longitudinal analysis of CCR6 expression measured by MFI on CD4 and CD8 T cells (Freidman test with Dunn's *post hoc* correction). **(E)** Gestation matched comparison of CCR6 expression on CD4 T cells between P4 treated and controls. **(F)** Longitudinal analysis of CCR6 expression on CD4 T cells from the RU486 group. **(G)** Longitudinal variation in HLA-DR expression on CD4 T cells in the P4-treated group. **(H)** Gestation-matched comparison of HLA-DR expression on CD4 T cells between P4 treated and controls. **(I)** Longitudinal analysis of HLA-DR expression on CD4 T cells from the RU486 group. Gestation at sampling is indicated: in pregnant controls (●) at <20^{+0} weeks ($N = 42$), 28 weeks ($N = 35$), 34 weeks ($N = 33$); and P4 treated pregnancies (○) at <20^{+0} weeks ($N = 15$), 28 weeks ($N = 11$), 34 weeks ($N = 11$), 36 weeks ($N = 10$). For RU486 treated ($N = 8$) symbols represent individual patients. Longitudinal data was analyzed with either one-way analysis of variance with Tukey's *post hoc* correction or Freidman test with Dunn's *post hoc* correction depending on the data distribution. *P* values are two tailed and significance is defined as $^*P < 0.05$ and $^{**}P < 0.01$.

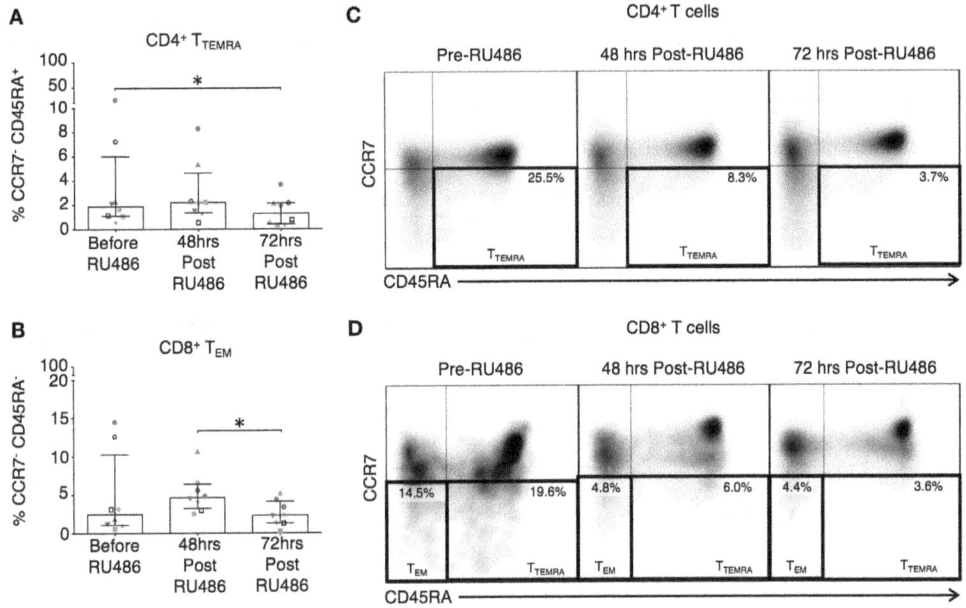

FIGURE 9 | RU486 treatment is associated with reduced proportions of CD4 and CD8 differentiated effector memory subtypes. **(A)** Longitudinal analysis of proportions of CD4$^+$CCR7$^-$CD45RA$^-$ T_{EM} and **(B)** CD8 T_{EM} (CCR7$^-$CD45RA$^-$) in RU486-treated ($N = 8$) symbols represent individual patients. *P* values are two tailed and significance is defined as $^*P < 0.05$, by Freidman test with Dunn's *post hoc* correction. Representative flow cytometry plots of **(C)** singlet CD4$^+$ lymphocytes co-expressing CCR7 and CD45RA is shown with percentages of T_{EM} cell, and **(D)** singlet CD8$^+$ lymphocytes co-expressing CCR7 and CD45RA is shown with percentages of T_{EM} and T_{TEMRA} cells. Populations were gated using isotype controls.

in non-pregnant women is approximately 15 versus 60 ng/ml in early and 180 ng/ml in late pregnancy, which represent a 4- and 12-fold increase, respectively (53, 54). This suggests that any changes due to menstrual variation in serum P4 are unlikely to compare to changes in pregnancy. In fact, in our previous work, we found that despite *in vitro* culture with P4, leukocyte PIBF expression in controls, at different stages in their menstrual cycle, did not equal those seen in pregnancy suggesting that neuro-endocrine differences are not the sole determinant of leukocyte phenotype in pregnancy (39). Therefore, in our study, peripheral blood samples were not controlled for phases of the menstrual cycle.

Serum concentrations of endogenous P4 increase throughout pregnancy and reach 175–636 nmol/l in the maternal circulation during the third trimester (53). Yet, as a potent endogenous suppressor of cytotoxic immune responses and regulator of cytokine secretion, our results suggest its effects decline after 34 weeks of pregnancy. Therefore, we expected the addition of exogenous P4, as well as modeling its withdrawal using RU486, would be noticeable until the end of the second trimester pregnancy and thereafter become less obvious. Previous studies have shown that, outside of pregnancy, P4 is antiproliferative and suppresses the production of the pro-inflammatory cytokines IFN-γ, TNF-α, while upregulating IL-4 in PBMC cultures with PHA, and that these effects are reversed by RU486 (1, 14). In addition, P4 has been shown to suppress cytotoxic T cell activity (12). Conversely, RU486 has been shown to increase uterine NK cytotoxicity (12, 55, 56). In human and animal models, P4 also has systemic and tissue specific anti-inflammatory effects, acting predominantly *via* the inhibition of NFκB and MAPK/AP-1 pathways (3, 57–59). However, in some disease states, P4 is less effective once pro-inflammatory processes are established, and this may be associated with a differential tissue expression of PR isoforms (60, 61). In fact, in myometrial tissue, this is thought to be one of

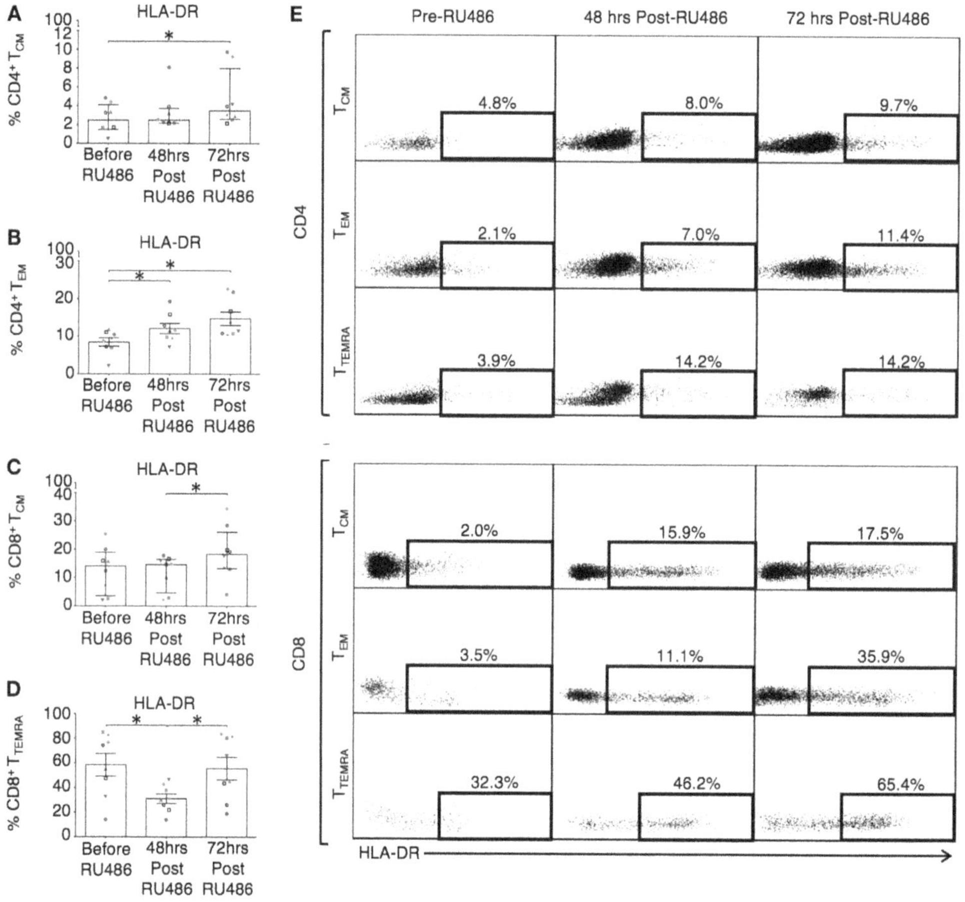

FIGURE 10 | Differentiated effector memory subtypes in RU486 treated have an increased expression of HLA-DR. **(A)** Longitudinal change in percentage expression of HLA-DR on: CD4 T_{CM} (Freidman test with Dunn's *post hoc* correction), **(B)** CD4 T_{EM} [one-way analysis of variance (ANOVA) with Tukey's *post hoc* correction], **(C)** CD8 T_{CM} (Freidman test with Dunn's *post hoc* correction), and **(D)** CD8 T_{TEMRA} (one-way ANOVA with Tukey's *post hoc* correction). *P* values are two tailed and significance is defined as $^*P < 0.05$. **(E)** Representative flow cytometry plots showing the percentage expression of HLA-DR on both CD4 and CD8 ($CCR7^+CD45RA^-$) T_{CM}, ($CCR7^-CD45RA^-$) T_{EM}, and ($CCR7^-CD45RA^+$) T_{TEMRA} subsets in PBMC from subjects receiving RU486 treatment. Memory $CD4^+$ and $CD8^+$ subset HLA-DR expression, gated with SSC on the vertical axis is shown. Populations were gated using isotype controls and percentages of HLA-DR expressing cells is indicated.

the contributors to the onset of term labor (62). We found that, in contrast to control pregnancies, P4 supplementation appeared to encourage a stable IFN-γ response that was significantly reduced when compared to gestation-matched controls. This occurred without any negative effect on longitudinal CD38 and CCR6 T-cell expression, which continued to increase despite exogenous P4 supplementation. Both receptors are important for inflammatory responses and cell migration. CD38 is characteristically raised in chronic inflammation and is associated with an enhanced ability to produce IFN-γ (63, 64). CCR6 is expressed on effector memory populations that contribute to recall responses (33). RU486 treatment had the opposite effect, with significant increases in IFN-γ responses posttreatment. These changes were statistically significant 72 h post RU486, which was post-delivery, rather than 48 h post treatment. However, altogether, our findings point to a P4 mediated effect rather than a consequence of delivery. P4 is known to negatively effect polyfunctional cytokine production from CD8 T cells and suppresses decidual lymphocyte cytotoxicity (12, 14). Granzyme B is primarily produced by activated CTLs and NKs cells and is, therefore, a useful surrogate marker for the functional activity of CTLs. Similar to the IFN-γ data, granzyme responses in the P4 treated group, when compared to gestation-matched controls at 34 weeks of pregnancy, were reduced; conversely, in the RU486 treated group, the response was increased, and these included responses against FEC peptide pool that incorperates CD8 specific epitopes. Although the latter results were significant post delivery, the control pregnancies did not show delivery was associated with any changes in the granzyme B response, suggesting that the differences are are most likely to be RU486 related.

Interestingly, although IL-10 and IL-4 responses in the P4 as well as in the RU486 treated groups were, on the whole, unaffected, suggesting the altered antigen-specific responses are not T_H2 or IL-10 driven. Our findings contradict murine models that have previously shown that in pregnancy, systemic and uterine Treg proportions as well as their suppressive activity is increased with P4 and blocked by RU486, but this increase does

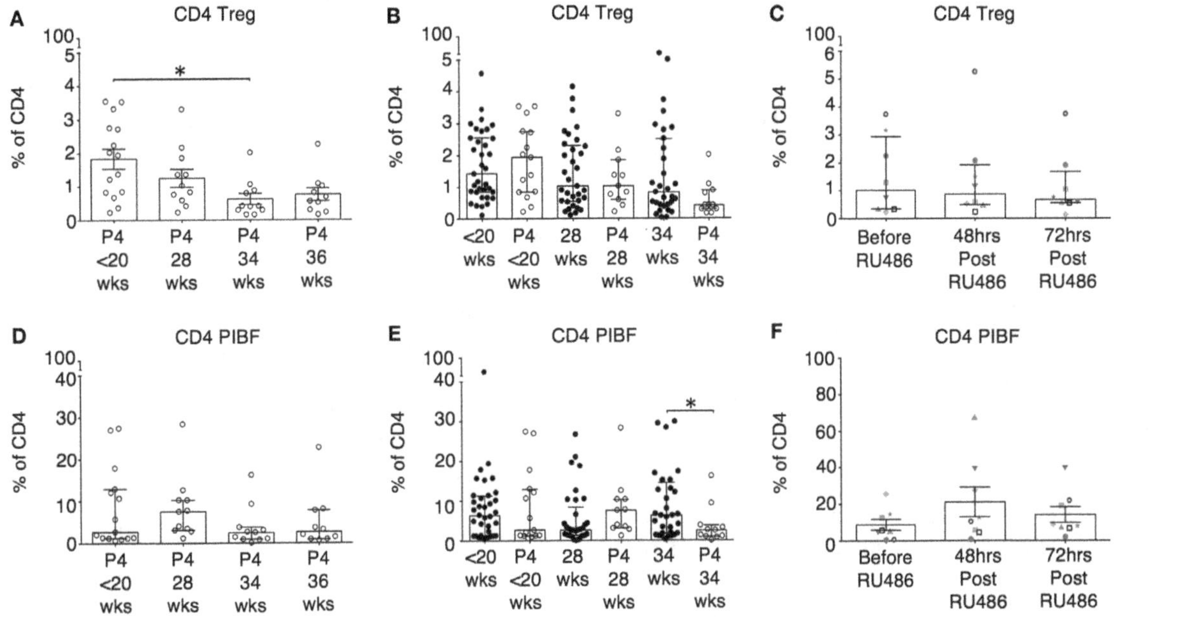

FIGURE 11 | The influence of P4 and RU486 on CD4+ regulatory T cell (Tregs) and P4-induced blocking factor (PIBF) expressing CD4+ T cells. **(A)** Longitudinal analysis of CD4 Treg proportions ($CD4^+CD45RO^+CD25^+CD127^{lo}$) in peripheral blood obtained from P4 treated patients. **(B)** Gestation-matched paired comparisons of Treg proportions in peripheral blood obtained from P4 treated versus untreated pregnant controls that were previously analyzed longitudinally in **Figure 3C**. **(C)** Longitudinal analysis of Treg proportions in peripheral blood obtained from RU486 treated pregnant patients. **(D)** Longitudinal analysis of PIBF expressing CD4 T cells in peripheral blood obtained from P4-treated patients. **(E)** Gestation matched paired comparisons of PIBF expressing CD4 T cells in peripheral blood obtained from P4 treated versus untreated pregnant controls (Unpaired Mann–Whitney *U* test). **(F)** Longitudinal analysis of PIBF expressing CD4 T cells in peripheral blood obtained from RU486-treated pregnant patients. Gestation at sampling is indicated: in pregnant controls (●) at $< 20^{+0}$ weeks (*N = 42*), 28 weeks (*N = 35*), 34 weeks (*N = 33*); and P4 treated pregnancies (′) at $<20^{+0}$ weeks (*N = 15*), 28 weeks (*N = 11*), 34 weeks (*N = 11*), 36 weeks (*N = 10*). For RU486 treated (*N = 8*) symbols represent individual patients. Longitudinal data were analyzed with either one-way ANOVA with Tukey's *post hoc* correction or Freidman test with Dunn's *post hoc* correction depending on the data distribution. *P* values are two tailed and significance is defined as $^*P < 0.05$.

not necessarily prevent spontaneous fetal loss (65). Schumacher et al. showed that in abortion-prone mice, although decidual Treg numbers increased following intra-peritoneal P4 administration, this did not result in greater fetal survival (66). It is possible that these Tregs may have been poorly functioning or that other pathways are more influential at improving fetal outcomes. Of note, the human equivalent doses (HED) of P4 used in both of these studies were either comparable or lower than the 400 mg P4 dose used in our study, and the RU486 HED (30 mg) used by Mao et al. was far less than that used in our study (200 mg) (65–67). Therefore, the different findings in their work compared to ours are surprising. All of the aforementioned murine studies analyzed the effects of P4 in early and mid pregnancy in mice, when the maternal response to the initial surge in fetal antigen is vital for ongoing pregnancy success. Therefore, expansion of potentially poorly functioning Tregs may not be sufficient to improve tolerance to fetal antigen. Interestingly, intravenous adoptive transfer of Tregs from normal pregnant to abortion prone mice at days 0–4 of pregnancy improves placentation and reduces reabsorption rates (68–70). However, miscarriage rates were not completely abrogated in these studies, and the same positive findings were not reproduced when the Tregs were isolated from non-pregnant mice (68–70). Our own results in pregnancy compared to non-pregnant controls showed an increased proportion of Tregs at baseline. However, we also found a longitudinal fall in Treg proportions with P4 supplementation. Mjösberg et al. have previously predicted such an effect, where, *in vitro*, P4 and 17β-estradiol reduced functionally suppressive CD4 Foxp3+ Tregs (71). Unfortunately, we did not investigate the suppressive activity of Tregs in this study, but the fall in number likely reflects the systemic anti-inflammatory effect of P4 and suggests pathways other than those involving Tregs are at play.

It is also worth noting that our unstimulated sera concentrations of IFN-γ, IL-1β, and IL-7 were significantly reduced pretreatment in the P4 group, and IFN-γ and IL-7 were also comparatively reduced at 28 weeks, suggesting that the effects were P4 related. These findings were not reciprocated in the RU486 group. The most likely confounder is that the P4-treated cohort represents patients at risk of premature delivery and so may have inherent immune differences. However, there were no other baseline differences between groups despite two of the patients delivering preterm at 34+ weeks of gestation immediately after stopping P4 treatment.

Our ELISpot results suggest that P4 may disrupt pro-inflammatory cell-mediated responses and its prolonged use is associated with suppressed antigen specific memory CTL responses, which are not fetal antigen specific. From our data, the latter effect does not seem to be driven by PIBF unlike in previous published reports (12, 72). In the P4-treated group, despite proportions of PIBF expressing CD4 T cells and cytotoxic

$CD16^{+}CD56^{lo}$ NK cells being reduced at 34 weeks of gestation, our RU486 data did not show any reciprocal changes. This is unusual as P4 has been shown to promote the production of PIBF from lymphocytes *in vitro via* PR (72). PIBF has a known anti-cytotoxic effect on NK cells, and this is thought to be by co-localizing in cytoplasmic granules and blocking degranulation (73, 74). Therefore, our results suggest that P4 supplementation in pregnancy has a limited effect on cellular PIBF expression, and consequently, that its effect on gestational length is independent of PIBF synthesis. It is likely that this is because P4 is acting *via* GR and thus the lack of opposite effects by RU486 may be due to different receptor-binding affinity (75, 76). Furthermore, GR binding may not always produce an immune suppressed affect. In transgenic rats, endogenous GR engagement is associated with an increase in activated and memory T cells (77). Regardless, our results showed suppressed IFN-γ responses, but we did not find any differences in memory T cell activation marker expression. This is in contrast to *in vitro* studies in animals, which have shown that in addition to inhibiting DC stimulation of naïve T cells in rats and memory CD8 IFN-γ production in mice, P4 reduces murine memory CD8 T cells during heterosubtypic influenza virus challenge (78–80). However, in the RU486 group, we found changes in MHC class II molecule expression on memory T cells that was highly suggestive of a reversal of pregnancy associated immune-modulation. The expression of HLA-DR increased on CD4 T_{EM} cells post RU486 treatment, and although the expression of HLA-DR was reduced on CD8 T_{TEMRA} cells, it subsequently increased 72 h post RU486. It is possible that CD8 T cells have a greater threshold for antigen exposure, and that the contributions of T_{EM} and T_{CM} cells can vary (81, 82). Furthermore, we show delivery in the presence of RU486 was associated with a fall in T_{TEMRA} and T_{EM} proportions, but with concurrent increases in HLA-DR expression. Surface MHC class II molecule expression on CD4 T cells corresponds to an improved ability for these cells to present antigen and regulate immune responses (83). Previously, murine data suggested that RU486 inhibits apoptosis of mature DC *via* GR and promotes HLA-DR expression on monocytes in humans (84, 85). Therefore, the effects of RU486 may be to initiate a rapid recovery of immune function as demonstrated by the ELISpot data, since, classically, memory T cells are highly responsive to recall antigens.

In conclusion, this study describes a novel method of examining the effects of P4 on the maternal immune system. Our data suggest that exogenous P4 reduces pro-inflammatory and cytotoxic T cell responses in pregnancy. It achieves this by a combination of effects on cell-mediated interactions, including altering memory T cell antigen sensitivity and regulating leukocyte migration. These effects are, in part, reversed with the use of RU486. Our results have identified which aspects of the maternal immune response are P4-regulated, as such modulation of these pathways may have potential as future therapeutic targets with the aim of modulating the maternal immune response to pregnancy. Future *in vivo* human work will help to key establish the cellular interactions at play during human pregnancy.

ETHICS STATEMENT

All subjects were recruited from Chelsea and Westminster Hospital, London, UK. This study was carried out in accordance with the recommendations of National Institute of Health Research (NIHR) Good Clinical Practise guidelines, and a NHS Research Ethics Committee. The protocol was approved by the National Research Ethics Service (NRES), London, UK committee as well as by Chelsea and Westminster NHS Trust, London, UK; Ref: 11/LO/0971. All subjects gave written informed consent in accordance with the Declaration of Helsinki.

AUTHOR CONTRIBUTIONS

NS, NI, and MJ had a substantial contribution to the conception and design of the project and its interpretation; were responsible for the acquisition, analysis, and interpretation of the data, and drafted the work. All authors contributed to revising of the manuscript and have approved the final version. All authors agreed to be accountable for all aspects of the work in ensuring that questions related to the accuracy or integrity of any part of the work are appropriately investigated and resolved.

ACKNOWLEDGMENTS

The authors thank medical statistician Dr. Sundhiya Mandalia for her input with data analysis and Mr. Alex Cocker for his help with aspects of the experimental work and during manuscript preparation. The authors also thank patients and staff at Chelsea and Westminster Hospital who participated in this study.

FUNDING

This work was funded by grants from Borne (charity number 1167073), and infrastructure support was provided by the National Institute of Health Research (NIHR) Imperial Biomedical Research Centre (BRC).

REFERENCES

1. Arck P, Hansen PJ, Mulac Jericevic B, Piccinni MP, Szekeres-Bartho J. Progesterone during pregnancy: endocrine-immune cross talk in mammalian species and the role of stress. *Am J Reprod Immunol* (2007) 58(3):268–79. doi:10.1111/j.1600-0897.2007.00512.x
2. Mesiano S. Myometrial progesterone responsiveness and the control of human parturition. *J Soc Gynecol Investig* (2004) 11(4):193–202. doi:10.1016/j.jsgi.2003.12.004
3. Tan H, Yi L, Rote NS, Hurd WW, Mesiano S. Progesterone receptor-A and -B have opposite effects on proinflammatory gene expression in human myometrial cells: implications for progesterone actions in human pregnancy

and parturition. *J Clin Endocrinol Metab* (2012) 97(5):E719–30. doi:10.1210/jc.2011-3251

4. Dosiou C, Hamilton AE, Pang Y, Overgaard MT, Tulac S, Dong J, et al. Expression of membrane progesterone receptors on human T lymphocytes and Jurkat cells and activation of G-proteins by progesterone. *J Endocrinol* (2008) 196(1):67–77. doi:10.1677/JOE-07-0317
5. Lei K, Chen L, Georgiou EX, Sooranna SR, Khanjani S, Brosens JJ, et al. Progesterone acts via the nuclear glucocorticoid receptor to suppress IL-1beta-induced COX-2 expression in human term myometrial cells. *PLoS One* (2012) 7(11):e50167. doi:10.1371/journal.pone.0050167
6. Li LB, Leung DYM, Hall CF, Goleva E. Divergent expression and function of glucocorticoid receptor β in human monocytes and T cells. *J Leukoc Biol* (2006) 79(4):818–27. doi:10.1189/jlb.0805466
7. Tomasicchio M, Avenant C, Du Toit A, Ray RM, Hapgood JP. The progestin-only contraceptive medroxyprogesterone acetate, but not norethisterone acetate, enhances HIV-1 Vpr-mediated apoptosis in human CD4+ T cells through the glucocorticoid receptor. *PLoS One* (2013) 8(5):e62895. doi:10.1371/journal.pone.0062895
8. Ugor E, Prenek L, Pap R, Berta G, Ernszt D, Najbauer J, et al. Glucocorticoid hormone treatment enhances the cytokine production of regulatory T cells by upregulation of Foxp3 expression. *Immunobiology* (2017) 223(4–5):422–31. doi:10.1016/j.imbio.2017.10.010
9. Engler JB, Kursawe N, Solano ME, Patas K, Wehrmann S, Heckmann N, et al. Glucocorticoid receptor in T cells mediates protection from autoimmunity in pregnancy. *Proc Natl Acad Sci U S A* (2017) 114(2):E181–90. doi:10.1073/pnas.1617115114
10. Areia A, Vale-Pereira S, Alves V, Rodrigues-Santos P, Moura P, Mota-Pinto A. Membrane progesterone receptors in human regulatory T cells: a reality in pregnancy. *BJOG* (2015) 122(11):1544–50. doi:10.1111/1471-0528.13294
11. Szekeres-Bartho J, Polgar B. PIBF: the double edged sword. Pregnancy and tumor. *Am J Reprod Immunol* (2010) 64(2):77–86. doi:10.1111/j.1600-0897.2010.00833.x
12. Laskarin G, Tokmadzic VS, Strbo N, Bogovic T, Szekeres-Bartho J, Randic L, et al. Progesterone induced blocking factor (PIBF) mediates progesterone induced suppression of decidual lymphocyte cytotoxicity. *Am J Reprod Immunol* (2002) 48(4):201–9. doi:10.1034/j.1600-0897.2002.01133.x
13. Ivanova-Todorova E, Mourdjeva M, Kyurkchiev D, Bochev I, Stoyanova E, Dimitrov R, et al. HLA-G expression is up-regulated by progesterone in mesenchymal stem cells. *Am J Reprod Immunol* (2009) 62(1):25–33. doi:10.1111/j.1600-0897.2009.00707.x
14. Lissauer D, Eldershaw SA, Inman CF, Coomarasamy A, Moss PA, Kilby MD. Progesterone promotes maternal-fetal tolerance by reducing human maternal T-cell polyfunctionality and inducing a specific cytokine profile. *Eur J Immunol* (2015) 45(10):2858–72. doi:10.1002/eji.201445404
15. Cohen RA, Check JH, Dougherty MP. Evidence that exposure to progesterone alone is a sufficient stimulus to cause a precipitous rise in the immunomodulatory protein the progesterone induced blocking factor (PIBF). *J Assist Reprod Genet* (2016) 33(2):221–9. doi:10.1007/s10815-015-0619-7
16. Wira CR, Rodriguez-Garcia M, Patel MV. The role of sex hormones in immune protection of the female reproductive tract. *Nat Rev Immunol* (2015) 15(4):217–30. doi:10.1038/nri3819
17. Loewendorf AI, Nguyen TA, Yesayan MN, Kahn DA. Normal human pregnancy results in maternal immune activation in the periphery and at the uteroplacental interface. *PLoS One* (2014) 9(5):e96723. doi:10.1371/journal.pone.0096723
18. Lissauer D, Piper K, Goodyear O, Kilby MD, Moss PA. Fetal-specific CD8+ cytotoxic T cell responses develop during normal human pregnancy and exhibit broad functional capacity. *J Immunol* (2012) 189(2):1072–80. doi:10.4049/jimmunol.1200544
19. Persson M, Ekerfelt C, Ernerudh J, Matthiesen L, Jenmalm M, Jonsson Y, et al. Increased circulating paternal antigen-specific IFN-gamma- and IL-4-secreting cells during pregnancy in allergic and non-allergic women. *J Reprod Immunol* (2008) 79(1):70–8. doi:10.1016/j.jri.2008.07.001
20. Kay AW, Fukuyama J, Aziz N, Dekker CL, Mackey S, Swan GE, et al. Enhanced natural killer-cell and T-cell responses to influenza A virus during pregnancy. *Proc Natl Acad Sci U S A* (2014) 111(40):14506–11. doi:10.1073/pnas.1416569111
21. Patas K, Engler JB, Friese MA, Gold SM. Pregnancy and multiple sclerosis: feto-maternal immune cross talk and its implications for disease activity. *J Reprod Immunol* (2013) 97(1):140–6. doi:10.1016/j.jri.2012.10.005
22. Hughes GC, Choubey D. Modulation of autoimmune rheumatic diseases by oestrogen and progesterone. *Nat Rev Rheumatol* (2014) 10(12):740–51. doi:10.1038/nrrheum.2014.144
23. Romero R, Yeo L, Miranda J, Hassan SS, Conde-Agudelo A, Chaiworapongsa T. A blueprint for the prevention of preterm birth: vaginal progesterone in women with a short cervix. *J Perinat Med* (2013) 41(1):27–44. doi:10.1515/jpm-2012-0272
24. Schober L, Radnai D, Schmitt E, Mahnke K, Sohn C, Steinborn A. Term and preterm labor: decreased suppressive activity and changes in composition of the regulatory T-cell pool. *Immunol Cell Biol* (2012) 90(10):935–44. doi:10.1038/icb.2012.33
25. Levy T, Gurevitch S, Bar-Hava I, Ashkenazi J, Magazanik A, Homburg R, et al. Pharmacokinetics of natural progesterone administered in the form of a vaginal tablet. *Hum Reprod* (1999) 14(3):606–10. doi:10.1093/humrep/14.3.606
26. Derhovanessian E, Solana R, Larbi A, Pawelec G. Immunity, ageing and cancer. *Immun Ageing* (2008) 5:11. doi:10.1186/1742-4933-5-11
27. Imami N, Hardy G, Burton C, Pires A, Pido-Lopez J, Moss R, et al. Immune responses and reconstitution in HIV-1 infected individuals: impact of anti-retroviral therapy, cytokines and therapeutic vaccination. *Immunol Lett* (2001) 79(1–2):63–76. doi:10.1016/S0165-2478(01)00267-X
28. Bailey T, Stark S, Grant A, Hartnett C, Tsang M, Kalyuzhny A. A multidonor ELISPOT study of IL-1 beta, IL-2, IL-4, IL-6, IL-13, IFN-gamma and TNF-alpha release by cryopreserved human peripheral blood mononuclear cells. *J Immunol Methods* (2002) 270(2):171–82. doi:10.1016/S0022-1759(02)00297-1
29. Duricki DA, Soleman S, Moon LD. Analysis of longitudinal data from animals with missing values using SPSS. *Nat Protoc* (2016) 11(6):1112–29. doi:10.1038/nprot.2016.048
30. Roederer M, Nozzi JL, Nason MC. SPICE: exploration and analysis of post-cytometric complex multivariate datasets. *Cytometry A* (2011) 79(2):167–74. doi:10.1002/cyto.a.21015
31. Quarona V, Zaccarello G, Chillemi A, Brunetti E, Singh VK, Ferrero E, et al. CD38 and CD157: a long journey from activation markers to multifunctional molecules. *Cytometry B Clin Cytom* (2013) 84(4):207–17. doi:10.1002/cyto.b.21092
32. Yamazaki T, Yang XO, Chung Y, Fukunaga A, Nurieva R, Pappu B, et al. CCR6 regulates the migration of inflammatory and regulatory T cells. *J Immunol* (2008) 181(12):8391–401. doi:10.4049/jimmunol.181.12.8391
33. Kondo T, Takata H, Takiguchi M. Functional expression of chemokine receptor CCR6 on human effector memory CD8+ T cells. *Eur J Immunol* (2007) 37(1):54–65. doi:10.1002/eji.200636251
34. Mahnke YD, Brodie TM, Sallusto F, Roederer M, Lugli E. The who's who of T-cell differentiation: human memory T-cell subsets. *Eur J Immunol* (2013) 43(11):2797–809. doi:10.1002/eji.201343751
35. Lim HW, Lee J, Hillsamer P, Kim CH. Human Th17 cells share major trafficking receptors with both polarized effector T cells and FOXP3+ regulatory T cells. *J Immunol* (2008) 180(1):122–9. doi:10.4049/jimmunol.180.1.122
36. Mellor-Heineke S, Villanueva J, Jordan MB, Marsh R, Zhang K, Bleesing JJ, et al. Elevated Granzyme B in cytotoxic lymphocytes is a signature of immune activation in hemophagocytic lymphohistiocytosis. *Front Immunol* (2013) 4:72. doi:10.3389/fimmu.2013.00072
37. Sallusto F, Lenig D, Forster R, Lipp M, Lanzavecchia A. Two subsets of memory T lymphocytes with distinct homing potentials and effector functions. *Nature* (1999) 401(6754):708–12. doi:10.1038/44385
38. Amodio G, Comi M, Tomasoni D, Gianolini ME, Rizzo R, LeMaoult J, et al. HLA-G expression levels influence the tolerogenic activity of human DC-10. *Haematologica* (2015) 100(4):548–57. doi:10.3324/haematol.2014.113803
39. Shah NM, Herasimtschuk AA, Boasso A, Benlahrech A, Fuchs D, Imami N, et al. Changes in T cell and dendritic cell phenotype from mid to late pregnancy are indicative of a shift from immune tolerance to immune activation. *Front Immunol* (2017) 8:1138. doi:10.3389/fimmu.2017.01138

40. Malavige GN, Jeewandara C, Alles KM, Salimi M, Gomes L, Kamaladasa A, et al. Suppression of virus specific immune responses by IL-10 in acute dengue infection. *PLoS Negl Trop Dis* (2013) 7(9):e2409. doi:10.1371/journal.pntd.0002409
41. Ramos NL, Sekikubo M, Kironde F, Mirembe F, Saaf M, Brauner A. The impact of vitamin D on the innate immune response to uropathogenic *Escherichia coli* during pregnancy. *Clin Microbiol Infect* (2015) 21(5):482.e1–7. doi:10.1016/j.cmi.2014.12.010
42. Kumar A, Madden DL, Nankervis GA. Humoral and cell-mediated immune responses to herpesvirus antigens during pregnancy – a longitudinal study. *J Clin Immunol* (1984) 4(1):12–7. doi:10.1007/BF00915281
43. Bishop CV, Xu F, Steinbach R, Ficco E, Hyzer J, Blue S, et al. Changes in immune cell distribution and their cytokine/chemokine production during regression of the rhesus macaque corpus luteum. *Biol Reprod* (2017) 96(6):1210–20. doi:10.1093/biolre/iox052
44. Lee S, Kim J, Jang B, Hur S, Jung U, Kil K, et al. Fluctuation of peripheral blood T, B, and NK cells during a menstrual cycle of normal healthy women. *J Immunol* (2010) 185(1):756–62. doi:10.4049/jimmunol.0904192
45. Lorenz TK, Heiman JR, Demas GE. Sexual activity modulates shifts in TH1/TH2 cytokine profile across the menstrual cycle: an observational study. *Fertil Steril* (2015) 104(6):1513–21.e4. doi:10.1016/j.fertnstert.2015.09.001
46. Arruvito L, Sanz M, Banham AH, Fainboim L. Expansion of CD4+CD25+and FOXP3+ regulatory T cells during the follicular phase of the menstrual cycle: implications for human reproduction. *J Immunol* (2007) 178(4):2572–8. doi:10.4049/jimmunol.178.4.2572
47. Faas M, Bouman A, Moesa H, Heineman MJ, de Leij L, Schuiling G. The immune response during the luteal phase of the ovarian cycle: a Th2-type response? *Fertil Steril* (2000) 74(5):1008–13. doi:10.1016/S0015-0282(00)01553-3
48. Priyanka HP, Sharma U, Gopinath S, Sharma V, Hima L, ThyagaRajan S. Menstrual cycle and reproductive aging alters immune reactivity, NGF expression, antioxidant enzyme activities, and intracellular signaling pathways in the peripheral blood mononuclear cells of healthy women. *Brain Behav Immun* (2013) 32:131–43. doi:10.1016/j.bbi.2013.03.008
49. Caggiula AR, Stoney CM, Matthews KA, Owens JF, Davis MC, Rabin BS. T-lymphocyte reactivity during the menstrual cycle in women. *Clin Immunol Immunopathol* (1990) 56(1):130–4. doi:10.1016/0090-1229(90)90177-R
50. Sulke AN, Jones DB, Wood PJ. Variation in natural killer activity in peripheral blood during the menstrual cycle. *Br Med J (Clin Res Ed)* (1985) 290(6472):884–6. doi:10.1136/bmj.290.6472.884
51. Lorenz TK, Heiman JR, Demas GE. Interactions among sexual activity, menstrual cycle phase, and immune function in healthy women. *J Sex Res* (2017) 21:1–9. doi:10.1080/00224499.2017.1394961
52. Rowe JH, Ertelt JM, Xin L, Way SS. Pregnancy imprints regulatory memory that sustains anergy to fetal antigen. *Nature* (2012) 490(7418):102–6. doi:10.1038/nature11462
53. Johansson ED. Plasma levels of progesterone in pregnancy measured by a rapid competitive protein binding technique. *Acta Endocrinol (Copenh)* (1969) 61(4):607–17.
54. Ledoux F, Genest J, Nowaczynski W, Kuchel O, Lebel M. Plasma progesterone and aldosterone in pregnancy. *Can Med Assoc J* (1975) 112(8):943–7.
55. Zhou F, Chen XY, Zhuang YL, Chen YZ, Huang LL. Low-dose mifepristone increases uterine natural killer cell cytotoxicity and perforin expression during the receptive phase. *Fertil Steril* (2011) 96(3):649–53. doi:10.1016/j.fertnstert.2011.06.074
56. Chen Y, Wang Y, Zhuang Y, Zhou F, Huang L. Mifepristone increases the cytotoxicity of uterine natural killer cells by acting as a glucocorticoid antagonist via ERK activation. *PLoS One* (2012) 7(5):e36413. doi:10.1371/journal.pone.0036413
57. Coronel MF, Raggio MC, Adler NS, De Nicola AF, Labombarda F, González SL. Progesterone modulates pro-inflammatory cytokine expression profile after spinal cord injury: implications for neuropathic pain. *J Neuroimmunol* (2016) 292:85–92. doi:10.1016/j.jneuroim.2016.01.011
58. Xue XT, Kou XX, Li CS, Bi RY, Meng Z, Wang XD, et al. Progesterone attenuates temporomandibular joint inflammation through inhibition of NF-κB pathway in ovariectomized rats. *Sci Rep* (2017) 7(1):15334. doi:10.1038/s41598-017-15285-w
59. Lei B, Mace B, Dawson HN, Warner DS, Laskowitz DT, James ML. Anti-inflammatory effects of progesterone in lipopolysaccharide-stimulated BV-2 microglia. *PLoS One* (2014) 9(7):e103969. doi:10.1371/journal.pone.0103969
60. Yuan Y, Shimizu I, Shen M, Aoyagi E, Takenaka H, Itagaki T, et al. Effects of estradiol and progesterone on the proinflammatory cytokine production by mononuclear cells from patients with chronic hepatitis C. *World J Gastroenterol* (2008) 14(14):2200–7. doi:10.3748/wjg.14.2200
61. Wu Y, Strawn E, Basir Z, Halverson G, Guo SW. Promoter hypermethylation of progesterone receptor isoform B (PR-B) in endometriosis. *Epigenetics* (2006) 1(2):106–11. doi:10.4161/epi.1.2.2766
62. Nadeem L, Shynlova O, Matysiak-Zablocki E, Mesiano S, Dong X, Lye S. Molecular evidence of functional progesterone withdrawal in human myometrium. *Nat Commun* (2016) 7:11565. doi:10.1038/ncomms11565
63. Cannizzo ES, Bellistrì GM, Casabianca A, Tincati C, Iannotti N, Barco A, et al. Immunophenotype and function of CD38-expressing CD4+ and CD8+ T cells in HIV-infected patients undergoing suppressive combination antiretroviral therapy. *J Infect Dis* (2015) 211(9):1511–3. doi:10.1093/infdis/jiu634
64. Sandoval-Montes C, Santos-Argumedo L. CD38 is expressed selectively during the activation of a subset of mature T cells with reduced proliferation but improved potential to produce cytokines. *J Leukoc Biol* (2005) 77(4):513–21. doi:10.1189/jlb.0404262
65. Mao G, Wang J, Kang Y, Tai P, Wen J, Zou Q, et al. Progesterone increases systemic and local uterine proportions of CD4+CD25+ Treg cells during mid-term pregnancy in mice. *Endocrinology* (2010) 151(11):5477–88. doi:10.1210/en.2010-0426
66. Schumacher A, Dauven D, Zenclussen AC. Progesterone-driven local regulatory T cell induction does not prevent fetal loss in the CBA/J×DBA/2J abortion-prone model. *Am J Reprod Immunol* (2017) 77:e12626. doi:10.1111/aji.12626
67. Nair AB, Jacob S. A simple practice guide for dose conversion between animals and human. *J Basic Clin Pharm* (2016) 7(2):27–31. doi:10.4103/0976-0105.177703
68. Woidacki K, Meyer N, Schumacher A, Goldschmidt A, Maurer M, Zenclussen AC. Transfer of regulatory T cells into abortion-prone mice promotes the expansion of uterine mast cells and normalizes early pregnancy angiogenesis. *Sci Rep* (2015) 5:13938. doi:10.1038/srep13938
69. Zenclussen AC, Gerlof K, Zenclussen ML, Sollwedel A, Bertoja AZ, Ritter T, et al. Abnormal T-cell reactivity against paternal antigens in spontaneous abortion: adoptive transfer of pregnancy-induced CD4+CD25+ T regulatory cells prevents fetal rejection in a murine abortion model. *Am J Pathol* (2005) 166(3):811–22. doi:10.1016/S0002-9440(10)62302-4
70. Yin Y, Han X, Shi Q, Zhao Y, He Y. Adoptive transfer of CD4+CD25+ regulatory T cells for prevention and treatment of spontaneous abortion. *Eur J Obstet Gynecol Reprod Biol* (2012) 161(2):177–81. doi:10.1016/j.ejogrb.2011.12.023
71. Mjosberg J, Svensson J, Johansson E, Hellstrom L, Casas R, Jenmalm MC, et al. Systemic reduction of functionally suppressive CD4dimCD25highFoxp3+ Tregs in human second trimester pregnancy is induced by progesterone and 17beta-estradiol. *J Immunol* (2009) 183(1):759–69. doi:10.4049/jimmunol.0803654
72. Ivanova-Todorova E, Kyurkchiev DS, Nalbanski A, Timeva T, Shterev A, Kyurkchiev SD. Production and characterization of a novel monoclonal antibody against progesterone-induced blocking factor (PIBF). *J Reprod Immunol* (2008) 78(2):94–101. doi:10.1016/j.jri.2007.12.001
73. Bogdan A, Berta G, Szekeres-Bartho J. PIBF positive uterine NK cells in the mouse decidua. *J Reprod Immunol* (2017) 119:38–43. doi:10.1016/j.jri.2016.12.001
74. Faust Z, Laskarin G, Rukavina D, Szekeres-Bartho J. Progesterone-induced blocking factor inhibits degranulation of natural killer cells. *Am J Reprod Immunol* (1999) 42(2):71–5.
75. Lin VC, Aw SE, Ng EH, Ng EH, Tan MG. Demonstration of mixed properties of RU486 in progesterone receptor (PR)-transfected MDA-MB-231 cells: a model for studying the functions of progesterone analogues. *Br J Cancer* (2001) 85(12):1978–86. doi:10.1054/bjoc.2001.2167
76. Zhang J, Tsai FT, Geller DS. Differential interaction of RU486 with the progesterone and glucocorticoid receptors. *J Mol Endocrinol* (2006) 37(1):163–73. doi:10.1677/jme.1.02089
77. van den Brandt J, Lühder F, McPherson KG, de Graaf KL, Tischner D, Wiehr S, et al. Enhanced glucocorticoid receptor signaling in T cells impacts thymocyte apoptosis and adaptive immune responses. *Am J Pathol* (2007) 170(3):1041–53. doi:10.2353/ajpath.2007.060804

78. Butts CL, Shukair SA, Duncan KM, Bowers E, Horn C, Belyavskaya E, et al. Progesterone inhibits mature rat dendritic cells in a receptor-mediated fashion. *Int Immunol* (2007) 19(3):287–96. doi:10.1093/intimm/dxl145
79. Yao Y, Li H, Ding J, Xia Y, Wang L. Progesterone impairs antigen-non-specific immune protection by CD8 T memory cells via interferon-γ gene hypermethylation. *PLoS Pathog* (2017) 13(11):e1006736. doi:10.1371/journal.ppat.1006736
80. Hall OJ, Nachbagauer R, Vermillion MS, Fink AL, Phuong V, Krammer F, et al. Progesterone-based contraceptives reduce adaptive immune responses and protection against sequential influenza A virus infections. *J Virol* (2017) 91:e02160-16. doi:10.1128/JVI.02160-16
81. Roberts AD, Ely KH, Woodland DL. Differential contributions of central and effector memory T cells to recall responses. *J Exp Med* (2005) 202(1):123–33. doi:10.1084/jem.20050137
82. Mehlhop-Williams ER, Bevan MJ. Memory CD8+ T cells exhibit increased antigen threshold requirements for recall proliferation. *J Exp Med* (2014) 211(2):345–56. doi:10.1084/jem.20131271
83. Holling TM, Schooten E, van Den Elsen PJ. Function and regulation of MHC class II molecules in T-lymphocytes: of mice and men. *Hum Immunol* (2004) 65(4):282–90. doi:10.1016/j.humimm.2004.01.005
84. Cao Y, Bender IK, Konstantinidis AK, Shin SC, Jewell CM, Cidlowski JA, et al. Glucocorticoid receptor translational isoforms underlie maturational stage-specific glucocorticoid sensitivities of dendritic cells in mice and humans. *Blood* (2013) 121(9):1553–62. doi:10.1182/blood-2012-05-432336
85. Kim OY, Monsel A, Bertrand M, Coriat P, Cavaillon JM, Adib-Conquy M. Differential down-regulation of HLA-DR on monocyte subpopulations during systemic inflammation. *Crit Care* (2010) 14(2):R61. doi:10.1186/cc8959

16

Human Miscarriage is Associated with Dysregulations in Peripheral Blood-Derived Myeloid Dendritic Cell Subsets

Stefanie Ehrentraut[1], Karoline Sauss[1], Romy Neumeister[2], Lydia Luley[1,3], Anika Oettel[3], Franziska Fettke[1,3], Serban-Dan Costa[3], Stefanie Langwisch[1], Ana Claudia Zenclussen[1] and Anne Schumacher[1]*

[1] *Health Campus Immunology, Infectiology and Inflammation (GC-I[3]), Experimental Obstetrics and Gynecology, Medical Faculty, Otto-von-Guericke University, Magdeburg, Germany,* [2] *Gynecologic Ambulance, Haldensleben, Germany,* [3] *University Women's Clinic, Otto-von-Guericke University, Magdeburg, Germany*

Correspondence:
Anne Schumacher
anne.schumacher@med.ovgu.de

Dendritic cells (DC) are critically involved in decisions related to the acceptance or rejection of the foreign fetal antigens by the maternal immune system. However, particularly for human peripheral blood DCs (PBDC), available literature is rather inconsistent and the factors regulating these cells are ill-defined. Here, we investigated the phenotype and functionality of different human PBDC subsets during normal and pathologic pregnancies and studied an involvement of human chorionic gonadotropin (hCG) in PBDC regulation. Peripheral blood samples were obtained from normal pregnant women in all three trimesters, from first trimester miscarriage patients and from healthy non-pregnant women. Samples were analyzed for plasma hCG levels, for regulatory T (Treg) cell numbers, for frequencies of total and mature plasmacytoid (PDC) and myeloid (MDC1 and MDC2) PBDC subsets and for their cytokine secretion. *In vitro* assays, culturing PDC, MDC1 or MDC2 in the presence of two trophoblast cell lines, placenta explant supernatants or two hCG preparations were performed. The Treg-inducing capability of hCG- or non-hCG-treated stimulated MDC1 was assessed. Total and mature MDC1 and MDC2 frequencies increased during the first and second trimester of normal pregnancy, respectively. Miscarriage was associated with a reduced MDC1 and an increased MDC2 activation profile. PDC were not altered neither during normal pregnancy progression nor during miscarriage. *In vitro*, the culture of isolated PBDC subsets in the presence of placenta-derived factors impaired the maturation of MDC1 and differentially affected PDC maturation. An inhibitory effect on MDC1 and PDC maturation was also proven for the urine-derived hCG preparation. Finally, we observed a Treg cell elevation during early normal pregnancy that was not present in miscarriages. Stimulated MDC1 induced Treg cells *in vitro*, however, hCG was not involved in this process. Our findings suggest that during normal pregnancy PBDC subsets are differentially regulated dependent on gestational age. Miscarriage seems to be associated with dysregulations in the myeloid PBDC subsets and with disturbances in Treg cell frequencies. Moreover, our results propose an interdependency between MDC1 and Treg cells during early pregnancy. hCG, although shown to impair MDC1 maturation, does not seem to be a key regulator of PBDC alterations during pregnancy.

Keywords: peripheral blood dendritic cells, plasmacytoid dendritic cells, myeloid dendritic cells, regulatory T cells, human chorionic gonadotropin, placenta factors, fetal tolerance, pregnancy

INTRODUCTION

Pregnancy is characterized by finely regulated immunological adaptions that allow the persistence of the foreign fetal antigens in the maternal womb. Notably, since Schmorl and colleagues in 1893 identified for the first time fetal cells at various maternal tissue sites (1), it became obvious that not only local immune cell populations residing directly at the fetal-maternal interface but also immune cell types circulating in the periphery get in direct contact to fetal structures and are able to react toward them. Thus, pregnancy-driven immunological adjustments take place locally and peripherally and dysregulations in uterine as well as circulating immune responses may interfere with normal pregnancy progression. Several studies implicated immune modulatory properties of placenta-derived factors suggesting that the fetal tissue itself regulates its surrounding environment (2). These factors include among others cytokines, growth factors and hormones and were reported to educate local and peripheral immune cells in such a way that they contribute to fetal tolerance and growth (3–9). Thereby, peripheral immune cell populations reportedly adapt their phenotype and functionality so to enter the fetal-maternal interface as "fetal-friendly" cells. However, the precise mechanisms how this is realized during pregnancy are still under investigation.

As one of the first immune cell types encountering fetal antigens, dendritic cells (DCs) possess the capacity to induce either immunity or tolerance toward the fetus (10). Their behavior highly depends on the maturation state and cytokine secretion pattern (10). In the human decidua, the presence of predominantly myeloid DCs possessing an immature phenotype and secreting anti-inflammatory cytokines was associated with fetal tolerance (11–14), while a mature DC phenotype could be associated with various pregnancy complications (15–18). By contrast, data referring to the distribution and the phenotype of peripheral blood DC (PBDC) subsets during normal and pathologic pregnancies are rather inconsistent which might be due to the different DC characterization strategies applied in the past (19–22). Moreover, most of the studies divided the total PBDC pool into two major subsets, one lymphoid, and one myeloid subset. However, in 2000 Dzionek and colleagues described the existence of three clearly defined PBDC subsets. Based on the expression of specific blood DC antigens (BDCA), the authors classified the total PBDC pool into one plasmacytoid (PDC) and two myeloid (MDC1 and MDC2) subsets (23). Later on, the Nomenclature Committee of the International Union of Immunological Societies approved this classification (24). Interestingly, the presence of the BDCA-defined DC subsets seems to be not restricted to the peripheral blood as Ban and colleagues were able to detect all three subsets in the human decidua during early normal pregnancy. Decidual BDCA-1^+ MDC1 and BDCA-3^+ MDC2 expressed low levels of the maturation markers CD86 and CD80 confirming an immature phenotype of local DCs during normal pregnancy (25). This finding gives rise to speculations about the origin of these cells. On the one hand, it can be assumed that BDCA-1^+ MDC1 and BDCA-3^+ MDC2 are part of the DC pool resident in the uterus and regulated locally once pregnancy arised. On the other hand, it can be hypothesized that both DC subsets immigrate from the peripheral blood stream into the fetal-maternal interface. In both cases, placenta-derived factors may contribute to the local regulation as well as to DC immigration (26–28). Zhao and colleagues suggested a participation of human placenta-produced factors in the differentiation process from blood-derived monocytes into decidual DCs. The authors further confirmed a tolerogenic phenotype of these differentiated DCs (29). Additionally, placental factors reaching the circulation may provoke alterations of PBDCs directly in the periphery. The pregnancy hormone human chorionic gonadotropin (hCG) may represent a good candidate to fulfill this function as it represents one, if not the first signal, provided by the fetal tissue to the mother and can be detected already 6–8 days following fertilization in the blood stream (30). Furthermore, there is evidence that hCG has the capability to modulate human PBDCs (20, 31, 32).

Here, we aimed to investigate the phenotype and functionality of PDC, MDC1, and MDC2 derived from human peripheral blood during normal and pathologic pregnancies. Moreover, we addressed a potential regulation of all PBDC subsets by placenta-derived factors with a specific focus on hCG.

METHODS

Sampling and Ethical Approval

Peripheral blood samples were obtained from healthy non-pregnant woman within the luteal phase of their menstrual cycle as well as from normal pregnant woman in all three trimesters and from first trimester miscarriage patients. Placental tissue from normal pregnant women and miscarriage patients was obtained by curettage during surgery. Sampling of blood and placental tissue was realized by physicians of the University Women's Clinic in Magdeburg, Germany after all subjects were informed in detail and gave their written consent. This study was carried out in accordance with the recommendations of ethic guidelines defined by the ethics board at the University of Magdeburg with written informed consent from all subjects.

TABLE 1 | Patient characteristics.

	Total number	Week of pregnancy	Age
***Ex vivo* analyses**			
Non-pregnant women	$n = 12$	N/A	24.82 ± 4.41
Normal pregnant women (I. Trimester)	$n = 20$	10.30 ± 1.39	25.95 ± 5.06
Normal pregnant women (II. Trimester)	$n = 14$	19.21 ± 3.97	28.36 ± 5.45
Normal pregnant women (III. Trimester)	$n = 18$	34.28 ± 3.38	30.06 ± 3.22
Miscarriage patients	$n = 20$	8.65 ± 1.11	30.70 ± 6.01
***In vitro* Assays**			
Non-pregnant women	$n = 6$	N/A	28.50 ± 4.15
Normal pregnant women (I. Trimester)	$n = 16$	9.81 ± 1.70	30.00 ± 5.97
Miscarriage patients (I. Trimester)	$n = 16$	8.69 ± 0.98	31.50 ± 4.85

All subjects gave written informed consent in accordance with the Declaration of Helsinki. The protocol was approved by the ethics board at the University of Magdeburg (study 28/08). Characteristics of all study subjects are displayed in **Table 1**.

Determination of hCG Isoforms in Plasma and Placenta Supernatants by ELISA Analysis

After tissue collection, 500 mg of placental tissue (explants) was cultured in 1 ml of RPMI 1640 (Thermo Fisher Scientific, Germany) supplemented with 3% of charcolized fetal bovine serum (FBS, PAN-Biotech, Germany) and 1% penicillin/streptomycin (Thermo Fisher Scientific, Germany) for 24 h. Afterwards, placenta explant supernatants were collected and analyzed for the concentration of either regular hCG, free β-hCG or hyperglycosylated hCG (H-hCG) by enzyme-linked immunosorbent assay (ELISA). The concentrations of all hCG isoforms were evaluated in the plasma fraction of all blood samples. Regular and free β-hCG were determined using kits from DRG systems, Germany whereas H-hCG concentrations were evaluated using a kit from My Biosource, USA. All steps were performed according to the manufacturer's instructions.

Isolation of MDC1, MDC2, or PDC From PBMCs

The cellular fraction from all blood samples was used to isolate peripheral blood mononuclear cells (PBMCs) by density gradient centrifugation using Ficoll-Paque™ (GE Healthcare, Sweden) under sterile conditions. Afterwards, MDC1, MDC2, or PDC were separately isolated from PBMCs of non-pregnant and normal pregnant women (I. trimester) as well as from miscarriage patients (I. trimester) by magnetic activated cell sorting. The following isolations kits from Miltenyi Biotec, Germany were applied: MDC1 (CD1c Dendritic Cell Isolation Kit, human); MDC2 (CD141 MicroBead Kit, human); and PDC (CD304 MicroBead Kit, human). All steps were performed under sterile conditions following the instructions given. Purities of isolated MDC1, MDC2 and PDC were above 95, 45, and 85%, respectively. After isolation, all PBDC subsets were cultured for 24 h in RPMI 1640 supplemented with 50 μM β-mercaptoethanol (Sigma Aldrich, Germany), 10% FBS (Biochrom, Germany) and 1% penicillin/streptomycin (dendritic cell medium; DCM).

Cytometric Bead Array (CBA) Analysis of Cytokine Secretion by MDC1, MDC2, and PDC

5×10^4 isolated MDC1, MDC2, or PDC from either normal pregnant women or miscarriage patients in their first trimester of pregnancy were cultured in DCM for 48 h. Following, cell supernatants were collected and analyzed for the levels of IL-1β, IL-6, IL-8, IL-10, and TNF by CBA using the TH1/TH2 Cytokine Kit from BD Biosciences, Germany. All steps were performed according to the instructions provided by the manufacturer. Measurements were conducted by using a 4-color FACSCalibur™ flow cytometer (BD Biosciences, Germany) and analyses were performed using FCAPArray software (BD Biosciences, Germany).

Assessment of PBDC Maturation Under Different Culture Conditions Involving Trophoblast Cell Lines, Placental Explant Supernatants or Purified hCG Preparations

For the following experiments, MDC1, MDC2, or PDC were isolated from PBMCs derived from healthy non-pregnant women in the luteal phase of their menstrual cycle. The maturation of all three PBDC subsets was induced by the addition of 10 ng/ml lipopolysaccharide (LPS) to the DCM. In each experimental setting, the maturation state was assessed after 24 h by determining the numbers of CD83-, CD86-, or HLA-DR-expressing MDC1, MDC2, or PDC. The appropriate gating strategy is displayed in **Supplementary Figure 1**.

In the first set of experiments, 1×10^4 MDC1, MDC2, or PDC were co-cultured with 3×10^4 JEG-3 cells (hCG-secreting human choriocarcinoma cell line) or SWAN-71 cells (non hCG-secreting human immortalized extravillious cytotrophoblast cell line). Therefore, both trophoblast cell lines were plated 1 day before starting the co-cultures to allow adherence to the culture plate. JEG-3 and SWAN-71 cells were cultured in Dulbecco's modified eagle medium (DMEM, Invitrogen, Germany) supplemented with 10% FBS, 1% penicillin/streptomycin, 100 nM MEM non-essential amino acids (Invitrogen, Germany), 1 mM sodium pyruvate (Sigma-Aldrich, Germany), and 10 mM hepes (Biochrom, Germany). Both cell lines were cultured at 37°C and 5% CO_2.

In the second set of experiments, 1×10^4 MDC1, MDC2, or PDC were cultured in placental explant supernatants enriched with DCM in a ratio 1:1. Placental explants were derived from normal pregnant women or miscarriage patients in their first trimester of pregnancy.

In the third set of experiments, 1×10^4 MDC1, MDC2, or PDC were treated with either 100IU/ml recombinant hCG (rhCG, Ovitrelle, Merck, Germany) or 250 IU/ml urine-derived hCG (uhCG, Sigma, Germany). The concentration of uhCG was chosen according to physiological hCG levels found in normal pregnant women during the first trimester (25-288IU/ml during gestation weeks 9–12 according to the *American Pregnancy*

Association) and rhCG concentration was chosen according to concentrations used for rhCG and other recombinant gonadotropins in previous studies (33, 34).

Assessment of Treg Cell Generation After Co-culture With hCG- or Non hCG-Treated MDC1

MDC1 were isolated from non-pregnant women, stimulated with 10 ng/ml LPS and cultured in the absence or presence of hCG (100 mIU/ml rhCG or 250IU/ml uhCG) for 24 h as described above. Afterwards, 1×10^4 MDC1 were co-cultured with 1×10^4 $CD4^{+}CD25^{-}$ T cells in DCM containing 10 ng/ml recombinant IL-2, 1 μg/ml anti-CD3 and 5 μg/ml anti-CD28 for another 24 h. $CD4^{+}CD25^{-}$ T cells were obtained from the same donors who provided the MDC1 by using the human $CD4^{+}CD25^{+}$ Regulatory T Cell Isolation Kit (Miltenyi Biotec, Germany). Frequencies of $CD4^{+}CD25^{high}Foxp3^{+}$ Treg cells were determined by flow cytometry using a 4-color FACSCalibur™ flow cytometer. The appropriate gating strategy is displayed in **Supplementary Figure 2**.

Flow Cytometry Analysis

To estimate the frequencies of total and mature MDC1, MDC2, and PDC within PBMCs from non-pregnant and normal pregnant women as well as from miscarriage patients, PBMCs were stained for distinct surface markers defining the different DC subsets and for the maturation markers CD83, CD86, and HLA-DR. Additionally, Treg cell frequencies were determined in all samples. Therefore, PBMCs were stained for the extracellular markers CD4 and CD25 as well as for the intracellular marker Foxp3. Briefly, PBMCs were washed in PBS containing 1% bovine serum albumin (BSA) and 0.1% sodium azide (flow cytometry (FC) buffer). Afterwards, staining for extracellular markers (1:100 antibody dilutions) was performed for 30 min at 4°C in the dark. Following another washing step in FC buffer, cells were fixed overnight using the fixation/permeabilization set from Thermo Fisher Scientific, Germany. For intracellular staining, PBMCs were washed in permeabilization buffer and then incubated for 30 min at 4°C in the dark in the staining solution (1:200 antibody dilution). After washing in permeabilization buffer, cells were resuspended in FC buffer and measured using a 4-color FACSCalibur flow cytometer. The appropriate gating strategy is displayed in **Supplementary Figure 3**. MDC1, MDC2, PDC, and T cells obtained from *in vitro* culture experiments were stained accordingly. The following antibodies were used: APC-conjugated anti-human CD303 (PDC, clone: AC144), APC-conjugated anti-human CD1c (MDC1, clone: AD5-8E7) or APC-conjugated anti-human CD141 (MDC2, clone: AD5-14H12); all purchased from Miltenyi Biotec, Germany. PE-Cy7-conjugated anti-human CD83 (clone: HB15e), FITC-conjugated anti-human CD86 (clone: FUN-1), PE-conjugated anti-human HLA-DR (clone: G46-6), FITC-conjugated anti-human CD4 (clone: OKT4), PerCp-Cy5.5-conjugated anti-human CD25 (clone: BC96), and AF647-conjugated anti-human Foxp3 (clone: 259D/C7); purchased from BioLegend, eBiosciences and BD Biosciences, Germany, respectively.

Data Analysis and Statistics

Data analysis and presentation were performed with GraphPad Prism 7.0 software (Statcon, Germany). Data are displayed as means plus standard deviation (S.D.) or standard error of the mean (S.E.M.). The total number of replicates is indicated in the figure legends for each specific data set. All data sets were tested for normality by using the Shapiro-Wilk test and parametric or non-parametric tests were used accordingly. Normal distributed data sets were analyzed by using One- or Two-Way-ANOVA followed by Tukey's or Dunn's multiple comparison test. Not normal distributed data sets were analyzed by applying the Mann-Whitney-*U*-test. For *in vitro* culture experiments, controls (LPS alone) were set as "1" and experimental groups (trophoblast co-cultures, placenta explant supernatants and hCG preparations) were calculated as fold change to controls.

RESULTS

Pregnancy Provokes Alterations in the Number of Total and Mature Myeloid PBDC Subsets

First, we wondered whether PBDC subsets would change depending on gestational age during normal pregnancy progression. All subsets represented minor populations within total PBMCs (PDC: 0.25–2.64%; MDC1: 0.07–3.87%; MDC2: 0.03–1.06%). Frequencies of total and mature PDC from normal pregnant women of all trimesters were not altered when compared to non-pregnant women (**Figures 1A,D**). However, we observed an increase in the frequencies of total MDC1 and MDC2 during the first and second trimester in normal pregnant women, respectively, as compared to non-pregnant individuals (**Figures 1B,C**). Accordingly, HLA-DR-expressing MDC1 as well as CD83 and CD86-expressing MDC2 were elevated at the same gestational ages (**Figures 1E,F**).

Miscarriage Is Associated With an Altered Profile of Both Myeloid PBDC Subsets

Next, we sought to determine whether similar alterations in both myeloid PBDC subsets could be observed in miscarriage patients. We found no augmentation of total MDC1 frequencies in patients suffering from abortions when compared to non-pregnant women and a significant diminution as compared to normal pregnant women (**Figure 2B**). Moreover, frequencies of HLA-DR-expressing MDC1 were reduced in miscarriage patients when compared to normal pregnant women (**Figure 2E**). However, this did not reach statistical significance. Notably, frequencies of total and mature MDC2 were significantly elevated in miscarriage patients as compared to non-pregnant and normal pregnant women (**Figures 2C,F**). This included CD83-, CD86- and HLA-DR-expressing MDC2 (**Figure 2F**). As for PDC, no significant changes could be detected in miscarriage patients, neither to normal pregnant women nor to non-pregnant individuals (**Figures 2A,D**).

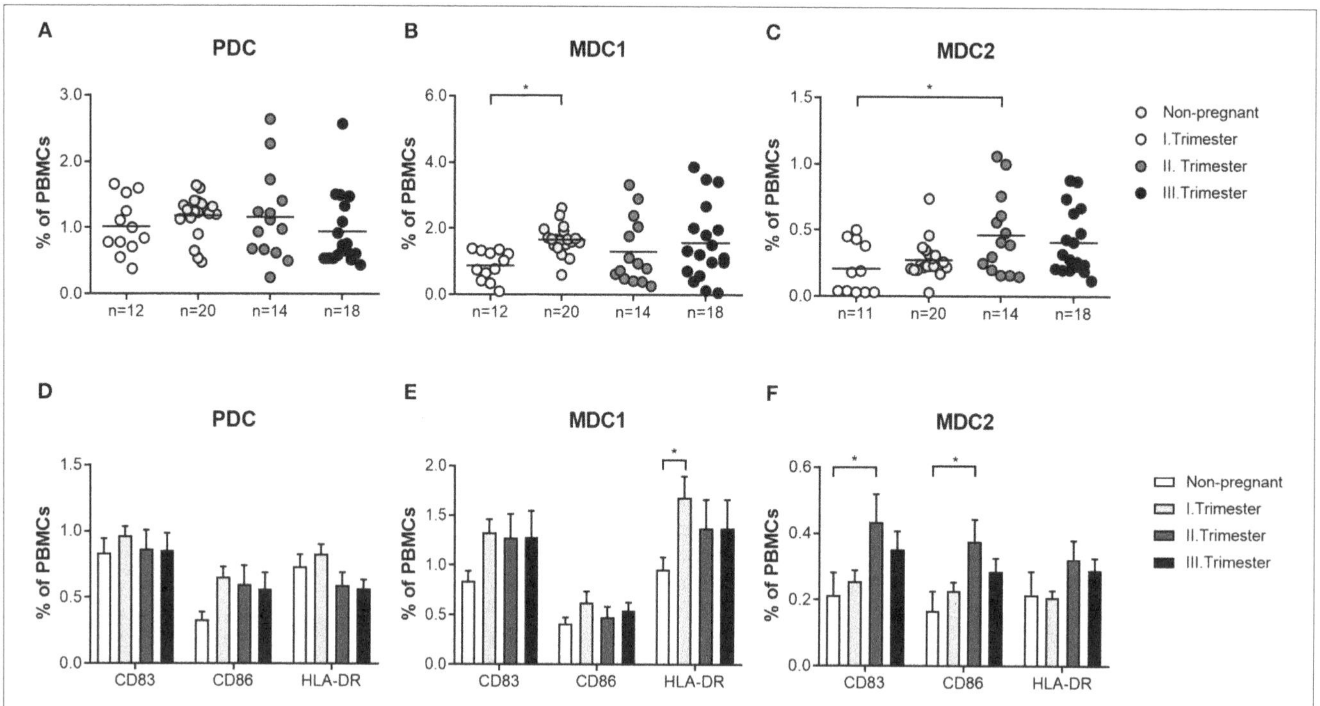

FIGURE 1 | The frequencies of total and mature MDC1 and MDC2 are altered depending on gestational age. PBMCs were isolated from normal pregnant women in all trimesters (n = 14–20) as well as from healthy non-pregnant women (n = 12) and stained for markers defining the distinct PBDC subsets and for the maturation markers CD83, CD86, and HLA-DR. The total frequencies of **(A)** PDC, **(B)** MDC1, and **(C)** MDC2 as well as the frequencies of mature **(D)** PDC, **(E)** MDC1, and **(F)** MDC2 were determined by flow cytometry. Statistical analysis was performed using One- or Two-Way-ANOVA followed by Tukey's multiple comparison test. $^*p \leq 0.05$.

Miscarriage Is Associated With a Disturbed Cytokine Secretion Capacity of the MDC1 Subset

Based on our findings, showing altered frequencies of total and mature MDC1 and MDC2 in miscarriage patients, we were curious whether both myeloid subsets would also possess a disturbed cytokine secretion profile. Therefore, we separately assessed the capacity to secrete cytokines of all PBDC subsets after their isolation from normal pregnant women or miscarriage patients. In agreement with our previous results, PDC from miscarriage patients secreted equal amounts of pro- and anti-inflammatory cytokines as the ones from normal pregnant women (**Figure 3A**). MDC1 from miscarriage patients had a significant reduced capacity to secrete IL-1β, IL-6, IL-10, and TNF (**Figure 3B**), while MDC2 from miscarriage patients did not behave differentially from MDC2 of normal pregnant women (**Figure 3C**). However, we have to admit that the purity of the MDC2 isolation was rather poor.

Miscarriage Is Associated With Reduced Peripheral and Local Levels of Different hCG Isoforms

As our results revealed changes during early normal pregnancy and predominantly in the MDC1 subset that could not be observed in pathologic pregnancies, we wondered whether placenta-derived factors might be responsible for the observed alterations. Here, we particularly focused on the pregnancy hormone hCG, known to be highly elevated during the first trimester. Analyses of plasma samples as well as placental explant supernatants exhibited significant diminished levels of regular hCG in plasma samples from miscarriage patients when compared to normal pregnant women but not in placental explant supernatants (**Table 2**). Even more interestingly, we found significant reduced levels of two other hCG isoforms, namely free β-hCG and H-hCG, in the plasma and the placenta supernatants from miscarriage patients (**Table 2**). Correlation analyses between all hCG isoforms and all PBDC subsets demonstrated a negative correlation between regular hCG or H-hCG and MDC2 but no correlation between free β-hCG and MDC2 (data not shown). Moreover, no correlations could be proven for all hCG isoforms and MDC1 or PDC (data not shown).

Placenta-Derived Factors Differentially Regulate the Maturation of PBDC Subsets

To determine whether placenta-derived factors and particularly hCG might be involved in PBDC alterations, we first co-cultured PDC, MDC1 or MDC2 with two different trophoblast cell lines and evaluated the effect on the maturation process. We chose one hCG-secreting trophoblast cell line (JEG-3) and one non hCG-secreting trophoblast cell line (SWAN-71). The presence of hCG-secreting JEG-3 cells contributed to an increase of CD83-expressing PDC but impaired an elevation

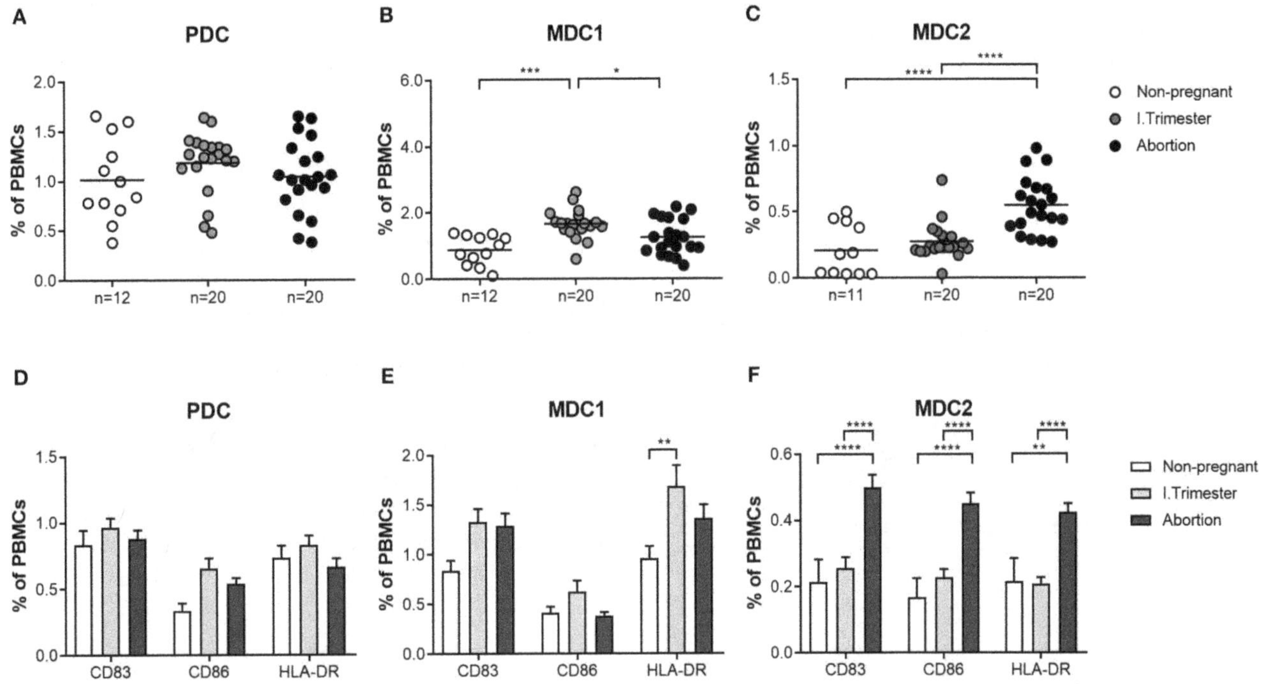

FIGURE 2 | The frequencies of total and mature MDC1 and MDC2 are altered in miscarriages. PBMCs were isolated from normal pregnant women and miscarriage patients in the first trimester ($n = 20$) as well as from healthy non-pregnant women ($n = 12$) and stained for markers defining the distinct PBDC subsets and for the maturation markers CD83, CD86, and HLA-DR. The total frequencies of **(A)** PDC, **(B)** MDC1, and **(C)** MDC2 as well as the frequencies of mature **(D)** PDC, **(E)** MDC1, and **(F)** MDC2 were determined by flow cytometry. Statistical analysis was performed using One- or Two-Way-ANOVA followed by Tukey's multiple comparison test. *$p \leq 0.05$, **$p \leq 0.01$, ***$p \leq 0.001$, ****$p \leq 0.0001$.

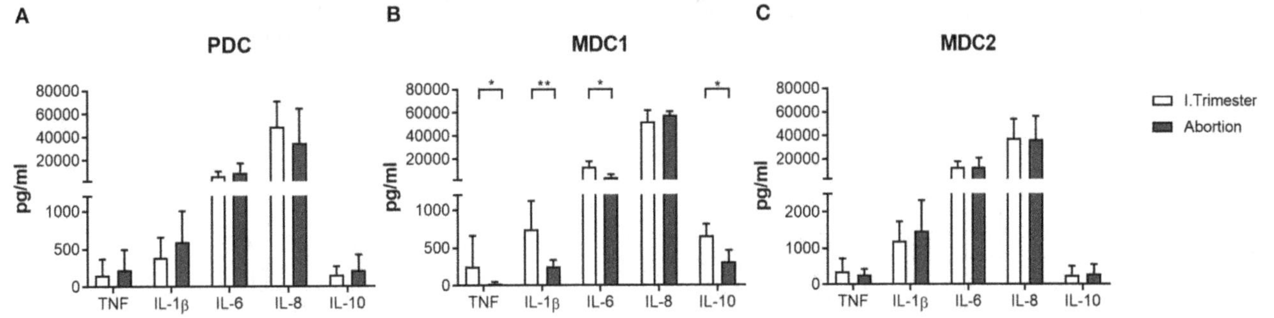

FIGURE 3 | MDC1 from miscarriages showed an altered cytokine profile. PDC, MDC1, or MDC2 were isolated from PBMCs of normal pregnant women and miscarriage patients in the first trimester ($n = 4–5$). All PBDC subsets were cultured for 48 h. Afterwards, cell culture supernatants were analyzed for the levels of different cytokines by CBArray. The concentration of TNF, IL-1β, IL-6, IL-8, and IL-10 produced by **(A)** PDC, **(B)** MDC1, and **(C)** MDC2 is displayed. Statistical analysis was performed using the Mann-Whitney-*U*-test. *$p \leq 0.05$, **$p \leq 0.01$.

of CD86- and HLA-DR-expressing MDC1 (**Figures 4A,B**). Non hCG-secreting SWAN-71 cells favored an augmentation of CD83- and CD86-expressing PDC and hampered an increase of HLA-DR-expressing MDC1 (**Figures 4A,B**). None of the cell lines significantly affected the maturation process of MDC2 (**Figure 4C**).

Secondly, we decided to culture each PBDC subsets with supernatants from placental explants derived from either normal pregnant women or miscarriage patients. Here, in addition to our co-cultures with the trophoblast cell lines, we studied a potential influence of soluble factors derived from primary trophoblast cells mimicking a more physiologic scenario. Besides, it is important to mention that placental explant supernatants contain a mixture of all hCG isoforms whereas JEG-3 cells almost exclusively secrete H-hCG. Unfortunately, most of our primary trophoblast cultures lose the ability to secrete hCG in culture and were therefore not suitable for these kind of experiments. Supernatants from miscarriage patients significantly hampered an augmentation of CD86-expressing PDC and HLA-DR-expressing MDC1 (**Figures 4D,E**), whereas supernatants from normal pregnant women had no effect on PDC and MDC1 (**Figures 4D,E**). Moreover, maturation of MDC2 was not influenced by the addition of placental explant supernatants (**Figure 4F**).

TABLE 2 | Miscarriage is associated with reduced levels of hCG isoforms.

	regular hCG (mIU/ml)	free β-hCG (pg/ml)	H-hCG (nmol/L)
Plasma			
I. Trimester	112855 ± 106610	43.63 ± 37.91	38.21 ± 43.43
Abortion	43840 ± 46906*	23.57 ± 22.56*	12.70 ± 5.43**
Placenta explants			
I. Trimester	175.60 ± 216.10	97.99 ± 42.48	198.40 ± 261.40
Abortion	252.30 ± 261.20	53.67 ± 54.53*	64.69 ± 92.57*

*Plasma and placenta explants from normal pregnant women and miscarriage patients in the first trimester (n = 15–20) were analyzed for the levels of different hCG isoforms by ELISA. Statistical analysis was performed using the Mann-Whitney-U-test. *p < 0.05 vs. I. Trimester; **p < 0.01 vs. I. Trimester.*

Thirdly, as our data were rather inconsistent with regard to a potential effect of hCG, we cultured PDC, MDC1, or MDC2 in the presence of two hCG preparations. We chose an rhCG preparation containing only intact regular hCG molecules and an uhCG preparation containing the broad variety of all hCG isoforms. We observed an impaired elevation of CD86-expressing PDC as well as CD83-, CD86-, and HLA-DR-expressing MDC1 when uhCG was added to the cultures (**Figures 4G,H**), whereas the presence of rhCG did not affect the maturation of PDC and MDC1 (**Figures 4G,H**). In line with our previous results, MDC2 maturation was not affected at all (**Figure 4I**). However, again we would like to point out that our MDC2 isolations suffered from a poor purity.

hCG Does Not Enhance MDC1-Induced Treg Generation

Own previous studies identified hCG as a factor driving Treg induction during early pregnancy (35). However, it is still a matter of debate through which pathways hCG

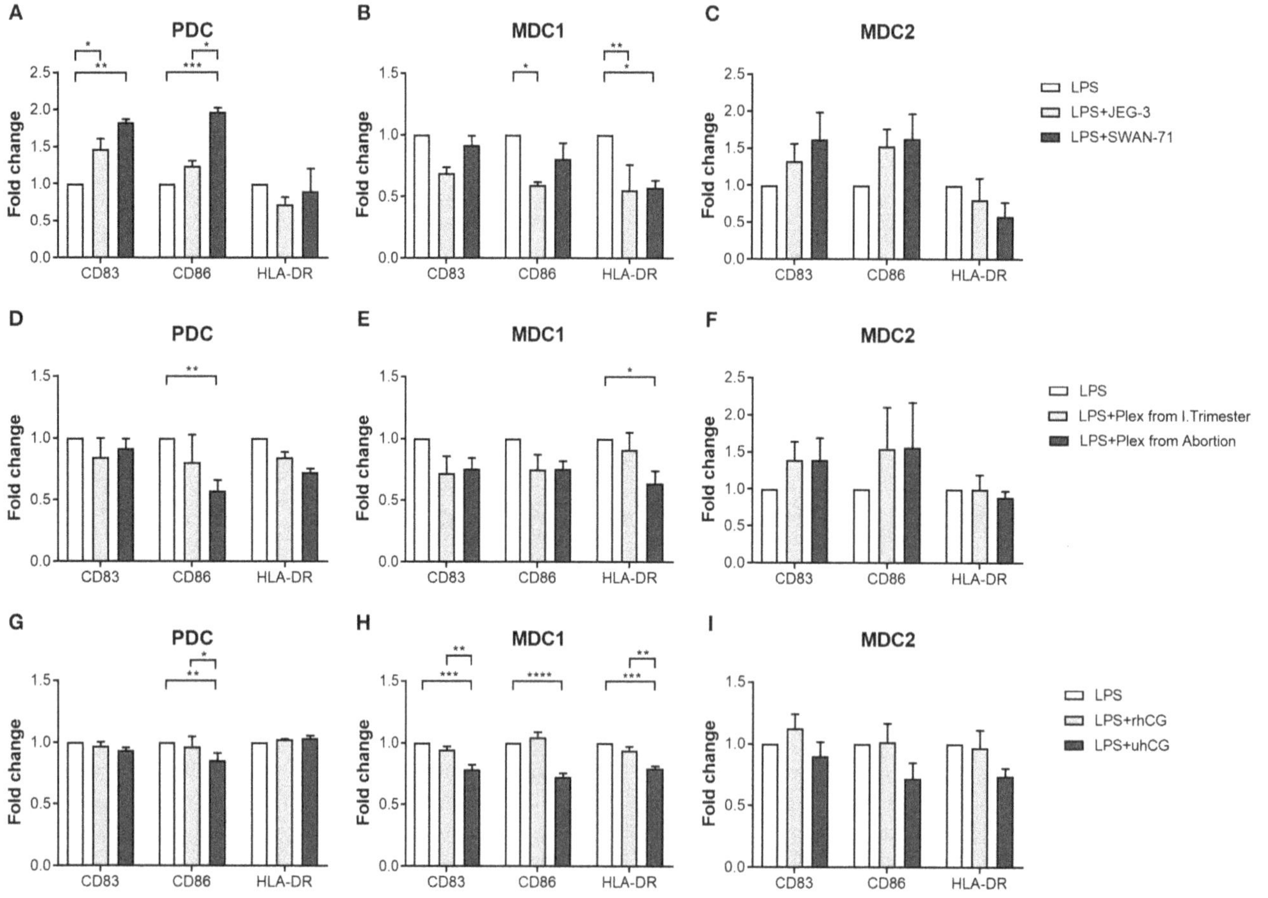

FIGURE 4 | PDC, MDC1 and MDC2 are differentially affected by placenta-derived factors. PDC, MDC1, or MDC2 were isolated from PBMCs of healthy non-pregnant women and cultured in the presence of **(A–C)** JEG-3 or SWAN-71 trophoblast cell lines ($n = 3$) **(D–F)**, supernatants of placental explants (Plex; $n = 4$) or **(G–I)** two hCG preparations [100 mIU/ml recombinant hCG (rhCG); 250IU/ml urine-derived (uhCG)]. The frequencies of mature **(A,D,G)** PDC, **(B,E,H)** MDC1, and **(C,F,I)** MDC2 were determined by flow cytometry. Statistical analysis was performed using Two-Way-ANOVA followed by Tukey's multiple comparison test. *$p \le 0.05$, **$p \le 0.01$, ***$p \le 0.001$, ****$p \le 0.0001$.

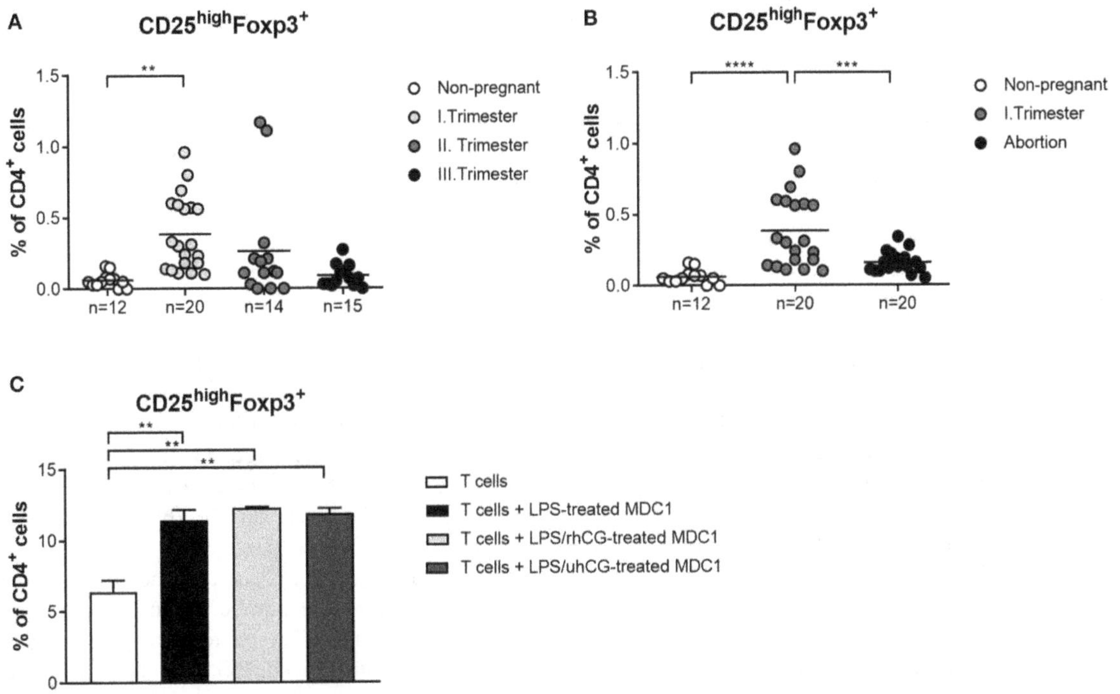

FIGURE 5 | MDC1 cells are able to induce Treg cells that are reduced in miscarriages. PBMCs were isolated from normal pregnant women in all trimesters (n = 14–20), from miscarriage patients in the first trimester (n = 20) as well as from healthy non-pregnant women (n = 12) and stained for Treg cell markers. Treg frequencies are shown for **(A)** normal pregnancy progression and for **(B)** miscarriage patients compared to normal and non-pregnant women. Moreover, MDC1 were isolated from non-pregnant women (n = 3), stimulated with 10 ng/ml LPS in the presence or absence of 100 mIU/ml recombinant hCG (rhCG) or 250IU/ml urine-derived hCG (uhCG) for 24 h and then co-cultured with $CD4^+CD25^-$ T cells derived from the same donors for another 24 h. **(C)** Treg frequencies were determined by flow cytometry. Statistical analysis was performed using One-Way-ANOVA followed by Dunn's multiple comparison test. $^{**}p \leq 0.01$, $^{***}p \leq 0.001$, $^{****}p \leq 0.0001$.

mediates its Treg-inducing properties. Here, we wondered whether an interdependency between Treg and PBDCs during early pregnancy exists and if hCG might represent the intermediate factor between both immune cell types. Therefore, we determined the frequencies of Treg during normal pregnancy progression as well as during miscarriage. $CD4^+CD25^{high}Foxp3^+$ Treg frequencies were significantly elevated in first trimester normal pregnant women when compared to non-pregnant women and declined during the second and third trimester (**Figure 5A**). Miscarriage patients had significantly reduced Treg frequencies as compared to normal pregnant women (**Figure 5B**). Notably, normal pregnancy-associated Treg alterations are in line with changes observed for MDC1 (**Figures 1B, 5A**). Moreover, miscarriage was characterized by lower Treg and MDC1 frequencies suggesting an interrelation between these two cell populations. To follow up this idea, we tested whether MDC1 possessed the ability to induce Treg *in vitro*. We pre-treated MDC1 with rhCG or uhCG to study a potential involvement of hCG in MDC1-mediated Treg induction. We confirmed the ability of MDC1 to induce Treg generation. However, pre-treatment with either rhCG or uhCG did not further enhance Treg numbers (**Figure 5C**).

DISCUSSION

Pregnancy can be considered as a remarkable challenge for the maternal immune system where a variety of immunological adaptions has to go hand in hand to guarantee the survival of the semi-allogeneic fetus. Hereby, not only local immune cell populations residing at the fetal-maternal interface but also immune cell types circulating through lymphoid tissues and the peripheral blood are aware of the foreign fetal antigens. Thus, pregnancy-driven immunological regulations take place in the proximity as well as in the distance of the fetal tissues and it is suggested that the fetus itself contributes to these regulatory processes by expressing and secreting immune modulating factors.

DCs are one of the major immune cell populations that are affected by pregnancy-driven alterations and on their part function as key regulators for other immune cells types. There is accumulating evidence that during normal human pregnancy progression myeloid DCs are the predominant DC population, locally as well as peripherally (11, 19, 20). Moreover, human decidual DCs adopt a tolerogenic profile by expressing an exclusive set of markers and possessing a reduced T cell stimulatory capacity (11, 12). PBDCs also undergo changes in their phenotype and functionality throughout normal human pregnancy. However, several studies presented different outcomes (19–22, 36) that might be partly explained by the combination of markers used to characterize the various PBDC subsets. Furthermore, the majority of the previous studies did not separately examine the frequencies of MDC1 and MDC2 but rather focused on one myeloid PBDC population. This kind of analysis may mask potential gestational-dependent alterations within distinct myeloid PBDC subsets.

Our current findings propose significant augmentations of total MDC1 and MDC2 during the first and second trimester of normal pregnancy, respectively, while total PDC remained unchanged at all trimesters. Likewise, we found elevations of mature myeloid PBDCs during the first and second trimester while the number of mature PDC was not altered. These observed gestational age-related changes in the number and functionality of PBDCs seem to be relevant to finely regulate the degree of alloreactive immune reactions. On the one hand, PBDCs have to be alert to systemic infections at any time while on the other hand ensure tolerance toward the fetal alloantigens. To overcome this paradoxical situation, it was proposed that PBDCs pass through an incomplete activation process during normal pregnancy enabling them to present fetal alloantigens without provoking overwhelming anti-fetal immune reactions. Moreover, there is evidence that PBDCs are involved in the induction of acquired thymic tolerance and it was suggested that incompletely activated PBDCs promote tolerance to fetal alloantigens by educating thymic T cells (19). Notably, the extent of DC activation seems to be decisive for pregnancy outcome as an over- or under-activation of PBDCs was associated with pregnancy complications such as pre-eclampsia, intrauterine growth retardation or miscarriage (18, 22). Our own findings support this idea, as we were able to demonstrate a significant lower number of mature MDC1 in miscarriage patients compared to normal pregnant women. Moreover, these cells had a reduced capacity to secrete cytokines suggesting an overall diminished potential to stimulate T cells. Our data suggest that also an underactivation of specific PBDC subsets may provoke fetal demise. Limited activation of MDC1 may result in a reduced potential to induce Treg cells that at first glance seems to be contradictory, as it is believed that predominantly DCs being in an immature or semi-mature state force Treg generation (37). However, Banerjee and colleagues proved that human myeloid DCs matured with a cocktail of inflammatory cytokines had the highest capability to induce Treg cells. Even myeloid DCs matured in the presence of LPS induced Treg cells to a greater extent than immature DCs (38). Our own data revealed that LPS-stimulated MDC1 supported the generation of Treg cells *in vitro*. Hence, we propose that during early stages of normal pregnancy, activated MDC1 enhance Treg cells in the periphery whereas underactivated MDC1 may lack the capacity for an adequate Treg induction. Our findings provide another explanation for the observed early Treg increment that is fundamental for fetal tolerance induction as reported earlier (39, 40) and again confirmed in our current study. Interestingly, MDC2 showed a completely different pattern when compared to MDC1 underlying the need to separately study the different myeloid PBDC subsets during pregnancy. Mature MDC2 were significantly augmented in miscarriage patients as compared to normal pregnant women. We assume that MDC1 and MDC2 overtake different functions at different gestational ages and that an over or underrepresentation of each subset at other pregnancy time points may be deleterious for pregnancy. According to a study by Hayashi and colleagues, MDC1 can be seen as TH1-promoting cells while MDC2 are rather TH2-promoting cells (41). As normal pregnancy begins with TH1-related immune responses (peri-implantation phase), changes to TH2-related immune responses (mid-gestation) and finally shifts back to TH1-related immune responses at the end of pregnancy (labor induction) (42), our data suggest a critical role for MDC1 during the first trimester and for MDC2 during the second trimester. Here, at specific pregnancy periods both myeloid PBDC subsets may keep the delicate balance between pro- and anti-inflammatory immune reactions that are required for maintenance of a normal pregnancy.

After confirming pregnancy-associated alterations in the PBDCs and particularly in the MDC1 subset, we wondered whether placental-derived factors might provoke these changes. Previous studies proposed various effects of placental factors on DCs from different origins (26, 43–46). Our own data revealed no remarkable effect of soluble factors derived from normal primary trophoblast cells on all PBDC subsets. In contrast, supernatants from miscarriage trophoblast cells and co-culture of PBDCs with the trophoblast cell lines JEG-3 and SWAN-71 profoundly affected the number of mature PDC and MDC1. Among the molecules suggested to participate in placenta-driven PBDC modulation are: HLA-G, TGF-β, and indoleamine-2,3 dioxygenase (46) as well as pregnancy hormones. The latter ones, due to their autocrine and paracrine modes of action, can affect resident cells at the fetal-maternal interface and distant cells in the periphery (47, 48). Segerer and colleagues confirmed an inhibitory effect of hCG on DC maturation while estrogen and progesterone did not have any impact (32). Interestingly, Della Bella and colleagues, although not concentrating on hCG-mediated effects, suggested this hormone to be involved in the incomplete activation of PBDC during human pregnancy (19). In our current study, the presence of uhCG impaired the maturation of MDC1 and affected the frequency of mature PDC while rhCG did not. This only partly reflects our previous results where we found an inhibitory effect of hCG on the MDC1 subset that was mainly mediated by rhCG. However, in this study, we did not separately examine each PBDC subset and interdependencies between PDC, MDC1 and MDC2 could therefore not be excluded (31). A limiting factor in the present study was the purity of the isolated MDC2 that could be achieved by magnetic cell isolation. According to the manufacturer's instructions in the manual of this specific MDC2 isolation kit, some MDC1, PDC and monocytes are co-enriched with MDC2. Thus, we cannot completely exclude an influence of these "contaminating" immune cell populations on a potential hCG-mediated effect on MDC2 and conclusions derived from our MDC2 data have to be considered with caution.

In contrast to our data, Yoshimura and colleagues exhibited a stimulatory effect of hCG on myeloid and plasmacytoid PBDCs including the maturation, the cytokine secretion and the T cell stimulatory capacity (20). This shows that data referring to an hCG-mediated function on PBDCs during pregnancy are still inconsistent and further studies are needed to finally clarify this issue. Particularly, the PBDC characterization strategy has to be standardized to make studies comparable. Moreover, equivalent hCG preparations should be applied or at least a clear definition of the preparation used in each study should be provided. Our own investigations let assume that the immunological effects of rhCG or uhCG differ in some aspects and we suggest that this might be due to the different composition of both preparations. While rhCG preparations only contain intact molecules of regular hCG, uhCG preparations comprise intact and nicked variants of all hCG isoforms that can be physiologically found during pregnancy. These hCG isoforms have been shown to possess distinct functions. Regular hCG primarily promotes *corpus luteal* progesterone production, induces cytotrophoblast differentiation and contributes to uterine angiogenesis whereas free-β hCG exerts growth-promoting activity and blocks apoptosis (49). H-hCG, together with regular hCG promotes angiogenesis of the uterine vasculature and represents a key factor for trophoblast invasion (50). Notably, H-hCG was reported to activate the TGF-β receptor (51) implicating a potential pathway through which this isoform may regulate immune cell activity. Although our analysis of the different plasma hCG isoforms revealed that miscarriage patients suffer from reduced levels of regular hCG; free-β hCG and H-hCG as well as from altered MDC1 and MDC2 frequencies, based on our *in vitro* assays we do not believe that hCG is causative for the PBDC changes associated with miscarriage. However, we suggest that hCG has the potential to affect the phenotype of the distinct PBDC subsets.

In conclusion, our findings suggest that during normal pregnancy progression PBDC subsets are differentially regulated depending on gestational age. Miscarriage seems to be associated with dysregulations in the frequencies and functionality of the myeloid PBDC subsets as well as with disturbances in Treg frequencies. In the light of our results, we further propose the existence of an interdependency between MDC1 and Treg cells during early pregnancy. hCG, although shown to correlate negatively with MDC2 frequencies and to impair MDC1 maturation, does not seem to be a key regulator of PBDC alterations during pregnancy.

ETHICS STATEMENT

This study was carried out in accordance with the recommendations of ethic guidelines defined by the ethics board at the University of Magdeburg with written informed consent from all subjects. All subjects gave written informed consent in accordance with the Declaration of Helsinki. The protocol was approved by the ethics board at the University of Magdeburg (study 28/08).

AUTHOR CONTRIBUTIONS

SE and KS performed and analyzed experiments. AS designed and supervised experiments. SE and AS prepared figures, interpreted data, and wrote the manuscript. S-DC, RN, LL, AO, and FF provided human sample material. SL and AZ critically revised the manuscript and provided financial support.

FUNDING

This present work was financed by a grant from the DFG to AS (SCHU 2905/3-1) and intramural funding to AZ. KS was supported by a grant from the Medical Faculty of the Otto-von-Guericke University (Kommission zur Förderung des wissenschaftlichen Nachwuchses).

REFERENCES

1. Lapaire O, Holzgreve W, Oosterwijk JC, Brinkhaus R, Bianchi DW. Georg Schmorl on trophoblasts in the maternal circulation. *Placenta.* (2007) 28:1–5. doi: 10.1016/j.placenta.2006.02.004
2. Mincheva-Nilsson L, Baranov V. Placenta-derived exosomes and syncytiotrophoblast microparticles and their role in human reproduction: immune modulation for pregnancy success. *Am J Reprod Immunol.* (2014) 72:440–57. doi: 10.1111/aji.12311
3. Petroff MG, Chen L, Phillips TA, Azzola D, Sedlmayr P, Hunt JS. B7 family molecules are favorably positioned at the human maternal-fetal interface. *Biol Reprod.* (2003) 68:1496–504. doi: 10.1095/biolreprod.102.010058
4. Ban Y, Zhao Y, Liu F, Dong B, Kong B, Qu X. Effect of indoleamine 2,3-dioxygenase expressed in HTR-8/SVneo cells on decidual NK cell cytotoxicity. *Am J Reprod Immunol.* (2016) 75:519–28. doi: 10.1111/aji.12481
5. Phillips TA, Ni J, Pan G, Ruben SM, Wei YF, Pace JL, et al. TRAIL (Apo-2L) and TRAIL receptors in human placentas: implications for immune privilege. *J Immunol.* (1999) 162:6053–9.
6. Phillips TA, Ni J, Hunt JS. Death-inducing tumour necrosis factor (TNF) superfamily ligands and receptors are transcribed in human placentae, cytotrophoblasts, placental macrophages and placental cell lines. *Placenta.* (2001) 22:663–72. doi: 10.1053/plac.2001.0703
7. Runic R, Lockwood CJ, Ma Y, Dipasquale B, Guller S. Expression of Fas ligand by human cytotrophoblasts: implications in placentation and fetal survival. *J Clin Endocrinol Metab.* (1996) 81:3119–22. doi: 10.1210/jcem.81.8.8768884
8. Denison FC, Kelly RW, Calder AA, Riley SC. Cytokine secretion by human fetal membranes, decidua and placenta at term. *Hum Reprod.* (1998) 13:3560–5. doi: 10.1093/humrep/13.12.3560
9. Ramhorst R, Fraccaroli L, Aldo P, Alvero AB, Cardenas I, Leirós CP, et al. Modulation and recruitment of inducible regulatory T cells by first trimester trophoblast cells. *Am J Reprod Immunol.* (2012) 67:17–27. doi: 10.1111/j.1600-0897.2011.01056.x
10. Bakdash G, Sittig SP, van Dijk T, Figdor CG, de Vries, I Jolanda M. The nature of activatory and tolerogenic dendritic cell-derived signal II. *Front Immunol.* (2013) 4:53. doi: 10.3389/fimmu.2013.00053
11. Gardner L, Moffett A. Dendritic cells in the human decidua. *Biol Reprod.* (2003) 69:1438–46. doi: 10.1095/biolreprod.103.017574
12. Kämmerer U, Eggert AO, Kapp M, McLellan AD, Geijtenbeek TBH, Dietl J, et al. Unique appearance of proliferating antigen-presenting cells expressing DC-SIGN (CD209) in the decidua of early human pregnancy. *Am J Pathol.* (2003) 162:887–96. doi: 10.1016/S0002-9440(10)63884-9

13. Amodio G, Mugione A, Sanchez AM, Viganò P, Candiani M, Somigliana E, et al. HLA-G expressing DC-10 and CD4+ T cells accumulate in human decidua during pregnancy. *Hum Immunol.* (2013) 74:406–11. doi: 10.1016/j.humimm.2012.11.031
14. Miyazaki S, Tsuda H, Sakai M, Hori S, Sasaki Y, Futatani T, et al. Predominance of Th2-promoting dendritic cells in early human pregnancy decidua. *J Leukoc Biol.* (2003) 74:514–22. doi: 10.1189/jlb.1102566
15. Qian ZD, Huang LL, Zhu XM. An immunohistochemical study of CD83- and CD1a-positive dendritic cells in the decidua of women with recurrent spontaneous abortion. *Eur J Med Res.* (2015) 20:2. doi: 10.1186/s40001-014-0076-2
16. Tirado-González I, Muñoz-Fernández R, Blanco O, Leno-Durán E, Abadía-Molina AC, Olivares EG. Reduced proportion of decidual DC-SIGN+ cells in human spontaneous abortion. *Placenta.* (2010) 31:1019–22. doi: 10.1016/j.placenta.2010.09.008
17. Askelund K, Liddell HS, Zanderigo AM, Fernando NS, Khong TY, Stone PR, et al. CD83(+) dendritic cells in the decidua of women with recurrent miscarriage and normal pregnancy. *Placenta.* (2004) 25:140–5. doi: 10.1016/S0143-4004(03)00182-6
18. Zhang W, Zhou Y, Ding Y. Lnc-DC mediates the over-maturation of decidual dendritic cells and induces the increase in Th1 cells in preeclampsia. *Am J Reprod Immunol.* (2017) 77:e12647. doi: 10.1111/aji.12647
19. Della Bella S, Giannelli S, Cozzi V, Signorelli V, Cappelletti M, Cetin I, et al. Incomplete activation of peripheral blood dendritic cells during healthy human pregnancy. *Clin Exp Immunol.* (2011) 164:180–92. doi: 10.1111/j.1365-2249.2011.04330.x
20. Yoshimura T, Inaba M, Sugiura K, Nakajima T, Ito T, Nakamura K, et al. Analyses of dendritic cell subsets in pregnancy. *Am J Reprod Immunol.* (2003) 50:137–45. doi: 10.1034/j.1600-0897.2003.00063.x
21. Ueda Y, Hagihara M, Okamoto A, Higuchi A, Tanabe A, Hirabayashi K, et al. Frequencies of dendritic cells (myeloid DC and plasmacytoid DC) and their ratio reduced in pregnant women: comparison with umbilical cord blood and normal healthy adults. *Hum Immunol.* (2003) 64:1144–51. doi: 10.1016/j.humimm.2003.08.342
22. Cappelletti M, Giannelli S, Martinelli A, Cetin I, Colombo E, Calcaterra F, et al. Lack of activation of peripheral blood dendritic cells in human pregnancies complicated by intrauterine growth restriction. *Placenta.* (2013) 34:35–41. doi: 10.1016/j.placenta.2012.10.016
23. Dzionek A, Fuchs A, Schmidt P, Cremer S, Zysk M, Miltenyi S, et al. BDCA-2, BDCA-3, and BDCA-4: three markers for distinct subsets of dendritic cells in human peripheral blood. *J Immunol.* (2000) 165:6037–46. doi: 10.4049/jimmunol.165.11.6037
24. Ziegler-Heitbrock L, Ancuta P, Crowe S, Dalod M, Grau V, Hart DN, et al. Nomenclature of monocytes and dendritic cells in blood. *Blood.* (2010) 116:74–80. doi: 10.1182/blood-2010-02-258558
25. Ban YL, Kong BH, Qu X, Yang QF, Ma YY. BDCA-1+, BDCA-2+ and BDCA-3+ dendritic cells in early human pregnancy decidua. *Clin Exp Immunol.* (2008) 151:399–406. doi: 10.1111/j.1365-2249.2007.03576.x
26. Guo PF, Du MR, Wu HX, Lin Y, Jin LP, Li DJ. Thymic stromal lymphopoietin from trophoblasts induces dendritic cell-mediated regulatory TH2 bias in the decidua during early gestation in humans. *Blood.* (2010) 116:2061–9. doi: 10.1182/blood-2009-11-252940
27. Vinketova K, Mourdjeva M, Oreshkova T. Human decidual stromal cells as a component of the implantation niche and a modulator of maternal immunity. *J Pregnancy.* (2016) 2016:8689436. doi: 10.1155/2016/8689436
28. Paparini D, Gori S, Grasso E, Scordo W, Calo G, Perez Leiros C, et al. Acetylcholine contributes to control the physiological inflammatory response during the peri-implantation period. *Acta Physiol.* (2015) 214:237–47. doi: 10.1111/apha.12494
29. Zhao L, Shao Q, Zhang Y, Zhang L, He Y, Wang L, et al. Human monocytes undergo functional re-programming during differentiation to dendritic cell mediated by human extravillous trophoblasts. *Sci Rep.* (2016) 6:20409. doi: 10.1038/srep20409
30. Chard T. Pregnancy tests: a review. *Hum Reprod.* (1992) 7:701–10. doi: 10.1093/oxfordjournals.humrep.a137722
31. Sauss K, Ehrentraut S, Zenclussen AC, Schumacher A. The pregnancy hormone human chorionic gonadotropin differentially regulates plasmacytoid and myeloid blood dendritic cell subsets. *Am J Reprod Immunol.* (2018) 79:e12837. doi: 10.1111/aji.12837
32. Segerer SE, Müller N, van Den Brandt J, Kapp M, Dietl J, Reichardt HM, et al. ORIGINAL ARTICLE: impact of female sex hormones on the maturation and function of human dendritic cells. *Am J Reprod Immunol.* (2009) 62:165–73. doi: 10.1111/j.1600-0897.2009.00726.x
33. Kawamata F, Nishihara H, Homma S, Kato Y, Tsuda M, Konishi Y, et al. Chorionic gonadotropin-β modulates epithelial-mesenchymal transition in colorectal carcinoma metastasis. *Am J Pathol.* (2018) 188:204–15. doi: 10.1016/j.ajpath.2017.08.034
34. Park KE, Ku S-Y, Jung KC, Liu HC, Kim YY, Kim YJ, et al. Effects of urinary and recombinant gonadotropins on *in vitro* maturation outcomes of mouse preantral follicles. *Reprod Sci.* (2013) 20:909–16. doi: 10.1177/1933719112468948
35. Poloski E, Oettel A, Ehrentraut S, Luley L, Costa SD, Zenclussen AC, et al. JEG-3 trophoblast cells producing human chorionic gonadotropin promote conversion of human CD4+FOXP3- T cells into CD4+FOXP3+ regulatory T cells and foster T cell suppressive activity. *Biol Reprod.* (2016) 94:106. doi: 10.1095/biolreprod.115.135541
36. Darmochwal-Kolarz D, Rolinski J, Tabarkiewicz J, Leszczynska-Gorzelak B, Buczkowski J, Wojas K, et al. Myeloid and lymphoid dendritic cells in normal pregnancy and pre-eclampsia. *Clin Exp Immunol.* (2003) 132:339–44. doi: 10.1046/j.1365-2249.2003.02136.x
37. Hubert P, Jacobs N, Caberg JH, Boniver J, Delvenne P. The cross-talk between dendritic and regulatory T cells: good or evil? *J Leukoc Biol.* (2007) 82:781–94. doi: 10.1189/jlb.1106694
38. Banerjee DK, Dhodapkar MV, Matayeva E, Steinman RM, Dhodapkar KM. Expansion of FOXP3high regulatory T cells by human dendritic cells (DCs) *in vitro* and after injection of cytokine-matured DCs in myeloma patients. *Blood.* (2006) 108:2655–61. doi: 10.1182/blood-2006-03-011353
39. Kwiatek M, Geca T, Krzyzanowski A, Malec A, Kwaśniewska A. Peripheral dendritic cells and CD4+CD25+Foxp3+ regulatory T cells in the first trimester of normal pregnancy and in women with recurrent miscarriage. *PLoS ONE.* (2015) 10:e0124747. doi: 10.1371/journal.pone.0124747
40. Schumacher A, Brachwitz N, Sohr S, Engeland K, Langwisch S, Dolaptchieva M, et al. Human chorionic gonadotropin attracts regulatory T cells into the fetal-maternal interface during early human pregnancy. *J Immunol.* (2009) 182:5488–97. doi: 10.4049/jimmunol.0803177
41. Hayashi Y, Ishii Y, Hata-Suzuki M, Arai R, Chibana K, Takemasa A, et al. Comparative analysis of circulating dendritic cell subsets in patients with atopic diseases and sarcoidosis. *Respir Res.* (2013) 14:29. doi: 10.1186/1465-9921-14-29
42. Mor G, Aldo P, Alvero AB. The unique immunological and microbial aspects of pregnancy. *Nat Rev Immunol.* (2017) 17:469–82. doi: 10.1038/nri.2017.64
43. Du M-R, Guo P-F, Piao H-L, Wang S-C, Sun C, Jin L-P, et al. Embryonic trophoblasts induce decidual regulatory T cell differentiation and maternal-fetal tolerance through thymic stromal lymphopoietin instructing dendritic cells. *J Immunol.* (2014) 192:1502–11. doi: 10.4049/jimmunol.1203425
44. Talayev VY, Matveichev AV, Lomunova MA, Talayeva MV, Tsaturov ME, Zaichenko IY, et al. The effect of human placenta cytotrophoblast cells on the maturation and T cell stimulating ability of dendritic cells *in vitro*. *Clin Exp Immunol.* (2010) 162:91–9. doi: 10.1111/j.1365-2249.2010.04149.x
45. MacDonald KPA, Munster DJ, Clark GJ, Dzionek A, Schmitz J, Hart DNJ. Characterization of human blood dendritic cell subsets. *Blood.* (2002) 100:4512–20. doi: 10.1182/blood-2001-11-0097
46. Salamone G, Fraccaroli L, Gori S, Grasso E, Paparini D, Geffner J, et al. Trophoblast cells induce a tolerogenic profile in dendritic cells. *Hum Reprod.* (2012) 27:2598–606. doi: 10.1093/humrep/des208
47. Schumacher A, Costa S-D, Zenclussen AC. Endocrine factors modulating immune responses in pregnancy. *Front Immunol.* (2014) 5:196. doi: 10.3389/fimmu.2014.00196
48. Uemura Y, Liu T-Y, Narita Y, Suzuki M, Matsushita S. 17β-Estradiol (E2) plus tumor necrosis factor-α induces a distorted maturation of human monocyte-derived dendritic cells and promotes their capacity

to initiate T-helper 2 responses. *Hum Immunol.* (2008) 69:149–57. doi: 10.1016/j.humimm.2008.01.017
49. Cole LA. hCG, the wonder of today's science. *Reprod. Biol Endocrinol.* (2012) 10:24. doi: 10.1186/1477-7827-10-24
50. Evans J. Hyperglycosylated hCG: a unique human implantation and invasion factor. *Am J Reprod Immunol.* (2016) 75:333–40. doi: 10.1111/aji.12459
51. Berndt S, Blacher S, Munaut C, Detilleux J, Perrier d'Hauterive S, Huhtaniemi I, et al. Hyperglycosylated human chorionic gonadotropin stimulates angiogenesis through TGF-β receptor activation. *FASEB J.* (2013) 27:1309–21. doi: 10.1096/fj.12-213686

17

Integrated Systems Biology Approach Identifies Novel Maternal and Placental Pathways of Preeclampsia

Nandor Gabor Than[1,2,3,4,5,6], Roberto Romero[1,2,7,8,9]*, Adi Laurentiu Tarca[1,2,3,10], Katalin Adrienna Kekesi[11], Yi Xu[1,2], Zhonghui Xu[1,2,12], Kata Juhasz[4], Gaurav Bhatti[1,2], Ron Joshua Leavitt[13], Zsolt Gelencser[4], Janos Palhalmi[4], Tzu Hung Chung[13], Balazs Andras Gyorffy[11], Laszlo Orosz[14], Amanda Demeter[4], Anett Szecsi[4], Eva Hunyadi-Gulyas[15], Zsuzsanna Darula[15], Attila Simor[11], Katalin Eder[16], Szilvia Szabo[4,17], Vanessa Topping[1,2], Haidy El-Azzamy[1,2], Christopher LaJeunesse[1,2], Andrea Balogh[1,2,4], Gabor Szalai[1,2,4], Susan Land[9], Olga Torok[14], Zhong Dong[1,2], Ilona Kovalszky[6], Andras Falus[16], Hamutal Meiri[18], Sorin Draghici[9,19], Sonia S. Hassan[1,2,3,20], Tinnakorn Chaiworapongsa[1,2,3], Manuel Krispin[13], Martin Knöfler[21], Offer Erez[1,2,3,22], Graham J. Burton[23], Chong Jai Kim[1,2,24,25], Gabor Juhasz[11] and Zoltan Papp[5]**

[1] Perinatology Research Branch, Eunice Kennedy Shriver National Institute of Child Health and Human Development, National Institutes of Health, United States Department of Health and Human Services, Bethesda, MD, United States, [2] Perinatology Research Branch, Eunice Kennedy Shriver National Institute of Child Health and Human Development, National Institutes of Health, United States Department of Health and Human Services, Detroit, MI, United States, [3] Department of Obstetrics and Gynecology, Wayne State University School of Medicine, Detroit, MI, United States, [4] Systems Biology of Reproduction Lendulet Research Group, Institute of Enzymology, Research Centre for Natural Sciences, Hungarian Academy of Sciences, Budapest, Hungary, [5] Maternity Private Department, Kutvolgyi Clinical Block, Semmelweis University, Budapest, Hungary, [6] First Department of Pathology and Experimental Cancer Research, Semmelweis University, Budapest, Hungary, [7] Department of Obstetrics and Gynecology, University of Michigan, Ann Arbor, MI, United States, [8] Department of Epidemiology and Biostatistics, Michigan State University, East Lansing, MI, United States, [9] Center for Molecular Medicine and Genetics, Wayne State University, Detroit, MI, United States, [10] Department of Computer Science, College of Engineering, Wayne State University, Detroit, MI, United States, [11] Laboratory of Proteomics, Department of Physiology and Neurobiology, ELTE Eotvos Lorand University, Budapest, Hungary, [12] Channing Division of Network Medicine, Brigham and Women's Hospital, Harvard University, Boston, MA, United States, [13] Zymo Research Corporation, Irvine, CA, United States, [14] Department of Obstetrics and Gynaecology, University of Debrecen, Debrecen, Hungary, [15] Institute of Biochemistry, Biological Research Centre, Hungarian Academy of Sciences, Szeged, Hungary, [16] Department of Genetics, Cell and Immunobiology, Semmelweis University, Budapest, Hungary, [17] Department of Morphology and Physiology, Semmelweis University, Budapest, Hungary, [18] TeleMarpe Ltd, Tel Aviv, Israel, [19] Department of Clinical and Translational Science, Wayne State University, Detroit, MI, United States, [20] Department of Physiology, Wayne State University School of Medicine, Detroit, MI, United States, [21] Department of Obstetrics and Gynecology, Medical University of Vienna, Vienna, Austria, [22] Department of Obstetrics and Gynecology, Soroka University Medical Center School of Medicine, Faculty of Health Sciences, Ben-Gurion University of the Negev, Beer Sheva, Israel, [23] Centre for Trophoblast Research, Department of Physiology, Development and Neuroscience, University of Cambridge, Cambridge, United Kingdom, [24] Department of Pathology, Wayne State University School of Medicine, Detroit, MI, United States, [25] Department of Pathology, Asan Medical Center, University of Ulsan, Seoul, South Korea

***Correspondence:**
Nandor Gabor Than
than.gabor@ttk.mta.hu;
Roberto Romero
prbchiefstaff@med.wayne.edu;
Zoltan Papp
pzorvosihetilap@maternity.hu

Preeclampsia is a disease of the mother, fetus, and placenta, and the gaps in our understanding of the complex interactions among their respective disease pathways preclude successful treatment and prevention. The placenta has a key role in the pathogenesis of the terminal pathway characterized by exaggerated maternal systemic inflammation, generalized endothelial damage, hypertension, and proteinuria. This *sine qua non* of preeclampsia may be triggered by distinct underlying mechanisms that occur at early stages of pregnancy and induce different phenotypes. To gain insights into these molecular pathways, we employed a systems biology approach and integrated different "omics," clinical, placental, and functional data from patients with distinct phenotypes of preeclampsia. First trimester maternal blood proteomics uncovered an altered abundance of proteins of the renin-angiotensin and immune systems, complement, and coagulation cascades in patients with term or preterm preeclampsia. Moreover, first trimester maternal blood from preterm preeclamptic patients *in vitro* dysregulated trophoblastic gene expression. Placental transcriptomics of women with preterm preeclampsia identified distinct gene modules associated with maternal or fetal disease. Placental "virtual" liquid biopsy showed that the dysregulation of these disease gene modules originates during the first trimester. *In vitro* experiments on hub transcription factors of these gene modules demonstrated that DNA hypermethylation in the regulatory region of *ZNF554* leads to gene down-regulation and impaired trophoblast invasion, while *BCL6* and *ARNT2* up-regulation sensitizes the trophoblast to ischemia, hallmarks of preterm preeclampsia. In summary, our data suggest that there are distinct maternal and placental disease pathways, and their interaction influences the clinical presentation of preeclampsia. The activation of maternal disease pathways can be detected in all phenotypes of preeclampsia earlier and upstream of placental dysfunction, not only downstream as described before, and distinct placental disease pathways are superimposed on these maternal pathways. This is a paradigm shift, which, in agreement with epidemiological studies, warrants for the central pathologic role of preexisting maternal diseases or perturbed maternal–fetal–placental immune interactions in preeclampsia. The description of these novel pathways in the "molecular phase" of preeclampsia and the identification of their hub molecules may enable timely molecular characterization of patients with distinct preeclampsia phenotypes.

Keywords: inflammation, ischemia, liquid biopsy, omics, placenta, pregnancy, systems biology, trophoblast invasion

INTRODUCTION

Preeclampsia, one of the most severe obstetrical complications affecting 5–8% of pregnant women (1–5), is a leading cause of maternal (4–15) and perinatal morbidity and mortality (6, 16–18). In addition, pathologic changes in the affected mothers and fetuses lead to a higher risk of subsequent metabolic and cardiovascular diseases later in life (8, 9, 11, 13, 19–23), further increasing healthcare costs. In spite of the severity of the problem, there is yet no early diagnosis of all forms of preeclampsia, and the current therapy is still based on the delivery of the placenta (2, 24), given the complexity of the disease and the lack of insight into the early perturbed molecular pathways.

Indeed, preeclampsia is a syndrome with heterogeneous etiology and a spectrum of phenotypes (**Figure 1**). It may affect women at varying gestational ages with different degrees of severity and consequences for the fetus (2, 25–31). The current classifications of preeclampsia are based upon its severity and the timing of clinical presentation, mostly dividing preeclampsia into preterm (<37 weeks) or term (≥37 weeks) and early-onset (<34 weeks) or late-onset (≥34 weeks) phenotypes (24, 26, 32–36). Preterm preeclampsia has a more severe clinical presentation and is often accompanied by fetal growth restriction compared to term preeclampsia (2, 25, 26, 29). However, severe maternal disease and fetal growth restriction may be observed in both term and preterm preeclampsia, and their presentation may not be associated with each other, suggesting that the clinical phenotype is the result of an interplay between various factors and disease pathways, also supported by observations in animal models (37).

A growing body of evidence offers support for the conclusion that the maldevelopment and/or dysfunction of distinct trophoblast lineages of the placenta have a central role in the pathogenesis of preeclampsia, and that the severity of the placental disease is subsequently reflected in the clinical phenotype of this syndrome. In the preclinical stage, extravillous trophoblast (EVT) development may be impaired, leading to EVT dysfunction, shallow trophoblast invasion, failure of the physiological transformation of the maternal spiral arteries, abnormal blood-flow to the placenta, and histological changes consistent with maternal vascular malperfusion (28, 30, 38–43). The frequency and severity of these lesions decrease from the preterm toward the term phenotype of preeclampsia (28, 33, 44–46) (**Figure 1**), mirrored by the decreasing prevalence of fetal growth restriction or the delivery of small-for-gestational age (SGA) neonates (47–53). Thus, EVT development is less frequently and extensively affected in late-onset preeclampsia, which constitutes about 90% of all cases (50, 54, 55).

In preterm preeclampsia, failure of the remodeling of the spiral arteries may lead to abnormal blood flow to the placenta and subsequently to placental structural damage and ischemic stress, villous trophoblast (VT) dysfunction and the release of

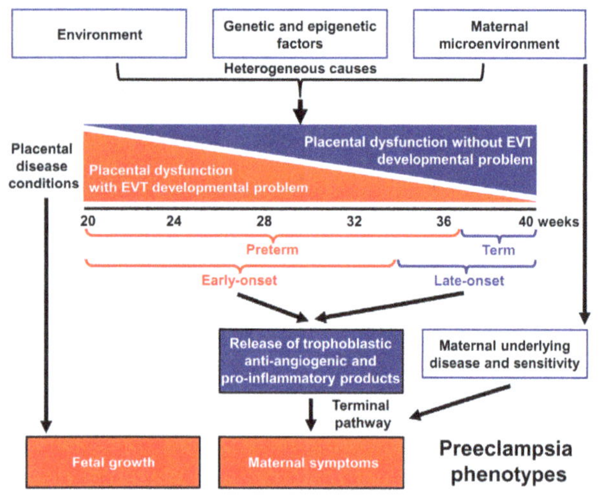

FIGURE 1 | Pathogenesis of preeclampsia. Preeclampsia is a syndrome with heterogeneous etiology and a spectrum of phenotypes. It may appear at varying gestational ages with different degrees of severity and involvement of the fetus. Preterm, especially early-onset preeclampsia generally has a more severe clinical presentation in the mother and is more often associated with the delivery of a growth-restricted neonate than term or late-onset preeclampsia. It is a multi-stage disease with the maldevelopment and/or dysfunction of distinct trophoblast lineages of the placenta at the center of the disease. Villous and extravillous trophoblast (EVT) development and/or function may be impaired in the preclinical stage, most extensively in preterm preeclampsia associated with fetal growth restriction. The resulting abnormal maternal spiral artery remodeling, fluctuating blood-flow, and ischemic stress lead to placental histological changes and the release of harmful substances from the placenta. As a consequence, the terminal pathway of preeclampsia, an exaggerated maternal systemic inflammatory and anti-angiogenic condition, occurs. The frequency and severity of placental developmental problems continuously decrease with advancing gestational age. In term forms, other stressors than maternal vascular malperfusion and placental ischemia may trigger placental stress, trophoblastic dysfunction, and the induction of the terminal pathway. Alternatively, the maternal endothelium may have an exaggerated sensitivity to factors released from a relatively normal placenta.

detrimental placental substances (e.g. anti-angiogenic factors, pro-inflammatory cytokines, and syncytiotrophoblast debris) into the maternal circulation (40, 41, 43, 56–66). As a consequence, the terminal pathway of preeclampsia, featuring an anti-angiogenic state and exaggerated maternal systemic inflammation, occurs in most cases, and its intensity correlates with the severity of preeclampsia, which may be coupled with damage to the maternal endothelium and to the kidneys, liver, and central nervous system during the clinical phase (21, 42, 43, 64, 67–72). VT development can also be impaired in preeclampsia (73–75), especially in the preterm form associated with SGA, where VT turnover is affected together with morphometric features (73, 76).

Term preeclampsia is characterized by a lesser magnitude of maternal systemic inflammatory and anti-angiogenic states (30, 37, 55–57, 61, 62, 77–92). This phenotype may result from different stressors other than maternal vascular malperfusion and ischemia of the placenta, which include various preexisting maternal disorders, such as obesity, chronic hypertension, diabetes, and metabolic, kidney, and autoimmune diseases (25, 93, 94). These stressors may still trigger placental stress and VT dysfunction (31, 91) and induce a maternal pro-inflammatory milieu. Alternatively, maternal endothelial dysfunction may result from an exaggerated sensitivity to factors released from the placenta (21, 25, 31, 95), which increases the risk of preeclampsia upon maternal genetic predisposition for cardiovascular disease (96, 97). Indeed, preeclampsia has a genetic predisposition with high heritability of both phenotypes, and it shares common risk alleles with coronary artery disease (98–104).

In spite of extensive research efforts, our understanding of the early pathologic pathways of preeclampsia has been limited given several obstacles. First, the complexity of the disease pathways and the heterogeneity of the syndrome have not been investigated in an integrative manner in both maternal and placental compartments throughout pregnancy. Second, it has been impossible to investigate the early placental disease pathways because of the invasive nature of placental biopsy and the limited information on placental functions obtained non-invasively. Consequently, an increasing number of high-dimensional studies aiming to detect molecular signatures of preeclampsia either in the placenta or in maternal blood have mostly targeted later stages of pregnancy, at a more advanced stage of placental development and pathology (105–143). Third, animal models of preeclampsia fail to mimic early placental pathways of preeclampsia due to the anatomical and physiological uniqueness of deep placentation in humans (144–147). Fourth, *in vitro* studies on human placental development and trophoblast functions are hindered by the lack of self-replicating trophoblast stem cells with the ability to differentiate into both VTs and EVTs (148–150).

Here, we used a systems biology approach that integrated various omics and targeted methods to investigate both placental and maternal compartments and most aspects of preeclampsia, including placental disease; fetal and maternal outcomes; environmental, maternal, microenvironmental, and epigenetic factors; and trophoblastic functions. In the first placental study, we performed extensive investigations of the placenta at histologic, transcriptomic, epigenetic, and protein levels to target molecular pathways at the center of the disease. Molecular changes were correlated with maternal and neonatal morbidities associated with preeclampsia to uncover placental pathways affecting either maternal or fetal wellbeing. In the second, maternal study, we employed maternal blood proteomics and "virtual" liquid biopsy of the placenta to reveal blood factors of maternal or placental origin that can reflect disease conditions in early pregnancy. In the third, trophoblast study, we utilized *in vitro* functional assays on the trophoblast to investigate hub transcription factors at the center of placental disease gene modules and to model their *in vivo* involvement in placental pathways associated with maternal or placental/fetal disease (**Figure 2**).

RESULTS

Placental Study

Alterations in the Placental Transcriptome in Preterm Preeclampsia

Given that the pathogenesis of preeclampsia has been implicated to originate from the placenta, we first aimed to investigate placental transcriptomic changes leading to placental dysfunction

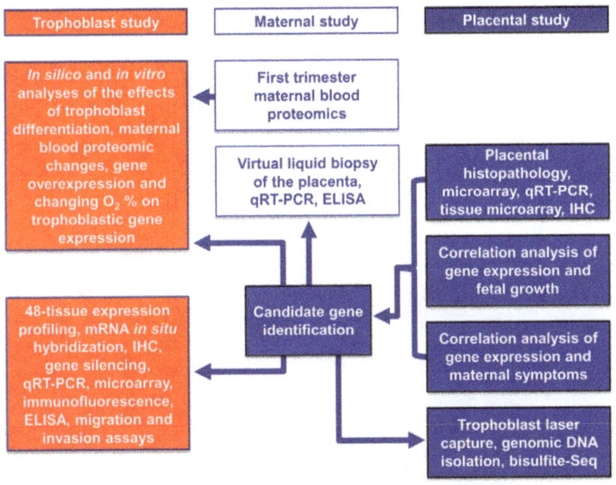

FIGURE 2 | Flow-chart of experimental procedures. The placental study included extensive histologic, transcriptomic, epigenetic, and protein level investigations of the placenta to target the molecular pathways in the center of disease. Molecular changes were correlated with disease outcomes in both mothers and babies to uncover placental pathways affecting either maternal or fetal wellbeing. The maternal study included first trimester maternal blood proteomics and "virtual" liquid biopsy of the placenta to reveal blood factors of maternal or placental origin that can reflect disease conditions in early pregnancy. In the trophoblast study, hub transcription factors in placental gene modules separately associated with maternal or placental/fetal disease were investigated with various *in vitro* methods to model *in vivo* disease pathways.

as well as regulatory networks involved in the pathologic pathways. The combined analysis of preterm preeclampsia cases and gestational age-matched controls (n = 17) in a Hungarian patient population (**Table 1**) in our placental microarray data (132) revealed 1,409 differentially expressed (DE) genes (Data S1 in Supplementary Material), which are involved in fundamental cellular processes, including blood pressure (BP) regulation, apoptosis, development, hormone secretion, metabolism, homeostasis, and signaling (**Figure 3A**). DE genes included 137 transcription regulatory genes and 38 predominantly placenta-expressed genes. This latter set of genes (n = 164, Data S2 in Supplementary Material), which was defined by BioGPS microarray data (n = 153) or expression data from separate studies in the lack of BioGPS data (n = 11) (151–153), was enriched among DE genes in preeclampsia [odds ratio (OR) = 3.4, $p = 6.9 \times 10^{-9}$]. This suggests that genes predominantly expressed by the placenta have pathologic and diagnostic significance in preeclampsia, a phenomenon indicated earlier by our targeted studies (153–155).

Subsequently, we investigated the genomic links among DE genes by searching for genomic regions associated with the observed placental transcriptomic changes. We found that Chr6 (OR = 1.54, $q = 1.6 \times 10^{-3}$) and Chr7 (OR = 1.42, q = 0.02) were particularly affected by these gene expression changes (Data S3 in Supplementary Material), while Chr19 (OR = 2.6, q = 0.02) was enriched in dysregulated transcription regulatory genes (Data S4 in Supplementary Material). Of interest, predominantly placenta-expressed genes were also enriched on Chr19 (OR = 2.5, q = 0.002) (Data S5 in Supplementary Material). **Figure 3B** shows the non-random genomic localization of DE genes in preterm preeclampsia and the pronounced gene dysregulation associated with Chr19. These results are consistent with the fact that Chr19 harbors large transcription regulatory gene families (156), and probably reflect its regulatory role in placental/trophoblastic gene expression and their dysregulation in preeclampsia.

TABLE 1 | Demographics of Hungarian women included in the placental microarray study.

Groups	Controls for preterm PE (n = 5)	Preterm PE (n = 12)
Maternal age (years)[b]	31.6 (31.5–34.3)	30.3 (26.1–35)
Primiparity[a]	40	66.7
Gestational age (weeks)[b]	31.0 (30.9–34.0)	31.2 (29.3–33.2)
Race[a]		
Caucasian	100	100
African-American	0	0
Other	0	0
Systolic BP (mmHg)[b]	120 (120–120)	163 (160–170)[c]
Diastolic BP (mmHg)[b]	80 (70–80)	100 (100–101)[c]
Proteinuria[a]	0	100[c]
Birthweight (g)[b]	1,990 (1,640–2,210)	1,065 (990–1,420)
Cesarean delivery[a]	100	100

BP, blood pressure; PE, preeclampsia.
[a]Percentage.
[b]Median (interquartile range).
[c]$p < 0.01$.

Alterations in Biological Processes and Regulatory Networks in Preterm Preeclampsia

Next, we aimed to identify functional links among DE genes by identifying gene co-expression network modules and hub transcription regulatory genes driving differential expression in the modules. Weighted co-expression network analysis (WGCNA) was conducted among DE genes resulting in the assignment of these into four major modules, labeled as M1 (green, n = 506), M2 (red, n = 442), M3 (blue, n = 381), and M4 (orange, n = 74) (**Figure 3C**; Data S1 in Supplementary Material). Most predominantly placenta-expressed genes belonged to modules M1 (n = 22 genes) and M2 (n = 12). Module M1 was enriched in down-regulated genes (OR = 1.88, $p = 2.59 \times 10^{-8}$), while module M2 was enriched in up-regulated genes (OR = 6.47, $p = 2.2 \times 10^{-16}$), suggesting the presence of distinct dysregulated gene-networks. Genes with predominant VT expression (14%) were mainly down-regulated, while genes with predominant EVT expression (9%) were mainly up-regulated even though both sets had the most members in module M1 (**Figure 3D**). These data suggested that the functions of both VT and EVT are strongly impacted in preterm preeclampsia, albeit in different ways.

Predominantly placenta-expressed genes, down-regulated in module M1, are regulators of fetal growth (*CSH1*, *HSD11B2*) (157, 158), metabolism (*ESRRG*) (159), estrogen synthesis (*HSD17B1*) (160), and immune functions (*LGALS14*) (153), some of which were reported to be down-regulated in preeclampsia (30, 91, 130, 155, 161, 162). Within this module, *ESRRG*, *POU5F1*, and *ZNF554* transcription regulatory genes had the highest number of significant correlations with predominantly placenta-expressed genes

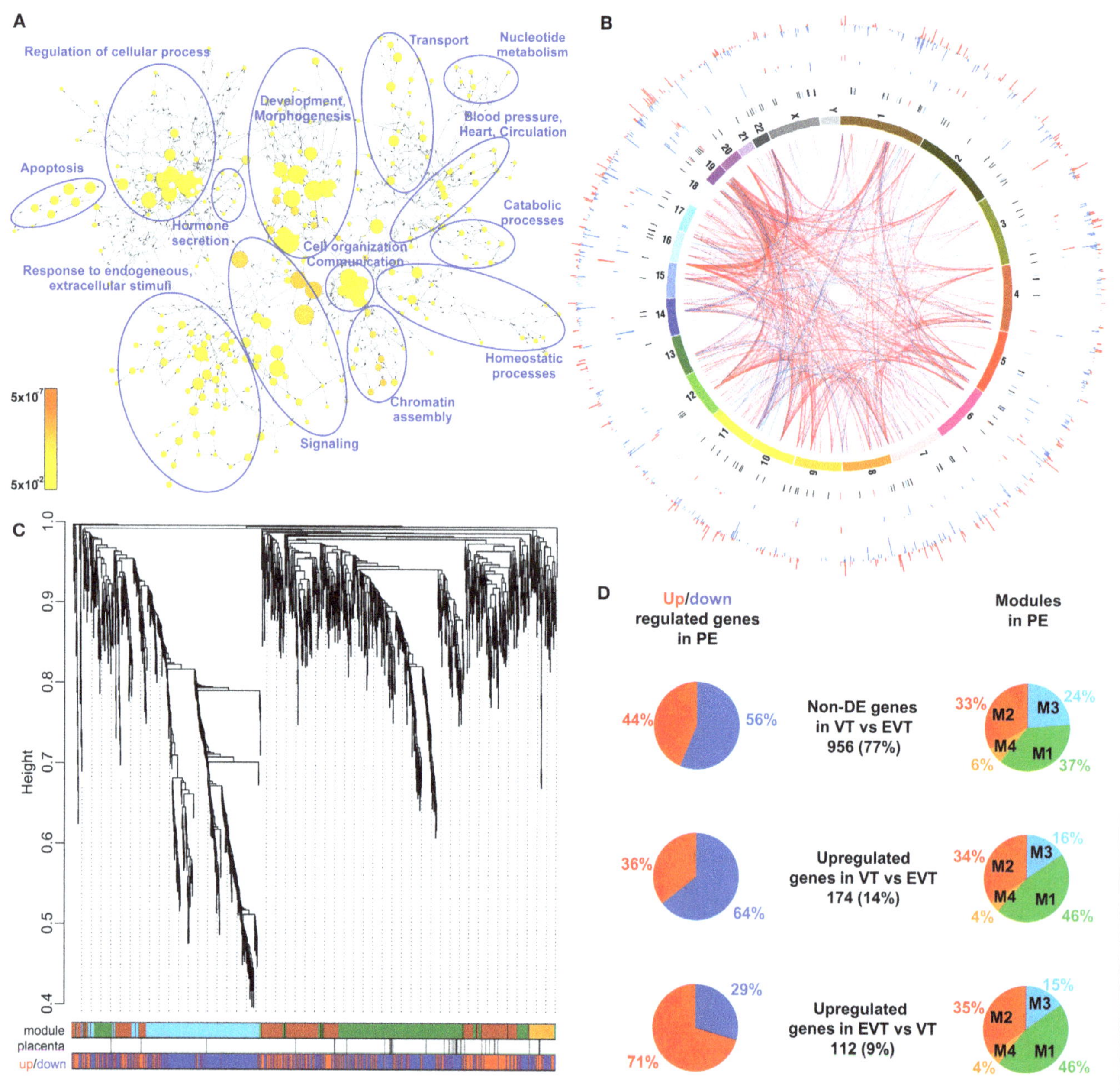

FIGURE 3 | Placental transcriptomic changes in preterm preeclampsia. **(A)** The network of biological processes enriched among differentially expressed (DE) genes. Circle sizes relate to the number of genes involved in the biological processes; colors refer to *p*-values according to the color code. Groups of the most enriched biological processes were circled and labeled. **(B)** Circos visualization of DE genes in preterm preeclampsia (PE). The inner circle shows chromosomes; curved lines represent correlation (red: positive; blue: negative) between transcription regulatory genes and their targets; the second circle shows genomic location of predominantly placenta-expressed genes (black lines: non-DE; red or blue lines: up- or down-regulated); third and fourth circles show the locations of DE transcription regulatory genes and their targets, respectively with blue (down-regulated) and red (up-regulated) bars. The height of the bars represents the magnitude of expression changes. **(C)** Dysregulated placental gene expression was characterized by four major disease gene modules within DE genes, marked with different colors. The height plotted on the *y*-axis represents distance metric. Of 38 predominantly placenta-expressed genes (black vertical lines), 33 belonged to the M1 (green, $n = 22$) and M2 (red, $n = 11$) modules. These modules were enriched in predominantly placenta-expressed genes and enriched in up-regulated (M2) or down-regulated (M1) genes marked under the modules with red or blue lines, respectively. **(D)** Pie charts depict the distribution of three gene sets among dysregulated genes or gene modules. Genes with similar expression in villous (VT) and extravillous trophoblast (EVT) had similar distribution among up- or down-regulated genes and in modules M1 and M2. Genes with up-regulation in VT compared to EVT were predominantly down-regulated in preeclampsia and positioned in module M1. Genes with up-regulation in EVT compared to VT were predominantly up-regulated in preeclampsia and positioned also in module M1.

and, hence, deemed as hub factors (Figure S1A in Supplementary Material). Of note, these transcription factors have been implicated in the regulation of stemness and differentiation (163, 164), pointing to the possible involvement of module M1 in the dysregulation of trophoblast differentiation in preterm preeclampsia. We selected *ZNF554* for functional studies, since it belongs to the

KRAB zinc finger family, crucial for early embryonic development and differentiation (165), and it may regulate genes in its co-expression network involved in biological processes affected by preeclampsia, such as development, chromatin assembly, signaling, adhesion, migration, and metabolism (Figure S1B in Supplementary Material).

In module M2, *FLT1,* which expresses sFlt-1, the main driver of BP elevation in the terminal pathway of preeclampsia (56, 90), was up-regulated. Moreover, module M2 genes were strongly overrepresented (OR = 29.9, $p = 6.54 \times 10^{-95}$) among genes that had correlated expression with mean arterial pressure (MAP) (Data S6 in Supplementary Material), suggesting a key role for this module in promoting hypertension. Within this module, *BCL6, BHLHE40,* and *ARNT2* had the highest correlation in gene expression with predominantly placenta-expressed genes, including *FLT1* (Figure S1A in Supplementary Material). Of note, these transcription regulatory hub genes are involved in hypoxia response. ARNT2 heterodimerizes with hypoxia-response regulator HIF-1α that is involved in trophoblast invasion and the pathogenesis of preeclampsia (166–169), and ARNT2 is a key regulator for adaption to hypoxic conditions at high altitudes, where the incidence of preeclampsia is much higher (16%) than at low altitude (170, 171). *BHLHE40* links immune and hypoxia-induced pathways (172). *BCL6,* a gene previously found to be up-regulated in the placenta in preterm preeclampsia, represses trophoblast differentiation and is regulated by stress-activated protein kinase signaling pathways (135, 173, 174). Our co-expression analysis revealed an enrichment of biological processes, such as differentiation, apoptosis, metabolism, signaling, and responses to stimuli including oxygen among genes co-expressed with *BCL6* (Figure S1C in Supplementary Material). Since *BCL6* is a key player in inflammation and oxygen-driven regulation of cell fate, we selected this gene for functional studies along with *ARNT2.*

The Association of Gene Modules With Clinical Parameters

Next, to validate the microarray results on a larger patient population ($n = 100$) comprised mostly of subjects of African-American origin presenting various phenotypes of preeclampsia (**Table 2**; Figure S2 in Supplementary Material), we selected 47 genes for qRT-PCR profiling of 100 placentas (**Table 3**), provided these genes were: (1) dysregulated genes with predominant placental and syncytiotrophoblastic expression, potentially encoding biomarkers; (2) dysregulated hub transcription regulatory genes that had a high co-expression with dysregulated, predominantly placenta-expressed genes in modules M1 and M2; and (3) non-dysregulated genes with roles in trophoblast differentiation, trophoblast-specific gene expression, or the pathogenesis of preeclampsia.

TABLE 2 | Demographics of American women included in the placental validation study.

Groups	Controls for preterm PE (n = 20)	Preterm PE (n = 20)	Preterm PE with SGA (n = 20)
Maternal age (years)[b]	22 (20–28.5)	23.5 (21–27)	22.5 (19.5–30)
Primiparity[a]	20	40	25
Gestational age (weeks)[b]	32.3 (28.2–34.9)	31.4 (29.6–33.6)	31.8 (29.7–34.4)
Race[a]			
Caucasian	5	10	10
African-American	95	90	90
Other	0	0	0
Systolic BP (mmHg)[b]	116 (110–125)	177 (166–187)[c]	171 (164–189)[c]
Diastolic BP (mmHg)[b]	65 (59–71)	105 (103–111)[c]	108 (94–118)[c]
Proteinuria[b]	0	3 (2–3)[c]	3 (3–3)[c]
Birthweight (g)[b]	1,635 (1,075–2,715)	1,488 (1,050–1,908)	1,173 (908-1,650)[d]
Birthweight percentile[b]	40.5 (31.9–53.4)	22.7 (18.3–32.9)[d]	6.7 (1–8.6)[c]
Cesarean delivery[a]	45	80[d]	75
Groups	**Controls for term PE (n = 20)**	**Term PE (n = 10)**	**Term PE with SGA (n = 10)**
Maternal age (years)[b]	22 (21–32)	19 (19–35)	26.5 (19–31)
Primiparity[a]	15	40	10
Gestational age (weeks)[b]	38.6 (38–39.1)	39.1 (38.6–39.6)	38.4 (37.3–38.9)
Race[a]			
Caucasian	15	0	0
African-American	80	100	100
Other	5	0	0
Systolic BP (mmHg)[b]	121 (111–134)	173 (165–178)[c]	169 (164–190)[c]
Diastolic BP (mmHg)[b]	70 (64–73)	106 (102–110)[c]	102 (97–104)[c]
Proteinuria[b]	0	3 (1–3)[c]	3 (1–3)[c]
Birthweight (g)[b]	3,215 (3,110–3,335)	3,123 (2,990–3,200)	2,405 (2,205–2,555)[c]
Birthweight percentile[b]	46 (37.2–63)	37.1 (28.5–48.8)	1.1 (1–3.5)[c]
Cesarean delivery[a]	55	40	20

BP, blood pressure; PE, preeclampsia; SGA, small-for-gestational age.

[a]*Percentage.*

[b]*Median (interquartile range).*

[c]$p < 0.001$.

[d]$p < 0.05$.

TABLE 3 | Genes included in the placental qRT-PCR validation study.

Gene symbol	DE genes in preterm PE (microarray)	Gene modules (microarray)	Hub TR genes in modules (microarray)	TR genes	PPE genes	DE genes in preterm PE (qRT-PCR)	DE genes in term PE (qRT-PCR)
ARNT2	Up	M2	M2	Yes	–	**Up**	–
BCL3	Up	M1	–	Yes	–	–	**Up**
BCL6	Up	M2	M2	Yes	–	**Up**	–
BTG2	Down	M2	–	Yes	–	**Down**	**Down**
CDKN1A	Down	M1	–	–	–	–	Up
CGB	Up	M4	–	–	Yes	–	**Up**
CLC	Up	M2	–	–	–	**Up**	**Up**
CLDN1	Down	M1	–	–	–	**Down**	**Down**
CRH	Up	M2	–	–	Yes	**Up**	–
CSH1	–	M1	–	–	Yes	Down	–
CYP19A1	–	–	–	Yes	Yes	–	–
DUSP1	Up	M2	–	–	–	**Up**	–
ENG	–	–	–	–	–	Up	Up
ERVFRDE1	–	–	–	–	Yes	–	–
ERVWE1	–	–	–	–	Yes	–	–
ESRRG	Down	M1	M1	Yes	Yes	**Down**	–
FBLN1	Down	M1	–	–	Yes	–	–
FLT1	Up	M2	–	–	–	**Up**	**Up**
GATA2	–	–	–	Yes	–	–	–
GCM1	–	–	–	Yes	Yes	Down	–
GH2	–	–	–	–	Yes	–	–
HLF	Down	M1	–	Yes	–	**Down**	–
HSD11B2	Down	M1	–	–	Yes	–	–
HSD17B1	Down	M1	–	–	Yes	**Down**	**Down**
IKBKB	Up	M1	–	–	–	–	–
INSL4	Up	M4	–	–	Yes	–	–
JUNB	Up	M2	–	Yes	–	**Up**	–
KIT	Up	M2	–	–	–	**Up**	–
LEP	Up	M2	–	–	Yes	**Up**	**Up**
LGALS13	–	–	–	–	Yes	Down	Down
LGALS14	Down	M1	–	–	Yes	**Down**	**Down**
LGALS16	–	–	–	–	Yes	–	–
LGALS17A	–	–	–	–	–	–	–
MAPK13	–	–	–	–	–	–	Up
NANOG	–	–	–	Yes	–	–	–
PAPPA	–	–	–	–	Yes	–	–
PAPPA2	Up	M2	–	–	Yes	**Up**	**Up**
PGF	–	–	–	–	Yes	–	–
PLAC1	Down	M1	–	–	Yes	**Down**	–
POU5F1	Up	M1	M1	Yes	–	–	–
SIGLEC6	Up	M2	–	–	Yes	**Up**	**Up**
TEAD3	–	–	–	Yes	Yes	–	Up
TFAM	Down	M3	–	Yes	–	–	Up
TFAP2A	–	–	–	Yes	Yes	–	–
TPBG	Up	M2	–	–	–	**Up**	**Up**
VDR	Up	M2	–	Yes	–	–	–
ZNF554	Down	M1	M1	Yes	–	**Down**	**Down**

PE, preeclampsia; DE, differentially expressed; TR, transcription regulatory; PPE, predominantly placenta-expressed.
Identical dysregulation in the validation cohort as in the microarray cohort is depicted in bold font.

As depicted in the heatmap representing qRT-PCR data for the 100 placentas and 47 genes (**Figure 4A**), validation data supported microarray experiments in terms of (1) differential expression of selected genes, (2) high correlation of genes within modules M1 and M2, and (3) separate dysregulation of modules M1 and M2 from each other. Comparison between preterm preeclampsia and gestational age-matched controls revealed that qRT-PCR data validated microarray results (differential or non-differential gene expression) for 33 of 47 genes (70%), and further confirmed the differential expression of four genes that were non-dysregulated in the microarray cohort (**Table 3**). As expected, the extent of changes in gene expression was less pronounced in term preeclampsia (**Table 3**; **Figure 4C**; Figure S3 in Supplementary Material). As a further confirmation, there was a strong correlation between qRT-PCR data as well as tissue microarray (TMA) and immunostaining results for selected proteins in module M2 (**Figures 4C–E**). The extent of dysregulation was larger in preterm phenotypes of preeclampsia than in term phenotypes, in agreement with the more severe placental pathology (44). Among transcription regulatory genes of module M1, *HLF* had strong down-regulation only in preterm preeclampsia while *ZNF554* was expressed at a lower

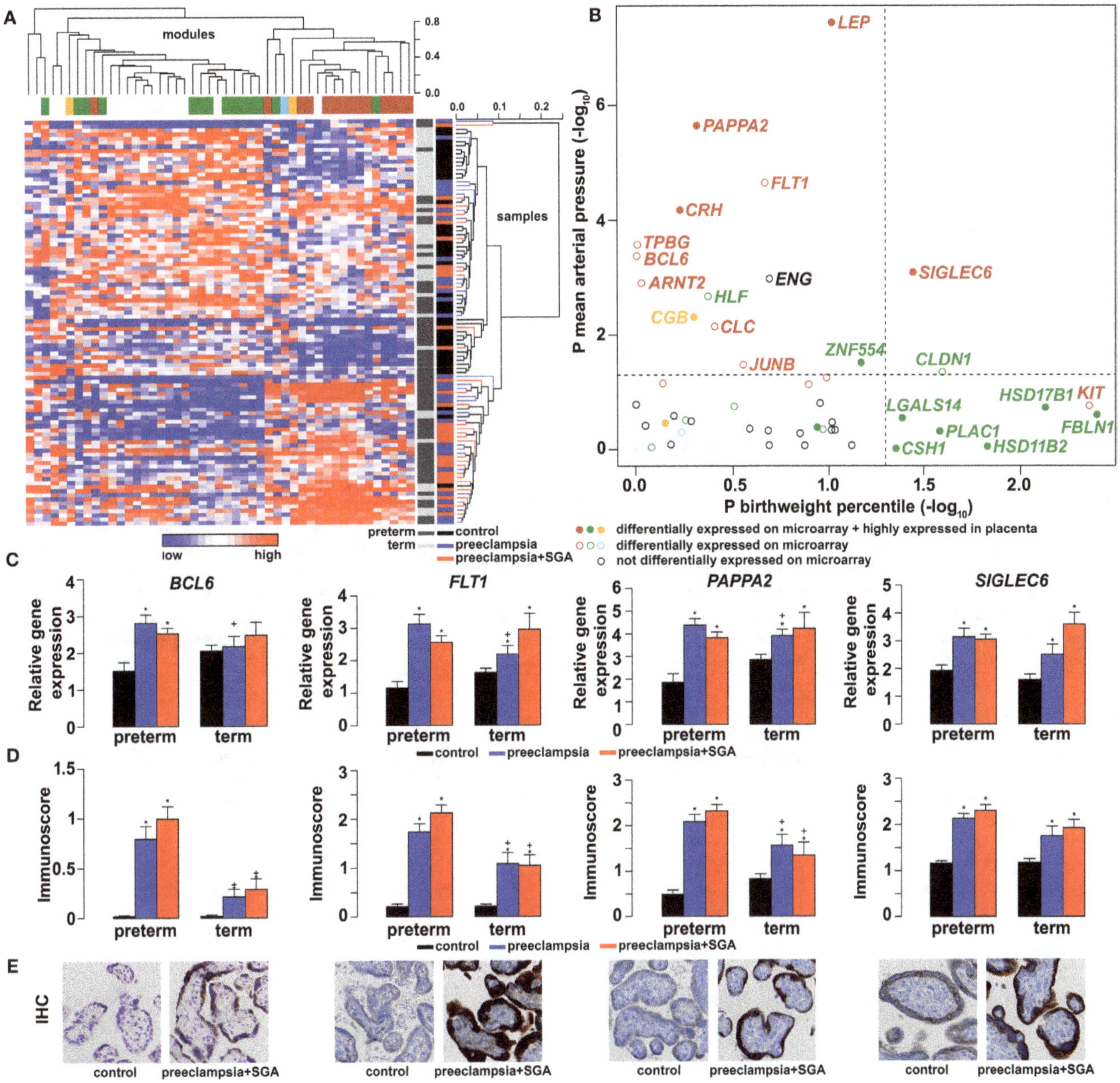

FIGURE 4 | Gene modules associated with blood pressure (BP) and birthweight (BW). **(A)** Hierarchical clustering of qRT-PCR data obtained with 100 samples and 47 genes. Pearson correlation was used for similarity analysis and average method for linkage calculation. Samples were colored according to patient groups and maturity status. M1 (green) and M2 (red) module genes and 34 of 60 samples from women with preeclampsia clustered together. **(B)** Association of gene expression with BP and BW. The significance p-values for these coefficients were plotted for all genes, colored according to module classification (black: not changed on the microarray). Filled circles represent predominantly placenta-expressed genes and dashed lines the significance threshold at $p = 0.05$. Seven of 9 genes related to BW belong to module M1, while 10 of 15 genes related to BP are from module M2. Gene expression **(C)** and protein immunostaining **(D)** of selected four genes in module M2 show similar patterns in the sub-groups of preeclampsia, and semi-quantitative immunoscorings validate gene expression data. Significant differences in preterm or term preeclampsia samples compared to gestational-age matched controls are shown with "*". When the change with preeclampsia in preterm samples was different from that in term samples, a "+" marks such an interaction. Comparisons for all genes are available in Figure S3 in Supplementary Material. **(E)** Representative images of the same placenta from a preterm control (left, 29 weeks) and a patient with preterm preeclampsia associated with SGA (right, 31 weeks) are shown for the immunostainings (hematoxylin counterstaining, 40× magnification).

level in all preeclampsia phenotypes (Figure S3 in Supplementary Material). Among the transcription regulatory genes in module M2, *ARNT2*, *BCL6*, and *JUNB* were highly expressed in preterm but not in term preeclampsia, suggesting that these might play a role only in the pathology of preterm cases (**Figure 4C**; Figure S3 in Supplementary Material). Overall, these data reflect the heterogeneous placental pathology and the more severely affected pathways in preterm preeclampsia.

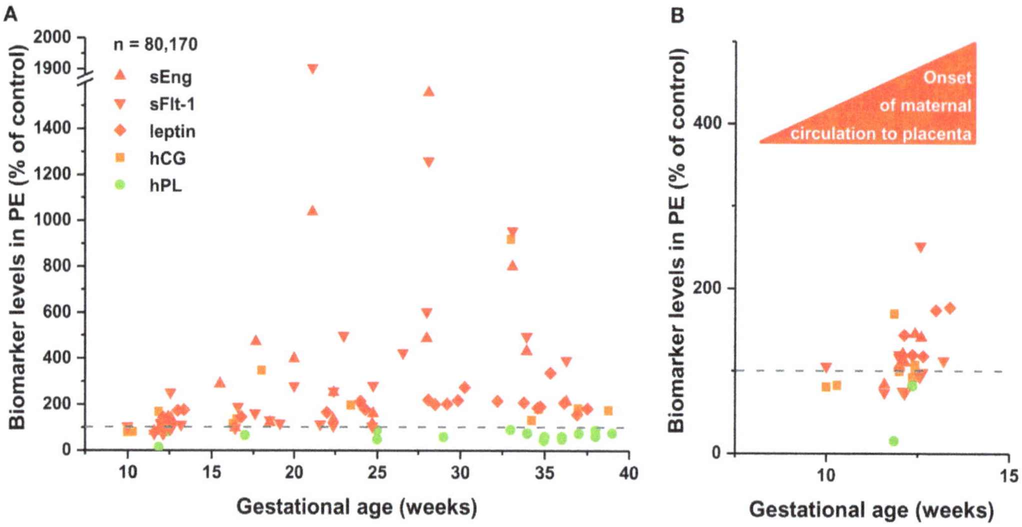

FIGURE 5 | The timing of gene module dysregulation in preterm preeclampsia. **(A)** A database of 80,170 measurements published in 61 reports (35, 61, 82, 88, 126, 178–233) was built for "virtual" liquid biopsy of the placenta in preterm preeclampsia with maternal blood levels of proteins with the highest expression in the placenta among all tissues [i.e. hCG, human placental lactogen (hPL), sEng, sFlt-1, and leptin]. Levels of these biomarkers in preterm preeclampsia were expressed as the percentage of control levels (dashed line) and were represented in scatter plots by different colors reflecting gene module classification. Based on qRT-PCR data, sEng belongs to module M2 (red). hPL (M1, green module) levels in preeclampsia were constantly below control levels during gestation, while the levels of module M2 biomarkers in preeclampsia had continuous elevation compared to control levels as a function of gestational age. **(B)** Analysis of first trimester data revealed the lower expression of all biomarkers in preeclampsia than in controls before the onset of maternal circulation, and the increasing expression of module M2 biomarkers in preeclampsia compared to controls after 12 weeks of gestation.

TABLE 4 | Demographics of Israeli women included in the maternal blood two-dimensional differential in-gel electrophoresis proteomics study.

Groups	Controls for preterm PE with SGA (n = 5)	Preterm PE with SGA (n = 5)	Controls for term PE (n = 5)	Term PE (n = 5)
Maternal age (years)[b]	30 (24–31)	29 (27–37)	29 (27–34)	26 (23–32)
Primiparity[a]	40	20	80	40
Gestational age at blood draw (weeks)[b]	10 (9–11)	8 (8–9)	8 (8–9)	9 (8–10)
Gestational age at delivery (weeks)[b]	39.7 (38.6–40.0)	34.9 (29.3–35.3)[d]	38.7 (38.6–41.0)	38.1 (38.0–38.1)
Race[a]				
Caucasian	100	100	100	100
African-American	0	0	0	0
Other	0	0	0	0
Systolic BP (mmHg)[b]	105 (104–110)	160 (150–165)[c]	110 (110–118)	150 (140–160)[c]
Diastolic BP (mmHg)[b]	60 (60–70)	100 (100–100)[c]	67 (63–68)	100 (90–100)[c]
Proteinuria[b]	0	4 (3–4)[c]	0	3 (3–4)[c]
Birthweight (g)[b]	2,955 (2,900–3,100)	1,720 (975–1,800)[c]	3,390 (3,270–3,600)	3,200 (3,150–3,210)
Cesarean delivery[a]	0	60[c]	60	40

BP, blood pressure; PE, preeclampsia; SGA, small-for-gestational age.
[a]Percentage.
[b]Median (interquartile range).
[c]$p < 0.05$ when compared to corresponding controls.
[d]$p < 0.001$ when compared to corresponding controls.

Because of the possible involvement of these two gene modules in distinct pathologic pathways, we correlated qRT-PCR data with maternal and fetal clinico-pathological indicators to further investigate their association (**Figure 4B**). This analysis showed that 7 of 9 genes related to the birthweight (BW) percentile were from module M1, while 10 of 15 genes related to BP were from module M2, confirming our observations with microarray data. Therefore, we decided to also refer to these as "M1-BW" and "M2-BP" modules. Of interest, the expression of most (9/14) M1 genes was negatively associated with the "maternal vascular malperfusion" score of the placenta, while the expression of most (10/14) M2 genes was positively correlated with this parameter (Data S7 in Supplementary Material). This observation fits well with the accepted concept that maternal vascular malperfusion of the placenta leads to oxidative stress (40, 41, 63, 175) and the increased placental expression of *FLT1* (63).

Maternal Study

Maternal Blood Reflects Gene Module Dysregulation in Preeclampsia

Next, we investigated whether placental gene module dysregulation can be detected in maternal blood and whether liquid biopsy

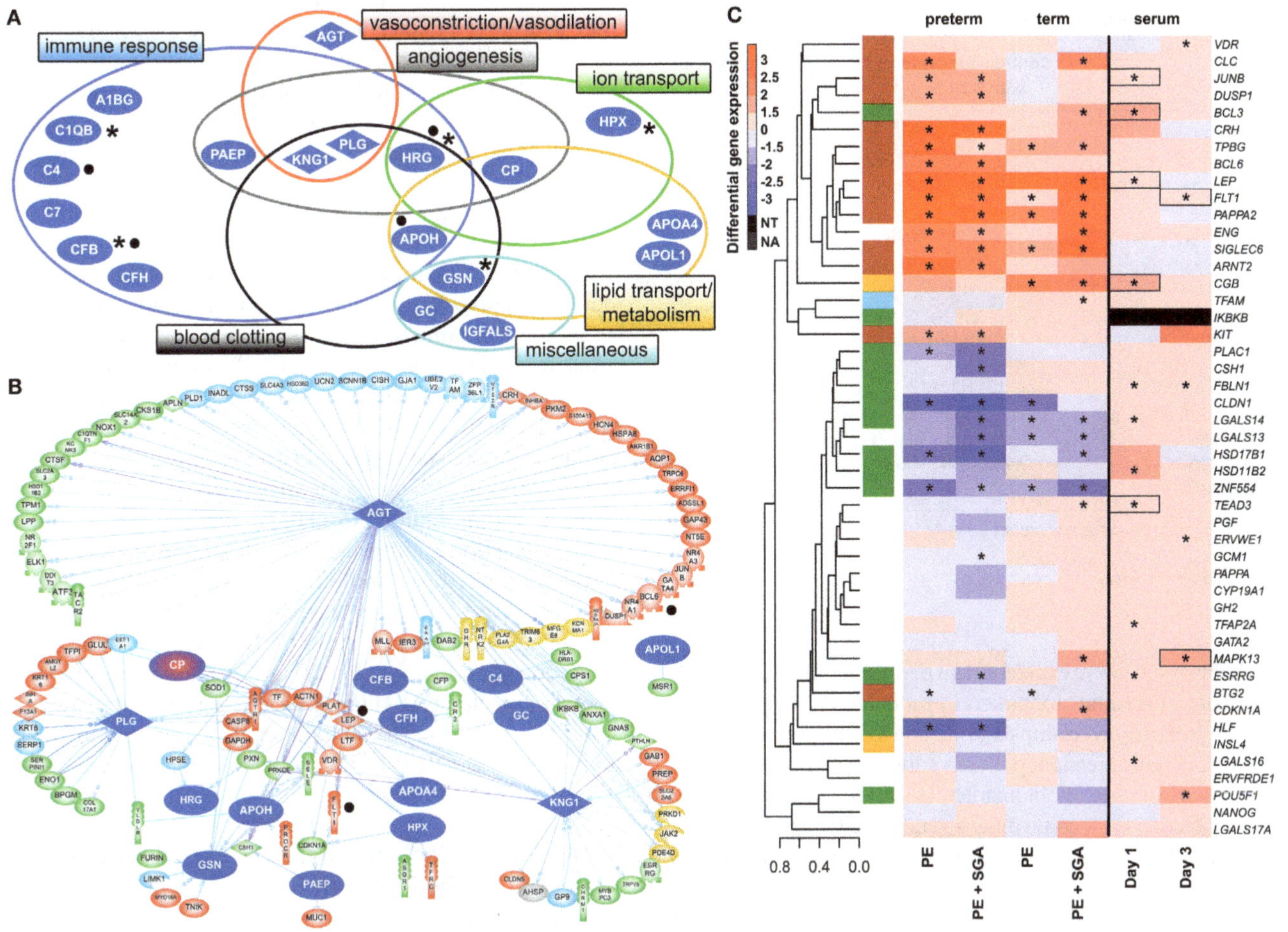

FIGURE 6 | Maternal blood proteomic changes and their effect on differentially expressed (DE) genes in preterm preeclampsia. **(A)** The 19 DE maternal serum proteins in preterm preeclampsia identified by two-dimensional differential in-gel electrophoresis could be classified into functional groups relevant for preeclampsia pathophysiology. Asterisks denote proteins reported by others to have the same direction differential abundance in the first trimester in patients developing preterm preeclampsia (126, 143, 239–241). Dots denote immune proteins that multiple reaction monitoring assays identified to have differential abundance in preterm preeclampsia in the same direction. **(B)** The 19 DE serum proteins have connections to 121 DE placental genes, among which 48 belong to module M2. Angiotensinogen has more connections than other proteins (OR = 1.9, $p = 4.9 \times 10^{-5}$), and the most connections to module M2 genes ($n = 35$); 77 of 86 connections of angiotensinogen have a directional effect toward the gene. Dots denote genes in connection to angiotensinogen found up-regulated in villous trophoblast (VT) upon treatment with first trimester serum from preeclamptic women. **(C)** Hierarchical clustering tree and heatmap representing differential placental gene expression in preeclampsia as in **Figure 4A**. The expression of the same genes (except *IKBKB*) was determined in primary VTs upon treatment with first trimester maternal serum. Serum from preeclamptic compared to control women induced the up-regulation of seven placental dysregulated genes (depicted with boxes) on the first and third days of VT differentiation, among which six were up-regulated in term and three in preterm preeclampsia. Stars depict significant changes, color bar encodes signed (up or down)-fold changes. Abbreviations: NA, not expressed; NT, not examined.

can be used to determine when the module dysregulation occurs. To study the relationship between placental gene expression and maternal biomarker concentrations, we selected predominantly placenta-expressed genes with the most differential expression in modules M1 (*CSH1*) or M2 (*LEP*), and correlated their placental expression levels with concentrations of their secreted protein products (hPL and leptin) in maternal blood collected in both first ($n = 12$) and third trimesters ($n = 19$) in a Hungarian patient population. Positive correlations were found between placental gene expression and maternal blood protein concentrations for both biomarkers in both trimesters (Figure S4 in Supplementary Material), suggesting that certain proteins in the maternal circulation reflect the placental expression of their encoding genes throughout pregnancy.

To detect disease-associated protein signatures of placental dysfunction in maternal blood, similar to plasma DNA tissue mapping for noninvasive prenatal assessments (176, 177), we performed "virtual" liquid biopsy of the placenta in preterm preeclampsia (Figure S5 in Supplementary Material; **Figure 5**). We identified five genes with predominant placental expression, which have products extensively investigated in maternal blood in preterm preeclampsia or in all cases of preeclampsia during all trimesters. From data of 61 reports (35, 61, 82, 88, 126, 178–233), we built a database of 80,170 measurements in which

TABLE 5 | Demographics of Hungarian women included in the maternal blood multiple reaction monitoring proteomics study.

Groups	Controls for preterm PE with SGA (n = 10)	Preterm PE with SGA (n = 5)
Maternal age (years)[b]	29.7 (28.9–31.5)	34.7 (28.6–35.1)
Primiparity[a]	20	80
Gestational age at blood draw (weeks)[b]	12.6 (12.6–12.8)	12.4 (12.4–13.0)
Gestational age at delivery (weeks)[b]	40.3 (39.9–40.8)	32.4 (26.4–34.0)[c]
Race[a]		
Caucasian	100	100
African-American	0	0
Other	0	0
Systolic BP (mmHg)[b]	124 (118–126)	170 (170–170)[c]
Diastolic BP (mmHg)[b]	75 (68–79)	100 (100–110)[c]
Proteinuria (g)[b]	0	3 (1–6)[c]
Birthweight (g)[b]	3,460 (3,308–3,623)	1,380 (790–1,450)[c]
Cesarean delivery[a]	30	100[c]

BP, blood pressure; PE, preeclampsia; SGA, small-for-gestational age.
[a]*Percentage.*
[b]*Median (interquartile range).*
[c]*$p < 0.05$.*

preeclampsia data were expressed as a percentage of average levels in controls. Regarding biomarkers in module M1, we found hPL levels in preterm preeclampsia to be consistently below control levels throughout pregnancy. This is substantiated by the down-regulation of another M1 biomarker, HSD17B1, in first trimester maternal blood (160), confirming a generalized down-regulation of M1 biomarkers in early pregnancy. By contrast, the levels of biomarkers in module M2 had constant elevation in preterm preeclampsia compared to controls during gestation. When analyzing only data collected in the first trimester, prior to the onset of maternal circulation to the placenta, levels of M1 and M2 biomarkers were lower in women with preeclampsia compared to controls, while after 12 weeks of gestation, following the opening of the intervillous spaces to maternal blood flow, patients had increasing levels of M2 biomarkers in maternal blood compared to controls. These findings offer support for the conclusion that placental transcriptomic changes typical for preeclampsia in the third trimester are rooted in the first trimester.

Altered Maternal Serum Proteome in Preeclampsia

Next, we investigated the maternal serum proteome in early pregnancy in distinct phenotypes of preeclampsia and the potential effects of proteomic changes on the placental transcriptome. Comparing samples from women with preterm preeclampsia associated with SGA and their respective controls from an Israeli patient population (n = 10, **Table 4**), 19 DE protein spots were identified and investigated by mass spectrometry. According to public data, many of these proteins have a role in immune response, complement and coagulation cascades, lipid transport and metabolism, angiogenesis, BP regulation, and ion transport (**Figure 6A**, Data S8 in Supplementary Material). Comparing samples from women with term preeclampsia and their respective controls from this Israeli patient population (n = 10, **Table 4**), 14 DE protein spots could be identified (Figure S6A; Data S8 in Supplementary Material). Many of the proteins found in these spots are the same as those found in preterm preeclampsia or function in the same pathways. Of note, these pathways and the 26 differentially abundant proteins identified in term and preterm preeclampsia had mostly been implicated in a later stage of preeclampsia (43, 101, 120, 234–238). We concluded that there is a common dysregulation of the maternal serum proteome in term and preterm preeclampsia; however, the extent of changes is larger in the latter, in agreement with the more fulminant and early pathogenesis.

Supporting our findings, five studies (126, 143, 239–241) found proteins with differential abundance in preterm preeclampsia in the same direction as our two-dimensional differential in-gel electrophoresis (2D-DIGE) study (**Figure 6A**). We also collected maternal blood specimens in the first trimester from a Hungarian patient population (n = 15, **Table 5**), and measured the concentrations of 10 immune proteins in patients with preterm preeclampsia associated with SGA and matched controls using liquid chromatography–mass spectrometry multiple reaction monitoring (MRM). In spite of the difference between the methods and ethnic background, MRM identified 4 of these 10 proteins as having differential abundance in the same direction as in the 2D-DIGE study, supporting the early pro-inflammatory changes in the maternal proteome in preterm preeclampsia (**Figure 6A**; Data S9 in Supplementary Material). MRM and proteomic evidence published to date supported 37% (7/19) of the proteomic changes detected by 2D-DIGE.

The *In Silico* Effects of Altered Maternal Serum Proteome on the Placenta

To reveal whether early proteomic changes in maternal blood may affect the placental transcriptome, placental DE genes with documented connections to DE proteins in maternal serum were identified by Pathway Studio. The 121 DE placental genes with connections to DE serum proteins in preterm preeclampsia were marginally over-represented by those from module M2 (48/121, OR = 1.4, p = 0.057). Angiotensinogen had the largest number of connections to DE genes including *FLT1* and *LEP* (n = 86, OR = 1.9, $p = 4.9 \times 10^{-5}$). This protein also had the largest number of connections to module M2 genes (n = 35), followed by plasminogen (n = 11) and kininogen-1 (n = 9), all involved in BP regulation (**Figure 6B**). These data were supported by the "renin-angiotensin signaling" as being a top pathway ($p = 1.28 \times 10^{-4}$) among the 35 angiotensinogen-connected DE genes (Data S10 in Supplementary Material). Similar results were obtained when analyzing connections between 116 DE placental genes and DE serum proteins in term preeclampsia (Figure S6B in Supplementary Material).

Trophoblast Study

The *In Vitro* Effects of an Altered Maternal Serum Proteome on the Trophoblast

Next, we aimed to study various factors implicated in the pathogenesis of preeclampsia in trophoblast models to determine whether these may drive the observed placental transcriptomic changes. Since the results noted above suggested that maternal serum proteins can influence the placental transcriptome, we

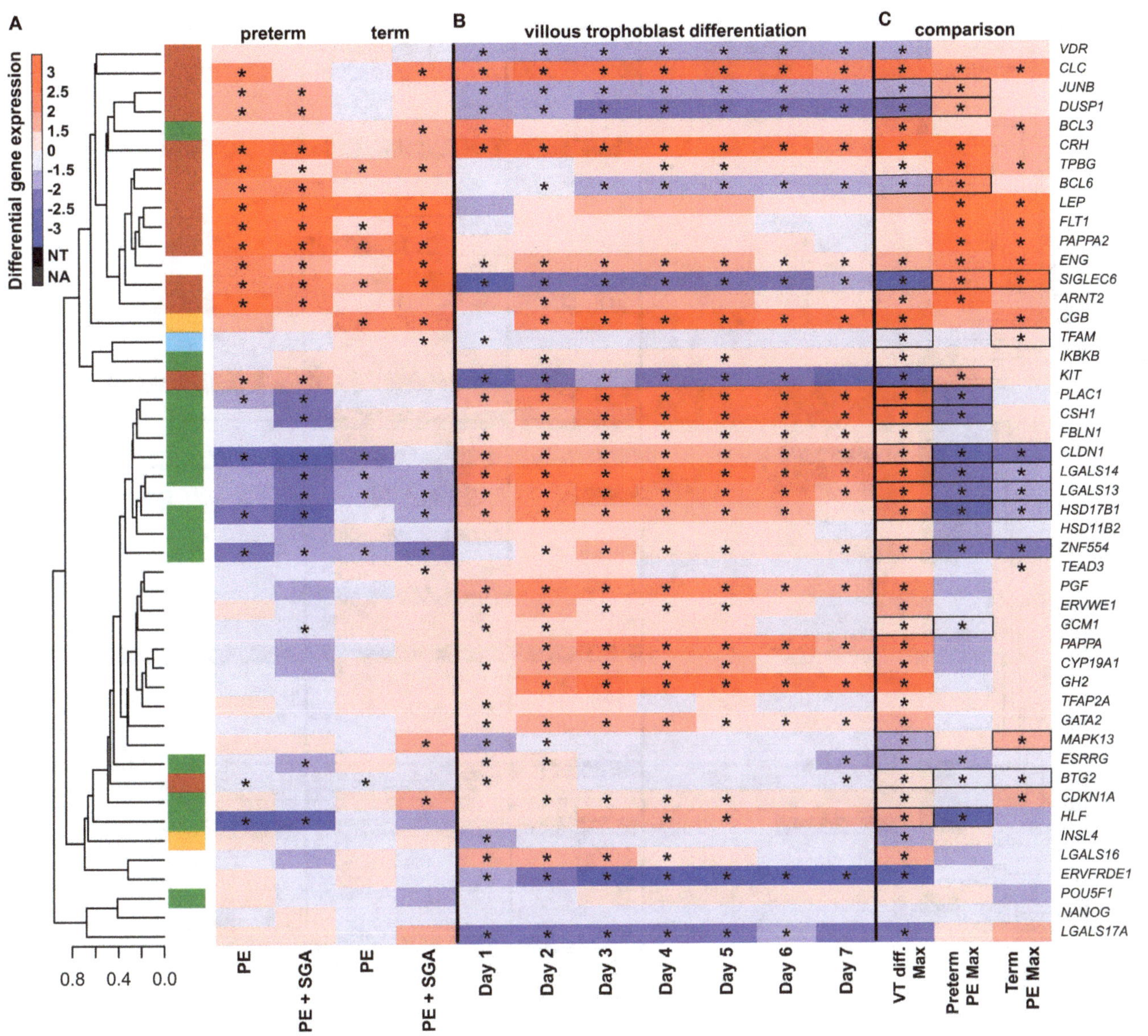

FIGURE 7 | The effect of trophoblast differentiation on differentially expressed genes in preeclampsia. **(A)** Hierarchical clustering tree of expression data for 47 genes in 100 placental specimens was augmented with a heatmap representing differential gene expression in term or preterm subgroups of preeclampsia. **(B)** Primary villous trophoblast (VT) differentiation time series expression data for 47 genes were depicted with a heatmap representing differential gene expression in each time point (days 1–7) compared to day 0. **(C)** Maximum expression values in the VT differentiation time series were presented alongside with maximum expression values in the placenta in preterm or term preeclampsia. Comparative visualization revealed the opposite-direction differential regulation of 17 genes in preeclampsia compared to VT differentiation as depicted with black boxes. Among these genes, 15 had this behavior in preterm preeclampsia and 9 in term preeclampsia ($p = 0.057$). In **(A–C)**, stars depict significant changes, color bar encodes signed (up or down)-fold changes. Abbreviations: NA, not expressed; NT, not examined.

first measured the effects of maternal blood from early pregnancy on trophoblastic gene expression. We treated primary VTs during differentiation with first trimester sera from women with preterm preeclampsia or normal pregnancy, and analyzed the expression of genes included in the placental validation study. Serum from preeclamptic women compared to controls induced up-regulation of seven placental DE genes on the first and third days of trophoblast differentiation, including *FLT1* and *LEP* (**Figure 6C**). Among these, six genes were up-regulated in the placenta in term and three in preterm preeclampsia. These results support *in silico* findings and suggest that maternal serum factors can up-regulate *FLT1* and may induce the terminal pathway.

The Effects of Altered VT Differentiation

Next, we examined whether disturbance in VT differentiation may be reflected in the placental gene expression signature in women with different preeclampsia phenotypes. Since there

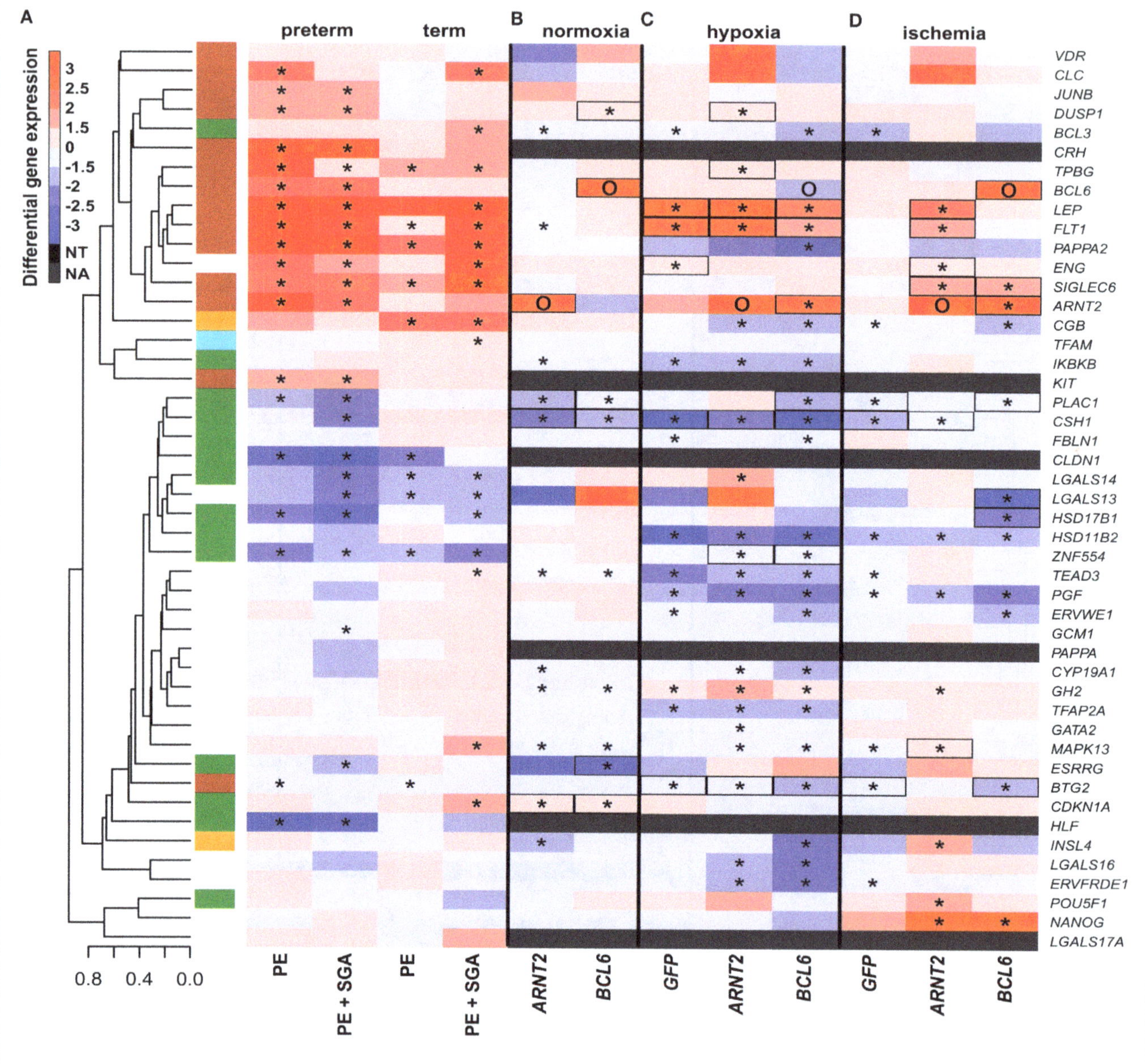

FIGURE 8 | The effect of O_2 levels, *BCL6* and *ARNT2* overexpression on differentially expressed genes in preeclampsia. **(A)** Hierarchical clustering tree and heatmap representing differential placental gene expression in preeclampsia. **(B)** The overexpression of *ARNT2* or *BCL6* in normoxic BeWo cells induced the dysregulation of three or five genes dysregulated in preeclampsia, respectively (boxed). **(C)** Hypoxia induced the dysregulation of five genes in BeWo cells also altered in preeclampsia. Hypoxia combined with *ARNT2* or *BCL6* overexpression led to the dysregulation of a large number of genes. **(D)** Ischemia induced the dysregulation of three genes in BeWo cells similar to preeclampsia. Ischemia combined with *ARNT2* or *BCL6* overexpression led to the dysregulation of 11 genes similar to preeclampsia. **(C,D)** Represents comparisons of gene expressions between hypoxia/ischemia vs. normoxia. In **(A–D)**, stars depict significant changes, "O" depicts "overexpressed," color bar encodes signed (up or down)-fold changes. Black boxes depict genes with similar expression changes *in vitro* as in the placenta in preeclampsia. Abbreviations: NA, not expressed; NT, not examined.

were no (n = 46) or subtle (n = 2) gestational age-dependent differences in the expression of selected target or housekeeping genes in third trimester control placentas in our microarray study (132), the comparison of placentas and trophoblasts from various gestational ages was deemed to be valid. Thus, we performed qRT-PCR profiling of primary VTs during 7 days of differentiation to reveal the dynamics in the expression of genes (**Figure 7B**), which we similarly profiled in the placenta (**Figure 7A**). We determined whether maximum expression change of selected genes during VT differentiation compared to day 0 inversely correlated with their maximum expression change in different preeclampsia phenotypes. We found that this was the case for 17 genes (**Figure 7C**), suggesting the delay or inhibition of VT differentiation-related expression change of these genes in preeclampsia. Among these 17 genes, 15 showed this behavior in preterm and 9 in term preeclampsia, suggesting that VT differentiation problems are more pronounced in preterm than in term preeclampsia ($p = 0.057$).

The Impact of Hypoxia, Ischemia, and Overexpression of *BCL6* and *ARNT2* on the Trophoblast

Subsequently, we tested how other factors implicated in preeclampsia pathogenesis, namely physiologic hypoxia (2% O_2) (167) or alternating hypoxic (1% O_2) and normoxic (20% O_2) conditions (ischemia) (40, 41, 242), in combination with the overexpression of hub transcription regulatory factors, may affect trophoblastic gene expression in a widely used BeWo cell trophoblast model. Two percent O_2 induced the dysregulation of only five genes, including *LEP* and *FLT1*, from the set of genes investigated in the placenta in preterm preeclampsia (**Figure 8C**), while alternating O_2 concentrations induced the dysregulation of only three genes (**Figure 8D**). Since hypoxia or ischemia alone did not induce similar transcriptomic changes in BeWo cells as seen in the placenta in preeclampsia, we examined how the overexpression of hub transcription regulatory genes in module M2 may modify the effects of these two conditions. Of note, 2% O_2 combined with *ARNT2* or *BCL6* overexpression led to the dysregulation of a large number of genes (**Figure 8C**). There were 9 genes (6 in the M2 and 3 in the M1 modules) dysregulated in BeWo cells, including *FLT1*, *ARNT2*, and *ZNF554*, similar to preeclampsia. Alternating O_2 concentrations combined with *ARNT2* or *BCL6* overexpression led to the dysregulation of 11 genes (5 in the M2 and 3 in the M1 modules), including *LEP*, *FLT1*, and *ENG*, similar to preeclampsia (**Figure 8D**). However, *ARNT2* or *BCL6* overexpression at normoxic conditions did not lead to substantial gene expression changes (**Figure 8B**), underlining the importance of gene–environment interactions. A permutation test showed that *BCL6* overexpression in ischemia mimicked overall expression changes of module M1 and M2 genes in preterm preeclampsia, while *ARNT2* overexpression in ischemia (and also in hypoxia) mimicked the up-regulation of module M2 genes in term and preterm preeclampsia (Data S11 in Supplementary Material). Since *BCL6* overexpression up-regulated *ARNT2* both in ischemia and hypoxia but not *vice versa*, we propose that *BCL6* is upstream of *ARNT2*. The up-regulation of these two transcription regulatory genes sensitize the trophoblast to ischemia, leading to the early dysregulation of modules M1 and M2, thus promoting preterm preeclampsia (Figure S7 in Supplementary Material).

Since none of the investigated conditions could up-regulate *BCL6*, we wondered whether *BCL6* overexpression might have an epigenetic background. Treating BeWo cells with 5-azacitidine down-regulated *BCL6*, supporting that its expression is regulated by DNA methylation in the trophoblast (Figure S8 in Supplementary Material). Of note, a recent study described the first intron of *BCL6* to be key in its overexpression in Burkitt lymphoma *via* altered DNA methylation (243). The Human Reference Epigenome Mapping Project revealed a differentially methylated region (DMR) in this intron in H1 embryonic stem cells as well as trophoblastic and neuronal cells derived from H1 cells, suggesting that this DMR may be differentially methylated in the trophoblast compared to other cells. To address whether this intronic region may be affected in the trophoblast in preeclampsia, we investigated DNA methylation in this region in primary VTs compared to cord blood cells collected from the same normal pregnancies. Bisulfite sequencing showed that Chr3:187,458,083-187,458,651 and Chr3:187,460,304-187,460,374 regions contain 12 hypermethylated CpGs in the trophoblasts compared to cord blood cells (Figures S8 and S9 in Supplementary Material). Further, we tested DNA methylation in this region in 100 placentas with qRT-PCR data including patients with preeclampsia after laser capturing VTs. Three CpGs (Chr3:187,458,095, Chr3:187,458,163, and Chr3:187,458,327) were differentially methylated in preeclampsia (Figure S10 in Supplementary Material), of which CpG Chr3:187,458,163 was differentially methylated in preterm preeclampsia, suggesting that this CpG may have a role in *BCL6* dysregulation in preeclampsia.

The Effects of *ZNF554* Down-Regulation in VTs

Next, we were interested in how the dysregulation of module M1 genes may play a role in preeclampsia pathology. Among hub genes of this module, *ZNF554* was of most interest due to the biological processes enriched in its co-expression network (Figure S1B in Supplementary Material), and also to its potential placenta- and preeclampsia-related regulation by transposable elements. This hypothesis was based on the fact that insertion of transposable elements into regulatory regions can lead to transcriptional changes, especially in the placenta (155, 244–247), and that the 5′ flanking region of *ZNF554* contains many LTR10A copies which had top enrichment among module M1 genes (OR = 17.4, $p = 1.27 \times 10^{-7}$; Data S12 in Supplementary Material). Of note, LTR10A drives placenta-specific expression of *NOS3* (248), and it may also have a similar effect on *ZNF554*. Indeed, *ZNF554* had the highest expression in the placenta in comparison to 47 other human tissues, which mostly had negligible *ZNF554* expression (**Figure 9A**).

Subsequent *in situ* hybridization (**Figure 9B**) and immunostaining (**Figure 9C**) of first and third trimester placentas of women with a normal pregnancy showed dominant *ZNF554* expression in the syncytiotrophoblast but not in the villous cytotrophoblast. Thus, we investigated *ZNF554* expression during VT differentiation, in which it was up-regulated similar to *CSH1* (**Figure 9D**), supporting that *ZNF554* expression is developmentally regulated in VTs. Of interest, ZNF554 immunostaining was faint in the syncytiotrophoblast in preeclampsia compared to controls (**Figures 9E,F**). To characterize the loss of syncytiotrophoblastic ZNF554 function, we silenced *ZNF554* in BeWo cells. At 74% *ZNF554* knock-down ($p = 5.24 \times 10^{-6}$) (**Figure 9G**), decreased nuclear and cytoplasmic ZNF554 immunostaining was found (**Figure 9H**). Microarray analyses of *ZNF554*-silenced cells revealed 123 DE genes (Data S13 in Supplementary Material) including 9 DE placental genes in preeclampsia, and the dysregulation of the "glycolysis/gluconeogenesis" pathway (OR = 7.8, $q = 0.06$) as well as 18 molecular functions including "RNA binding" (down) and "activin binding" (up) (**Figure 9I**; Data S14 in Supplementary Material). The up-regulation of *FSTL3* was confirmed by qRT-PCR (2.7-fold, $p < 0.001$) (**Figure 9J**). *FSTL3* encodes a secreted glycoprotein that

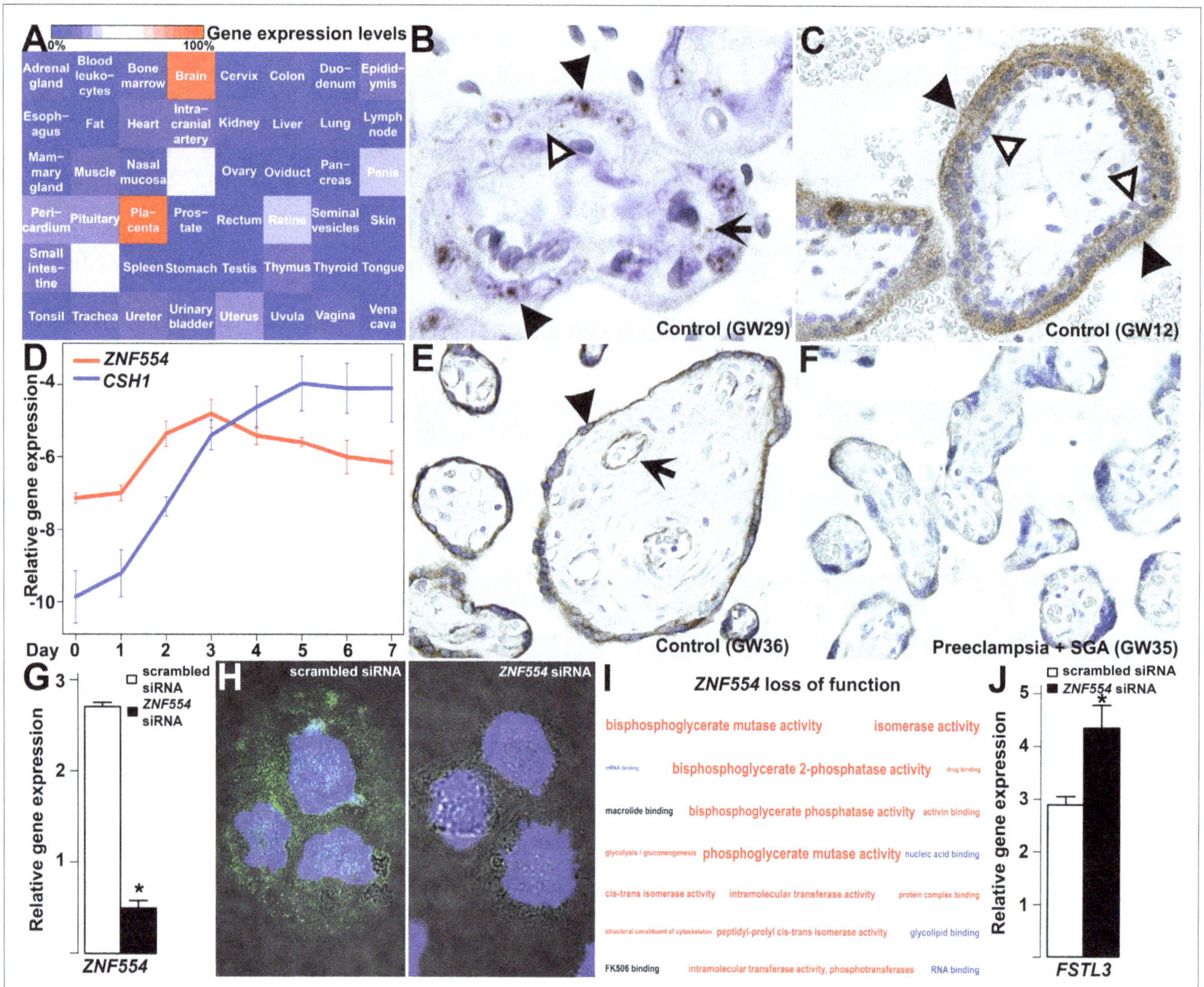

FIGURE 9 | *ZNF554* down-regulation in the villous trophoblast (VT) in preeclampsia. **(A)** Tissue qRT-PCR array revealed the highest *ZNF554* expression in the placenta among 48 human tissues. Color code depicts gene expression levels relative to that of the placenta (100%). **(B)** *In situ* hybridization of a third trimester control placenta (GW29) and **(C)** immunohistochemistry of a first trimester placenta (GW12) shows mainly syncytiotrophoblastic *ZNF554* expression (hematoxylin counterstaining, 1,400 and 400x magnifications, respectively). Black or white arrowheads depict syncytiotrophoblast or cytotrophoblast, while black arrow depicts fetal endothelium, respectively. **(D)** qRT-PCR revealed that *ZNF554* expression is up-regulated during VT differentiation in parallel with *CSH1*. **(E,F)** ZNF554 immunopositivity was faint in the syncytiotrophoblast in preeclampsia [**(F)**, GW35] compared to gestational-age matched controls [**(E)**, GW36] (hematoxylin counterstaining, 400x magnifications). Arrow and arrowhead depict syncytiotrophoblast and villous endothelium, respectively. **(G)** *ZNF554* mRNA expression was 74% lower in *ZNF554*-silenced BeWo cells compared to controls used for the microarrays ($p = 5.24 \times 10^{-6}$). **(H)** Nuclear and cytoplasmic ZNF554 immunofluorescence decreased in BeWo cells treated with *ZNF554* siRNA compared to control cells (3,500x magnifications). **(I)** Molecular functions and one Kyoto Encyclopedia of Genes and Genomes (KEGG) pathway (glycolysis/gluconeogenesis) affected in *ZNF554*-silenced BeWo cells. Colors denote the proportions of up- or down-regulated genes (red: >0.5 up-regulated; blue:>0.5 down-regulated; black: 0.5–0.5 up- and down-regulated). Letter sizes represent the minus $\log_{10}$ of *p*-values of the given functions or pathway. **(J)** qRT-PCR validated *FSTL3* up-regulation (2.7-fold, $p < 0.001$) in BeWo cells upon *ZNF554* knock-down.

inactivates activin and other TGFβ ligands (249). It is involved in the regulation of EVT invasion (250, 251) and its placental up-regulation is associated with low BW in preeclampsia (252). This finding confirms that the dysregulation of *ZNF554* may have key downstream effects on the pathogenesis of preeclampsia.

The Effects of *ZNF554* Down-Regulation in EVTs

We supposed that *ZNF554* may also affect EVTs, since its expression in EVTs was detected in first and third trimester maternal decidua (**Figures 10A–D**), and ZNF554-positive intraluminal and endovascular trophoblasts were found in the wall of transformed spiral arteries (**Figure 10B**). In preterm preeclampsia, ZNF554 immunostaining of EVTs was weaker than in controls (**Figures 10C,D**). To characterize the loss of ZNF554 function in EVTs, we silenced *ZNF554* in trophoblastic HTR8/SVneo cells (253). At 87% knock-down ($p < 0.001$) (**Figure 10E**), we observed decreased nuclear and cytoplasmic ZNF554 immunostaining (**Figure 10F**). Microarray analysis

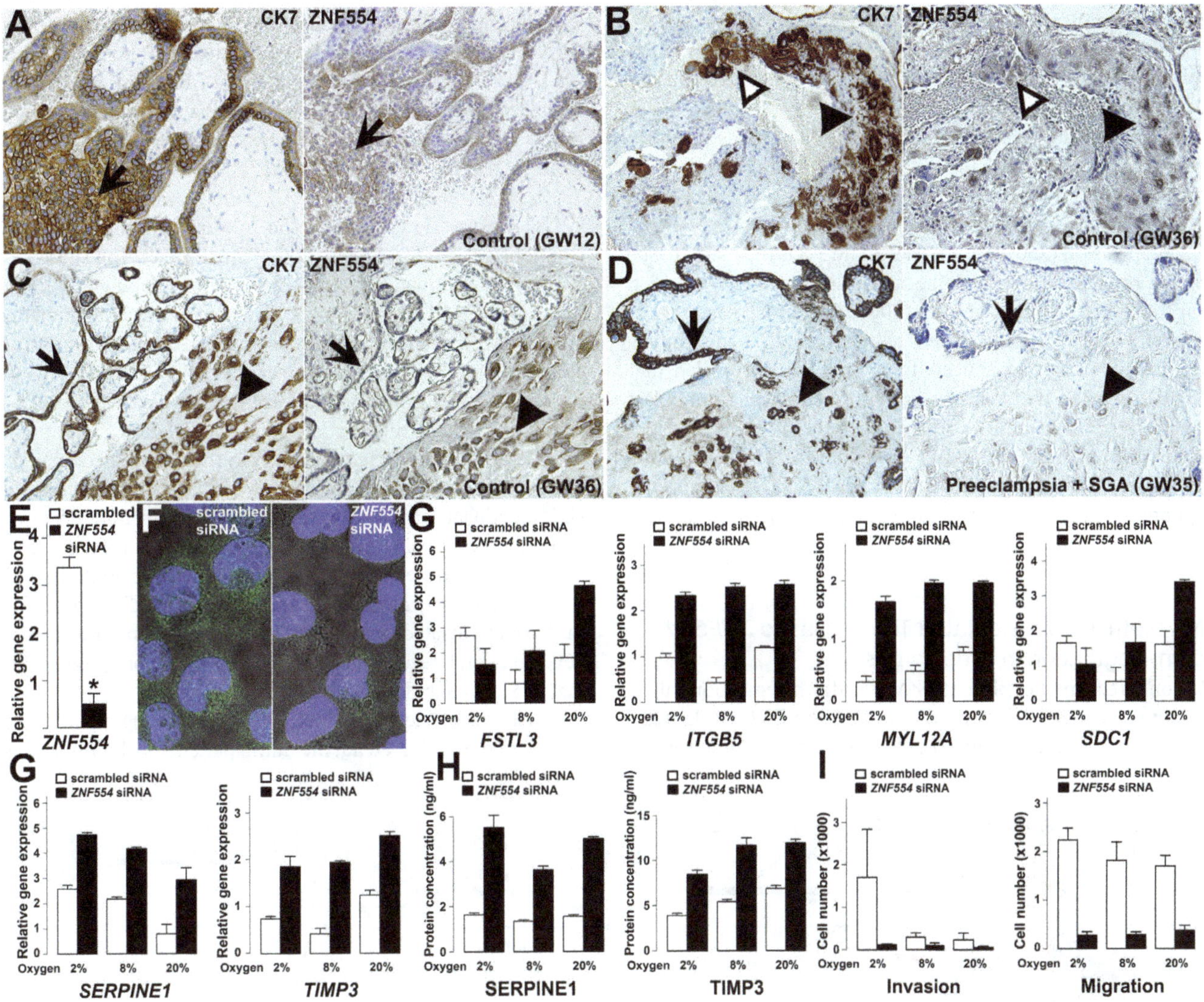

FIGURE 10 | *ZNF554* down-regulation in extravillous trophoblasts (EVTs) in preeclampsia. **(A)** EVTs in trophoblastic columns and **(B)** endovascular and intraluminal trophoblasts in the myometrium were immunostained for cytokeratin-7 (left) and ZNF554 (right). Arrows depict the direction of trophoblast invasion, black and white arrowheads point to EVTs in the wall and lumen of the spiral artery, respectively (serial sections, hematoxylin counterstaining, 200x magnifications). ZNF554 immunostaining in EVTs (arrowheads) and syncytiotrophoblast (arrows) was weaker in **(D)** preeclampsia than in **(C)** controls (serial sections, hematoxylin counterstaining, 200x magnifications). **(E)** *ZNF554* mRNA expression decreased to 13% upon knock-down ($p < 0.001$), **(F)** ZNF554 immunofluorescence was weaker in the nucleus and cytoplasm of *ZNF554*-silenced (left) than of control (right) HTR8/SVneo cells (3,500x magnifications). **(G)** The dysregulation of selected genes upon *ZNF554* knock-down was confirmed by qRT-PCR. **(H)** Plasminogen activator inhibitor-1 (PAI-1 / SERPINE1) and TIMP-3 proteins were increasingly secreted from *ZNF554*-silenced cells. **(I)** *ZNF554*-silenced cells had remarkably decreased invasive (left) and migratory (right) characteristics. O_2 concentrations are shown below the bars.

of *ZNF554*-silenced cells showed 185 DE genes (Data S15 in Supplementary Material) including 18 DE placental genes in preeclampsia. Gene ontology (GO) analysis revealed 16 molecular functions dysregulated, including "cyclin-dependent protein kinase regulator activity," "metalloendopeptidase inhibitor activity," and "insulin-like growth factor binding." The 67 enriched biological processes included "regulation of growth," "smooth muscle cell migration," "smooth muscle cell-matrix adhesion," and "response to oxygen levels," all relevant to trophoblast invasion and placental pathology of preeclampsia (Data S16 in Supplementary Material).

qRT-PCR confirmed the dysregulation of eight DE genes. Two genes (*CDKN1A*, *STK40*) are involved in the regulation of cell proliferation and differentiation (254, 255), and proliferation assays showed that *ZNF554* knock-down decreased cell proliferation in HTR8/SVneo cells slightly after 48 h (-14%, $p = 0.02$) (Figure S11 in Supplementary Material). Six genes (*FSTL3*, *ITGB5*, *MYL12A*, *SDC1*, *SERPINE1*, and *TIMP3*) encode proteins involved in cell adhesion, migration, invasion, and angiogenesis (**Figure 10G**). Since EVTs move through an environment with changing O_2 levels, we used O_2 concentrations for conditions relevant for endovascular (8%) and interstitial (2%) trophoblast invasion besides standard cell cultures (20%). The effect of *ZNF554* knockdown was significant regardless of O_2 levels on four genes (*ITGB5*, *MYL12A*, *SERPINE1*, and *TIMP3*), while there was an interaction between O_2 levels and *ZNF554* silencing on two genes (*FSTL3* and *SDC1*) (**Figure 10G**).

The up-regulation of SERPINE1 (PAI-1) and tissue inhibitor of metalloproteinases-3 (TIMP-3) was also confirmed at the protein level in supernatants of *ZNF554*-silenced cells (**Figure 10H**). Both proteins have an inhibitory function on trophoblast migration and invasion (250, 256, 257), and TIMP-3 is the major tissue metalloproteinase inhibitor at the maternal–fetal interface, which is up-regulated in preeclampsia (106, 258, 259). These results suggested that *ZNF554*-silenced cells have reduced migratory and invasive functions. Indeed, functional assays revealed that *ZNF554* silencing had a strong inhibitory effect on trophoblast migration ($p = 1.9 \times 10^{-10}$) regardless of the O_2 concentration, and also on invasion ($p < 0.001$), especially at 2% O_2 concentration (**Figure 10I**). These data corroborated that *ZNF554* supports trophoblast invasion *via* modulating a set of key genes that are involved in this process.

DNA Methylation-Mediated Trophoblastic *ZNF554* Down-Regulation in Preeclampsia

We wondered whether placental *ZNF554* down-regulation might have an epigenetic background, given that the *ZNF554* flanking region contains several transposable elements, including several Alus, which are generally hypomethylated in germ cells and the placenta (260, 261), while their hypermethylation leading to altered gene expression may be detected in preeclampsia (262, 263). Thus, the down-regulation of *ZNF554* expression in the placenta of patients with preeclampsia may also be reflected in the DNA methylation of the transposable elements in its 5′ flanking region.

The treatment of BeWo cells with 5-azacitidine increased *ZNF554* expression, showing the role of DNA methylation in trophoblastic *ZNF554* regulation (**Figure 11A**). The subsequent search in the Human Reference Epigenome Mapping Project data revealed a DMR located in the AluY, which was hypomethylated in H1 embryonic stem cells and H1-derived trophoblasts compared to H1-derived neuronal cells (**Figure 11B**). This was of interest, since AluY is a retrotransposon evolved recently in primates, and its differential DNA methylation supports the expression of other gene transcripts in the placenta compared to somatic tissues (264). These data prompted us to investigate the DNA methylation in this genomic region in primary VTs and cord blood cells collected from the same normal pregnancies. In fact, bisulfite sequencing showed that the AluY, similarly to the AluSq2, is heavily methylated in cord blood cells compared to the hypomethylated trophoblast, suggesting its importance in the developmental regulation of *ZNF554* expression (**Figure 11B**; Figure S12 in Supplementary Material).

Further, we tested DNA methylation in this region in 100 placentas with qRT-PCR data, including patients with preeclampsia

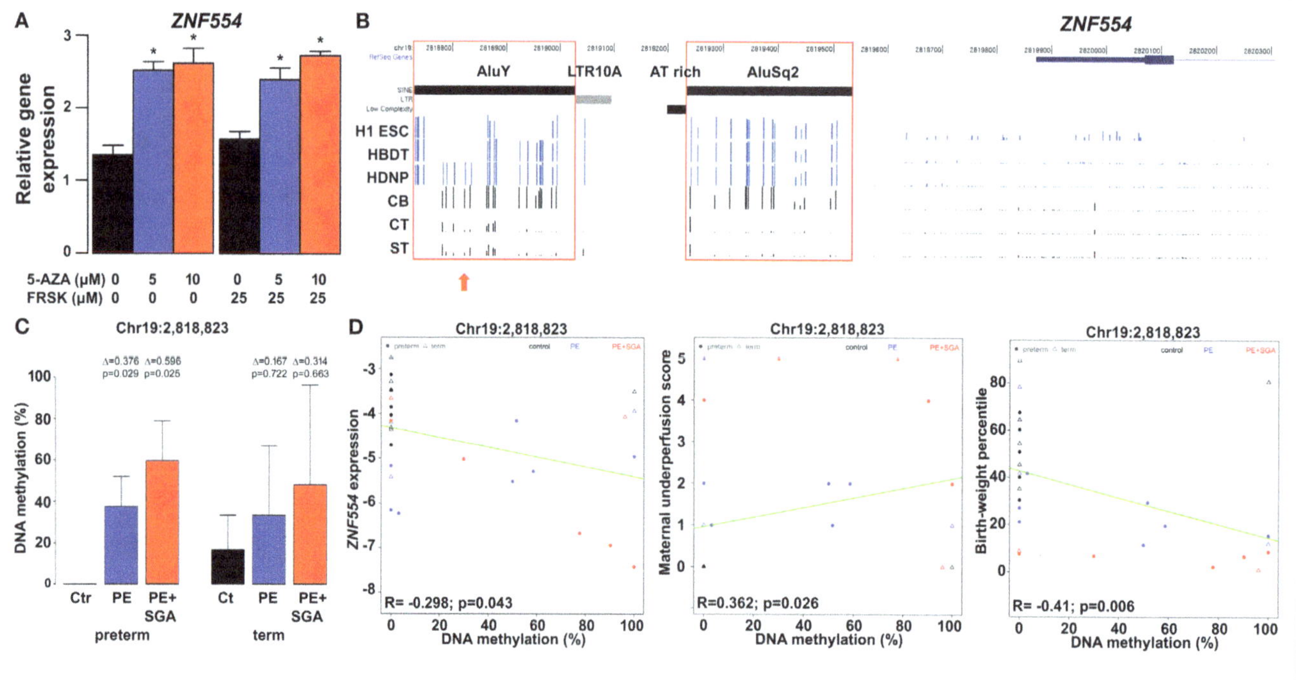

FIGURE 11 | The effect of trophoblastic DNA methylation on *ZNF554* expression and clinical parameters in preeclampsia. **(A)** Increased *ZNF554* expression in BeWo cells upon treatment with 5-azacitidine (5-AZA) irrespective of forskolin (FRSK) co-treatment. **(B)** *Upper three lanes*: whole genome bisulfite sequencing data of *ZNF554* 5′ flanking region from the Human Reference Epigenome Mapping Project. H1 ESC, H1 embryonic stem cell; HBDT, H1 BMP4-derived trophoblast; and HDNP, H1-derived neuronal progenitor. *Lower three lanes:* bisulfite sequencing data from this study. Abbreviations: CB, cord blood cell; CT, cytotrophoblast; ST, syncytiotrophoblast. *Red boxes:* AluY and AluSq2 are heavily methylated in cord blood cells and hypomethylated in trophoblasts. *Red arrow:* CpG Chr19:2,818,823. **(C)** CpG Chr19:2,818,823 was differentially methylated in trophoblasts in preterm preeclampsia ± SGA. **(D)** Correlation was observed between Chr19:2,818,823 CpG methylation and *ZNF554* expression, maternal vascular malperfusion score of the placenta, and birthweight percentile.

after laser capture of the VTs. Bisulfite sequencing of the trophoblastic DNA revealed four CpGs on AluY (Chr19:2,818,823, Chr19:2,818,864, Chr19:2,818,868, and Chr19:2,818,876) hypomethylated in controls but hypermethylated in preterm preeclampsia, with highest methylation in cases associated with SGA (**Figure 11C**; Figure S13 in Supplementary Material). Importantly, we found correlations between Chr19:2,818,823 CpG methylation and *ZNF554* expression ($R = -0.30$, $p = 0.04$), maternal vascular underperfusion score of the placenta ($R = 0.36$, $p = 0.03$), and BW percentile ($R = -0.41$, $p < 0.01$) (**Figure 11D**). These data collectively provide evidence that the hypermethylation of certain CpGs in AluY in the trophoblast may result in low *ZNF554* expression, impaired trophoblast invasion, preeclampsia, and fetal growth restriction.

DISCUSSION

The placenta has a key role in the pathogenesis of the terminal pathway of preeclampsia, which may be triggered by discrete disease pathways at early stages of pregnancy, leading to the development of different preeclampsia phenotypes. In this study, an integrated systems biology approach was employed to gain insights into these complex pathways, given that this strategy offered the ultimate analytic solution to investigate and understand the complex disease pathways of the syndrome of preeclampsia (265–268). We incorporated "omics," clinical, placental, and functional data from patients with distinct phenotypes of preeclampsia. We employed molecular network-based approaches to identify networks and modules of genes or proteins that are perturbed in the placenta and the maternal circulation of women with preeclampsia.

Our placental transcriptomics study identified 1,409 DE genes involved in many biological processes (e.g. BP regulation, apoptosis, development, hormone secretion, metabolism, and signaling) that were previously implicated in the pathogenesis of preterm preeclampsia by other placental transcriptomics studies (105, 110, 111, 113, 114, 116, 117, 122, 123, 125, 127, 128, 130, 131, 134, 137, 269–272). Despite the differences in patient populations, design, or methodologies between these studies, many DE genes on our list have also been found by other groups. Indeed, from the 40-gene meta-signature that characterized the significant intersection of DE genes from independent placental gene signatures in preeclampsia in the meta-analysis of Kleinrouweler et al. (135), our microarray and qRT-PCR studies found 26 (65%) to be DE in preterm preeclampsia. Of note, 16 of these 26 genes belong to module M2, while only six to the M1 module. This supports our observation that the dysregulation of module M2 is associated with BP elevation, the maternal disease condition required for patient inclusion into these studies. The weaker involvement of module M1 genes in the meta-signature may reflect the heterogeneity of preeclampsia transcriptomics studies regarding fetal (growth restriction) and placental disease conditions. Our microarray study was homogeneous for preterm preeclampsia cases with low BW and placental disease, while only a couple of other studies had this rigor. To overcome the inconsistency of smaller placental transcriptomics studies, Leavey et al. (140, 142) employed advanced bioinformatics methods to aggregate microarray datasets across multiple platforms to generate large datasets of patient samples. Unsupervised clustering of these datasets revealed three distinct molecular subclasses of preeclampsia. Among these, the "canonical" subclass, which is associated with the differential expression of our module M2 genes, was characteristic for preterm preeclampsia and consistent with stress response to poor oxygenation, further supporting our findings. However, our discovery on the two major dysregulated placental disease gene modules and their hub transcription regulatory genes, separately associated with maternal or fetal disease pathways, are novel (**Figure 12**).

Functional assays on hub transcription factors of these two disease gene modules demonstrated that *ZNF554* (M1) down-regulation leads to impaired trophoblast invasion, while *BCL6* and *ARNT2* (M2) overexpression sensitizes the trophoblast to ischemia, which are hallmarks in the pathogenesis of preterm preeclampsia. In the "ZNF554" pathway, hypermethylation of AluY in the *ZNF554 5′* flanking region inhibits gene expression, leading to impaired trophoblast invasion, placental vascular malperfusion, and low BW. In the "BCL6-ARNT2" pathway, which is activated only in preterm preeclampsia, ischemic stress of the trophoblast coupled with *BCL6* and *ARNT2* overexpression increases *FLT1* expression. This then eventually promotes the anti-angiogenic state, hypertension (37, 56, 57, 61, 62, 83), and the early onset of this syndrome (Figure S7 in Supplementary Material).

The perturbed placental disease gene modules in preterm preeclampsia can be detected by liquid biopsy in maternal blood in the early stages of pregnancy. Indeed, we detected the down-regulation of M1 and M2 disease gene module biomarkers in these patients during the first trimester. Of interest, the up-regulation of module M2 biomarkers can be detected after the establishment of maternal circulation in the intervillous space. These findings support the observation that placental transcriptomic changes, typical for preterm preeclampsia observed in the third trimester, are rooted in the first trimester. The positive correlation of gene expression in module M1 with BW and in module M2 with BP suggests that M1 genes may be biomarkers for placental and fetal growth and development while M2 genes can serve as biomarkers for placental stress.

First trimester maternal blood proteomics uncovered the altered abundance of proteins of the renin–angiotensin and immune systems as well as complement and coagulation cascades in patients who subsequently developed both preterm and term preeclampsia. The same proteins and pathways were found to be dysregulated in maternal blood in later stages of preeclampsia by other proteomics studies (108, 115, 118–120, 126, 129, 133, 136, 138, 139, 143); however, ours is the first revealing their dysregulation at an earlier stage of pregnancy when there is no or minimal direct connection between the placenta and the maternal circulation (273).

From these dysregulated maternal serum proteins, *in silico* analysis pointed to candidates, which may drive trophoblastic transcriptomic changes, and corroborated earlier findings on angiotensinogen/angiotensin II in driving hypertension indirectly through *FLT1* up-regulation in addition to its direct effects (91, 274). Moreover, *in vitro* functional assays revealed that altered maternal serum proteome in the first trimester can affect the trophoblastic transcriptome and up-regulate *FLT1*.

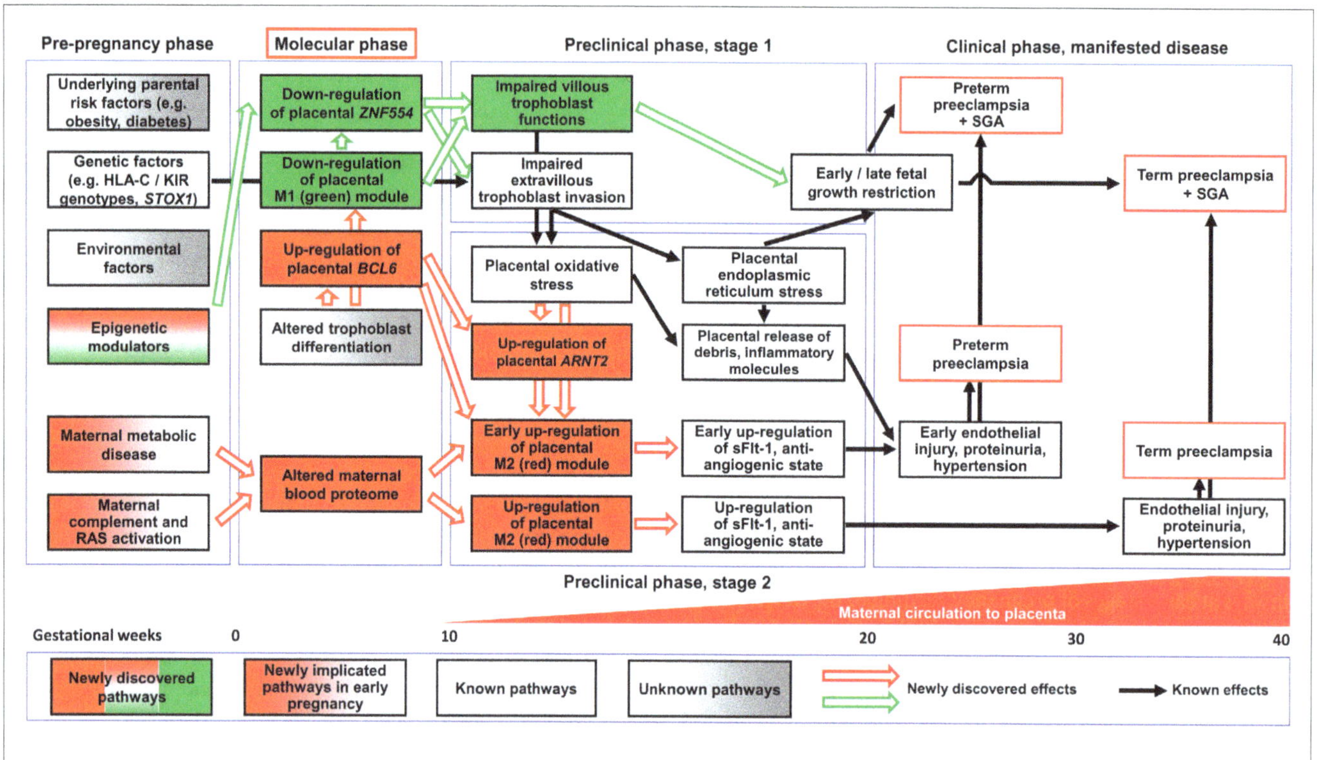

FIGURE 12 | Pathologic pathways in preeclampsia. *Maternal pathways:* alterations in the maternal blood proteome, including systemic inflammatory changes, can be observed in both preterm and term preeclampsia before the maternal circulation of the placenta has been established, supporting the observation that maternal factors have a key role in triggering early disease pathways. Later, these alterations can induce trophoblastic functional changes leading to the up-regulation of module M2 genes, the overproduction of sFlt-1, and an anti-angiogenic state through a trajectory that does not necessarily affect fetal growth. *Placental pathways:* altered differentiation of the trophoblast leads to the dysregulation of module M1 genes and hub factors in module M2. The down-regulation of *ZNF554* and module M1 genes involved in the regulation of fetal growth and metabolism imply impaired villous trophoblast (VT) functions besides abnormal extravillous trophoblast (EVT) invasion. The up-regulation of the *BCL6-ARNT2* pathway sensitizes the trophoblast to ischemia and increases *FLT1* expression after the maternal circulation to the placenta has been established. These changes are observed only in preterm preeclampsia, suggesting that this placental pathway promotes the early development of preeclampsia. The interplay of these molecular pathways leads to the complex pathogenesis of preeclampsia. Abbreviations: RAS, renin-angiotensin system; SGA, small-for-gestational age.

This is in agreement with reports indicating that maternal blood factors in preeclampsia can induce trophoblastic soluble endoglin overexpression and the development of preeclampsia-like symptoms in mice (85, 275).

Remarkably, most of the dysregulated maternal serum proteins in the first trimester in both preterm (11 of 19) and term (7 of 14) preeclampsia are implicated in immune functions (**Figure 6**; Figure S6 in Supplementary Material), suggesting a critical role for immune pathways and inflammation in the early pathogenesis of both phenotypes of preeclampsia. This is consistent with clinical, epidemiological, and immunological evidence showing that: (1) preeclampsia has multiple risk factors (e.g. dyslipidemia, hypertension, insulin resistance, and obesity) characterized by heightened inflammation (29, 276); (2) the combination of inhibitory decidual NK (dNK) cell killer immunoglobulin-like receptor and the fetal HLA-C2 genotype increases the susceptibility to preeclampsia due to the loss of activating interactions between trophoblasts and dNK cells at early stages of placentation (168, 277–283); (3) an altered local immune regulation and a shift toward the pro-inflammatory macrophage phenotype promotes a pro-inflammatory milieu in the maternal decidua in preeclampsia (284, 285); (4) an imbalance between Th1/Th2/Th17/Treg cells in preeclampsia leads to failure of maternal–fetal tolerance mechanisms (286–289); and (5) complement system activation in preeclampsia leads to the activation of innate immune cells and placental damage (101, 234, 236, 237, 290–292). The role of inflammation in early preeclampsia disease pathways is also supported by *in vivo* studies showing that bacterial endotoxin administration to pregnant rats induces placentation defects and symptoms consistent with preeclampsia (293–298).

Overall, our data show that there are distinct maternal and placental disease pathways, and their interaction influences the clinical presentation of preeclampsia. The activation of maternal disease pathways can be detected in both preterm and term preeclampsia earlier and upstream of placental dysfunction, not only downstream as described before (43), and distinct placental disease pathways are superimposed on these maternal pathways. This is a paradigm shift in our understanding of preeclampsia, which in agreement with epidemiological studies (25, 31) warrants for the central pathologic role of preexisting maternal diseases or perturbed maternal–fetal–placental immune interactions in preeclampsia.

The superimposed placental disease pathways differ between preterm and term preeclampsia. For preterm preeclampsia, our functional data suggest that placental disease pathways are partly originated from altered trophoblast differentiation, which is followed by trophoblastic stress, induced by perturbed maternal blood proteome factors and/or ischemia after the onset of maternal circulation to the placenta. Our data are consistent with recent views indicating that defects in trophoblast proliferation, differentiation, invasion, and plugging are associated with defective decidualization (299), decidual inflammation (300), and the disturbance in endometrial-trophoblast dialog during the peri-conception (301) period. Abnormal trophoblast invasion and plugging will subsequently lead to the aberrant onset of maternal circulation (273) and malperfusion, causing placental oxidative stress in preterm preeclampsia (175, 273, 302). On the other hand, maternal disease pathways induce mainly placental dysfunction without maldevelopment in term preeclampsia. This is substantiated by the differences observed in the maternal proteome, placental transcriptome, and trophoblastic DNA methylation between term and preterm preeclampsia in our study. Moreover, this is also consistent with the major differences between these two preeclampsia phenotypes in etiology (31), placental histopathology (28, 33, 44–46), and stress levels (303) as well as clinical presentation (2, 25, 26, 29, 304).

Our findings are very timely in the light of recent clinical research showing that the administration of aspirin before 16 weeks of gestation to pregnant women at risk for preeclampsia prevents the preterm phenotype of this syndrome (24, 305–309). Thus, the anti-inflammatory and anti-platelet actions of aspirin (308–311) may ameliorate the early pro-inflammatory disease pathways leading to placental maldevelopment in preterm preeclampsia. Based on our discovery of these novel disease pathways and their hub molecules, we propose a "molecular phase" of preeclampsia (**Figure 12**), where early pathologic events can already be detected by maternal blood biomarkers, offering non-invasive diagnostics of maternal and placental disease pathways. Biomarkers of these disease pathways may open new venues for the molecular characterization of patients destined to develop preeclampsia, using multi-biomarker profiles that support preventive approaches for patients with distinct preeclampsia phenotypes.

MATERIALS AND METHODS

Placental Study

Placental Microarray Study

Study Groups and Clinical Definitions

Placental tissue and maternal blood samples were collected from Caucasian women at the First Department of Obstetrics and Gynaecology, Semmelweis University in Budapest, Hungary as described previously (132). Pregnancies were dated according to ultrasound scans between 8 and 12 weeks of gestation. Patients with multiple pregnancies or fetuses having congenital or chromosomal abnormalities were excluded. The collection and investigation of human clinical samples were approved by the Health Science Board of Hungary. Written informed consent was obtained from women prior to sample collection, and the experiments conformed to the principles set out in the World Medical Association Declaration of Helsinki and the Department of Health and Human Services Belmont Report. Specimens and data were stored anonymously.

Women were enrolled in the following groups: (1) preterm severe preeclampsia, with or without HELLP (hemolysis, elevated liver enzymes, low platelets) syndrome ($n = 12$) and (2) preterm controls ($n = 5$) (**Table 1**). Preeclampsia was defined according to the criteria set by the American College of Obstetricians and Gynecologists (1), and subdivided into preterm (<37 weeks) or term (≥37 weeks) groups. Severe preeclampsia was defined according to Sibai et al. (2). Preterm controls had no medical complications, clinical or histological signs of chorioamnionitis, and delivered neonates with a BW appropriate-for-gestational age (AGA) (312). SGA was defined as neonatal BW below the 10th percentile for gestational age. Cesarean delivery was performed in all cases due to severe symptoms as well as in all controls due to previous Cesarean delivery or malpresentation.

Placental Tissue and Maternal Blood Collection

Placental tissue specimens were processed immediately after delivery as described previously (132). For the microarray study, 1 × 1 cm villous tissue samples were excised from central cotyledons close to the umbilical cord to reduce the possible bias due to regional differences in gene expression (313, 314). These tissue blocks were then dissected from the choriodecidua on dry ice, snap-frozen, and stored at −80°C. For histopathologic evaluations, five representative tissue blocks were taken from each placenta to include central and peripheral cotyledons and the maternal side of the placenta with the fetal membranes. These blocks were embedded in paraffin after fixation in 10% neutral-buffered formalin (FFPE). Maternal blood samples were obtained at the time of admission into the delivery room; aliquots of maternal sera and plasma were stored at −80°C.

Histopathologic Evaluation of the Placentas

Placental specimens were examined according to a standard protocol, describing the topography and size of macroscopic lesions. Four micrometer sections were cut from the five FFPE blocks and mounted on SuperFrost/Plus slides (Fisherbrand, UK). After deparaffinization, slides were rehydrated, stained with hematoxylin and eosin, and examined in 10 randomly chosen microscopic fields using bright-field light microscopy by a pathologist blinded to the clinical information. Macroscopic and microscopic lesions were defined according to published criteria (315–317).

Placental Total RNA Isolation and Microarray Experiments

Tissues were homogenized using a ThermoSavant FastPrep FP120 Homogenizer (Thermo Scientific, Wilmington, DE, USA) with Lysing MatrixD (MP Biomedicals, Illkirch, France). Total RNA was isolated using RNeasy Fibrous Tissue Mini Kit (QIAGEN GmbH, Hilden, Germany), quantified with NanoDrop 1000 (Thermo Scientific), and assessed by Agilent 2100 Bioanalyzer (Matriks AS, Oslo, Norway). Total RNAs were labeled, and Cy3-RNAs were fragmented and hybridized to the Whole Human Genome Oligo Microarray G4112A (Agilent Technologies, Santa Clara, CA, USA) on an Agilent scanner, and processed with Agilent Feature Extraction software v9.5 according to the manufacturer's guidelines.

Data Analysis

Demographics data were compared by the Fisher's exact test and Mann–Whitney test using SPSS version 12.0 (SPSS Inc., Chicago, IL, USA). Microarray data analysis was performed using the R statistical language and environment[1] following the MIAME guidelines and methodologies described previously (318). Microarray expression intensities were background corrected using the "minimum" method in the "backgroundCorrect" function of the "limma" package (319). After $\log_2$ transformation, data were quantile-normalized. From the 41,093 probesets on the array, 93 were removed before differential expression analysis, lacking annotation in the array definition file (Agilent Technologies). Subsequently, an expression filter was applied to retain probesets with intensity greater than $\log_2(50)$ in at least two samples, yielding a final matrix of 30,027 probesets (15,939 unique genes). Differential gene expression was assessed using linear models including adjustment for batch effects, with coefficient evaluation *via* moderated *t*-tests. *P*-values were adjusted using the false discovery rate (FDR) method and Benjamini–Hochberg correction to compute *q*-values. Since there were no differences among patient groups in maternal age or ethnic background, we did not adjust for these parameters. Target gene Entrez IDs for the probesets were determined using the R package "hgu4112a.db." For probesets without annotation in the package, Entrez IDs were taken from the array definition file (Agilent Technologies). Probesets remaining un-annotated (without Entrez ID and/or gene symbol) were removed from further analysis. Probesets were defined as DE ($n = 1{,}409$) if they had a $q \leq 0.2$ and a fold-change ≥ 1.5 (Data S1 in Supplementary Material).

From the DE genes in preeclampsia, those encoding for proteins with functions in transcription regulation ($n = 137$) were identified using the Metacore (GeneGo Inc., Saint Joseph, MI, USA) and GeneCards v3[2] databases.

We downloaded the human U133A/GNF1H microarray data on 79 human tissues, cells, and cell lines from the Symatlas/BioGPS database (151) to identify human genes with predominant placental expression. A probeset was defined as having predominant placental expression if its placental expression was (1) $\geq 1{,}000$ fluorescence units; (2) six times higher than the median value in 78 other tissue and cell sources; and (3) two times higher than its expression in the tissue with the second highest expression. The resulting 215 probesets corresponded to 153 unique genes. Eleven additional genes that were not present on the microarray platform used by Symatlas/BioGPS (Affymetrix, Santa Clara, CA, USA) were added to this list based on previously published evidence of placenta-specific expression (151–153) (Data S2 in Supplementary Material). Of the 164 predominantly placenta-expressed genes, 157 were present in our placental microarray data. These genes were tested for enrichment in DE genes compared to all genes on the array (1,409 of 15,939) using the Fisher's exact test.

The expression levels of DE genes in EVT compared to VT lineages were analyzed by retrieving published microarray datasets (320–322) and reanalyzing expression data. Raw Affymetrix GeneChip Human Genome U133A 2.0 Array data from Bilban et al. (320) and Tilburgs et al. (322) was downloaded from GEO (GSE9773) and ArrayExpress (E-MATB-3217) respectively, and was processed with the *"affy"* (323) and *"limma"* (324) packages of Bioconductor.[3] After RMA normalization, log-fold changes were calculated. Processed Illumina Human HT-12 V3 BeadArray data from Apps et al. (321) was downloaded from ArrayExpress (E-MATB-429), and then log-fold changes were calculated.

Chromosomal locations for all genes tested on the Agilent array were obtained from the R package "org.Hs.eg.db." Of the 15,939 unique and 1,409 DE genes on the array, 15,935 and 1,408 could be assigned to chromosomes, respectively. Mapping the microarray probesets on the Affymetrix human U133A/GNF1H chips to ENTREZ identifiers was performed using the Bioconductor "hgu133a.db" and "hgfocus.db" packages (325, 326). Chromosomal locations of the resulting list of genes were obtained from the package "org.Hs.eg.db" and from the National Center for Biotechnology Information for the 11 additional genes (327). Enrichment analyses for chromosomes among predominantly placenta-expressed genes, DE genes and DE genes encoding for transcriptional regulators (Data S3–S5 in Supplementary Material) were tested by the Fisher's exact test. Chromosomal locations of these genes were visualized by Circos (328).

Weighted gene co-expression network analysis (329, 330) was applied on the 1,409 DE genes across 17 samples to identify distinct regulatory modules and prioritize candidate genes for qRT-PCR validation. A gene pair-wise similarity (absolute Pearson correlation) matrix was first computed, then soft-thresholded by raising it to the power of 10 (chosen based on the scale-free topology criterion) to obtain an adjacency matrix. The topology overlap matrix (TOM) was then derived from the adjacency matrix. The topology overlap (331) measures the node interconnectedness within a network and was generalized to WGCNA (329). This measure defines the similarity between the two genes based on both correlations within themselves and outside other genes. Gene distance matrix was defined as 1-TOM and used for average linkage hierarchical clustering. A hybrid dynamic tree-cutting method (332) was applied to obtain modules (tree clusters).

Gene modules identified with this approach were further tested for enrichment in DE genes using the Fisher's exact test. Transcription regulatory genes expressed at high levels (average $\log_2$ intensity >9) and co-expressed (absolute Pearson coefficient >0.7) with the most genes among DE genes were treated as candidates for hub genes in the module. Hub genes then were selected based on the number and strength of their Pearson co-expression partners as well as their and their networks' biological activities. The networks of biological processes enriched among genes co-expressed with hub factors modules were created by BINGO and visualized with Cytoscape.

Enrichment analysis of transposable elements present in the 10,000 bp upstream region of DE genes was performed separately for the M1 (green) and the M2 (red) modules in preeclampsia versus all genes present on the microarray using the Fisher's exact

[1] www.r-project.org.
[2] www.genecards.org.

[3] www.bioconductor.org.

test. The locations of transposable elements and their families and classes were obtained from the "RepeatMasker" table of the UCSC Table Browser.[4] *P*-values <0.05 were considered significant.

Placental Validation Study

Study Groups and Clinical Definitions

Third trimester placentas (n = 100) collected predominantly from African-American women were retrieved from the Bank of Biological Specimens of the Perinatology Research Branch (Detroit, MI, USA). Pregnancies were dated according to ultrasound scans between 8 and 12 weeks. Patients with multiple pregnancies or fetuses having congenital or chromosomal abnormalities were excluded. The use of biological specimens and clinical data for research purposes was approved by the Wayne State University Human Investigation Committee and the Institutional Review Board of the *Eunice Kennedy Shriver* National Institute of Child Health and Human Development (NICHD, NIH, DHHS). Written informed consent was obtained from women prior to sample collection, and the experiments conformed to the principles set out in the World Medical Association Declaration of Helsinki and the Department of Health and Human Services Belmont Report. Specimens and data were stored anonymously.

The following homogenous patient groups were selected from a cohort: (1) preterm severe preeclampsia (n = 20); (2) preterm severe preeclampsia associated with SGA (n = 20); (3) preterm controls (n = 20); (4) term severe preeclampsia (n = 10); (5) term severe preeclampsia associated with SGA (n = 10); and (6) term controls (n = 20). Term controls, consisting of normal pregnant women with (n = 10) or without (n = 10) labor, and preterm controls with preterm labor and delivery had no medical complications or clinical or histological signs of chorioamnionitis, and delivered an AGA neonate (333) (**Table 2**; Figure S2 in Supplementary Material).

Labor was defined by the presence of regular uterine contractions at a frequency of at least two contractions every 10 min with cervical changes resulting in delivery (334). Preeclampsia was defined according to the criteria set by the American College of Obstetricians and Gynecologists (1) and was subdivided into preterm (<37 weeks) or term (≥37 weeks) groups. Severe preeclampsia was defined according to Sibai et al. (2). SGA was defined as neonatal BW below the 10th percentile for gestational age (333). Cesarean delivery was performed in cases due to severe symptoms and in controls due to previous Cesarean delivery or malpresentation.

Placental Tissue Collection

Third trimester placental tissue specimens (n = 100) were processed immediately after delivery. For histopathologic evaluations, representative tissue blocks were taken from each placenta to include central and peripheral cotyledons, maternal side of the placenta, fetal membranes, and the umbilical cord. These blocks were embedded in paraffin after fixation in 10% neutral-buffered formalin (FFPE). Villous tissue blocks from central cotyledons were selected for TMA. For gene expression studies, systematic random sampling (335) was used to obtain villous tissues to reduce the possible bias due to regional gene expression differences (313, 314). Excised tissue blocks were homogenized and mixed in TRIzol reagent (Life Technologies), snap-frozen with liquid N_2, and stored at −80°C.

Histopathologic Evaluation of the Placentas

Placental specimens (n = 100) were examined according to a standard protocol, describing the topography and size of macroscopic lesions. Five μm sections were cut from the representative FFPE tissue blocks, stained with hematoxylin and eosin, and examined using bright-field light microscopy by two anatomic pathologists blinded to the clinical information. Histopathologic changes of the placenta were defined according to published criteria proposed by the Perinatal Section of the Society for Pediatric Pathology (336). "Maternal vascular malperfusion score" was calculated by summing the number of pathologic lesions consistent with this lesion category (46, 336) present in a given placenta.

Placental Total RNA Isolation and qRT-PCR

Total RNA was isolated from snap-frozen third trimester placental villous tissues (n = 100) with TRIzol reagent (Life Technologies) and RNeasy kit (QIAGEN, Valencia, CA, USA) according to the manufacturers' recommendations. The 28S/18S ratios and the RNA integrity numbers were assessed using an Agilent Bioanalyzer 2100, and RNA concentrations were measured with NanoDrop 1000. Total RNA (500 ng) was reverse transcribed with the High Capacity cDNA Reverse Transcription Kit using random hexamers (Applied Biosystems, Foster City, CA, USA). TaqMan Assays (Applied Biosystems; **Table 3**, Data S17 in Supplementary Material) were used for high-throughput gene expression profiling on the Biomark qRT-PCR system (Fluidigm, San Francisco, CA, USA) according to the manufacturers' instructions.

Placental TMA Construction, Immunohistochemistry, and Immunoscoring

Tissue microarrays were constructed from central tissue blocks of third trimester FFPE placentas (n = 100) as described earlier (337). Briefly, three 20 × 35 mm recipient blocks were made of Paraplast X-Tra tissue embedding media (Fisher Scientific, Pittsburgh, PA, USA). One mm diameter cores from tissue blocks were transferred in triplicate into recipient paraffin blocks using an automated tissue arrayer (Beecher Instruments, Inc., Silver Spring, MD, USA). Five μm sections cut from TMAs were placed on silanized slides and stained with antibodies and reagents (Data S18 in Supplementary Material) either on Ventana Discovery or Leica BOND-MAX autostainers.

Tissue microarray immunostainings were semi-quantitatively scored by three examiners blinded to the clinical information with an immunoreactive score modified from a previously published one (154). Immunostaining intensity was graded as follows: 0 = negative, 1 = weak, 2 = intermediate, and 3 = strong. All villi in a random field of each of the three cores were evaluated by all examiners, and scores within each core were averaged to represent the target protein quantity of that core. Thus, each

[4]http://genome.ucsc.edu/.

placenta had three scores corresponding to the three cores examined.

Data Analysis

Demographics data were compared by the Fisher's exact test and Mann–Whitney test using SPSS version 12.0 (SPSS). All other data were analyzed in the R statistical environment (see text footnote 1).

Placental qRT-PCR. Data were analyzed using the $\Delta\Delta$Ct method. Data were first normalized to the reference gene (*RPLPO*), and the batch effect was adjusted through calibrator samples. Log_2 mRNA relative concentrations were obtained for each sample as $-\Delta Ct_{(gene)} = Ct_{(RPLPO)} - Ct_{(gene)}$. The surrogate gene expression values ($-\Delta Ct_{gene}$) were used to perform a hierarchical clustering with 1-Pearson correlation distance and average linkage. Between-group comparisons (in which groups were predefined based on the clinical characteristics of the patients) were performed by fitting a linear model on $-\Delta$Ct values, using the group variable indicator and the maturity status of the fetus (term vs. preterm) as covariates while allowing for an interaction effect (**Figure 4**; Figure S3 in Supplementary Material).

Histopathology. The association between qRT-PCR gene expression and the "maternal vascular malperfusion" score was tested using a linear model. *P*-values of <0.05 were considered significant.

TMA Immunoscoring. Group comparisons using immunoscores were conducted in the same way as for the qRT-PCR data (**Figure 4**).

Correlation of Clinical Parameters and Placental Gene Expression

Data Analysis

To reveal whether the expression of any gene on the microarray was correlated with MAP while controlling for BW, a linear model (y~MAP + BW + Batch) was fit for every gene on the array, in which y represents gene expression, and the dependent variables represent MAP, BW, and batch, respectively. A moderated t-test was used to obtain p-values, which then were adjusted using the FDR method and Benjamini–Hochberg correction for multiple testing. Significance was determined using a $q \leq 0.2$. Gene modules were also tested for the enrichment in genes with their expression correlated with MAP using the Fisher's exact test (Data S6 in Supplementary Material).

In the qRT-PCR validation study, we extended our analysis to include all 100 patients to test for the association between gene expression and mean arterial BP as well as BW percentile while adjusting for gestational age. All variables were treated as continuous. *P*-values of <0.05 were considered significant (**Figure 4**).

Genomic DNA Methylation Analysis of the Trophoblast

Laser Capture Microdissection

Fifteen μm sections were cut from snap-frozen placentas that were also used for qRT-PCR expression profiling ($n = 100$) on 2 μm Glass Foiled PEN slides (Leica Microsystems). The trophoblast layer of 300–350 villi in each specimen was laser captured by a Leica DM6000B microscope (Leica Microsystems) into 0.5 ml microcentrifuge tubes. The captured material was digested with Proteinase K (PicoPure DNA Extraction Kit, Applied Biosystems) at 56°C by overnight incubation. Digestions were stopped at 95°C, and samples were stored at −70°C until DNA isolation.

Genomic DNA Isolation

Genomic DNA was isolated from laser captured VTs ($n = 100$), from primary VTs ($n = 3$) collected for functional studies described below, and from respective umbilical cord blood leukocytes ($n = 3$) taken from the same pregnancies. The EZ1 Advanced Nucleic Acid Isolation System using EZ1 DNA Tissue and EZ1 DNA Blood Kits (QIAGEN) were utilized for DNA isolation, and DNA samples were quantified with Quantifiler Human DNA Quantification Kit (Applied Biosystems) according to the manufacturers' instructions.

Primer Design and Validation

The methylation status of CpGs in human H1 embryonic stem cells, H1-derived trophoblast cultured cells, and H1-derived neuronal progenitor cultured cells obtained by whole-genome shotgun bisulfite sequencing (University of California, San Diego, USA; UCSD Human Reference Epigenome Mapping Project) were visualized by the Epigenome Browser[5] and used for the selection of regions of interest. Primer design, targeted amplification, and sequencing were conducted using the targeted sequencing service protocol of Zymo Research Corporation. For targeted bisulfite sequencing, 30 primer pairs were designed and validated. Primers were synthesized by Integrated DNA Technologies, Inc., (Coralville, IA, USA) and underwent quality control, which included duplicate testing for specific amplification of 1 ng bisulfite DNA using bisulfite converted human DNA. Quality control criteria included robust and specific amplification (Cp values <40 cycles and CV <10% for duplicates) of the bisulfite primers on a LightCycler 480 real-time qRT-PCR instrument (Roche Diagnostics Corp. Indianapolis, IN, USA).

Bisulfite Conversion, Multiplex Amplification, Bar-Coding and Adapterization PCR, and Next-Generation Sequencing

Genomic DNA samples from laser captured VTs, primary VTs, and umbilical cord blood cells as well as control samples were subjected to sodium bisulfite treatment using the EZ DNA Methylation-Direct Kit (Zymo Research Corporation). For non-methylated control, human DNA was extracted and purified with Quick-gDNA Miniprep Kit (Zymo Research Corporation) from the HCT116 cell line (American Type Culture Collection, Manassas, VA, USA), which is double knock-out for both DNA methyltransferases DNMT1 (−/−) and DNMT3b (−/−), and thus contains a low level (<5%) of DNA methylation. For methylated control, human DNA was purified similarly from the HCT116 cell line and was enzymatically methylated at all cytosine positions comprising CG dinucleotides by CpG Methylase (Zymo Research Corporation).

[5]www.epigenomebrowser.org.

Bisulfite-treated samples and 30 validated primer pairs were subjected to targeted amplification on the 48.48 Access Array System (Fluidigm), using the targeted sequencing service protocol of Zymo Research Corporation. Fluidigm's protocols were used for sample loading, harvesting, and pooling, 1:100 dilution of amplicon pools for each sample, and for amplification using barcoded adapter-linkers (Fluidigm). Reactions were cleaned up using the DNA Clean and Concentrator-5 (Zymo Research Corporation), and products were normalized by concentration and pooled. The sequencing library was denatured, diluted, and sequenced with a 150-base paired-end run on the MiSeq Benchtop Sequencer (Illumina) according to Illumina's protocols.

Sequence Alignment and Data Analysis

Sequence reads from bisulfite-treated libraries were identified using standard Illumina base-calling software, and then analyzed using a Zymo Research Corporation proprietary analysis pipeline. Residual cytosines (Cs) in each read were first converted to thymines (Ts), with each such conversion noted for subsequent analysis. Reads were aligned by Bismark, a Bowtie-based alignment tool for bisulfite converted reads.[6] The number of mismatches in the induced alignment was then counted between the unconverted read and reference, ignoring cases in which a T in the unconverted read was matched to a C in the unconverted reference. For a given read, only the best scored alignment was kept. If there were more than one best read, then only one was kept arbitrarily. The methylation level of each sampled cytosine was estimated as the number of reads reporting a C, divided by the total number of reads reporting a C or T. CpGs with coverage of less than four reads were removed from the analysis. The developed sensitive and robust bisulfite sequencing assays yielded a median total sequencing read of 533 (range: 30–1,725) per CpG in the trophoblast-fetal blood cell comparison and a median total sequencing read of 136 (range: 4–2,609) per CpG in the clinical sample comparison.

Multiple sequencing counts (total and methylated) were summed for each sample at each CpG site, and samples with a total count <4 were dropped from the analysis. The mean methylation ratio in each group was computed for genomic visualization. In the comparison of methylation levels between trophoblasts and cord blood cells, a group sample size of two was considered as a minimum. In order to fit the count data, we used a generalized linear model of Poisson distribution with log link. When all samples in any of the two groups being compared had zero methylation counts, the maximum likelihood estimation of the Poisson model went to infinity. In such cases, the Student's t-test was used alternatively. P-values and the group difference in methylation ratios were included above the bar plots in Figures S9 and S12 in the Supplementary Material. For comparisons of methylation levels between the clinical groups, only comparisons with a minimum group sample size of four were considered, and the Wilcoxon rank-sum test was used. P-values and the group difference in methylation ratios were included above the bar plots in **Figure 11** as well as Figures S10 and S13 in the Supplementary Material. Differential methylation was considered to be mild, moderate, or strong when the p-value was <0.05 and the difference in methylation ratios was ≥0.125, ≥0.25, or ≥0.5, respectively. The correlation between methylation levels on each CpG in clinical samples and various demographical, clinical, or histopathological variables were evaluated by Kendall's tau statistics. Correlation coefficients and p-values were plotted in the scatter plots. A Kendall's tau $p < 0.05$ was considered significant.

[6] http://www.bioinformatics.babraham.ac.uk/projects/download.html#bismark.

Maternal Study

"Virtual" Liquid Biopsy of the Placenta in Preterm Preeclampsia

Sample Collection

First trimester placentas and maternal blood samples were collected from healthy Caucasian women undergoing termination of pregnancy ($n = 12$), and processed at the Maternity Clinic and Semmelweis University in Budapest, Hungary. Villous tissues were dissected from the choriodecidua on dry ice and stored at −80°C. Aliquots of maternal sera and plasma were stored at −80°C.

Pregnancies were dated according to ultrasound scans between 5 and 13 weeks of gestation. Patients with multiple pregnancies were excluded. The collection and investigation of human clinical samples were approved by the Health Science Board of Hungary. Written informed consent was obtained from women prior to sample collection, and the experiments conformed to the principles set out in the World Medical Association Declaration of Helsinki and the Department of Health and Human Services Belmont Report. Specimens and data were stored anonymously.

Placental Total RNA Isolation and qRT-PCR

Total RNA was isolated from snap-frozen first trimester placental villous tissues ($n = 12$) with Direct-zol RNA MiniPrep Kit (Zymo Research Corporation) according to the manufacturer's recommendations. The 28S/18S ratios and the RNA integrity numbers were assessed using an Agilent Bioanalyzer 2100 (Agilent Technologies), and RNA concentrations were measured with NanoDrop 1000. Total RNA (500 ng) was reverse transcribed with the qScript cDNA Synthesis Kit (Quanta Biosciences, Gaithersburg, MD, USA). TaqMan Assays (Applied Biosystems; Data S17 in Supplementary Material) were used for expression profiling on the StepOnePlus Real-Time PCR System (Applied Biosystems).

Enzyme-Linked Immunosorbent Assays

Concentrations of leptin and human placental lactogen (hPL) in first ($n = 12$) and third ($n = 19$) trimester maternal blood samples were measured with sensitive and specific immunoassays (Leptin ELISA Kit, Abnova, Taipei City, Taiwan; Human Placental Lactogen ELISA Kit, Alpco, Salem, NH, USA) according to the manufacturers' instructions. Standard curves were generated, and sample assay values were extrapolated. The sensitivities of the assays were <4.4 ng/ml (leptin) and <550 ng/ml (hPL).

Correlation Analysis of Placental Gene Expressions and Maternal Plasma Protein Concentrations

Placental gene expression was measured with either microarray on third trimester samples or qRT-PCR on first trimester samples as described above. Maternal plasma protein concentrations were measured with the above-described immunoassays on respective blood samples taken from the same patients on the day of either delivery or termination of pregnancy. Correlations between placental gene expression and maternal plasma concentrations of gene product proteins were calculated with the Pearson method and visualized on scatter plots (Figure S4 in Supplementary Material).

Publication Search, Database Build, and "Virtual" Liquid Biopsy of the Placenta

To detect disease-associated protein signatures of placental dysfunction in maternal blood, similar to plasma DNA tissue mapping for noninvasive prenatal, cancer, and transplantation assessments (176), we performed "virtual" liquid biopsy of the placenta. Briefly, human microarray data on 79 human tissues and cells were downloaded from the BioGPS database, which was used for the generation of placenta enrichment scores (placental expression/mean expression in 78 other tissues and cells). Five genes (*CGB3*, *CSH1*, *ENG*, *FLT1*, and *LEP*) with enrichment scores between 1.4 and 1,490 were selected based on a literature search due to the extensive investigations of their gene products in maternal blood in preeclampsia (Figure S5 in Supplementary Material). Next, an extensive PubMed search was conducted for first trimester maternal blood protein measurements of these five gene products in patients who developed preeclampsia later in pregnancy. Altogether, 61 scientific reports were identified that met the inclusion criteria, which contained data for 80,170 measurements (35, 61, 82, 88, 126, 178–233). These reports were used to build a database for the "virtual" liquid biopsy. In this database, biomarker levels in preterm preeclampsia were expressed as the percentage of control levels as a function of gestational age. Then, the correlations of control percentage values with gestational age were evaluated using the Pearson method. Scatterplots were used to visualize data (Figure S5 in Supplementary Material; **Figure 5**).

Maternal Serum Proteomics Discovery Study

Study Groups, Clinical Definitions, and Sample Collection

Women were enrolled in a prospective, longitudinal, and multicenter study (196) in prenatal community clinics of the Maccabi Healthcare Services, Israel. Pregnancies were dated according to the last menstrual period and verified by first trimester ultrasound. Patients with multiple pregnancies or fetuses having congenital or chromosomal abnormalities were excluded. The collection and investigation of human clinical samples were approved by the Maccabi Institutional Review Board. Written informed consent was obtained from women prior to sample collection, and the experiments conformed to the principles set out in the World Medical Association Declaration of Helsinki and the Department of Health and Human Services Belmont Report. Specimens and data were stored anonymously.

Preeclampsia was defined according to the criteria set by the International Society for the Study of Hypertension in Pregnancy (338) and was subdivided into preterm (<37 weeks) or term (≥37 weeks) groups. Severe preeclampsia was defined by Sibai et al. (2). SGA was defined as neonatal BW below the 10th percentile for gestational age. Healthy controls had no medical or obstetric complications and delivered a neonate with a BW appropriate for gestational age.

Peripheral blood samples were obtained by venipuncture in the first trimester from women who subsequently developed preterm severe preeclampsia ($n = 5$) and term severe preeclampsia ($n = 5$) as well as healthy controls ($n = 10$) matched for gestational age at blood draw (**Table 4**). Blood samples were allowed to clot and were then centrifuged at $10,000 \times g$ for 10 min to separate and collect sera. Serum samples were stored in aliquots at −20°C in the Maccabi Central Laboratory until shipped on dry ice to Hungary.

Sample Preparations, Immunodepletion of High-Abundance Serum Proteins

Sera were immunodepleted at Biosystems International Ltd., (Debrecen, Hungary) for 14 highly abundant serum proteins on an Agilent 1100 HPLC system using Multiple Affinity Removal LC Column-Human 14 (Agilent Technologies) according to the manufacturer's protocol. To improve the resolution of 2D gels, immunodepleted serum samples were lyophilized, delipidated, and salt-depleted at the Proteomics Laboratory of the Eotvos Lorand University (Budapest, Hungary) (339). The delipidated and salt-depleted plasma protein samples were dissolved in lysis buffer, and their pH was adjusted to 8.0.

Fluorescent Labeling and 2D-DIGE

Protein concentrations of the immunodepleted, desalted, and delipidated serum samples were between 2 and 4 μg/μl as determined with PlusOne 2D Quant Kit (GE Healthcare, Little Chalfont, United Kingdom). Samples were equalized for protein content, and then 5 μg of each protein sample was labeled with a CyDye DIGE Fluor Labeling kit for Scarce Samples (saturation dye) (GE Healthcare) according to the manufacturer's instructions. Individual samples from cases ($n = 2 \times 5$) and controls ($n = 2 \times 5$) were labeled with Cy5. An internal standard reference sample was pooled from equal amounts (2.5 μg) of all individual samples in this experimental set and was labeled with Cy3. Then, 5 μg of each Cy5-labeled individual sample was merged with 5 μg of the Cy3-labeled reference sample, and these 20 mixtures were run in 2 × 10 gels simultaneously. Briefly, labeled proteins were dissolved in isoelectric focusing (IEF) buffer and were rehydrated passively onto 24 cm immobilized non-linear pH gradient (IPG) strips (pH 3–10, GE Healthcare) for at least 14 h at room temperature. After rehydration, the IPG strips were subjected to the first dimension of IEF for 24 h to attain a total of 80 kVh. Focused proteins were reduced by equilibrating with a buffer containing 1% mercaptoethanol for 20 min. After reduction, IPG strips were loaded onto 10% polyacrylamide gels (24 × 20 cm) and SDS-PAGE was conducted at 12W/gel in the second dimension. Then, gels were scanned in a Typhoon TRIO + scanner (GE Healthcare) using appropriate lasers and filters with the photomultiplier tube biased at 600V. Images in different channels were overlaid using selected colors, and the differences were visualized using Image Quant software (GE Healthcare). Differential protein expression analysis was performed using the differential in-gel analysis and biological variance analysis (BVA) modules of the DeCyder 6.0 software package (GE Healthcare).

Identification of DE Protein Spots

The internal standard reference sample representative of every protein present in all experiments was loaded equally in all gels and thus provided an average image for the normalization of individual samples. The determination of the relative abundance of the fluorescent signal between internal standards across all gels provided standardization between the gels, removing experimental variations and reducing gel-to-gel variations. According to the standard proteomic protocol, the threshold for differential expression was set at 1.05-fold minimum fold-change (340). A p-value was determined for each protein spot using the Student's t-test by the BVA module of the DeCyder software. A p-value of <0.05 was considered statistically significant.

Sample Preparation, Fluorescent Labeling, and Preparative 2D-DIGE

The density of spots in the case of Colloidal Coomassie Blue labeling depends only on the concentration of protein in the sample; however, the density of the spots in the case of saturation dye labeling also depends on the number of cysteines of the labeled proteins because the saturation dye labeling method labels all available cysteines on each protein. This results in the same pattern with different density among samples on the analytical and the preparative gels, rendering identification more difficult. To eliminate this problem for the exact identification of proteins in spots of interest, preparative 2D gel electrophoresis was performed using CyDye saturation fluorescent labeling and Colloidal Coomassie Blue labeling in the same gel. A total of 800 μg of proteins per each of the two gels was run. Following electrophoresis, gels were scanned in a Typhoon TRIO + scanner as described above, the significantly altered spots were matched among the "master" analytical and the fluorescent preparative gel images using the BVA module of the DeCyder 6.0 software package. The resolved protein spots were visualized by the Colloidal Coomassie Blue G-250 staining protocol. Individual spots of interest were excised from the gels based on the comparison of the matched images.

In-Gel Digestion, Liquid Chromatography–Tandem Mass Spectrometry (LC–MS/MS)

The excised protein spots were analyzed at the Proteomics Research Group of the Biological Research Center of the Hungarian Academy of Sciences (Szeged, Hungary); the detailed protocol is described in http://ms-facility.ucsf.edu/ingel.html. Briefly, salts, SDS, and Coomassie brilliant blue dye were washed out, disulfide bridges were reduced with dithiothreitol, and then free sulfhydryls were alkylated with iodoacetamide. Digestion with side-chain protected porcine trypsin (Promega, Madison, WI, USA) proceeded at 37°C for 4 h. The resulting peptides were extracted from the gel using 1% formic acid in 50% acetonitrile; then the samples were dried down and dissolved in 0.1% formic acid.

Samples were analyzed on an Eldex nanoHPLC system online coupled to a 3D ion trap tandem mass spectrometer (LCQ Fleet, Thermo Scientific) in "triple play" data-dependent acquisition mode, where MS acquisitions were followed by CID analyses on computer-selected multiply charged ions. HPLC conditions included in-line trapping onto a nanoACQUITY UPLC trapping column (Symmetry, C18 5 μm, 180 μm × 20 mm; and 15 μl/min with 3% solvent B) followed by a linear gradient of solvent B (5–60% in 35 min, flow rate: 300 nl/min, where solvent A was 0.1% formic acid in water and solvent B was 0.1% formic acid in acetonitrile) on a Waters Atlantis C18 Column (3 μm, 75 μm × 100 mm).

Database Search and Data Interpretation

Raw data files were converted into Mascot generic files (*.mgf) with the Mascot Distiller software v2.1.1.0 (Matrix Science Inc, London, UK). The resulting peak lists were searched against a human subdatabase of the non-redundant protein database of the NCBI (NCBInr, Bethesda, MD, USA) in MS/MS ion search mode on an in-house Mascot server v2.2.04 using Mascot Daemon software v2.2.2 (Matrix Science Inc). Monoisotopic masses with peptide mass tolerance of ±0.6 Da and fragment mass tolerance of ±1 Da were submitted. Trypsin with up to two missed cleavages was specified as an enzyme. Carbamidomethylation of cysteines was set as fixed modification, and acetylation of protein N-termini, methionine oxidation, and pyroglutamic acid formation from peptide N-terminal glutamine residues were permitted as variable modifications. Acceptance criterion was set to at least two significant (peptide score >40, $p < 0.05$) individual peptides per protein. Localization of identified peptides in the core protein sequences was visually analyzed in order to identify potential protein split products.

Biological functions of the altered serum proteins were retrieved from Pathway Studio 9.0 software (Ariadne Genomics Inc., Rockville, MD, USA), and from the open-access GO database[7] (**Figure 6**; Figure S6 and Data S8 in Supplementary Material). To elucidate possible interactions between the altered serum proteins and placental genes in the microarray data, bioinformatics analysis was performed using the same software. Molecular networks between the changed serum proteins in preterm ($n = 19$) or term preeclampsia ($n = 14$) and DE placental genes annotated in the GO database ($n = 1{,}142$) were built separately with a non-linear literature processing search engine, and the resulting connections were manually validated by reading full-text publications (**Figure 6**; Figure S6 in Supplementary Material). The Fisher's exact test was used to test for the enrichment of the connections between the altered serum proteins and (1) DE genes in individual modules, taking the connections between the proteins and DE genes in all modules as a background; and (2) DE placental genes, taking the connections between the proteins and all genes tested on the array as a background. To reveal the pathways enriched among the DE genes connected to angiotensinogen, the Ingenuity Pathway Analysis software (QIAGEN, Redwood City, Redwood City, CA, USA) was used, which utilizes Fisher's exact test and Benjamini–Hochberg correction for multiple testing for the analyses. Statistical significance was set at $q < 0.01$ (Data S10 in Supplementary Material).

[7] http://www.geneontology.org/.

Maternal Serum Proteomics Validation Pilot Study

Study Groups, Clinical Definitions, and Sample Collection

Caucasian women were enrolled in a prospective study at the Department of Obstetrics and Gynaecology of the University of Debrecen and at the Andras Josa Teaching Hospital in Nyiregyhaza, Hungary. Pregnancies were dated according to ultrasound scans between 8 and 14 weeks of gestation. Patients with multiple pregnancies or fetuses having congenital or chromosomal abnormalities were excluded. The collection and investigation of human clinical samples were approved by the Regional Ethics Committee of the University of Debrecen. Written informed consent was obtained from women prior to sample collection, and the experiments conformed to the principles set out in the World Medical Association Declaration of Helsinki and the Department of Health and Human Services Belmont Report. Specimens and data were stored anonymously.

Women were included in the following groups: (1) preterm severe preeclampsia with SGA ($n = 5$) and (2) controls ($n = 10$). Women were matched for gestational age at blood draw (**Table 5**). Preeclampsia was defined according to the criteria set by the American College of Obstetricians and Gynecologists (1) and was subdivided into preterm (<37 weeks) or term (≥37 weeks) groups. Severe preeclampsia was defined according to Sibai et al. (2). SGA was defined as neonatal BW below the 10th percentile for gestational age. Healthy controls had no medical or obstetric complications and delivered a neonate with a BW appropriate for gestational age.

Peripheral blood samples were obtained by venipuncture in the first trimester. Plasma samples were separated by double centrifugation for 10 min. Samples were stored in aliquots at −80°C.

Sample Preparations

All solvents were HPLC-grade from Sigma-Aldrich (St. Louis, MO, USA) and all chemicals, where not stated otherwise, were obtained from Sigma-Aldrich. Frozen plasma samples were thawed and denatured with denaturing buffer (Biognosys AG; Schlieren, Switzerland). Samples were alkylated using alkylation solution (Biognosys). Subsequently, samples were digested overnight with sequencing grade modified trypsin (Promega; Madison, WI, USA) at a protein:protease ratio of 50:1. C18 cleanup for mass spectrometry was carried out according to the manufacturer's instructions using C18 Micro Spin columns (Nest Group Inc.; Southborough, MA, USA). Peptides were dried down to complete dryness using a SpeedVac system. Dried peptides were redissolved with LC solvent A (1% acetonitrile in water with 0.1% formic acid). Final peptide concentrations were determined for all samples by 280 nm measurement (Spectrostar^{NANO}, BMG Labtech, Offenburg, Germany). Samples were spiked with PlasmaDive™ (Biognosys) reference peptides mix at known concentrations.

LC–MRM Measurements and Data Analysis

Peptides (1 μg per sample, corresponding to injection of 0.0259 μl of initial plasma sample) were injected to a self-packed C18column [75 μm inner diameter and 10 cm column length, New Objective (Woburn, MA, USA); column material was Magic AQ, 3 μm particle size, and 200Å pore size from Michrom] on a ThermoScientific EASY-nLC1000 nano-liquid chromatography system. LC–MRM assays were measured on a ThermoScientific TSQ Vantage triple quadrupole mass spectrometer equipped with a standard nano-electrospray source. The LC gradient for LC–MRM was 6–40% solvent B (85% acetonitrile in water with 0.1% formic acid) for 30 min followed by 40–94% solvent B for 2 min and 94% solvent B for 8 min (total gradient length was 40 min). A subset of Biognosys' PlasmaDive™ MRM Panel of 10 peptides representing 10 proteins (Data S9 in Supplementary Material) was used for the measurements of 10 altered proteins involved in immune responses. For the quantification of the peptides across samples, the TSQ Vantage was operated in scheduled MRM mode with an acquisition window length of 5 min. The LC eluent was electrosprayed at 1.9 kV and Q1/Q3 were operated at unit resolution (0.7 Da). Signal processing and data analysis were carried out using SpectroDive™ 8.0—Biognosys' software for multiplexed MRM/PRM data analysis based on mProphet (341). A q-value filter of 1% was applied.

Because of the small sample size of this pilot study, statistical simulations were carried out to predict power and significance in the extended validation study by multiple permutation testing. The probability of significant differences between the two groups was estimated by a paired t-test and the Mann–Whitney test. For both, $p < 0.05$ was taken as criteria to count successful simulations. The number of successful simulations was calculated for different sample sizes ($n = 10$ or 100) and repeats of simulations ($n = 10, 100$, or 1,000). The simulated significance level at $p < 0.05$ was accepted if the number of successful simulations was >25% (**Figure 6**; Data S9 in Supplementary Material).

Publication Search

An extensive PubMed search was conducted for first trimester maternal blood protein measurements of the DE proteins found by 2D-DIGE. Altogether five scientific reports were identified that met the inclusion criteria (126, 143, 239–241). **Figure 6** depicts biomarkers with the same direction differential abundance in preterm preeclampsia in published data as in 2D-DIGE assays.

Trophoblast Study

In Vitro Modeling of Placental Disease Pathways

Database Search and Data Analysis

To build optimal *in vitro* cellular models of trophoblastic disease, an extensive PubMed search was first conducted for similar assays. Since no human trophoblastic stems cells were yet available that would enable a natural proliferative trophoblastic pool with differentiation potential into villous or extravillous lineages, choriocarcinoma-derived trophoblastic cell lines or immortalized EVTs were mostly used for such purposes. Our search revealed BeWo cells (342) and HTR8/SVneo cells (253) as the increasingly most accepted cell model systems based on 1,500 published articles.

Primary VT Differentiation

For *in vitro* trophoblast experiments, placentas ($n = 6$) were collected prospectively at the Perinatology Research Branch (NICHD, NIH, DHHS) from normal pregnant women at term who delivered an AGA neonate with Cesarean section.

Cytotrophoblasts were isolated from these placentas by the modified method of Kliman et al. (343). Briefly, 100 g villous tissues were cut, rinsed in PBS, and sequentially digested with Trypsin (0.25%; Life Technologies, Grand Island, NY, USA) and DNAse I (60 U/ml; Sigma-Aldrich) for 90 min at 37°C. Dispersed cells were filtered through 100 μm Falcon nylon mesh cell strainers (BD Biosciences, San Jose, CA, USA), and then erythrocytes were lysed with 5 ml NH_4Cl solution (Stemcell Technologies, Vancouver, BC, Canada). Washed and resuspended cells were layered over 20–50% Percoll gradients and centrifuged for 20 min at 1,200 × *g*. Trophoblast containing bands were collected and non-trophoblastic cells were excluded by negative selection using anti-CD9 (20 μg/ml) and anti-CD14 (20 μg/ml) mouse monoclonal antibodies (R&D Systems, Minneapolis, MN, USA), MACS anti-mouse IgG microbeads, and MS columns (Miltenyi Biotec, Auburn, CA, USA). Then, primary VTs were plated on a collagen-coated 12-well plate (BD Biosciences; 3×10^6 cells/well) in Iscove's modified Dulbecco's medium (IMDM; Life Technologies) supplemented with 10% fetal bovine serum (FBS) and 1% penicillin/streptomycin (P/S). To test the effect of trophoblast differentiation on selected genes' expression, primary trophoblasts were kept in IMDM containing 5% non-pregnant human serum (SeraCare, Milford, MA, USA) and 1% P/S. The medium was replenished every 24 h, and cells were harvested for total RNA every 24 h between days 1 and 7.

The Effect of Maternal Serum on Trophoblastic Gene Expression

Villous trophoblasts were isolated from normal term placentas and plated as described above. To test the effect of preeclampsia serum on VTs at two time points of differentiation, VTs were kept in IMDM containing 1% P/S and 10% first trimester maternal sera from control or preeclamptic women. Medium was replenished after 48 h, and cells were harvested for total RNA either 24 or 72 h after the start of the human serum treatment. All experiments were run in triplicate.

The Effect of Oxygen Levels, BCL6, and ARNT2 Overexpression on Trophoblastic Gene Expression

BeWo cells (American Type Culture Collection) were incubated in a T-25 flask or 6-well plate with Ham's F12-K medium (Life Technologies) supplemented with 10% FBS and 1% P/S in a humidified incubator (5% CO_2, 20% O_2) at 37°C until reaching 50–80% confluence. To test the effect of *ARNT2* or *BCL6* overexpression on gene expression, cells were transiently transfected with *ARNT2, BCL6*, or control (GFP) vectors. Briefly, 4 μg expression plasmid (OriGene Technologies, Inc., Rockville, MD, USA) and 12 μl FuGENE HD transfection reagent (Promega) were mixed with 180 μl Ham's F12-K medium (10% FBS, 1% P/S), incubated at RT for 15 min and added to cell cultures with 1.8 ml medium in each well of 6-well plate. Twenty-four hours after transfection, cells were split into three treatment groups and kept under either normoxic (20% O_2), hypoxic (2% O_2), or ischemic (1% and 20% O_2 alternating for 6 h) conditions in an Oxycycler C42 (BioSpherix, Lacona, NY, USA) for 48 h before cell harvest. This study setup followed the generally accepted view in reproductive sciences that ~2% O_2 concentration represents physiologic hypoxia at the implantation site and that placental development occurs under physiologic hypoxia in the first trimester (242, 344).

Total RNA Isolation and qRT-PCR

Total RNA was isolated from primary VTs on days 0–7 of differentiation and from BeWo cell cultures with TRIzol reagent (Life Technologies) and RNeasy kit (QIAGEN) according to the manufacturers' recommendations. The 28S/18S ratios and the RNA integrity numbers were assessed using an Agilent Bioanalyzer 2100; RNA concentrations were measured with NanoDrop 1000. Total RNA (500 ng) was reverse transcribed with High Capacity cDNA Reverse Transcription Kit using random hexamers (Applied Biosystems). TaqMan Assays (Applied Biosystems; Data S17 in Supplementary Material) were used for high-throughput gene expression profiling on the Biomark qRT-PCR system (Fluidigm) according to the manufacturers' instructions.

Data Analysis

qRT-PCR. Data were analyzed using the ΔΔCt method. Data were first normalized to the reference gene (*RPLPO*), and $\log_2$ mRNA relative concentrations were obtained for each sample as $-\Delta Ct_{(gene)} = Ct_{(RPLPO)} - Ct_{(gene)}$.

Primary Trophoblast Differentiation. The overall changes in gene expression during the 7 days of differentiation were analyzed by comparing the mean expressions on a given day versus Day 0. The highest fold change for a given gene was defined as the maximum of the daily expression differences during the 7-day time-period. Significant differences were defined by a paired *t*-test ($p < 0.05$) (**Figure 7**).

Serum Treatment of Primary Trophoblast. Gene expression data were analyzed using the Student's *t*-test to compare the effect of preeclampsia serum with the effect of control serum on gene expression at Days 1 and 3 of trophoblast differentiation. *P*-values of <0.05 were considered significant (**Figure 6**).

BeWo Cell Transfections. Gene expression data were analyzed to compare the effect of *ARNT2* or *BCL6* overexpression with the effect of control vector overexpression on gene expression in normoxic conditions using a one-way ANOVA model. The same model was used to assess the differential effect of *ARNT2, BCL6*, or *GFP* overexpression on gene expression in hypoxic or ischemic conditions vs. normoxia. *P*-values of <0.05 were considered significant (**Figure 8**).

A *permutation test* was used to measure the statistical significance of the matching between differential gene expression patterns in *in vitro* and *in vivo* conditions. Genes were discretized into three states, i.e. up-regulated (UP), down-regulated (DN), or unchanged (NS). For each gene in the two conditions, a score of 1 was assigned for a perfect match of UP/UP or DN/DN, 0 for a neutral match of NS/NS, −1 for a perfect mismatch of UP/DN or DN/UP, and −0.5 for all other patterns. The matching score for any pair of conditions was computed as the sum of all scores for each individual gene. The significance of the scores was assessed *via* a permutation on the class labels. Permutations were exhaustive when feasible, otherwise limited to a random sample of 5,000 (Data S11 in Supplementary Material).

Evaluation of Placental/Trophoblastic Expression and Function of ZNF554

Tissue qRT-PCR Array Expression Profiling

TaqMan assays for *ZNF554* and *RPLP0* (Data S17 in Supplementary Material) were run in triplicate for expression profiling of the Human Major Tissue qPCR Array (OriGene Technologies) that contains cDNAs from 48 different pooled tissues.

mRNA In Situ Hybridization

In situ hybridization on third trimester FFPE placental tissues ($n = 6$) retrieved from the Bank of Biological Specimens of the Perinatology Research Branch was carried out using the RNAscope 2.0 FFPE Assay–Brown (Advanced Cell Diagnostics, Hayward, CA, USA) on a HybEZ Hybridization System (**Figure 9**). Briefly, tissue sections were incubated with *ZNF554* target probe (Cat.No.: 423831, Advanced Cell Diagnostics) for 2 h at 40°C. After rinsing with 1× Wash Buffer, slides underwent a six-step amplification procedure at 40°C and were washed with 1× Wash Buffer between amplification steps. Chromogenic detection was performed using a 1:1 mixture of Brown-A and Brown-B solutions. Slides were counterstained with hematoxylin, dehydrated in graded ethanol, and mounted in xylene.

Immunohistochemistry

Third trimester placentas were retrieved from the Bank of Biological Specimens of the Perinatology Research Branch. First trimester placentas were collected from healthy Caucasian women undergoing termination of pregnancy and processed at the Maternity Clinic and Semmelweis University in Budapest, Hungary as described above. Five µm sections of first and third trimester FFPE placental tissues ($n = 15$) were placed on silanized slides and stained using anti-ZNF554 or anti-cytokeratin-7 antibodies as well as reagents listed in Data S18 (Supplementary Material) either on Ventana Discovery (Ventana Medical Systems, Inc, Tucson, AZ, USA) or Leica BOND-MAX (Leica Microsystems, Wetzlar, Germany) autostainers (**Figures 9** and **10**).

Primary VT Differentiation

The experimental procedures were embedded in the study on VT differentiation as described above (**Figure 9**).

BeWo Cell Cultures

BeWo cells were incubated in a T-25 flask or 6-well plate with Ham's F12-K medium (Life Technologies) supplemented with 10% FBS and 1% P/S in a humidified incubator (5% CO_2, 20% O_2) at 37°C until reaching 50–80% confluence.

To test the effect of *ZNF554* knockdown on gene expression, cells were treated either with 100 nM *ZNF554* siRNA (Ambion-Life Technologies, Foster City, CA, USA) or 100 nM scrambled (control) siRNA (Ambion) using X-tremeGENE siRNA transfection reagent (Roche, Mississauga, ON, Canada), and incubated at 37°C in 2 ml serum-free Opti-MEM (Gibco-Life Technologies) medium. After 6 h, the medium was replaced with 2 ml Ham's F12-K medium supplemented with 10% FBS. After 48 h, cells were collected for RNA isolation, microarray, and qRT-PCR as well as confocal microscopy (**Figure 9**).

To test the effect of DNA methylation on gene expression, BeWo cells were treated with 5 or 10 µM 5-azacitidine (Sigma-Aldrich), and control cells with DMSO. This experiment was also performed when both 5-azacitidine-treated and control cells received 25 µM forskolin (Sigma-Aldrich) to induce syncytialization. After 24 h incubation, cells were harvested for RNA isolation and qRT-PCR. The experiment was performed in six replicates (**Figure 11**; Figure S8 in Supplementary Material).

HTR8/SVneo Cell Cultures

HTR8/SVneo EVT cells (kindly provided by Dr. Charles H. Graham, Queen's University, Kingston, Ontario, Canada) were incubated in a 6-well plate with RPMI-1640 medium (Gibco-Life Technologies) supplemented with 10% FBS and 1% P/S in a humidified incubator (5% CO_2, 20% O_2) at 37°C until reaching 50% confluence.

To test the effect of *ZNF554* knockdown on gene expression and functions, cells were treated either with 100 nM *ZNF554* siRNA or 100 nM scrambled (control) siRNA as described for BeWo cells. After 6 h, the medium was replaced with 2 ml RPMI-1640 medium (Gibco-Life Technologies) supplemented with 10% FBS. On the following day, cells were kept in various O_2 concentrations (2, 8, or 20%) in an Oxycycler C42. Cells were collected for functional assays after 24 h, while cells were collected for RNA isolation, microarray, qRT-PCR, or confocal microscopy and their supernatants for ELISA after 48 h. Cell cultures were used for cell proliferation assays after 0, 24, and 48 h.

Total RNA Isolation, Microarray, and qRT-PCR

Total RNA was isolated from BeWo and HTR8/SVneo cell cultures with TRIzol reagent (Life Technologies) and RNeasy kit (QIAGEN, Valencia, CA, USA) according to the manufacturers' recommendations. The 28S/18S ratios and the RNA integrity numbers were assessed using an Agilent Bioanalyzer 2100; RNA concentrations were measured with NanoDrop 1000. DNase-treated RNA from BeWo and HTR8/SVneo cells (500 ng) was amplified and biotin-labeled with the Illumina TotalPrep RNA Amplification Kit (Ambion-Life Technologies). Labeled cRNAs were hybridized to a HumanHT-12v4 Expression BeadChip (Illumina, Inc., San Diego, CA). BeadChips were imaged using a BeadArray Reader (Illumina, Inc.), and raw data were obtained with BeadStudio Software V.3.4.0 (Illumina, Inc.). Total RNA (500 ng) was also reverse transcribed with High Capacity cDNA Reverse Transcription Kit using random hexamers (Applied Biosystems, Foster City, CA, USA). TaqMan Assays (Applied Biosystems; Data S17 in Supplementary Material) were used for high-throughput gene expression profiling on the Biomark qRT-PCR system (Fluidigm, San Francisco, CA, USA) according to the manufacturers' instructions.

Confocal Microscopy

ZNF554 knock-down and control BeWo and HTR8/SVneo cells cultured in 6-well plate were detached with 0.05% Trypsin-EDTA (Life Technologies), washed, and resuspended in PBS, and then 4×10^4 cells were cytospined to Superfrost Plus slides (Fisher

Scientific). Then, cells were fixed with 4% paraformaldehyde (Electron Microscopy Sciences, Hatfield, PA, USA), blocked with Protein Block (Dako North America, Inc., Carpinteria, CA, USA), and immunostained with anti-ZNF554 mouse polyclonal antibody (1:100 dilution, overnight; Abnova, Taipei City, Taiwan) and an AlexaFluor-488 goat anti-mouse antibody (1:1,000 dilution; Life Technologies). Cells were mounted with ProLong Gold antifade reagent with 4',6-diamidino-2-phenylindole (DAPI; Life Technologies), followed by confocal microscopy using a Leica TCS SP5 MP spectral confocal system (Leica Microsystems) (**Figures 9** and **10**).

Enzyme-Linked Immunosorbent Assays

Concentrations of human plasminogen activator inhibitor-1 (PAI-1) and TIMP-3 in HTR8/SVneo cell culture supernatants were measured with sensitive and specific immunoassays (Human PAI-1 ELISA Kit, Invitrogen; TIMP-3 Human ELISA Kit, Abcam Inc., Cambridge, MA, USA) according to the manufacturers' instructions. Standard curves were generated, and sample assay values were extrapolated. The sensitivities of the assays were <30 pg/mL (PAI-1) and <2 pg/ml (TIMP-3) (**Figure 10**).

Cell Proliferation Assays

Cell cultures of control and *ZNF554* siRNA treated HTR8/SVneo cells were assayed using the CellTiter 96 Aqueous Non-radioactive Cell Proliferation Assay (Promega) according to the manufacturer's instructions (Figure S11 in Supplementary Material).

Migration Assay

The migratory capacity of HTR8/SVneo cells was examined with 8μm-pore transwell inserts (Corning, NY, USA) inserted in a 12-well plate described previously (345). After transfection with *ZNF554* or scrambled siRNAs for 24 h, 5×10^5 HTR8/SVneo cells were plated in the upper chambers in a serum-free RPMI-1640 medium, whereas the lower chambers contained an RPMI-1640 medium supplemented with 10% FBS. After incubation for 36 h in 2, 8, or 20% O_2 concentrations, cells on the upper side of the membranes were removed by cotton swab, and the inserts were fixed in methanol for 10 min at RT and washed once with PBS. Then, the membranes were cut out and mounted on Superfrost Plus slides (Fisher Scientific) with ProLong Gold antifade reagent with DAPI. Comprehensive images of each membrane were taken using a Leica TCS SP5 MP spectral confocal system. The number of invaded cells was quantified using Image-Pro Premier v9.0.2 (Media Cybernetics, Inc., Rockville, MD, USA). The experiment was performed in six replicates (**Figure 10**).

Matrigel Invasion Assay

The invasiveness of HTR8/SVneo cells was examined with a Matrigel invasion assay using 8 μm-pore cell culture inserts (BD Biosciences) pre-coated with Matrigel (125 ng/ml; BD Biosciences) and inserted in a 24-well plate described previously (345). After transfection with *ZNF554* or scrambled siRNAs for 24 h, 2×10^5 cells were plated in the upper chambers in a serum-free RPMI-1640 medium, whereas an RPMI-1640 medium supplemented with 10% FBS was added to the lower chambers. After incubation for 48 h in 2, 8, or 20% O_2 concentrations, cells on the Matrigel side of the membranes were removed by cotton swab, and the membranes were processed as in the migration assay. Comprehensive images taken using the Leica TC5 SP5 spectral confocal system were quantified using Image-Pro Plus 6.2 (Media Cybernetics, Inc.). The experiment was performed in triplicate (**Figure 10**).

Data Analysis

Tissue qRT-PCR Array. The expression of *ZNF554* relative to *RPLP0* in the placenta was compared to 47 other human tissues using the Student's *t*-test. *P*-values of <0.05 were considered significant (**Figure 9**).

The Student's *t*-test was used to evaluate *ZNF554* knock-down efficiency and the effect of *ZNF554* knock-down on gene expression in BeWo and HTR8/SVneo cells (**Figures 9** and **10**).

BeWo and HTR8/SVneo Cell Microarray. Data were analyzed using the Bioconductor packages in R (346) following the MIAME guidelines and methodologies described previously (318). Raw microarray gene expression data were normalized by a quantile normalization approach. A moderated *t*-test was used to select DE genes using a cutoff of >1.5 fold-change and $q < 0.1$. GO analysis and pathway analysis using the Kyoto Encyclopedia of Genes and Genomes (KEGG) pathway database were also performed.

HTR8/SVneo Cell qRT-PCR, Immunoassay, Cell Proliferation, Migration, and Invasion. qRT-PCR data were analyzed using the ΔΔCt method relative to *RPLP0* expression. The Student's *t*-test was used to evaluate *ZNF554* knock-down efficiency in HTR8/SVneo cells and the effect of *ZNF554* knock-down on gene expression and cell proliferation. A linear model was built to quantify the effects of *ZNF554* knock-down and various O_2 concentrations on the gene expression and protein secretion of HTR8/SVneo cells as well as on their migratory and invasive capacity. O_2 concentration was treated as a continuous variable, and the interaction between *ZNF554* knock-down and O_2 concentrations was retained in the model when the coefficient was significant. *P*-values of <0.05 were considered significant (**Figure 10**).

ETHICS STATEMENT

The collection and use of human biological specimens and clinical data for research purposes were approved by the Health Science Board of Hungary, the Institutional Review Board of the *Eunice Kennedy Shriver* National Institute of Child Health and Human Development (NICHD, NIH, DHHS), the Wayne State University Human Investigation Committee, the Maccabi Institutional Review Board, and the Regional Ethics Committee of the University of Debrecen. Written informed consent was obtained from women prior to sample collection, and the experiments conformed to the principles set out in the World Medical Association Declaration of Helsinki and the Department of Health and Human Services Belmont Report. Specimens and data were stored anonymously.

AUTHOR CONTRIBUTIONS

NGT conceptualized study and designed research. NGT, KAK, YX, KJ, RJL, EH-G, ZsD, AS, KE, SzSz, VT, HE-A, CL, AB, GSz, SL, and ZD performed research. NGT, RR, ALT, ZX, LO, OT, HM, SD, SSH, THC, CJK, and ZP contributed new reagents/analytic tools/clinical specimens. NGT, RR, ALT, KAK, YX, ZX, KJ, GB, ZsG, JP, THC, BAGy, AD, ASz, ZsD, GSz, IK, AF, MKr, MKn, OE, GJB, CJK, GJ, and ZP analyzed and interpreted data. All authors contributed to manuscript writing and approved the paper.

ACKNOWLEDGMENTS

We thank Brad Baker, Ryan Cantarella, Po Jen Chiang, Stella DeWar, Sandy Field, Hong Meng, Olesya Plazyo, Russ Price, Theodore Price, Gerardo Rodriguez, Dayna Sheldon, Sivasakthy Sivalogan, Rona Wang (Perinatology Research Branch), Matthew Hess, Daniel Lott, Tara Reinholz (Wayne State University), Katalin Karaszi, Barbara Kocsis-Deak, Edit Zabolai (Semmelweis University), and Istvan Kurucz (Biosystems International) for their assistance, Gergely Szakacs, Professor Peter Zavodszky (Hungarian Academy of Sciences), Petronella Hupuczi (Maternity Private Department), Professor Sinuhe Hahn, Simona Rossi (University of Basel), Professor Douglas Ruden (Wayne State University) and Geza Ambrus-Aikelin (Jecure Therapeutics) for helpful discussions, Maureen McGerty and Sara Tipton (Wayne State University) for critical reading of the manuscript.

FUNDING

This research was supported by: the Perinatology Research Branch, Division of Obstetrics and Maternal-Fetal Medicine, Division of Intramural Research, *Eunice Kennedy Shriver* National Institute of Child Health and Human Development, National Institutes of Health, US Department of Health and Human Services (NICHD/NIH/DHHS); Federal funds from NICHD/NIH/DHHS under Contract No. HHSN275201300006C; European Union FP6 grant Pregenesys-037244; Hungarian Academy of Sciences Momentum grant LP2014-7/2014; Hungarian National Research, Development and Innovation Fund grant FIEK_16-1-2016-0005; Hungarian National Science Fund grant OTKA K124862; and Zymo Research Corporation. The funders had no role in study design, data collection and analysis, decision to publish, or preparation of the manuscript.

SUPPLEMENTARY MATERIAL

FIGURE S1 | Hub transcription regulatory genes in the M1 and M2 modules and their interaction network. **(A)** Co-expression matrix of transcription regulatory genes and predominantly placenta-expressed genes in the M1 and M2 modules. Within the M1 (green) module, *ESRRG*, *POU5F1*, and *ZNF554* transcription regulatory genes correlated most strongly with predominantly placenta-expressed genes. *ESRRG* and *ZNF554* had the most correlation with *CSH1* and *HSD11B2*, genes strongly implicated in fetal growth. Within the M2 (red) module, *BCL6*, *BHLHE40*, and *ARNT2* transcription regulatory genes were correlated most strongly with predominantly placenta-expressed genes. *BCL6* and *ARNT2* had the most correlation with *FLT1*. Heatmap represents Pearson coefficients. **(B,C)** The networks of biological processes enriched among genes dysregulated in preeclampsia and co-expressed with hub factors in M1 (*ZNF554*) and M2 (*BCL6*) modules were visualized with the BINGO module of Cytoscape. Sizes of the circles relate to the number of genes involved in the biological processes and colors refer to *p*-values. The groups of most enriched biological processes were manually circled and labeled. The color code depicts *p*-values.

FIGURE S2 | Clinical characteristics in the transcriptomic validation study groups. Blood pressure, birth weight, and gestational age data from the 100 pregnant women included in the validation study show that preeclampsia phenotypes are heterogeneous, underlining the complex pathways of disease in preeclampsia.

FIGURE S3 | Placental gene expression changes in various phenotypes of preeclampsia detected by qRT-PCR. Data represent gene expressions relative to *RPLP0* measured across 100 placentas. In each bar plot (mean ± SE), the left and right panels show significant differences ("*") in preterm and term preeclampsia associated with or without SGA samples compared to gestational age-matched controls, respectively. Changes in preterm preeclampsia samples significantly different to changes in term preeclampsia samples are indicated by "+".

FIGURE S4 | The correlation between placental gene expression and maternal plasma protein concentration. Placental *LEP* and *CSH1* gene expression was either measured with microarrays in the third trimester or with qRT-PCR in the first trimester. Maternal plasma leptin and serum human placental lactogen protein concentrations were measured with ELISA. Third trimester placental microarray data were correlated with ELISA data from maternal blood samples collected at the time of delivery from the same patients. qRT-PCR data from placentas taken from first trimester terminations were correlated with ELISA data from blood samples collected at the time of the procedure from the same patients. Correlations were investigated with the Pearson method and visualized on scatter plots. The two investigated genes' expression and their protein products' concentrations correlated both in the first and third trimesters.

FIGURE S5 | The timing of gene module dysregulation in preterm preeclampsia. **(A)** Human microarray data on 79 human tissues and cells downloaded from the BioGPS database was used for the generation of placenta enrichment scores (placental expression/mean expression in 78 other tissues and cells). Five genes with scores between 1.4 and 1,490 were selected based on literature search due to the extensive investigations of their gene products in maternal blood in preeclampsia. Colors depict gene module involvement. **(B–F)** The 80,170 measurements for five gene products published in 61 scientific reports (35, 61, 82, 88, 126, 178–233) were used for the virtual liquid biopsy of the placenta in preterm preeclampsia. Biomarker levels in preterm preeclampsia were expressed as the percentage of control levels (dotted lines) throughout pregnancy. Percentage values were represented in the scatter plots by different colors reflecting gene module classification. Based on qRT-PCR data, sEng belongs to M2 (red) module. The number of measurements, the Pearson correlation values for biomarker levels, and gestational age as well as corresponding *p*-values are depicted for each biomarker.

FIGURE S6 | Maternal blood proteomic changes in term preeclampsia and their effect on differentially expressed (DE) genes in the placenta. **(A)** The 14 DE maternal serum proteins in term preeclampsia belong to six functional groups. **(B)** These 14 proteins have connections with 116 DE placental genes, among which 46 belong to the M2 (red) module. Angiotensinogen has more connections than other proteins (OR = 2.5, $p = 1.6 \times 10^{-8}$) and the most with M2 (red) module genes ($n = 35$). Seventy seven of 86 connections of angiotensinogen have a directional effect toward the gene.

FIGURE S7 | Summary of functional experiments on module M2. Epigenetic changes to the trophoblast and abnormal trophoblast differentiation lead to a general down-regulation of gene expression and the up-regulation of hub factors in module M2 (e.g. *BCL6*). After placental circulation has been established and placental ischemic stress occurs, the up-regulation of *BCL6* sensitizes the trophoblast to ischemia by inducing *ARNT2* up-regulation and downstream increase of expression of *FLT1*, *ENG*, *LEP*, leading to the placental release of pro-inflammatory and anti-angiogenic gene products. This pathway is only observed in preterm preeclampsia, suggesting that the dysregulation of this placental pathway promotes the early development of preeclampsia. The alterations in maternal blood proteome can induce trophoblastic functional changes leading to the up-regulation of module M2 genes, the overproduction of sFlt-1 and an anti-angiogenic state through a trajectory that does not necessarily affect fetal growth.

FIGURE S8 | DNA methylation regulates *BCL6* expression in the trophoblast. **(A)** Decreased *BCL6* expression was observed in BeWo cells upon treatment with 5-azacitidine (5-AZA) irrespective of Forskolin (FRSK) co-treatment. **(B)** Upper three lanes: whole genome bisulfite sequencing data of *BCL6* first intron from the Human Reference Epigenome Mapping Project. H1 ESC; H1 embryonic stem cell; HBDT, H1 BMP4-derived trophoblast; and HDNP, H1-derived neuronal progenitor. Lower three lanes: bisulfite sequencing data in this study. Abbreviations: CB, cord blood cell; CT, cytotrophoblast; ST, syncytiotrophoblast. Red box: differentially methylated region; red arrow: CpG Chr3:187458163.

FIGURE S9 | DNA methylation levels at individual CpGs in *BCL6* in the trophoblast and umbilical cord blood cells. DNA methylation levels (0–100%) at individual CpGs in *BCL6* in umbilical cord blood cells (CB), cytotrophoblasts (CT), and differentiated syncytiotrophoblasts (ST) are depicted in the bar plots that represent means and SEs. Umbilical cord blood cells and cytotrophoblasts were obtained from the same fetuses. The genomic coordinates of the CpGs, the group differences (CB vs. CT; CT vs. ST) in mean DNA methylation levels and the *p*-values are shown above the bar plots. The number of samples analyzed with methylation reads above the threshold are shown below the bar plots (only comparisons with a group sample size of minimum two were considered). Differential methylation was claimed to be mild, moderate, or strong when the p-value was <0.05 and the difference in methylation level was ≥0.125, ≥0.25, or ≥0.5, respectively.

FIGURE S10 | DNA methylation levels at individual CpGs in *BCL6* in the trophoblast in controls and in cases of preeclampsia. DNA methylation levels (0–100%) at individual CpGs in *BCL6* in laser captured trophoblasts are depicted in the bar plots that represent means and SEs. The genomic coordinates of the CpGs, the group differences (compared preterm or term controls) in DNA methylation levels and the *p*-values are shown above the bar plots. The number of samples analyzed with methylation reads above the threshold are shown below the bar plots (only comparisons with a group sample size of minimum four were considered). Differential methylation was claimed to be mild, moderate, or strong when the p-value was <0.05 and the difference in methylation level was ≥0.125, ≥0.25, or ≥0.5, respectively. Preterm (left) and term (right) groups of patients were analyzed separately. Abbreviations: PE, preeclampsia; PE + SGA, preeclampsia associated with small-for-gestational age.

FIGURE S11 | The effect of *ZNF554* knock-down on cell proliferation in HTR8/SVneo extravillous trophoblastic cells. **(A)** Cell proliferation assays showed that *ZNF554* knock-down slightly but significantly decreased (−14%, $p = 0.02$) cell proliferation rate in HTR8/SVneo extravillous trophoblastic cells after 48 h. *Y*-axis depicts viable cell number, *X*-axis shows incubation time. **(B)** The differential expression of *CDKN1A* (cyclin-dependent kinase inhibitor 1A) and *STK40* (serine/threonine kinase 40), genes involved in the regulation of cell cycle, upon *ZNF554* knock-down was confirmed by qRT-PCR.

FIGURE S12 | DNA methylation levels at individual CpGs in *ZNF554* in the trophoblast and umbilical cord blood cells. DNA methylation levels (0–100%) at individual CpGs in *ZNF554* in umbilical cord blood cells (CB), cytotrophoblasts (CT), and differentiated syncytiotrophoblasts (ST) are depicted in the bar plots that represent means and SEs. Umbilical cord blood cells and CT were obtained from the same fetuses. The genomic coordinates of the CpGs, the group differences (CB vs. CT; CT vs. ST) in mean methylation levels and the *p*-values are shown above the bar plots. The number of samples analyzed with methylation reads above the threshold are shown below the bar plots (only comparisons with a group sample size of minimum two were considered). Differential methylation was claimed to be mild, moderate, or strong when the p-value was <0.05 and the difference in methylation level was ≥0.125, ≥0.25, or ≥0.5, respectively.

FIGURE S13 | DNA methylation levels at individual CpGs in *ZNF554* in the trophoblast in controls and in cases of preeclampsia. DNA methylation levels (0–100%) at individual CpGs in *ZNF554* in laser captured trophoblasts are depicted in the bar plots that represent means and SEs. The genomic coordinates of the CpGs, the group differences (compared preterm or term controls) in methylation levels, and the *p*-values are shown above the bar plots. The number of samples analyzed with methylation reads above the threshold are shown below the bar plots (only comparisons with a group sample size of minimum four were considered). Differential methylation was claimed to be mild, moderate, or strong when the p-value was <0.05 and the difference in methylation level was ≥0.125, ≥0.25, or ≥0.5, respectively. Preterm (left) and term (right) groups of patients were analyzed separately. Abbreviations: PE, preeclampsia; PE + SGA, preeclampsia associated with SGA.

DATA S1 | Genes differentially expressed in the placenta in preterm preeclampsia.

DATA S2 | Predominantly placenta-expressed genes.

DATA S3 | The enrichment of differentially expressed genes on chromosomes.

DATA S4 | The enrichment of differentially expressed transcription regulatory genes on chromosomes.

DATA S5 | The enrichment of predominantly placenta-expressed genes on chromosomes.

DATA S6 | Genes associated with blood pressure.

DATA S7 | The association of gene expression with placental pathology.

DATA S8 | Maternal blood proteomic changes in preeclampsia—two-dimensional differential in-gel electrophoresis.

DATA S9 | Maternal blood proteomic changes in preeclampsia—multiple reaction monitoring.

DATA S10 | Placental pathways enriched among the differentially expressed genes connected to angiotensinogen.

DATA S11 | Permutation test of functional experiments.

DATA S12 | Enrichment of transposable elements in genes within the M1 and M2 gene modules.

DATA S13 | Genes differentially expressed in ZNF554-silenced BeWo cells.

DATA S14 | Enrichment analysis of ZNF554-silenced BeWo cells.

DATA S15 | Genes differentially expressed in ZNF554-silenced HTR8/SVneo cells.

DATA S16 | Enrichment analysis of ZNF554-silenced HTR8/SVneo cells.

DATA S17 | TaqMan assays.

DATA S18 | Immunostaining conditions and antibodies.

REFERENCES

1. ACOG Committee on Practice Bulletins–Obstetrics. ACOG practice bulletin. Diagnosis and management of preeclampsia and eclampsia. Number 33, January 2002. *Obstet Gynecol* (2002) 99(1):159–67.
2. Sibai B, Dekker G, Kupferminc M. Pre-eclampsia. *Lancet* (2005) 365(9461):785–99. doi:10.1016/S0140-6736(05)71003-5
3. Wallis AB, Saftlas AF, Hsia J, Atrash HK. Secular trends in the rates of preeclampsia, eclampsia, and gestational hypertension, United States, 1987-2004. *Am J Hypertens* (2008) 21(5):521–6. doi:10.1038/ajh.2008.20
4. Kuklina EV, Ayala C, Callaghan WM. Hypertensive disorders and severe obstetric morbidity in the United States. *Obstet Gynecol* (2009) 113(6):1299–306. doi:10.1097/AOG.0b013e3181a45b25
5. Hutcheon JA, Lisonkova S, Joseph KS. Epidemiology of pre-eclampsia and the other hypertensive disorders of pregnancy. *Best Pract Res Clin Obstet Gynaecol* (2011) 25(4):391–403. doi:10.1016/j.bpobgyn.2011.01.006
6. Paruk F, Moodley J. Maternal and neonatal outcome in early- and late-onset pre-eclampsia. *Semin Neonatol* (2000) 5(3):197–207. doi:10.1053/siny.2000.0023
7. MacKay AP, Berg CJ, Atrash HK. Pregnancy-related mortality from preeclampsia and eclampsia. *Obstet Gynecol* (2001) 97(4):533–8. doi:10.1097/00006250-200104000-00011
8. Smith GC, Pell JP, Walsh D. Pregnancy complications and maternal risk of ischaemic heart disease: a retrospective cohort study of 129,290 births. *Lancet* (2001) 357(9273):2002–6. doi:10.1016/S0140-6736(00)05112-6
9. Bellamy L, Casas JP, Hingorani AD, Williams DJ. Pre-eclampsia and risk of cardiovascular disease and cancer in later life: systematic review and meta-analysis. *BMJ* (2007) 335(7627):974. doi:10.1136/bmj.39335.385301.BE
10. Berg CJ, Mackay AP, Qin C, Callaghan WM. Overview of maternal morbidity during hospitalization for labor and delivery in the United States: 1993-1997 and 2001-2005. *Obstet Gynecol* (2009) 113(5):1075–81. doi:10.1097/AOG.0b013e3181a09fc0
11. Stekkinger E, Zandstra M, Peeters LL, Spaanderman ME. Early-onset preeclampsia and the prevalence of postpartum metabolic syndrome. *Obstet Gynecol* (2009) 114(5):1076–84. doi:10.1097/AOG.0b013e3181b7b242
12. Schutte JM, Steegers EA, Schuitemaker NW, Santema JG, de Boer K, Pel M, et al. Rise in maternal mortality in the Netherlands. *BJOG* (2010) 117(4):399–406. doi:10.1111/j.1471-0528.2009.02382.x
13. Adams T, Yeh C, Bennett-Kunzier N, Kinzler WL. Long-term maternal morbidity and mortality associated with ischemic placental disease. *Semin Perinatol* (2014) 38(3):146–50. doi:10.1053/j.semperi.2014.03.003
14. Lisonkova S, Sabr Y, Mayer C, Young C, Skoll A, Joseph KS. Maternal morbidity associated with early-onset and late-onset preeclampsia. *Obstet Gynecol* (2014) 124(4):771–81. doi:10.1097/AOG.0000000000000472
15. Ozimek JA, Eddins RM, Greene N, Karagyozyan D, Pak S, Wong M, et al. Opportunities for improvement in care among women with severe maternal morbidity. *Am J Obstet Gynecol* (2016) 215(4):e1–6. doi:10.1016/j.ajog.2016.05.022
16. Hnat MD, Sibai BM, Caritis S, Hauth J, Lindheimer MD, MacPherson C, et al. Perinatal outcome in women with recurrent preeclampsia compared with women who develop preeclampsia as nulliparas. *Am J Obstet Gynecol* (2002) 186(3):422–6. doi:10.1067/mob.2002.120280
17. Madazli R, Yuksel MA, Imamoglu M, Tuten A, Oncul M, Aydin B, et al. Comparison of clinical and perinatal outcomes in early- and late-onset preeclampsia. *Arch Gynecol Obstet* (2014) 290(1):53–7. doi:10.1007/s00404-014-3176-x
18. Sarno L, Maruotti GM, Saccone G, Sirico A, Mazzarelli LL, Martinelli P. Pregnancy outcome in proteinuria-onset and hypertension-onset preeclampsia. *Hypertens Pregnancy* (2015) 34(3):284–90. doi:10.3109/10641955.2015.1015731
19. Barker DJ. Fetal nutrition and cardiovascular disease in later life. *Br Med Bull* (1997) 53(1):96–108. doi:10.1093/oxfordjournals.bmb.a011609
20. Irgens HU, Reisaeter L, Irgens LM, Lie RT. Long term mortality of mothers and fathers after pre-eclampsia: population based cohort study. *BMJ* (2001) 323(7323):1213–7. doi:10.1136/bmj.323.7323.1213
21. Powe CE, Levine RJ, Karumanchi SA. Preeclampsia, a disease of the maternal endothelium: the role of antiangiogenic factors and implications for later cardiovascular disease. *Circulation* (2011) 123(24):2856–69. doi:10.1161/CIRCULATIONAHA.109.853127
22. Clifton VL, Stark MJ, Osei-Kumah A, Hodyl NA. The feto-placental unit, pregnancy pathology and impact on long term maternal health. *Placenta* (2012) 33(Suppl):S37–41. doi:10.1016/j.placenta.2011.11.005
23. Chen CW, Jaffe IZ, Karumanchi SA. Pre-eclampsia and cardiovascular disease. *Cardiovasc Res* (2014) 101(4):579–86. doi:10.1093/cvr/cvu018
24. Chaiworapongsa T, Chaemsaithong P, Korzeniewski SJ, Yeo L, Romero R. Pre-eclampsia part 2: prediction, prevention and management. *Nat Rev Nephrol* (2014) 10(9):531–40. doi:10.1038/nrneph.2014.103
25. Ness RB, Roberts JM. Heterogeneous causes constituting the single syndrome of preeclampsia: a hypothesis and its implications. *Am J Obstet Gynecol* (1996) 175(5):1365–70. doi:10.1016/S0002-9378(96)70056-X
26. von Dadelszen P, Magee LA, Roberts JM. Subclassification of preeclampsia. *Hypertens Pregnancy* (2003) 22(2):143–8. doi:10.1081/PRG-120021060
27. Di Renzo GC. The great obstetrical syndromes. *J Matern Fetal Neonatal Med* (2009) 22(8):633–5. doi:10.1080/14767050902866804
28. Brosens I, Pijnenborg R, Vercruysse L, Romero R. The "great obstetrical syndromes" are associated with disorders of deep placentation. *Am J Obstet Gynecol* (2011) 204(3):193–201. doi:10.1016/j.ajog.2010.08.009
29. Than NG, Vaisbuch E, Kim CJ, Mazaki-Tovi S, Erez O, Yeo L, et al. Early-Onset Preeclampsia and HELLP Syndrome: an Overview. In: Preedy VR, editor. *Handbook of Growth and Growth Monitoring in Health and Disease.* New York: Springer (2012). p. 1867–1891.
30. Chaiworapongsa T, Chaemsaithong P, Yeo L, Romero R. Pre-eclampsia part 1: current understanding of its pathophysiology. *Nat Rev Nephrol* (2014) 10(8):466–80. doi:10.1038/nrneph.2014.102
31. Myatt L, Roberts JM. Preeclampsia: syndrome or disease? *Curr Hypertens Rep* (2015) 17(11):83. doi:10.1007/s11906-015-0595-4
32. Vatten LJ, Skjaerven R. Is pre-eclampsia more than one disease? *BJOG* (2004) 111(4):298–302. doi:10.1111/j.1471-0528.2004.00071.x
33. Sebire NJ, Goldin RD, Regan L. Term preeclampsia is associated with minimal histopathological placental features regardless of clinical severity. *J Obstet Gynaecol* (2005) 25(2):117–8. doi:10.1080/014436105400041396
34. Valensise H, Vasapollo B, Gagliardi G, Novelli GP. Early and late preeclampsia: two different maternal hemodynamic states in the latent phase of the disease. *Hypertension* (2008) 52(5):873–80. doi:10.1161/HYPERTENSIONAHA.108.117358
35. Akolekar R, Syngelaki A, Sarquis R, Zvanca M, Nicolaides KH. Prediction of early, intermediate and late pre-eclampsia from maternal factors, biophysical and biochemical markers at 11-13 weeks. *Prenat Diagn* (2011) 31(1):66–74. doi:10.1002/pd.2660
36. Tranquilli AL, Brown MA, Zeeman GG, Dekker G, Sibai BM. The definition of severe and early-onset preeclampsia. Statements from the International Society for the Study of Hypertension in Pregnancy (ISSHP). *Pregnancy Hypertens* (2013) 3(1):44–7. doi:10.1016/j.preghy.2012.11.001
37. Szalai G, Romero R, Chaiworapongsa T, Xu Y, Wang B, Ahn H, et al. Full-length human placental sFlt-1-e15a isoform induces distinct maternal phenotypes of preeclampsia in mice. *PLoS One* (2015) 10:e0119547. doi:10.1371/journal.pone.0119547
38. Brosens IA, Robertson WB, Dixon HG. The role of the spiral arteries in the pathogenesis of preeclampsia. *Obstet Gynecol Annu* (1972) 1:177–91.
39. Burton GJ, Jauniaux E. Placental oxidative stress: from miscarriage to preeclampsia. *J Soc Gynecol Investig* (2004) 11(6):342–52. doi:10.1016/j.jsgi.2004.03.003
40. Burton GJ, Woods AW, Jauniaux E, Kingdom JC. Rheological and physiological consequences of conversion of the maternal spiral arteries for uteroplacental blood flow during human pregnancy. *Placenta* (2009) 30(6):473–82. doi:10.1016/j.placenta.2009.02.009
41. Burton GJ, Yung HW, Cindrova-Davies T, Charnock-Jones DS. Placental endoplasmic reticulum stress and oxidative stress in the pathophysiology of unexplained intrauterine growth restriction and early onset preeclampsia. *Placenta* (2009) 30(Suppl A):S43–8. doi:10.1016/j.placenta.2008.11.003
42. Roberts JM, Hubel CA. The two stage model of preeclampsia: variations on the theme. *Placenta* (2009) 30(Suppl A):S32–7. doi:10.1016/j.placenta.2008.11.009
43. Redman CW, Sargent IL. Immunology of pre-eclampsia. *Am J Reprod Immunol* (2010) 63(6):534–43. doi:10.1111/j.1600-0897.2010.00831.x
44. Moldenhauer JS, Stanek J, Warshak C, Khoury J, Sibai B. The frequency and severity of placental findings in women with preeclampsia are gestational age

dependent. *Am J Obstet Gynecol* (2003) 189(4):1173–7. doi:10.1067/S0002-9378(03)00576-3

45. van der Merwe JL, Hall DR, Wright C, Schubert P, Grove D. Are early and late preeclampsia distinct subclasses of the disease – what does the placenta reveal? *Hypertens Pregnancy* (2010) 29(4):457–67. doi:10.3109/10641950903572282
46. Ogge G, Chaiworapongsa T, Romero R, Hussein Y, Kusanovic JP, Yeo L, et al. Placental lesions associated with maternal underperfusion are more frequent in early-onset than in late-onset preeclampsia. *J Perinat Med* (2011) 39(6):641–52. doi:10.1515/JPM.2011.098
47. Odegard RA, Vatten LJ, Nilsen ST, Salvesen KA, Austgulen R. Preeclampsia and fetal growth. *Obstet Gynecol* (2000) 96(6):950–5. doi:10.1097/00006250-200012000-00016
48. Yu CK, Khouri O, Onwudiwe N, Spiliopoulos Y, Nicolaides KH. Fetal medicine foundation second-trimester screening G. Prediction of pre-eclampsia by uterine artery Doppler imaging: relationship to gestational age at delivery and small-for-gestational age. *Ultrasound Obstet Gynecol* (2008) 31(3):310–3. doi:10.1002/uog.5252
49. Eskild A, Romundstad PR, Vatten LJ. Placental weight and birthweight: does the association differ between pregnancies with and without preeclampsia? *Am J Obstet Gynecol* (2009) 201(6):e1–5. doi:10.1016/j.ajog.2009.06.003
50. Lisonkova S, Joseph KS. Incidence of preeclampsia: risk factors and outcomes associated with early- versus late-onset disease. *Am J Obstet Gynecol* (2013) 209(6):e1–12. doi:10.1016/j.ajog.2013.08.019
51. Espinoza J, Lee W, Martin SR, Belfort MA. Customized growth curves for identification of large-for-gestational age neonates in pre-eclamptic women. *Ultrasound Obstet Gynecol* (2014) 43(2):165–9. doi:10.1002/uog.12518
52. Rasmussen S, Irgens LM, Espinoza J. Maternal obesity and excess of fetal growth in pre-eclampsia. *BJOG* (2014) 121(11):1351–7. doi:10.1111/1471-0528.12677
53. Verlohren S, Melchiorre K, Khalil A, Thilaganathan B. Uterine artery Doppler, birth weight and timing of onset of pre-eclampsia: providing insights into the dual etiology of late-onset pre-eclampsia. *Ultrasound Obstet Gynecol* (2014) 44(3):293–8. doi:10.1002/uog.13310
54. Kenneth L, Hall DR, Gebhardt S, Grove D. Late onset preeclampsia is not an innocuous condition. *Hypertens Pregnancy* (2010) 29(3):262–70. doi:10.3109/10641950902777697
55. Soto E, Romero R, Kusanovic JP, Ogge G, Hussein Y, Yeo L, et al. Late-onset preeclampsia is associated with an imbalance of angiogenic and anti-angiogenic factors in patients with and without placental lesions consistent with maternal underperfusion. *J Matern Fetal Neonatal Med* (2012) 25(5):498–507. doi:10.3109/14767058.2011.591461
56. Maynard SE, Min JY, Merchan J, Lim KH, Li J, Mondal S, et al. Excess placental soluble fms-like tyrosine kinase 1 (sFlt1) may contribute to endothelial dysfunction, hypertension, and proteinuria in preeclampsia. *J Clin Invest* (2003) 111(5):649–58. doi:10.1172/JCI17189
57. Chaiworapongsa T, Romero R, Espinoza J, Bujold E, Kim YM, Goncalves LF, et al. Evidence supporting a role for blockade of the vascular endothelial growth factor system in the pathophysiology of preeclampsia. Young Investigator Award. *Am J Obstet Gynecol* (2004) 190(6):1541–7. doi:10.1016/j.ajog.2004.03.043
58. Matthiesen L, Berg G, Ernerudh J, Ekerfelt C, Jonsson Y, Sharma S. Immunology of preeclampsia. *Chem Immunol Allergy* (2005) 89:49–61. doi:10.1159/000087912
59. Redman CW, Sargent IL. Latest advances in understanding preeclampsia. *Science* (2005) 308(5728):1592–4. doi:10.1126/science.1111726
60. Goswami D, Tannetta DS, Magee LA, Fuchisawa A, Redman CW, Sargent IL, et al. Excess syncytiotrophoblast microparticle shedding is a feature of early-onset pre-eclampsia, but not normotensive intrauterine growth restriction. *Placenta* (2006) 27(1):56–61. doi:10.1016/j.placenta.2004.11.007
61. Levine RJ, Lam C, Qian C, Yu KF, Maynard SE, Sachs BP, et al. Soluble endoglin and other circulating antiangiogenic factors in preeclampsia. *N Engl J Med* (2006) 355(10):992–1005. doi:10.1056/NEJMoa055352
62. Venkatesha S, Toporsian M, Lam C, Hanai J, Mammoto T, Kim YM, et al. Soluble endoglin contributes to the pathogenesis of preeclampsia. *Nat Med* (2006) 12(6):642–9. doi:10.1038/nm1429
63. Cindrova-Davies T. Gabor Than Award lecture 2008: pre-eclampsia - from placental oxidative stress to maternal endothelial dysfunction. *Placenta* (2009) 30(Suppl A):S55–65. doi:10.1016/j.placenta.2008.11.020
64. Gupta AK, Hasler P, Holzgreve W, Gebhardt S, Hahn S. Induction of neutrophil extracellular DNA lattices by placental microparticles and IL-8 and their presence in preeclampsia. *Hum Immunol* (2005) 66(11):1146–54. doi:10.1016/j.humimm.2005.11.003
65. Lai Z, Kalkunte S, Sharma S. A critical role of interleukin-10 in modulating hypoxia-induced preeclampsia-like disease in mice. *Hypertension* (2011) 57(3):505–14. doi:10.1161/HYPERTENSIONAHA.110.163329
66. Kumar A, Begum N, Prasad S, Agarwal S, Sharma S. IL-10, TNF-alpha & IFN-gamma: potential early biomarkers for preeclampsia. *Cell Immunol* (2013) 283(1–2):70–4. doi:10.1016/j.cellimm.2013.06.012
67. Roberts JM, Taylor RN, Musci TJ, Rodgers GM, Hubel CA, McLaughlin MK. Preeclampsia: an endothelial cell disorder. *Am J Obstet Gynecol* (1989) 161(5):1200–4. doi:10.1016/0002-9378(89)90665-0
68. Maynard S, Epstein FH, Karumanchi SA. Preeclampsia and angiogenic imbalance. *Annu Rev Med* (2008) 59:61–78. doi:10.1146/annurev.med.59.110106.214058
69. Vaisbuch E, Whitty JE, Hassan SS, Romero R, Kusanovic JP, Cotton DB, et al. Circulating angiogenic and antiangiogenic factors in women with eclampsia. *Am J Obstet Gynecol* (2011) 204(2):e1–9. doi:10.1016/j.ajog.2010.08.049
70. Hahn S, Giaglis S, Hoesli I, Hasler P. Neutrophil NETs in reproduction: from infertility to preeclampsia and the possibility of fetal loss. *Front Immunol* (2012) 3:362.:362. doi:10.3389/fimmu.2012.00362
71. Stoikou M, Grimolizzi F, Giaglis S, Schafer G, van Breda SV, Hoesli IM, et al. Gestational diabetes mellitus is associated with altered neutrophil activity. *Front Immunol* (2017) 8:702. doi:10.3389/fimmu.2017.00702
72. Bereczki D Jr. Pregnancy and acute ischemic stroke. *Orv Hetil* (2016) 157(20):763–6. doi:10.1556/650.2016.30421
73. Myatt L. Role of placenta in preeclampsia. *Endocrine* (2002) 19(1):103–11. doi:10.1385/ENDO:19:1:103
74. Roberts JM, Escudero C. The placenta in preeclampsia. *Pregnancy Hypertens* (2012) 2(2):72–83. doi:10.1016/j.preghy.2012.01.001
75. Sibley CP. Treating the dysfunctional placenta. *J Endocrinol* (2017) 234(2):R81–97. doi:10.1530/JOE-17-0185
76. Mayhew TM. A stereological perspective on placental morphology in normal and complicated pregnancies. *J Anat* (2009) 215(1):77–90. doi:10.1111/j.1469-7580.2008.00994.x
77. Levine RJ, Maynard SE, Qian C, Lim KH, England LJ, Yu KF, et al. Circulating angiogenic factors and the risk of preeclampsia. *N Engl J Med* (2004) 350(7):672–83. doi:10.1056/NEJMoa031884
78. Chaiworapongsa T, Romero R, Kim YM, Kim GJ, Kim MR, Espinoza J, et al. Plasma soluble vascular endothelial growth factor receptor-1 concentration is elevated prior to the clinical diagnosis of pre-eclampsia. *J Matern Fetal Neonatal Med* (2005) 17(1):3–18. doi:10.1080/14767050400028816
79. Maynard SE, Venkatesha S, Thadhani R, Karumanchi SA. Soluble Fms-like tyrosine kinase 1 and endothelial dysfunction in the pathogenesis of preeclampsia. *Pediatr Res* (2005) 57(5 Pt 2):1R–7R. doi:10.1203/01.PDR.0000159567.85157.B7
80. Vatten LJ, Eskild A, Nilsen TI, Jeansson S, Jenum PA, Staff AC. Changes in circulating level of angiogenic factors from the first to second trimester as predictors of preeclampsia. *Am J Obstet Gynecol* (2007) 196(3):e1–6. doi:10.1016/j.ajog.2006.10.909
81. Wikstrom AK, Larsson A, Eriksson UJ, Nash P, Norden-Lindeberg S, Olovsson M. Placental growth factor and soluble FMS-like tyrosine kinase-1 in early-onset and late-onset preeclampsia. *Obstet Gynecol* (2007) 109(6):1368–74. doi:10.1097/01.AOG.0000264552.85436.a1
82. Crispi F, Llurba E, Dominguez C, Martin-Gallan P, Cabero L, Gratacos E. Predictive value of angiogenic factors and uterine artery Doppler for early- versus late-onset pre-eclampsia and intrauterine growth restriction. *Ultrasound Obstet Gynecol* (2008) 31(3):303–9. doi:10.1002/uog.5184
83. Romero R, Nien JK, Espinoza J, Todem D, Fu W, Chung H, et al. A longitudinal study of angiogenic (placental growth factor) and anti-angiogenic (soluble endoglin and soluble vascular endothelial growth factor receptor-1) factors in normal pregnancy and patients destined to develop preeclampsia and deliver a small for gestational age neonate. *J Matern Fetal Neonatal Med* (2008) 21(1):9–23. doi:10.1080/14767050701830480
84. Chaiworapongsa T, Romero R, Kusanovic JP, Mittal P, Kim SK, Gotsch F, et al. Plasma soluble endoglin concentration in pre-eclampsia is associated with an increased impedance to flow in the maternal and fetal circulations. *Ultrasound Obstet Gynecol* (2010) 35(2):155–62. doi:10.1002/uog.7491

85. Kalkunte S, Boij R, Norris W, Friedman J, Lai Z, Kurtis J, et al. Sera from preeclampsia patients elicit symptoms of human disease in mice and provide a basis for an in vitro predictive assay. *Am J Pathol* (2010) 177(5):2387–98. doi:10.2353/ajpath.2010.100475
86. Agarwal I, Karumanchi SA. Preeclampsia and the anti-angiogenic state. *Pregnancy Hypertens* (2011) 1(1):17–21. doi:10.1016/j.preghy.2010.10.007
87. Kumasawa K, Ikawa M, Kidoya H, Hasuwa H, Saito-Fujita T, Morioka Y, et al. Pravastatin induces placental growth factor (PGF) and ameliorates preeclampsia in a mouse model. *Proc Natl Acad Sci U S A* (2011) 108(4):1451–5. doi:10.1073/pnas.1011293108
88. Myatt L, Clifton RG, Roberts JM, Spong CY, Wapner RJ, Thorp JM Jr., et al. Can changes in angiogenic biomarkers between the first and second trimesters of pregnancy predict development of pre-eclampsia in a low-risk nulliparous patient population? *BJOG* (2013) 120(10):1183–91. doi:10.1111/1471-0528.12128
89. Allen RE, Rogozinska E, Cleverly K, Aquilina J, Thangaratinam S. Abnormal blood biomarkers in early pregnancy are associated with preeclampsia: a meta-analysis. *Eur J Obstet Gynecol Reprod Biol* (2014) 182:194–201. doi:10.1016/j.ejogrb.2014.09.027
90. Szalai G, Xu Y, Romero R, Chaiworapongsa T, Xu Z, Chiang PJ, et al. *In vivo* experiments reveal the good, the bad and the ugly faces of sFlt-1 in pregnancy. *PLoS One* (2014) 9(11):e110867. doi:10.1371/journal.pone.0110867
91. Redman CW, Sargent IL, Staff AC. IFPA senior award lecture: making sense of pre-eclampsia – Two placental causes of preeclampsia? *Placenta* (2014) 35(Suppl):S20–5. doi:10.1016/j.placenta.2013.12.008
92. Hahn S, Lapaire O, Than NG. Biomarker development for presymptomatic molecular diagnosis of preeclampsia: feasible, useful or even unnecessary? *Expert Rev Mol Diagn* (2015) 15:617–29. doi:10.1586/14737159.2015.1025757
93. Eastabrook G, Brown M, Sargent I. The origins and end-organ consequence of pre-eclampsia. *Best Pract Res Clin Obstet Gynaecol* (2011) 25(4):435–47. doi:10.1016/j.bpobgyn.2011.01.005
94. Vaisbuch E, Mazaki-Tovi S. Preeclampsia, portliness, and perturbation of adipose tissue function-are we beginning to connect the Dots? *Am J Hypertens* (2017) 30(6):559–60. doi:10.1093/ajh/hpx040
95. Scioscia M, Karumanchi SA, Goldman-Wohl D, Robillard PY. Endothelial dysfunction and metabolic syndrome in preeclampsia: an alternative viewpoint. *J Reprod Immunol* (2015) 108:42–7. doi:10.1016/j.jri.2015.01.009
96. Kupferminc MJ, Eldor A, Steinman N, Many A, Bar-Am A, Jaffa A, et al. Increased frequency of genetic thrombophilia in women with complications of pregnancy. *N Engl J Med* (1999) 340(1):9–13. doi:10.1056/NEJM199901073400102
97. van Dijk M, Oudejans C. (Epi)genetics of pregnancy-associated diseases. *Front Genet* (2013) 4:180. doi:10.3389/fgene.2013.00180
98. Valenzuela FJ, Perez-Sepulveda A, Torres MJ, Correa P, Repetto GM, Illanes SE. Pathogenesis of preeclampsia: the genetic component. *J Pregnancy.* (2012) 2012:632732. doi:10.1155/2012/632732
99. McGinnis R, Steinthorsdottir V, Williams NO, Thorleifsson G, Shooter S, Hjartardottir S, et al. Variants in the fetal genome near FLT1 are associated with risk of preeclampsia. *Nat Genet* (2017) 49(8):1255–60. doi:10.1038/ng.3895
100. Majander KK, Villa PM, Kivinen K, Kere J, Laivuori H. A follow-up linkage study of finnish pre-eclampsia families identifies a new fetal susceptibility locus on chromosome 18. *Eur J Hum Genet* (2013) 21(9):1024–6. doi:10.1038/ejhg.2013.6
101. Lokki AI, Kaartokallio T, Holmberg V, Onkamo P, Koskinen LLE, Saavalainen P, et al. Analysis of complement C3 gene reveals susceptibility to severe preeclampsia. *Front Immunol* (2017) 8:589. doi:10.3389/fimmu.2017.00589
102. Lokki AI, Daly E, Triebwasser M, Kurki MI, Roberson EDO, Happola P, et al. Protective low-frequency variants for preeclampsia in the Fms related tyrosine kinase 1 gene in the finnish population. *Hypertension* (2017) 70(2):365–71. doi:10.1161/HYPERTENSIONAHA.117.09406
103. Johnson MP, Brennecke SP, East CE, Goring HH, Kent JW Jr., Dyer TD, et al. Genome-wide association scan identifies a risk locus for preeclampsia on 2q14, near the inhibin, beta B gene. *PLoS One* (2012) 7(3):e33666. doi:10.1371/journal.pone.0033666
104. Johnson MP, Brennecke SP, East CE, Dyer TD, Roten LT, Proffitt JM, et al. Genetic dissection of the pre-eclampsia susceptibility locus on chromosome 2q22 reveals shared novel risk factors for cardiovascular disease. *Mol Hum Reprod* (2013) 19(7):423–37. doi:10.1093/molehr/gat011
105. Reimer T, Koczan D, Gerber B, Richter D, Thiesen HJ, Friese K. Microarray analysis of differentially expressed genes in placental tissue of pre-eclampsia: up-regulation of obesity-related genes. *Mol Hum Reprod* (2002) 8(7):674–80. doi:10.1093/molehr/8.7.674
106. Pang ZJ, Xing FQ. Expression profile of trophoblast invasion-associated genes in the pre-eclamptic placenta. *Br J Biomed Sci* (2003) 60(2):97–101. doi:10.1080/09674845.2003.11783682
107. Tsoi SC, Cale JM, Bird IM, Kay HH. cDNA microarray analysis of gene expression profiles in human placenta: up-regulation of the transcript encoding muscle subunit of glycogen phosphorylase in preeclampsia. *J Soc Gynecol Investig* (2003) 10(8):496–502. doi:10.1016/S1071-5576(03)00154-0
108. Watanabe H, Hamada H, Yamada N, Sohda S, Yamakawa-Kobayashi K, Yoshikawa H, et al. Proteome analysis reveals elevated serum levels of clusterin in patients with preeclampsia. *Proteomics* (2004) 4(2):537–43. doi:10.1002/pmic.200300565
109. Gack S, Marme A, Marme F, Wrobel G, Vonderstrass B, Bastert G, et al. Preeclampsia: increased expression of soluble ADAM 12. *J Mol Med (Berl).* (2005) 83(11):887–96. doi:10.1007/s00109-005-0714-9
110. Heikkila A, Tuomisto T, Hakkinen SK, Keski-Nisula L, Heinonen S, Yla-Herttuala S. Tumor suppressor and growth regulatory genes are overexpressed in severe early-onset preeclampsia – an array study on case-specific human preeclamptic placental tissue. *Acta Obstet Gynecol Scand* (2005) 84(7):679–89. doi:10.1111/j.0001-6349.2005.00814.x
111. Soleymanlou N, Jurisica I, Nevo O, Ietta F, Zhang X, Zamudio S, et al. Molecular evidence of placental hypoxia in preeclampsia. *J Clin Endocrinol Metab* (2005) 90(7):4299–308. doi:10.1210/jc.2005-0078
112. Vaiman D, Mondon F, Garces-Duran A, Mignot TM, Robert B, Rebourcet R, et al. Hypoxia-activated genes from early placenta are elevated in preeclampsia, but not in intra-uterine growth retardation. *BMC Genomics* (2005) 6:111. doi:10.1186/1471-2164-6-111
113. Hansson SR, Chen Y, Brodszki J, Chen M, Hernandez-Andrade E, Inman JM, et al. Gene expression profiling of human placentas from preeclamptic and normotensive pregnancies. *Mol Hum Reprod* (2006) 12(3):169–79. doi:10.1093/molehr/gal011
114. Zhou R, Zhu Q, Wang Y, Ren Y, Zhang L, Zhou Y. Genomewide oligonucleotide microarray analysis on placentae of pre-eclamptic pregnancies. *Gynecol Obstet Invest* (2006) 62(2):108–14. doi:10.1159/000092857
115. Herse F, Dechend R, Harsem NK, Wallukat G, Janke J, Qadri F, et al. Dysregulation of the circulating and tissue-based renin-angiotensin system in preeclampsia. *Hypertension* (2007) 49(3):604–11. doi:10.1161/01.HYP.0000257797.49289.71
116. Nishizawa H, Pryor-Koishi K, Kato T, Kowa H, Kurahashi H, Udagawa Y. Microarray analysis of differentially expressed fetal genes in placental tissue derived from early and late onset severe pre-eclampsia. *Placenta* (2007) 28(5–6):487–97. doi:10.1016/j.placenta.2006.05.010
117. Enquobahrie DA, Meller M, Rice K, Psaty BM, Siscovick DS, Williams MA. Differential placental gene expression in preeclampsia. *Am J Obstet Gynecol* (2008) 199(5):566–511. doi:10.1016/j.ajog.2008.04.020
118. Blankley RT, Gaskell SJ, Whetton AD, Dive C, Baker PN, Myers JE. A proof-of-principle gel-free proteomics strategy for the identification of predictive biomarkers for the onset of pre-eclampsia. *BJOG* (2009) 116(11):1473–80. doi:10.1111/j.1471-0528.2009.02283.x
119. Blumenstein M, Prakash R, Cooper GJ, North RA. Aberrant processing of plasma vitronectin and high-molecular-weight kininogen precedes the onset of preeclampsia. *Reprod Sci* (2009) 16(12):1144–52. doi:10.1177/1933719109342756
120. Blumenstein M, McMaster MT, Black MA, Wu S, Prakash R, Cooney J, et al. A proteomic approach identifies early pregnancy biomarkers for preeclampsia: novel linkages between a predisposition to preeclampsia and cardiovascular disease. *Proteomics* (2009) 9(11):2929–45. doi:10.1002/pmic.200800625
121. Cox B, Kotlyar M, Evangelou AI, Ignatchenko V, Ignatchenko A, Whiteley K, et al. Comparative systems biology of human and mouse as a tool to guide the modeling of human placental pathology. *Mol Syst Biol* (2009) 5:279. doi:10.1038/msb.2009.37
122. Sitras V, Paulssen RH, Gronaas H, Leirvik J, Hanssen TA, Vartun A, et al. Differential placental gene expression in severe preeclampsia. *Placenta* (2009) 30(5):424–33. doi:10.1016/j.placenta.2009.01.012

123. Winn VD, Gormley M, Paquet AC, Kjaer-Sorensen K, Kramer A, Rumer KK, et al. Severe preeclampsia-related changes in gene expression at the maternal-fetal interface include sialic acid-binding immunoglobulin-like lectin-6 and pappalysin-2. *Endocrinology* (2009) 150(1):452–62. doi:10.1210/en.2008-0990
124. Centlow M, Hansson SR, Welinder C. Differential proteome analysis of the preeclamptic placenta using optimized protein extraction. *J Biomed Biotechnol* (2010) 2010:458748. doi:10.1155/2010/458748
125. Hoegh AM, Borup R, Nielsen FC, Sorensen S, Hviid TV. Gene expression profiling of placentas affected by pre-eclampsia. *J Biomed Biotechnol* (2010) 2010:787545. doi:10.1155/2010/787545
126. Rasanen J, Girsen A, Lu X, Lapidus JA, Standley M, Reddy A, et al. Comprehensive maternal serum proteomic profiles of preclinical and clinical preeclampsia. *J Proteome Res* (2010) 9(8):4274–81. doi:10.1021/pr100198m
127. Centlow M, Wingren C, Borrebaeck C, Brownstein MJ, Hansson SR. Differential gene expression analysis of placentas with increased vascular resistance and pre-eclampsia using whole-genome microarrays. *J Pregnancy* (2011) 2011:472354. doi:10.1155/2011/472354
128. Kang JH, Song H, Yoon JA, Park DY, Kim SH, Lee KJ, et al. Preeclampsia leads to dysregulation of various signaling pathways in placenta. *J Hypertens* (2011) 29(5):928–36. doi:10.1097/HJH.0b013e328344a82c
129. Liu C, Zhang N, Yu H, Chen Y, Liang Y, Deng H, et al. Proteomic analysis of human serum for finding pathogenic factors and potential biomarkers in preeclampsia. *Placenta* (2011) 32(2):168–74. doi:10.1016/j.placenta.2010.11.007
130. Nishizawa H, Ota S, Suzuki M, Kato T, Sekiya T, Kurahashi H, et al. Comparative gene expression profiling of placentas from patients with severe pre-eclampsia and unexplained fetal growth restriction. *Reprod Biol Endocrinol* (2011) 9:107. doi:10.1186/1477-7827-9-107
131. Tsai S, Hardison NE, James AH, Motsinger-Reif AA, Bischoff SR, Thames BH, et al. Transcriptional profiling of human placentas from pregnancies complicated by preeclampsia reveals disregulation of sialic acid acetylesterase and immune signalling pathways. *Placenta* (2011) 32(2):175–82. doi:10.1016/j.placenta.2010.11.014
132. Varkonyi T, Nagy B, Fule T, Tarca AL, Karaszi K, Schonleber J, et al. Microarray profiling reveals that placental transcriptomes of early-onset HELLP syndrome and preeclampsia are similar. *Placenta* (2011) 32(Suppl):S21–9. doi:10.1016/j.placenta.2010.04.014
133. Kolla V, Jeno P, Moes S, Lapaire O, Hoesli I, Hahn S. Quantitative proteomic (iTRAQ) analysis of 1st trimester maternal plasma samples in pregnancies at risk for preeclampsia. *J Biomed Biotechnol* (2012) 2012:305964. doi:10.1155/2012/305964
134. Lapaire O, Grill S, Lalevee S, Kolla V, Hosli I, Hahn S. Microarray screening for novel preeclampsia biomarker candidates. *Fetal Diagn Ther* (2012) 31(3):147–53. doi:10.1159/000337325
135. Kleinrouweler CE, van Uitert M, Moerland PD, Ris-Stalpers C, van der Post JA, Afink GB. Differentially expressed genes in the pre-eclamptic placenta: a systematic review and meta-analysis. *PLoS One* (2013) 8(7):e68991. doi:10.1371/journal.pone.0068991
136. Liu LY, Yang T, Ji J, Wen Q, Morgan AA, Jin B, et al. Integrating multiple 'omics' analyses identifies serological protein biomarkers for preeclampsia. *BMC Med* (2013) 11:236. doi:10.1186/1741-7015-11-236
137. Moslehi R, Mills JL, Signore C, Kumar A, Ambroggio X, Dzutsev A. Integrative transcriptome analysis reveals dysregulation of canonical cancer molecular pathways in placenta leading to preeclampsia. *Sci Rep* (2013) 3:2407. doi:10.1038/srep02407
138. Myers JE, Tuytten R, Thomas G, Laroy W, Kas K, Vanpoucke G, et al. Integrated proteomics pipeline yields novel biomarkers for predicting preeclampsia. *Hypertension* (2013) 61(6):1281–8. doi:10.1161/HYPERTENSIONAHA.113.01168
139. Wen Q, Liu LY, Yang T, Alev C, Wu S, Stevenson DK, et al. Peptidomic identification of serum peptides diagnosing preeclampsia. *PLoS One* (2013) 8(6):e65571. doi:10.1371/journal.pone.0065571
140. Leavey K, Bainbridge SA, Cox BJ. Large scale aggregate microarray analysis reveals three distinct molecular subclasses of human preeclampsia. *PLoS One* (2015) 10(2):e0116508. doi:10.1371/journal.pone.0116508
141. van Uitert M, Moerland PD, Enquobahrie DA, Laivuori H, van der Post JA, Ris-Stalpers C, et al. Meta-analysis of placental transcriptome data identifies a novel molecular pathway related to preeclampsia. *PLoS One* (2015) 10(7):e0132468. doi:10.1371/journal.pone.0132468
142. Leavey K, Benton SJ, Grynspan D, Kingdom JC, Bainbridge SA, Cox BJ. Unsupervised placental gene expression profiling identifies clinically relevant subclasses of human preeclampsia. *Hypertension* (2016) 68(1):137–47. doi:10.1161/HYPERTENSIONAHA.116.07293
143. Kolialexi A, Tsangaris GT, Sifakis S, Gourgiotis D, Katsafadou A, Lykoudi A, et al. Plasma biomarkers for the identification of women at risk for early-onset preeclampsia. *Expert Rev Proteomics* (2017) 14(3):269–76. doi:10.1080/14789450.2017.1291345
144. Wildman DE, Chen C, Erez O, Grossman LI, Goodman M, Romero R. Evolution of the mammalian placenta revealed by phylogenetic analysis. *Proc Natl Acad Sci U S A* (2006) 103(9):3203–8. doi:10.1073/pnas.0511344103
145. Carter AM. Comparative studies of placentation and immunology in non-human primates suggest a scenario for the evolution of deep trophoblast invasion and an explanation for human pregnancy disorders. *Reproduction* (2011) 141:391–6. doi:10.1530/REP-10-0530
146. Carter AM, Pijnenborg R. Evolution of invasive placentation with special reference to non-human primates. *Best Pract Res Clin Obstet Gynaecol* (2011) 25:249–57. doi:10.1016/j.bpobgyn.2010.10.010
147. McGowen MR, Erez O, Romero R, Wildman DE. The evolution of embryo implantation. *Int J Dev Biol* (2014) 58(2–4):155–61. doi:10.1387/ijdb.140020dw
148. Horii M, Li Y, Wakeland AK, Pizzo DP, Nelson KK, Sabatini K, et al. Human pluripotent stem cells as a model of trophoblast differentiation in both normal development and disease. *Proc Natl Acad Sci U S A* (2016) 113(27):E3882–91. doi:10.1073/pnas.1604747113
149. Yabe S, Alexenko AP, Amita M, Yang Y, Schust DJ, Sadovsky Y, et al. Comparison of syncytiotrophoblast generated from human embryonic stem cells and from term placentas. *Proc Natl Acad Sci U S A* (2016) 113(19):E2598–607. doi:10.1073/pnas.1601630113
150. Chang CW, Parast MM. Human trophoblast stem cells: real or not real? *Placenta* (2017) 60(Suppl 1):S57–60. doi:10.1016/j.placenta.2017.01.003
151. Su AI, Wiltshire T, Batalov S, Lapp H, Ching KA, Block D, et al. A gene atlas of the mouse and human protein-encoding transcriptomes. *Proc Natl Acad Sci U S A* (2004) 101(16):6062–7. doi:10.1073/pnas.0400782101
152. Rawn SM, Cross JC. The evolution, regulation, and function of placenta-specific genes. *Annu Rev Cell Dev Biol* (2008) 24:159–81. doi:10.1146/annurev.cellbio.24.110707.175418
153. Than NG, Romero R, Goodman M, Weckle A, Xing J, Dong Z, et al. A primate subfamily of galectins expressed at the maternal-fetal interface that promote immune cell death. *Proc Natl Acad Sci U S A* (2009) 106(24):9731–6. doi:10.1073/pnas.0903568106
154. Than NG, Abdul RO, Magenheim R, Nagy B, Fule T, Hargitai B, et al. Placental protein 13 (galectin-13) has decreased placental expression but increased shedding and maternal serum concentrations in patients presenting with preterm pre-eclampsia and HELLP syndrome. *Virchows Arch* (2008) 453(4):387–400. doi:10.1007/s00428-008-0658-x
155. Than NG, Romero R, Xu Y, Erez O, Xu Z, Bhatti G, et al. Evolutionary origins of the placental expression of chromosome 19 cluster galectins and their complex dysregulation in preeclampsia. *Placenta* (2014) 35(11):855–65. doi:10.1016/j.placenta.2014.07.015
156. Grimwood J, Gordon LA, Olsen A, Terry A, Schmutz J, Lamerdin J, et al. The DNA sequence and biology of human chromosome 19. *Nature* (2004) 428(6982):529–35. doi:10.1038/nature02399
157. Murphy VE, Zakar T, Smith R, Giles WB, Gibson PG, Clifton VL. Reduced 11beta-hydroxysteroid dehydrogenase type 2 activity is associated with decreased birth weight centile in pregnancies complicated by asthma. *J Clin Endocrinol Metab* (2002) 87(4):1660–8. doi:10.1210/jc.87.4.1660
158. Mannik J, Vaas P, Rull K, Teesalu P, Rebane T, Laan M. Differential expression profile of growth hormone/chorionic somatomammotropin genes in placenta of small- and large-for-gestational-age newborns. *J Clin Endocrinol Metab* (2010) 95(5):2433–42. doi:10.1210/jc.2010-0023
159. Poidatz D, Dos Santos E, Brule A, De Mazancourt P, Dieudonne MN. Estrogen-related receptor gamma modulates energy metabolism target genes in human trophoblast. *Placenta* (2012) 33(9):688–95. doi:10.1016/j.placenta.2012.06.002
160. Ohkuchi A, Ishibashi O, Hirashima C, Takahashi K, Matsubara S, Takizawa T, et al. Plasma level of hydroxysteroid (17-beta) dehydrogenase 1 in the second trimester is an independent risk factor for predicting preeclampsia after adjusting for the effects of mean blood pressure, bilateral notching and

plasma level of soluble fms-like tyrosine kinase 1/placental growth factor ratio. *Hypertens Res* (2012) 35(12):1152–8. doi:10.1038/hr.2012.109
161. Hertig A, Liere P, Chabbert-Buffet N, Fort J, Pianos A, Eychenne B, et al. Steroid profiling in preeclamptic women: evidence for aromatase deficiency. *Am J Obstet Gynecol* (2010) 203(5):477–9. doi:10.1016/j.ajog.2010.06.011
162. Ishibashi O, Ohkuchi A, Ali MM, Kurashina R, Luo SS, Ishikawa T, et al. Hydroxysteroid (17-beta) dehydrogenase 1 is dysregulated by miR-210 and miR-518c that are aberrantly expressed in preeclamptic placentas: a novel marker for predicting preeclampsia. *Hypertension* (2012) 59(2):265–73. doi:10.1161/HYPERTENSIONAHA.111.180232
163. Kumar P, Mendelson CR. Estrogen-related receptor gamma (ERRgamma) mediates oxygen-dependent induction of aromatase (CYP19) gene expression during human trophoblast differentiation. *Mol Endocrinol* (2011) 25(9):1513–26. doi:10.1210/me.2011-1012
164. Gupta R, Ezashi T, Roberts RM. Squelching of ETS2 transactivation by POU5F1 silences the human chorionic gonadotropin CGA subunit gene in human choriocarcinoma and embryonic stem cells. *Mol Endocrinol* (2012) 26(5):859–72. doi:10.1210/me.2011-1146
165. Groner AC, Meylan S, Ciuffi A, Zangger N, Ambrosini G, Denervaud N, et al. KRAB-zinc finger proteins and KAP1 can mediate long-range transcriptional repression through heterochromatin spreading. *PLoS Genet* (2010) 6(3):e1000869. doi:10.1371/journal.pgen.1000869
166. Maltepe E, Keith B, Arsham AM, Brorson JR, Simon MC. The role of ARNT2 in tumor angiogenesis and the neural response to hypoxia. *Biochem Biophys Res Commun* (2000) 273(1):231–8. doi:10.1006/bbrc.2000.2928
167. Nevo O, Soleymanlou N, Wu Y, Xu J, Kingdom J, Many A, et al. Increased expression of sFlt-1 in in vivo and in vitro models of human placental hypoxia is mediated by HIF-1. *Am J Physiol Regul Integr Comp Physiol* (2006) 291(4):R1085–93. doi:10.1152/ajpregu.00794.2005
168. Rosario GX, Konno T, Soares MJ. Maternal hypoxia activates endovascular trophoblast cell invasion. *Dev Biol* (2008) 314(2):362–75. doi:10.1016/j.ydbio.2007.12.007
169. Chakraborty D, Cui W, Rosario GX, Scott RL, Dhakal P, Renaud SJ, et al. HIF-KDM3A-MMP12 regulatory circuit ensures trophoblast plasticity and placental adaptations to hypoxia. *Proc Natl Acad Sci U S A* (2016) 113(46):E7212–21. doi:10.1073/pnas.1612626113
170. Palmer SK, Moore LG, Young D, Cregger B, Berman JC, Zamudio S. Altered blood pressure course during normal pregnancy and increased preeclampsia at high altitude (3100 meters) in Colorado. *Am J Obstet Gynecol* (1999) 180(5):1161–8. doi:10.1016/S0002-9378(99)70611-3
171. Bigham AW, Lee FS. Human high-altitude adaptation: forward genetics meets the HIF pathway. *Genes Dev* (2014) 28(20):2189–204. doi:10.1101/gad.250167.114
172. Ivanov SV, Salnikow K, Ivanova AV, Bai L, Lerman MI. Hypoxic repression of STAT1 and its downstream genes by a pVHL/HIF-1 target DEC1/STRA13. *Oncogene* (2007) 26(6):802–12. doi:10.1038/sj.onc.1209842
173. Moriyama M, Yamochi T, Semba K, Akiyama T, Mori S. BCL-6 is phosphorylated at multiple sites in its serine- and proline-clustered region by mitogen-activated protein kinase (MAPK) in vivo. *Oncogene* (1997) 14(20):2465–74. doi:10.1038/sj.onc.1201084
174. Muschol-Steinmetz C, Jasmer B, Kreis NN, Steinhauser K, Ritter A, Rolle U, et al. B-cell lymphoma 6 promotes proliferation and survival of trophoblastic cells. *Cell Cycle* (2016) 15(6):827–39. doi:10.1080/15384101.2016.1149273
175. Hansson SR, Naav A, Erlandsson L. Oxidative stress in preeclampsia and the role of free fetal hemoglobin. *Front Physiol* (2014) 5:516. doi:10.3389/fphys.2014.00516
176. Sun K, Jiang P, Chan KC, Wong J, Cheng YK, Liang RH, et al. Plasma DNA tissue mapping by genome-wide methylation sequencing for noninvasive prenatal, cancer, and transplantation assessments. *Proc Natl Acad Sci U S A* (2015) 112(40):E5503–12. doi:10.1073/pnas.1508736112
177. Nagy B, Csanadi Z, Poka R. The importance of "free" nucleic acids in the non-invasive diagnostics. *Orv Hetil* (2016) 157(48):1900–9. doi:10.1556/650.2016.30621
178. Lindberg BS, Nilsson BA. Human placental lactogen (HPL) levels in abnormal pregnancies. *J Obstet Gynaecol Br Commonw* (1973) 80(12):1046–53. doi:10.1111/j.1471-0528.1973.tb02978.x
179. Ergüler E, Özel N, Ergüler G, Kücükoglu E. Human placental lactogen levels in preeclampsia-eclampsia. *Gaizan Üniv Tip Fakült Derg* (1993) 4:237–41.
180. Luckas M, Hawe J, Meekins J, Neilson J, Walkinshaw S. Second trimester serum free beta human chorionic gonadotrophin levels as a predictor of pre-eclampsia. *Acta Obstet Gynecol Scand* (1998) 77(4):381–4. doi:10.1034/j.1600-0412.1998.770404.x
181. Mise H, Sagawa N, Matsumoto T, Yura S, Nanno H, Itoh H, et al. Augmented placental production of leptin in preeclampsia: possible involvement of placental hypoxia. *J Clin Endocrinol Metab* (1998) 83(9):3225–9. doi:10.1210/jc.83.9.3225
182. Gökdeniz R, Arigulogu E, Bazoglu N, Balat Ö. Elevated serum b-hCG levels in severe preeclampsia. *Turk J Med Sci* (2000) 30:43–5.
183. Bartha JL, Romero-Carmona R, Escobar-Llompart M, Comino-Delgado R. The relationships between leptin and inflammatory cytokines in women with pre-eclampsia. *BJOG* (2001) 108(12):1272–6. doi:10.1111/j.1471-0528.2001.00284.x
184. Bersinger NA, Odegard RA. Second- and third-trimester serum levels of placental proteins in preeclampsia and small-for-gestational age pregnancies. *Acta Obstet Gynecol Scand* (2004) 83(1):37–45. doi:10.1111/j.1600-0412.2004.00277.x
185. Ning Y, Williams MA, Muy-Rivera M, Leisenring WM, Luthy DA. Relationship of maternal plasma leptin and risk of pre-eclampsia: a prospective study. *J Matern Fetal Neonatal Med* (2004) 15(3):186–92. doi:10.1080/14767050410001668293
186. Kharfi A, Giguere Y, De Grandpre P, Moutquin JM, Forest JC. Human chorionic gonadotropin (hCG) may be a marker of systemic oxidative stress in normotensive and preeclamptic term pregnancies. *Clin Biochem* (2005) 38(8):717–21. doi:10.1016/j.clinbiochem.2005.04.011
187. Spencer K, Yu CK, Cowans NJ, Otigbah C, Nicolaides KH. Prediction of pregnancy complications by first-trimester maternal serum PAPP-A and free beta-hCG and with second-trimester uterine artery Doppler. *Prenat Diagn* (2005) 25(10):949–53. doi:10.1002/pd.1251
188. Spencer K, Yu CK, Savvidou M, Papageorghiou AT, Nicolaides KH. Prediction of pre-eclampsia by uterine artery Doppler ultrasonography and maternal serum pregnancy-associated plasma protein-A, free beta-human chorionic gonadotropin, activin A and inhibin A at 22 + 0 to 24 + 6 weeks' gestation. *Ultrasound Obstet Gynecol* (2006) 27(6):658–63. doi:10.1002/uog.2676
189. Banzola I, Farina A, Concu M, Sekizawa A, Purwosunu Y, Strada I, et al. Performance of a panel of maternal serum markers in predicting pre-eclampsia at 11-15 weeks' gestation. *Prenat Diagn* (2007) 27(11):1005–10. doi:10.1002/pd.1821
190. Ouyang Y, Chen H, Chen H. Reduced plasma adiponectin and elevated leptin in pre-eclampsia. *Int J Gynaecol Obstet* (2007) 98(2):110–4. doi:10.1016/j.ijgo.2007.04.021
191. Rana S, Karumanchi SA, Levine RJ, Venkatesha S, Rauh-Hain JA, Tamez H, et al. Sequential changes in antiangiogenic factors in early pregnancy and risk of developing preeclampsia. *Hypertension* (2007) 50(1):137–42. doi:10.1161/HYPERTENSIONAHA.107.087700
192. Zwahlen M, Gerber S, Bersinger NA. First trimester markers for pre-eclampsia: placental vs. non-placental protein serum levels. *Gynecol Obstet Invest* (2007) 63(1):15–21. doi:10.1159/000094672
193. De Vivo A, Baviera G, Giordano D, Todarello G, Corrado F, D'Anna R. Endoglin, PlGF and sFlt-1 as markers for predicting pre-eclampsia. *Acta Obstet Gynecol Scand* (2008) 87(8):837–42. doi:10.1080/00016340802253759
194. Diab AE, El-Behery MM, Ebrahiem MA, Shehata AE. Angiogenic factors for the prediction of pre-eclampsia in women with abnormal midtrimester uterine artery Doppler velocimetry. *Int J Gynaecol Obstet* (2008) 102(2):146–51. doi:10.1016/j.ijgo.2008.02.016
195. Erez O, Romero R, Espinoza J, Fu W, Todem D, Kusanovic JP, et al. The change in concentrations of angiogenic and anti-angiogenic factors in maternal plasma between the first and second trimesters in risk assessment for the subsequent development of preeclampsia and small-for-gestational age. *J Matern Fetal Neonatal Med* (2008) 21(5):279–87. doi:10.1080/14767050802034545
196. Gonen R, Shahar R, Grimpel YI, Chefetz I, Sammar M, Meiri H, et al. Placental protein 13 as an early marker for pre-eclampsia: a prospective longitudinal study. *BJOG* (2008) 115(12):1465–72. doi:10.1111/j.1471-0528.2008.01902.x
197. Kang JH, Farina A, Park JH, Kim SH, Kim JY, Rizzo N, et al. Down syndrome biochemical markers and screening for preeclampsia at first and second trimester: correlation with the week of onset and the severity. *Prenat Diagn* (2008) 28(8):704–9. doi:10.1002/pd.1997
198. Stepan H, Geipel A, Schwarz F, Kramer T, Wessel N, Faber R. Circulatory soluble endoglin and its predictive value for preeclampsia in second-trimester

pregnancies with abnormal uterine perfusion. *Am J Obstet Gynecol* (2008) 198(2):175–6. doi:10.1016/j.ajog.2007.08.052

199. Durkovic J, Mandic B. Human placental lactogen in the third trimester of pregnancy. *J Med Biochem* (2009) 28(2):97–100. doi:10.2478/v10011-009-0003-1
200. El-Baradie SM, Mahmoud M, Makhlouf HH. Elevated serum levels of interleukin-15, interleukin-16, and human chorionic gonadotropin in women with preeclampsia. *J Obstet Gynaecol Can* (2009) 31(2):142–8. doi:10.1016/S1701-2163(16)34098-1
201. Kim YN, Lee DS, Jeong DH, Sung MS, Kim KT. The relationship of the level of circulating antiangiogenic factors to the clinical manifestations of preeclampsia. *Prenat Diagn* (2009) 29(5):464–70. doi:10.1002/pd.2203
202. Kusanovic JP, Romero R, Chaiworapongsa T, Erez O, Mittal P, Vaisbuch E, et al. A prospective cohort study of the value of maternal plasma concentrations of angiogenic and anti-angiogenic factors in early pregnancy and midtrimester in the identification of patients destined to develop preeclampsia. *J Matern Fetal Neonatal Med* (2009) 22(11):1021–38. doi:10.3109/14767050902994754
203. Stepan H, Ebert T, Schrey S, Reisenbuchler C, Bluher M, Stumvoll M, et al. Preliminary report: Serum levels of retinol-binding protein 4 in preeclampsia. *Metabolism* (2009) 58(3):275–7. doi:10.1016/j.metabol.2008.10.001
204. Foidart JM, Munaut C, Chantraine F, Akolekar R, Nicolaides KH. Maternal plasma soluble endoglin at 11-13 weeks' gestation in pre-eclampsia. *Ultrasound Obstet Gynecol* (2010) 35(6):680–7. doi:10.1002/uog.7621
205. Gaber K, Hamdy E, Hanafy A. Soluble endoglin as a new marker for prediction of pre-eclampsia in early pregnancy. *Middle East Fertil Soc J* (2010) 15(1):42–6. doi:10.1016/j.mefs.2010.03.009
206. Masuyama H, Segawa T, Sumida Y, Masumoto A, Inoue S, Akahori Y, et al. Different profiles of circulating angiogenic factors and adipocytokines between early- and late-onset pre-eclampsia. *BJOG* (2010) 117(3):314–20. doi:10.1111/j.1471-0528.2009.02453.x
207. Papastefanou I, Samolis S, Panagopoulos P, Tagia M, Bale C, Kouskoukis A, et al. Correlation between maternal first trimester plasma leptin levels and birth weight among normotensive and preeclamptic women. *J Matern Fetal Neonatal Med* (2010) 23(12):1435–43. doi:10.3109/14767051003678283
208. Stepan H, Kralisch S, Klostermann K, Schrey S, Reisenbuchler C, Verlohren M, et al. Preliminary report: circulating levels of the adipokine vaspin in gestational diabetes mellitus and preeclampsia. *Metabolism* (2010) 59(7):1054–6. doi:10.1016/j.metabol.2009.11.001
209. Wortelboer EJ, Koster MP, Cuckle HS, Stoutenbeek PH, Schielen PC, Visser GH. First-trimester placental protein 13 and placental growth factor: markers for identification of women destined to develop early-onset pre-eclampsia. *BJOG* (2010) 117(11):1384–9. doi:10.1111/j.1471-0528.2010.02690.x
210. Dayal M, Gupta P, Manju V, Ghosh UK, Bhargava A. Role of second trimester maternal serum markers as predictor of preeclampsia. *J Obstet Gynecol India* (2011) 61(1):38–41.
211. Stepan H, Philipp A, Roth I, Kralisch S, Jank A, Schaarschmidt W, et al. Serum levels of the adipokine chemerin are increased in preeclampsia during and 6 months after pregnancy. *Regul Pept* (2011) 168(1–3):69–72. doi:10.1016/j.regpep.2011.03.005
212. Youssef A, Righetti F, Morano D, Rizzo N, Farina A. Uterine artery Doppler and biochemical markers (PAPP-A, PIGF, sFlt-1, P-selectin, NGAL) at 11 + 0 to 13 + 6 weeks in the prediction of late (> 34 weeks) pre-eclampsia. *Prenat Diagn* (2011) 31(12):1141–6. doi:10.1002/pd.2848
213. Nanda S, Akolekar R, Acosta IC, Wierzbicka D, Nicolaides KH. Maternal serum leptin at 11-13 weeks gestation in normal and pathological pregnancies. *Metabolic Synd.* (2012) 1:113. doi:10.4172/2167-0943.1000113
214. Perni U, Sison C, Sharma V, Helseth G, Hawfield A, Suthanthiran M, et al. Angiogenic factors in superimposed preeclampsia: a longitudinal study of women with chronic hypertension during pregnancy. *Hypertension* (2012) 59(3):740–6. doi:10.1161/HYPERTENSIONAHA.111.181735
215. Diguisto C, Le Gouge A, Piver E, Giraudeau B, Perrotin F. Second-trimester uterine artery Doppler, PlGF, sFlt-1, sEndoglin, and lipid-related markers for predicting preeclampsia in a high-risk population. *Prenat Diagn* (2013) 33(11):1070–4. doi:10.1002/pd.4198
216. Hassan MF, Rund NM, Salama AH. An elevated maternal plasma soluble fms-Like tyrosine kinase-1 to placental growth factor ratio at midtrimester is a useful predictor for preeclampsia. *Obstet Gynecol Int* (2013) 2013:202346. doi:10.1155/2013/202346
217. Keikkala E, Vuorela P, Laivuori H, Romppanen J, Heinonen S, Stenman UH. First trimester hyperglycosylated human chorionic gonadotrophin in serum - a marker of early-onset preeclampsia. *Placenta* (2013) 34(11):1059–65. doi:10.1016/j.placenta.2013.08.006
218. Stepan H, Richter J, Kley K, Kralisch S, Jank A, Schaarschmidt W, et al. Serum levels of growth arrest specific protein 6 are increased in preeclampsia. *Regul Pept* (2013) 182:7–11. doi:10.1016/j.regpep.2012.12.013
219. Suri S, Muttukrishna S, Jauniaux E. 2D-Ultrasound and endocrinologic evaluation of placentation in early pregnancy and its relationship to fetal birthweight in normal pregnancies and pre-eclampsia. *Placenta* (2013) 34(9):745–50. doi:10.1016/j.placenta.2013.05.003
220. Villa PM, Hamalainen E, Maki A, Raikkonen K, Pesonen AK, Taipale P, et al. Vasoactive agents for the prediction of early- and late-onset pre-eclampsia in a high-risk cohort. *BMC Pregnancy Childbirth* (2013) 13:110. doi:10.1186/1471-2393-13-110
221. Begum Z, Ara I, Tanira S, Keya K. The association between serum beta-human chorionic gonadotropin and preeclampsia. *J Dhaka Med Coll.* (2014) 23(1):89–93.
222. Camejo MI, Casart YC. Relation between human chorionic gonadotropin and thyroid hormones in preeclampsia. *Open Access Library J* (2014) 1:e652. doi:10.4236/oalib.1100652
223. Kulmala L, Phupong V. Combination of plasma-soluble fms-like tyrosine kinase 1 and uterine artery Doppler for the prediction of preeclampsia in cases of elderly gravida. *Hypertens Res* (2014) 37(6):538–42. doi:10.1038/hr.2014.27
224. Salimi S, Farajian-Mashhadi F, Naghavi A, Mokhtari M, Shahrakipour M, Saravani M, et al. Different profile of serum leptin between early onset and late onset preeclampsia. *Dis Markers* (2014) 2014:628476. doi:10.1155/2014/628476
225. Tobinaga CM, Torloni MR, Gueuvoghlanian-Silva BY, Pendeloski KP, Akita PA, Sass N, et al. Angiogenic factors and uterine Doppler velocimetry in early- and late-onset preeclampsia. *Acta Obstet Gynecol Scand* (2014) 93(5):469–76. doi:10.1111/aogs.12366
226. Crovetto F, Figueras F, Triunfo S, Crispi F, Rodriguez-Sureda V, Dominguez C, et al. First trimester screening for early and late preeclampsia based on maternal characteristics, biophysical parameters, and angiogenic factors. *Prenat Diagn* (2015) 35(2):183–91. doi:10.1002/pd.4519
227. Kalinderis M, Papanikolaou A, Kalinderi K, Vyzantiadis TA, Ioakimidou A, Tarlatzis BC. Serum levels of leptin and IP-10 in preeclampsia compared to controls. *Arch Gynecol Obstet* (2015) 292(2):343–7. doi:10.1007/s00404-015-3659-4
228. Rahman S, Zahoor AS. Serum leptin levels as a marker for severity of pre-eclampsia. *KJMS.* (2015) 8(1):85–8.
229. Taylor BD, Ness RB, Olsen J, Hougaard DM, Skogstrand K, Roberts JM, et al. Serum leptin measured in early pregnancy is higher in women with preeclampsia compared with normotensive pregnant women. *Hypertension* (2015) 65(3):594–9. doi:10.1161/HYPERTENSIONAHA.114.03979
230. Karampas GA, Eleftheriades MI, Panoulis KC, Rizou MD, Haliassos AD, Metallinou DK, et al. Prediction of pre-eclampsia combining NGAL and other biochemical markers with Doppler in the first and/or second trimester of pregnancy. A pilot study. *Eur J Obstet Gynecol Reprod Biol* (2016) 205:153–7. doi:10.1016/j.ejogrb.2016.08.034
231. Mohamed FA, El-Salam MA, Al-Nori MA, Asser T, Ismail Y. Uterine artery diastolic notch and serum leptin assay for prediction of pre-eclampsia. *Med J Cairo Univ* (2016) 84(2):251–6.
232. Poveda NE, Garces MF, Ruiz-Linares CE, Varon D, Valderrama S, Sanchez E, et al. Serum adipsin levels throughout normal pregnancy and preeclampsia. *Sci Rep* (2016) 6:20073. doi:10.1038/srep20073
233. Song Y, Gao J, Qu Y, Wang S, Wang X, Liu J. Serum levels of leptin, adiponectin and resistin in relation to clinical characteristics in normal pregnancy and preeclampsia. *Clin Chim Acta* (2016) 458:133–7. doi:10.1016/j.cca.2016.04.036
234. Rampersad R, Barton A, Sadovsky Y, Nelson DM. The C5b-9 membrane attack complex of complement activation localizes to villous trophoblast injury in vivo and modulates human trophoblast function in vitro. *Placenta* (2008) 29(10):855–61. doi:10.1016/j.placenta.2008.07.008
235. Zhou CC, Zhang Y, Irani RA, Zhang H, Mi T, Popek EJ, et al. Angiotensin receptor agonistic autoantibodies induce pre-eclampsia in pregnant mice. *Nat Med* (2008) 14(8):855–62. doi:10.1038/nm.1856

236. Girardi G, Prohaszka Z, Bulla R, Tedesco F, Scherjon S. Complement activation in animal and human pregnancies as a model for immunological recognition. *Mol Immunol* (2011) 48(14):1621–30. doi:10.1016/j.molimm.2011.04.011
237. Lokki AI, Heikkinen-Eloranta J, Jarva H, Saisto T, Lokki ML, Laivuori H, et al. Complement activation and regulation in preeclamptic placenta. *Front Immunol* (2014) 5:312. doi:10.3389/fimmu.2014.00312
238. Kouser L, Madhukaran SP, Shastri A, Saraon A, Ferluga J, Al-Mozaini M, et al. Emerging and novel functions of complement protein C1q. *Front Immunol* (2015) 6:317. doi:10.3389/fimmu.2015.00317
239. Bolin M, Wikstrom AK, Wiberg-Itzel E, Sundstrom-Poromaa I, Axelsson O, Thilaganathan B, et al. Prediction of preterm preeclampsia by combining histidine-rich glycoprotein and uterine artery Doppler in early pregnancy. *Pregnancy Hypertens* (2011) 1(3–4):282–3. doi:10.1016/j.preghy.2011.08.081
240. Tannetta DS, Redman CW, Sargent IL. Investigation of the actin scavenging system in pre-eclampsia. *Eur J Obstet Gynecol Reprod Biol* (2014) 172:32–5. doi:10.1016/j.ejogrb.2013.10.022
241. Anderson UD, Gram M, Ranstam J, Thilaganathan B, Kerstrom B, Hansson SR. Fetal hemoglobin, alpha1-microglobulin and hemopexin are potential predictive first trimester biomarkers for preeclampsia. *Pregnancy Hypertens* (2016) 6(2):103–9. doi:10.1016/j.preghy.2016.02.003
242. Burton GJ. Oxygen, the Janus gas; its effects on human placental development and function. *J Anat* (2009) 215(1):27–35. doi:10.1111/j.1469-7580.2008.00978.x
243. Lai AY, Fatemi M, Dhasarathy A, Malone C, Sobol SE, Geigerman C, et al. DNA methylation prevents CTCF-mediated silencing of the oncogene BCL6 in B cell lymphomas. *J Exp Med* (2010) 207(9):1939–50. doi:10.1084/jem.20100204
244. Lynch VJ, Leclerc RD, May G, Wagner GP. Transposon-mediated rewiring of gene regulatory networks contributed to the evolution of pregnancy in mammals. *Nat Genet* (2011) 43(11):1154–9. doi:10.1038/ng.917
245. Emera D, Wagner GP. Transposable element recruitments in the mammalian placenta: impacts and mechanisms. *Brief Funct Genomics* (2012) 11(4):267–76. doi:10.1093/bfgp/els013
246. Chuong EB, Rumi MA, Soares MJ, Baker JC. Endogenous retroviruses function as species-specific enhancer elements in the placenta. *Nat Genet* (2013) 45(3):325–9. doi:10.1038/ng.2553
247. Lynch VJ, Nnamani MC, Kapusta A, Brayer K, Plaza SL, Mazur EC, et al. Ancient transposable elements transformed the uterine regulatory landscape and transcriptome during the evolution of mammalian pregnancy. *Cell Rep* (2015) 10(4):551–61. doi:10.1016/j.celrep.2014.12.052
248. Huh JW, Ha HS, Kim DS, Kim HS. Placenta-restricted expression of LTR-derived NOS3. *Placenta* (2008) 29(7):602–8. doi:10.1016/j.placenta.2008.04.002
249. Schneyer A, Schoen A, Quigg A, Sidis Y. Differential binding and neutralization of activins A and B by follistatin and follistatin like-3 (FSTL-3/FSRP/FLRG). *Endocrinology* (2003) 144(5):1671–4. doi:10.1210/en.2002-0203
250. Knofler M, Pollheimer J. Human placental trophoblast invasion and differentiation: a particular focus on Wnt signaling. *Front Genet* (2013) 4:190. doi:10.3389/fgene.2013.00190
251. Li Y, Klausen C, Cheng JC, Zhu H, Leung PC. Activin A, B, and AB increase human trophoblast cell invasion by up-regulating N-cadherin. *J Clin Endocrinol Metab* (2014) 99(11):E2216–25. doi:10.1210/jc.2014-2118
252. Pryor-Koishi K, Nishizawa H, Kato T, Kogo H, Murakami T, Tsuchida K, et al. Overproduction of the follistatin-related gene protein in the placenta and maternal serum of women with pre-eclampsia. *BJOG* (2007) 114(9):1128–37. doi:10.1111/j.1471-0528.2007.01425.x
253. Graham CH, Hawley TS, Hawley RG, MacDougall JR, Kerbel RS, Khoo N, et al. Establishment and characterization of first trimester human trophoblast cells with extended lifespan. *Exp Cell Res* (1993) 206(2):204–11. doi:10.1006/excr.1993.1139
254. Steinman RA. Cell cycle regulators and hematopoiesis. *Oncogene* (2002) 21(21):3403–13. doi:10.1038/sj.onc.1205325
255. Zhang J, Zhang J, Zhao C, Shen R, Guo X, Li C, et al. Analysis of transcription factor Stk40 expression and function during mouse pre-implantation embryonic development. *Mol Med Rep* (2014) 9(2):535–40. doi:10.3892/mmr.2013.1828
256. Huber AV, Saleh L, Bauer S, Husslein P, Knofler M. TNFalpha-mediated induction of PAI-1 restricts invasion of HTR-8/SVneo trophoblast cells. *Placenta* (2006) 27(2–3):127–36. doi:10.1016/j.placenta.2005.02.012
257. Prutsch N, Fock V, Haslinger P, Haider S, Fiala C, Pollheimer J, et al. The role of interleukin-1beta in human trophoblast motility. *Placenta* (2012) 33(9):696–703. doi:10.1016/j.placenta.2012.05.008
258. Bass KE, Li H, Hawkes SP, Howard E, Bullen E, Vu TK, et al. Tissue inhibitor of metalloproteinase-3 expression is upregulated during human cytotrophoblast invasion in vitro. *Dev Genet* (1997) 21(1):61–7. doi:10.1002/(SICI)1520-6408(1997)21:1<61::AID-DVG7>3.0.CO;2-6
259. Giudice LC. Genes associated with embryonic attachment and implantation and the role of progesterone. *J Reprod Med* (1999) 44(2 Suppl):165–71.
260. Hellmann-Blumberg U, Hintz MF, Gatewood JM, Schmid CW. Developmental differences in methylation of human Alu repeats. *Mol Cell Biol* (1993) 13(8):4523–30. doi:10.1128/MCB.13.8.4523
261. Price EM, Cotton AM, Penaherrera MS, McFadden DE, Kobor MS, Robinson W. Different measures of "genome-wide" DNA methylation exhibit unique properties in placental and somatic tissues. *Epigenetics* (2012) 7(6):652–63. doi:10.4161/epi.20221
262. Gimenez J, Montgiraud C, Oriol G, Pichon JP, Ruel K, Tsatsaris V, et al. Comparative methylation of ERVWE1/syncytin-1 and other human endogenous retrovirus LTRs in placenta tissues. *DNA Res* (2009) 16(4):195–211. doi:10.1093/dnares/dsp011
263. Li F, Karlsson H. Expression and regulation of human endogenous retrovirus W elements. *APMIS* (2016) 124(1–2):52–66. doi:10.1111/apm.12478
264. Macaulay EC, Weeks RJ, Andrews S, Morison IM. Hypomethylation of functional retrotransposon-derived genes in the human placenta. *Mamm Genome* (2011) 22(11–12):722–35. doi:10.1007/s00335-011-9355-1
265. Wang K, Lee I, Carlson G, Hood L, Galas D. Systems biology and the discovery of diagnostic biomarkers. *Dis Markers* (2010) 28(4):199–207. doi:10.3233/DMA-2010-0697
266. Loscalzo J, Barabasi AL. Systems biology and the future of medicine. *Syst Biol Med.* (2011) 3(6):619–27. doi:10.1002/wsbm.144
267. Vidal M, Cusick ME, Barabasi AL. Interactome networks and human disease. *Cell* (2011) 144(6):986–98. doi:10.1016/j.cell.2011.02.016
268. Hood L, Balling R, Auffray C. Revolutionizing medicine in the 21st century through systems approaches. *Biotechnol J* (2012) 7(8):992–1001. doi:10.1002/biot.201100306
269. Junus K, Centlow M, Wikstrom AK, Larsson I, Hansson SR, Olovsson M. Gene expression profiling of placentae from women with early- and late-onset pre-eclampsia: down-regulation of the angiogenesis-related genes ACVRL1 and EGFL7 in early-onset disease. *Mol Hum Reprod* (2012) 18(3):146–55. doi:10.1093/molehr/gar067
270. Song Y, Liu J, Huang S, Zhang L. Analysis of differentially expressed genes in placental tissues of preeclampsia patients using microarray combined with the Connectivity Map database. *Placenta* (2013) 34(12):1190–5. doi:10.1016/j.placenta.2013.09.013
271. Louwen F, Muschol-Steinmetz C, Friemel A, Kampf AK, Tottel E, Reinhard J, et al. Targeted gene analysis: increased B-cell lymphoma 6 in preeclamptic placentas. *Hum Pathol* (2014) 45(6):1234–42. doi:10.1016/j.humpath.2014.02.002
272. Kaartokallio T, Cervera A, Kyllonen A, Laivuori K, Kere J, Laivuori H, et al. Gene expression profiling of pre-eclamptic placentae by RNA sequencing. *Sci Rep* (2015) 5:14107. doi:10.1038/srep14107
273. Jauniaux E, Watson AL, Hempstock J, Bao YP, Skepper JN, Burton GJ. Onset of maternal arterial blood flow and placental oxidative stress. A possible factor in human early pregnancy failure. *Am J Pathol* (2000) 157(6):2111–22. doi:10.1016/S0002-9440(10)64849-3
274. Xiong Y, Liebermann DA, Holtzman EJ, Jeronis S, Hoffman B, Geifman-Holtzman O. Preeclampsia-associated stresses activate Gadd45a signaling and sFlt-1 in placental explants. *J Cell Physiol* (2013) 228(2):362–70. doi:10.1002/jcp.24139
275. Aoki Y, Yamamoto T, Fumihisa C, Nakamura A, Asanuma A, Suzuki M. Effect on the production of soluble endoglin from human choriocarcinoma cells by preeclampsia sera. *Am J Reprod Immunol* (2012) 67(5):413–20. doi:10.1111/j.1600-0897.2011.01086.x
276. Savoia C, Schiffrin EL. Inflammation in hypertension. *Curr Opin Nephrol Hypertens* (2006) 15(2):152–8. doi:10.1097/01.mnh.0000203189.57513.76
277. Hanna J, Wald O, Goldman-Wohl D, Prus D, Markel G, Gazit R, et al. CXCL12 expression by invasive trophoblasts induces the specific migration of

CD16- human natural killer cells. *Blood* (2003) 102(5):1569–77. doi:10.1182/blood-2003-02-0517

278. Hanna J, Goldman-Wohl D, Hamani Y, Avraham I, Greenfield C, Natanson-Yaron S, et al. Decidual NK cells regulate key developmental processes at the human fetal-maternal interface. *Nat Med* (2006) 12(9):1065–74. doi:10.1038/nm1452
279. Moffett A, Loke C. Immunology of placentation in eutherian mammals. *Nat Rev Immunol* (2006) 6(8):584–94. doi:10.1038/nri1897
280. Sargent IL, Borzychowski AM, Redman CW. NK cells and human pregnancy – an inflammatory view. *Trends Immunol* (2006) 27(9):399–404. doi:10.1016/j.it.2006.06.009
281. Moffett A, Hiby SE. How does the maternal immune system contribute to the development of pre-eclampsia? *Placenta* (2007) 28(Suppl A):S51–6. doi:10.1016/j.placenta.2006.11.008
282. Chakraborty D, Rumi MA, Soares MJ. NK cells, hypoxia and trophoblast cell differentiation. *Cell Cycle* (2012) 11(13):2427–30. doi:10.4161/cc.20542
283. Xiong S, Sharkey AM, Kennedy PR, Gardner L, Farrell LE, Chazara O, et al. Maternal uterine NK cell-activating receptor KIR2DS1 enhances placentation. *J Clin Invest* (2013) 123(10):4264–72. doi:10.1172/JCI68991
284. Kliman HJ, Sammar M, Grimpel YI, Lynch SK, Milano KM, Pick E, et al. Placental protein 13 and decidual zones of necrosis: an immunologic diversion that may be linked to preeclampsia. *Reprod Sci* (2012) 19(1):16–30. doi:10.1177/1933719111424445
285. Faas MM, Spaans F, De Vos P. Monocytes and macrophages in pregnancy and pre-eclampsia. *Front Immunol* (2014) 5:298. doi:10.3389/fimmu.2014.00298
286. Saito S, Sakai M. Th1/Th2 balance in preeclampsia. *J Reprod Immunol* (2003) 59(2):161–73. doi:10.1016/S0165-0378(03)00045-7
287. Saito S, Sakai M, Sasaki Y, Nakashima A, Shiozaki A. Inadequate tolerance induction may induce pre-eclampsia. *J Reprod Immunol* (2007) 76(1–2):30–9. doi:10.1016/j.jri.2007.08.002
288. Sasaki Y, Darmochwal-Kolarz D, Suzuki D, Sakai M, Ito M, Shima T, et al. Proportion of peripheral blood and decidual CD4(+) CD25(bright) regulatory T cells in pre-eclampsia. *Clin Exp Immunol* (2007) 149(1):139–45. doi:10.1111/j.1365-2249.2007.03397.x
289. Saito S. Th17 cells and regulatory T cells: new light on pathophysiology of preeclampsia. *Immunol Cell Biol* (2010) 88(6):615–7. doi:10.1038/icb.2010.68
290. Ahmed A, Singh J, Khan Y, Seshan SV, Girardi G. A new mouse model to explore therapies for preeclampsia. *PLoS One* (2010) 5(10):e13663. doi:10.1371/journal.pone.0013663
291. Singh J, Ahmed A, Girardi G. Role of complement component C1q in the onset of preeclampsia in mice. *Hypertension* (2011) 58(4):716–24. doi:10.1161/HYPERTENSIONAHA.111.175919
292. Girardi G. Complement activation, a threat to pregnancy. *Semin Immunopathol* (2018) 40(1):103–11. doi:10.1007/s00281-017-0645-x
293. Faas MM, Schuiling GA, Baller JF, Visscher CA, Bakker WW. A new animal model for human preeclampsia: ultra-low-dose endotoxin infusion in pregnant rats. *Am J Obstet Gynecol* (1994) 171(1):158–64. doi:10.1016/0002-9378(94)90463-4
294. Santner-Nanan B, Peek MJ, Khanam R, Richarts L, Zhu E, Fazekas de St Groth B, et al. Systemic increase in the ratio between Foxp3+ and IL-17-producing CD4+ T cells in healthy pregnancy but not in preeclampsia. *J Immunol* (2009) 183(11):7023–30. doi:10.4049/jimmunol.0901154
295. Lin F, Zeng P, Xu Z, Ye D, Yu X, Wang N, et al. Treatment of Lipoxin A(4) and its analogue on low-dose endotoxin induced preeclampsia in rat and possible mechanisms. *Reprod Toxicol* (2012) 34(4):677–85. doi:10.1016/j.reprotox.2012.09.009
296. Cotechini T, Komisarenko M, Sperou A, Macdonald-Goodfellow S, Adams MA, Graham CH. Inflammation in rat pregnancy inhibits spiral artery remodeling leading to fetal growth restriction and features of preeclampsia. *J Exp Med* (2014) 211(1):165–79. doi:10.1084/jem.20130295
297. Huang Q, Liu L, Hu B, Di X, Brennecke SP, Liu H. Decreased seizure threshold in an eclampsia-like model induced in pregnant rats with lipopolysaccharide and pentylenetetrazol treatments. *PLoS One* (2014) 9(2):e89333. doi:10.1371/journal.pone.0089333
298. Xue P, Zheng M, Gong P, Lin C, Zhou J, Li Y, et al. Single administration of ultra-low-dose lipopolysaccharide in rat early pregnancy induces TLR4 activation in the placenta contributing to preeclampsia. *PLoS One* (2015) 10(4):e0124001. doi:10.1371/journal.pone.0124001
299. Garrido-Gomez T, Dominguez F, Quinonero A, Diaz-Gimeno P, Kapidzic M, Gormley M, et al. Defective decidualization during and after severe preeclampsia reveals a possible maternal contribution to the etiology. *Proc Natl Acad Sci U S A* (2017) 114(40):E8468–77. doi:10.1073/pnas.1706546114
300. Staff AC, Redman CW. IFPA award in placentology lecture: preeclampsia, the decidual battleground and future maternal cardiovascular disease. *Placenta* (2014) 35(Suppl):S26–31. doi:10.1016/j.placenta.2013.12.003
301. Ruane PT, Berneau SC, Koeck R, Watts J, Kimber SJ, Brison DR, et al. Apposition to endometrial epithelial cells activates mouse blastocysts for implantation. *Mol Hum Reprod* (2017) 23(9):617–27. doi:10.1093/molehr/gax043
302. Burton GJ, Jauniaux E. The cytotrophoblastic shell and complications of pregnancy. *Placenta* (2017) 60:134–9. doi:10.1016/j.placenta.2017.06.007
303. Yung HW, Atkinson D, Campion-Smith T, Olovsson M, Charnock-Jones DS, Burton GJ. Differential activation of placental unfolded protein response pathways implies heterogeneity in causation of early- and late-onset pre-eclampsia. *J Pathol* (2014) 234(2):262–76. doi:10.1002/path.4394
304. Sonek J, Krantz D, Carmichael J, Downing C, Jessup K, Haidar Z, et al. First-trimester screening for early and late preeclampsia using maternal characteristics, biomarkers, and estimated placental volume. *Am J Obstet Gynecol* (2018) 218(1):e1–13. doi:10.1016/j.ajog.2017.10.024
305. Sibai BM, Caritis SN, Thom E, Klebanoff M, McNellis D, Rocco L, et al. Prevention of preeclampsia with low-dose aspirin in healthy, nulliparous pregnant women. The National Institute of Child Health and Human Development Network of Maternal-Fetal Medicine Units. *N Engl J Med* (1993) 329(17):1213–8. doi:10.1056/NEJM199310213291701
306. Bujold E, Roberge S, Lacasse Y, Bureau M, Audibert F, Marcoux S, et al. Prevention of preeclampsia and intrauterine growth restriction with aspirin started in early pregnancy: a meta-analysis. *Obstet Gynecol* (2010) 116(2 Pt 1):402–14. doi:10.1097/AOG.0b013e3181e9322a
307. Roberge S, Giguere Y, Villa P, Nicolaides K, Vainio M, Forest JC, et al. Early administration of low-dose aspirin for the prevention of severe and mild preeclampsia: a systematic review and meta-analysis. *Am J Perinatol* (2012) 29(7):551–6. doi:10.1055/s-0032-1310527
308. Roberge S, Villa P, Nicolaides K, Giguere Y, Vainio M, Bakthi A, et al. Early administration of low-dose aspirin for the prevention of preterm and term preeclampsia: a systematic review and meta-analysis. *Fetal Diagn Ther* (2012) 31(3):141–6. doi:10.1159/000336662
309. Rolnik DL, Wright D, Poon LC, O'Gorman N, Syngelaki A, de Paco Matallana C, et al. Aspirin versus placebo in pregnancies at high risk for preterm pre-eclampsia. *N Engl J Med* (2017) 377(7):613–22. doi:10.1056/NEJMoa1704559
310. Atallah A, Lecarpentier E, Goffinet F, Doret-Dion M, Gaucherand P, Tsatsaris V. Aspirin for prevention of preeclampsia. *Drugs* (2017) 77(17):1819–31. doi:10.1007/s40265-017-0823-0
311. Cadavid AP. Aspirin: the mechanism of action revisited in the context of pregnancy complications. *Front Immunol* (2017) 8:261. doi:10.3389/fimmu.2017.00261
312. Papp C, Szabo G, Toth-Pal E, Papp Z. Fetal growth rate and its variations 1988/89. *Orv Hetil* (1991) 132(34):1865–70.
313. Wyatt SM, Kraus FT, Roh CR, Elchalal U, Nelson DM, Sadovsky Y. The correlation between sampling site and gene expression in the term human placenta. *Placenta* (2005) 26(5):372–9. doi:10.1016/j.placenta.2004.07.003
314. Burton GJ, Sebire NJ, Myatt L, Tannetta D, Wang YL, Sadovsky Y, et al. Optimising sample collection for placental research. *Placenta* (2014) 35(1):9–22. doi:10.1016/j.placenta.2013.11.005
315. Langston C, Kaplan C, Macpherson T, Manci E, Peevy K, Clark B, et al. Practice guideline for examination of the placenta: developed by the Placental Pathology Practice Guideline Development Task Force of the College of American Pathologists. *Arch Pathol Lab Med* (1997) 121(5):449–76.
316. Hargitai B, Marton T, Cox PM. Best practice no 178. Examination of the human placenta. *J Clin Pathol* (2004) 57(8):785–92. doi:10.1136/jcp.2003.014217
317. Redline RW, Boyd T, Campbell V, Hyde S, Kaplan C, Khong TY, et al. Maternal vascular underperfusion: nosology and reproducibility of placental reaction patterns. *Pediatr Dev Pathol* (2004) 7(3):237–49. doi:10.1007/s10024-003-8083-2
318. Tarca AL, Romero R, Draghici S. Analysis of microarray experiments of gene expression profiling. *Am J Obstet Gynecol* (2006) 195(2):373–88. doi:10.1016/j.ajog.2006.07.001

319. Smyth GK. Limma: linear models for microarray data. In: Gentleman R, Carey V, Dudoit S, Irizarry R, Huber W editors. *Bioinformatics and Computational Biology Solutions using R and Bioconductor*. New York: Springer (2005). p. 397–420.
320. Bilban M, Haslinger P, Prast J, Klinglmuller F, Woelfel T, Haider S, et al. Identification of novel trophoblast invasion-related genes: heme oxygenase-1 controls motility via peroxisome proliferator-activated receptor gamma. *Endocrinology* (2009) 150(2):1000–13. doi:10.1210/en.2008-0456
321. Apps R, Sharkey A, Gardner L, Male V, Trotter M, Miller N, et al. Genome-wide expression profile of first trimester villous and extravillous human trophoblast cells. *Placenta* (2011) 32(1):33–43. doi:10.1016/j.placenta.2010.10.010
322. Tilburgs T, Crespo AC, van der Zwan A, Rybalov B, Raj T, Stranger B, et al. Human HLA-G+ extravillous trophoblasts: Immune-activating cells that interact with decidual leukocytes. *Proc Natl Acad Sci U S A* (2015) 112(23):7219–24. doi:10.1073/pnas.1507977112
323. Gautier L, Cope L, Bolstad BM, Irizarry RA. affy – analysis of affymetrix GeneChip data at the probe level. *Bioinformatics* (2004) 20(3):307–15. doi:10.1093/bioinformatics/btg405
324. Ritchie ME, Phipson B, Wu D, Hu Y, Law CW, Shi W, et al. limma powers differential expression analyses for RNA-sequencing and microarray studies. *Nucleic Acids Res* (2015) 43(7):e47. doi:10.1093/nar/gkv007
325. Carlson S, Falcon S, Pages H, Li N. *hgfocus.db: Affymetrix Human Genome Focus Array annotation data (chip hgfocus). R package version 2.2.11.* (2005).
326. Carlson S, Falcon S, Pages H, Li N. *hgu133a.db: Affymetrix Human Genome U133 Set annotation data (chip hgu133a). R package version 2.2.11.* (2005).
327. Carlson S, Falcon S, Pages H, Li N. *org.Hs.eg.db: Genome wide annotation for Human. R package version 2.2.11.* (2005).
328. Krzywinski M, Schein J, Birol I, Connors J, Gascoyne R, Horsman D, et al. Circos: an information aesthetic for comparative genomics. *Genome Res* (2009) 19(9):1639–45. doi:10.1101/gr.092759.109
329. Zhang B, Horvath S. A general framework for weighted gene co-expression network analysis. *Stat Appl Genet Mol Biol* (2005) 4:Article17. doi:10.2202/1544-6115.1128
330. Langfelder P, Horvath S. WGCNA: an R package for weighted correlation network analysis. *BMC Bioinformatics* (2008) 9:559. doi:10.1186/1471-2105-9-559
331. Ravasz E, Somera AL, Mongru DA, Oltvai ZN, Barabasi AL. Hierarchical organization of modularity in metabolic networks. *Science* (2002) 297(5586):1551–5. doi:10.1126/science.1073374
332. Langfelder P, Zhang B, Horvath S. Defining clusters from a hierarchical cluster tree: the dynamic tree cut package for R. *Bioinformatics* (2008) 24(5):719–20. doi:10.1093/bioinformatics/btm563
333. Alexander GR, Himes JH, Kaufman RB, Mor J, Kogan M. A United States national reference for fetal growth. *Obstet Gynecol* (1996) 87(2):163–8. doi:10.1016/0029-7844(95)00386-X
334. Than NG, Kim SS, Abbas A, Han YM, Hotra J, Tarca AL, et al. Chorioamnionitis and increased galectin-1 expression in PPROM – an anti-inflammatory response in the fetal membranes? *Am J Reprod Immunol* (2008) 60(4):298–311. doi:10.1111/j.1600-0897.2008.00624.x
335. Mayhew TM. Taking tissue samples from the placenta: an illustration of principles and strategies. *Placenta* (2008) 29(1):1–14. doi:10.1016/j.placenta.2007.05.010
336. Redline RW, Heller D, Keating S, Kingdom J. Placental diagnostic criteria and clinical correlation – a workshop report. *Placenta* (2005) 26(Suppl A):S114–7. doi:10.1016/j.placenta.2005.02.009
337. Richani K, Romero R, Kim YM, Cushenberry E, Soto E, Han YM, et al. Tissue microarray: an effective high-throughput method to study the placenta for clinical and research purposes. *J Matern Fetal Neonatal Med* (2006) 19(8):509–15. doi:10.1080/14767050600852718
338. Brown MA, Lindheimer MD, de Swiet M, van Assche A, Moutquin JM. The classification and diagnosis of the hypertensive disorders of pregnancy: statement from the International Society for the Study of Hypertension in Pregnancy (ISSHP). *Hypertens Pregnancy* (2001) 20(1):IX–XIV. doi:10.1081/PRG-100104165
339. Santos-Gonzalez M, Gomez DC, Navas P, Villalba JM. Modifications of plasma proteome in long-lived rats fed on a coenzyme Q10-supplemented diet. *Exp Gerontol* (2007) 42(8):798–806. doi:10.1016/j.exger.2007.04.013
340. Marouga R, David S, Hawkins E. The development of the DIGE system: 2D fluorescence difference gel analysis technology. *Anal Bioanal Chem* (2005) 382(3):669–78. doi:10.1007/s00216-005-3126-3
341. Reiter L, Rinner O, Picotti P, Huttenhain R, Beck M, Brusniak MY, et al. mProphet: automated data processing and statistical validation for large-scale SRM experiments. *Nat Methods* (2011) 8(5):430–5. doi:10.1038/nmeth.1584
342. Pattillo RA, Gey GO, Delfs E, Mattingly RF. Human hormone production in vitro. *Science* (1968) 159(3822):1467–9. doi:10.1126/science.159.3822.1467
343. Kliman HJ, Nestler JE, Sermasi E, Sanger JM, Strauss JF III. Purification, characterization, and in vitro differentiation of cytotrophoblasts from human term placentae. *Endocrinology* (1986) 118(4):1567–82. doi:10.1210/endo-118-4-1567
344. Mohyeldin A, Garzon-Muvdi T, Quinones-Hinojosa A. Oxygen in stem cell biology: a critical component of the stem cell niche. *Cell Stem Cell* (2010) 7(2):150–61. doi:10.1016/j.stem.2010.07.007
345. Fu J, Lv X, Lin H, Wu L, Wang R, Zhou Z, et al. Ubiquitin ligase cullin 7 induces epithelial-mesenchymal transition in human choriocarcinoma cells. *J Biol Chem* (2010) 285(14):10870–9. doi:10.1074/jbc.M109.004200
346. Gentleman RC, Carey VJ, Bates DM, Bolstad B, Dettling M, Dudoit S, et al. Bioconductor: open software development for computational biology and bioinformatics. *Genome Biol* (2004) 5(10):R80. doi:10.1186/gb-2004-5-10-r80

Permissions

All chapters in this book were first published by Frontiers; hereby published with permission under the Creative Commons Attribution License or equivalent. Every chapter published in this book has been scrutinized by our experts. Their significance has been extensively debated. The topics covered herein carry significant findings which will fuel the growth of the discipline. They may even be implemented as practical applications or may be referred to as a beginning point for another development.

The contributors of this book come from diverse backgrounds, making this book a truly international effort. This book will bring forth new frontiers with its revolutionizing research information and detailed analysis of the nascent developments around the world.

We would like to thank all the contributing authors for lending their expertise to make the book truly unique. They have played a crucial role in the development of this book. Without their invaluable contributions this book wouldn't have been possible. They have made vital efforts to compile up to date information on the varied aspects of this subject to make this book a valuable addition to the collection of many professionals and students.

This book was conceptualized with the vision of imparting up-to-date information and advanced data in this field. To ensure the same, a matchless editorial board was set up. Every individual on the board went through rigorous rounds of assessment to prove their worth. After which they invested a large part of their time researching and compiling the most relevant data for our readers.

The editorial board has been involved in producing this book since its inception. They have spent rigorous hours researching and exploring the diverse topics which have resulted in the successful publishing of this book. They have passed on their knowledge of decades through this book. To expedite this challenging task, the publisher supported the team at every step. A small team of assistant editors was also appointed to further simplify the editing procedure and attain best results for the readers.

Apart from the editorial board, the designing team has also invested a significant amount of their time in understanding the subject and creating the most relevant covers. They scrutinized every image to scout for the most suitable representation of the subject and create an appropriate cover for the book.

The publishing team has been an ardent support to the editorial, designing and production team. Their endless efforts to recruit the best for this project, has resulted in the accomplishment of this book. They are a veteran in the field of academics and their pool of knowledge is as vast as their experience in printing. Their expertise and guidance has proved useful at every step. Their uncompromising quality standards have made this book an exceptional effort. Their encouragement from time to time has been an inspiration for everyone.

The publisher and the editorial board hope that this book will prove to be a valuable piece of knowledge for researchers, students, practitioners and scholars across the globe.

List of Contributors

Daiane Cristine Martins Ronchi, Mineia Alessandra Scaranello Malaquias, Patrícia Zadorosnei Rebutini, Letícia Arianne Panini do Carmo, Plínio Cézar Neto, Emily Scaranello Marini, Amanda Prokopenko, Seigo Nagashima and Lúcia de Noronha
Laboratory of Experimental Pathology, Postgraduate Program of Health Sciences, School of Medicine, Pontifícia Universidade Católica do Paraná, Curitiba, Brazil

Camila Zanluca and Claudia Nunes Duarte dos Santos
Molecular Virology Laboratory, Instituto Carlos Chagas, Fundação Oswaldo Cruz, Curitiba, Brazil

Nele Twisselmann, Annika Hartz and Christoph Härtel
Department of Pediatrics, University of Lübeck and University Medical Center Schleswig-Holstein, Lübeck, Germany

Yannic C. Bartsch
Laboratories of Immunology and Antibody Glycan Analysis, Institute for Nutrition Medicine, University of Lübeck and University Medical Center Schleswig-Holstein, Lübeck, Germany

Julia Pagel
Department of Pediatrics, University of Lübeck and University Medical Center Schleswig-Holstein, Lübeck, Germany
Department of Infectious Diseases and Microbiology, University of Lübeck and University Medical Center Schleswig-Holstein, Lübeck, Germany

Christian Wieg
Department of Neonatology, Hospital Aschaffenburg-Alzenau, Aschaffenburg, Germany

Marc Ehlers
Laboratories of Immunology and Antibody Glycan Analysis, Institute for Nutrition Medicine, University of Lübeck and University Medical Center Schleswig-Holstein, Lübeck, Germany
Airway Research Center North (ARCN), German Center for Lung Research (DZL), University of Lübeck, Lübeck, Germany

Bruno Vinicius Santos Valiate
Department of Biochemistry and Immunology, Institute of Biological Sciences, Universidade Federal de Minas Gerais, Belo Horizonte, Brazil
Center for Drug Research and Development of Pharmaceuticals, Institute of Biological Sciences, Universidade Federal de Minas Gerais, Belo Horizonte, Brazil

Fernanda Martins Marim and Mauro Martins Teixeira
Department of Biochemistry and Immunology, Institute of Biological Sciences, Universidade Federal de Minas Gerais, Belo Horizonte, Brazil
Research Group in Arboviral Diseases, Institute of Biological Sciences, Universidade Federal de Minas Gerais, Belo Horizonte, Brazil
Center for Drug Research and Development of Pharmaceuticals, Institute of Biological Sciences, Universidade Federal de Minas Gerais, Belo Horizonte, Brazil

Danielle Cunha Teixeira
Research Group in Arboviral Diseases, Institute of Biological Sciences, Universidade Federal de Minas Gerais, Belo Horizonte, Brazil
Center for Drug Research and Development of Pharmaceuticals, Institute of Biological Sciences, Universidade Federal de Minas Gerais, Belo Horizonte, Brazil

Celso Martins Queiroz-Junior and Vivian Vasconcelos Costa
Research Group in Arboviral Diseases, Institute of Biological Sciences, Universidade Federal de Minas Gerais, Belo Horizonte, Brazil
Center for Drug Research and Development of Pharmaceuticals, Institute of Biological Sciences, Universidade Federal de Minas Gerais, Belo Horizonte, Brazil
Departament of Morphology, Institute of Biological Sciences, Universidade Federal de Minas Gerais, Belo Horizonte, Brazil

Jose Carlos Alves-Filho and Thiago Mattar Cunha
Center for Research in Inflammatory Diseases (CRID), Department of Pharmacology, Ribeirao Preto Medical School, Universidade de São Paulo, Ribeirão Preto, Brazil

Robert Dantzer
Department of Symptom Research, The University of Texas MD Anderson Cancer Center, Houston, TX, United States

Antonio Lucio Teixeira
Department of Psychiatry and Behavioral Sciences, McGovern Medical Houston, The University of Texas Health Science Center at Houston, Houston, TX, United States

Hidetoshi Mezawa
Department of Pediatrics, The Jikei University School of Medicine, Tokyo, Japan

Mai Okuyama and Mitsuyoshi Urashima
Division of Molecular Epidemiology, The Jikei University School of Medicine, Tokyo, Japan
Department of Pediatrics, The Jikei University School of Medicine, Tokyo, Japan

Toshinao Kawai
Division of Immunology, National Center for Child Health and Development, Tokyo, Japan

Arianna S. Moss and Jean K. Lim
Department of Microbiology, Icahn School of Medicine at Mount Sinai, New York, NY, United States

Joshua A. Acklin and Julia A. Brown
Department of Microbiology, Icahn School of Medicine at Mount Sinai, New York, NY, United States
Graduate School of Biomedical Sciences, Icahn School of Medicine at Mount Sinai, New York, NY, United States

Javier D. Cattle
Department of Epidemiology, Mailman School of Public Health, Columbia University, New York, NY, United States

Gregory A. Foster, David Krysztof and Susan L. Stramer
Scientific Affairs, American Red Cross, Gaithersburg, MD, United States

Sarah A. Robertson, Ella S. Green, Alison S. Care, Lachlan M. Moldenhauer, Simon C. Barry and Gustaaf Dekker
Robinson Research Institute and Adelaide Medical School, University of Adelaide, Adelaide, SA, Australia

Jelmer R. Prins
University Medical Center Groningen, Groningen, Netherlands

M. Louise Hull
Women's and Children's Hospital, Adelaide, SA, Australia

Laura Sánchez García and Adelina Pellicer
Neonatology Department, Biomedical Research Foundation-IDIPAZ, La Paz University Hospital, Madrid, Spain

Natalia Gómez-Torres, Irma Castro, Claudio Alba and Juan Miguel Rodríguez Gómez
Nutrition and Food Science Department, Complutense University, Madrid, Spain

Fernando Cabañas
Neonatology Department, Quironsalud Madrid University Hospital and Quironsalud San José Hospital, Biomedical Research Foundation-IDIPAZ, La Paz University Hospital, Madrid, Spain

Raquel González-Sánchez and Manuela López-Azorín
Neonatology Department, Quironsalud Madrid University Hospital and Quironsalud San José Hospital, Madrid, Spain

M. Teresa Moral-Pumarega and Diana Escuder-Vieco
Neonatology Department, 12 Octubre University Hospital, Madrid, Spain

Esther Cabañes-Alonso
Neonatology Department and Regional Human Milk Bank, 12 Octubre University Hospital, Madrid, Spain

Sayaka Tsuda, Akitoshi Nakashima, Tomoko Shima and Shigeru Saito
Department of Obstetrics and Gynecology, University of Toyama, Toyama, Japan

Zachary W. Berkebile, Dira S. Putri, Mark R. Schleiss and Craig J. Bierle
Department of Pediatrics, Division of Pediatric Infectious Diseases, University of Minnesota, Minneapolis, MN, United States

Juan E. Abrahante
Informatics Institute, University of Minnesota, Minneapolis, MN, United States

Davis M. Seelig
Department of Veterinary Clinical Sciences, University of Minnesota, Minneapolis, MN, United States

Natascha Köstlin-Gille, Stefanie Dietz, Julian Schwarz, Bärbel Spring, Christian F. Poets and Christian Gille
Department of Neonatology, Tuebingen University Children's Hospital, Tuebingen, Germany

Jan Pauluschke-Fröhlich
Department of Obstetrics and Gynecology, Tuebingen, Germany

Cherley Borba Vieira Andrade, Victoria Regina de Siqueira Monteiro, Hanailly Ribeiro Gomes, Ronny Paiva Campos Sousa, Veronica Muller de Oliveira Nascimento, Flavia Fonseca Bloise and Tania Maria Ortiga-Carvalho
Institute of Biophysics Carlos Chagas Filho, Federal University of Rio de Janeiro, Rio de Janeiro, Brazil

Sharton Vinicius Antunes Coelho and Luciana Barros Arruda
Institute of Microbiology Paulo de Góes, Federal University of Rio de Janeiro, Rio de Janeiro, Brazil

Stephen Giles Matthews
Department of Physiology, Faculty of Medicine, University of Toronto, Toronto, ON, Canada
Department of Obstetrics & Gynecology, Faculty of Medicine, University of Toronto, Toronto, ON, Canada
Department of Medicine, Faculty of Medicine, University of Toronto, Toronto, ON, Canada
Lunenfeld-Tanenbaum Research Institute, Mount Sinai Hospital, Toronto, ON, Canada

Enrrico Bloise
Department of Morphology, Federal University of Minas Gerais, Belo Horizonte, Brazil

Anita van der Zwan, Ellen M. W. van der Meer-Prins, Paula P. M. C. van Miert, Heleen van den Heuvel, Jacqueline D. H. Anholts, Dave L. Roelen, Frans H. J. Claas and Sebastiaan Heidt
Department of Immunohematology and Blood Transfusion, Leiden University Medical Center, Leiden, Netherlands

Sayaka Tsuda, Xiaoxin Zhang, Tomoko Shima, Akemi Ushijima, Kei Tsuda and Shigeru Saito
Department of Obstetrics and Gynecology, University of Toyama, Toyama, Japan

Hiroshi Hamana
Department of Innovative Cancer Immunotherapy, Graduate School of Medicine and Pharmaceutical Sciences (Medicine), University of Toyama, Toyama, Japan

Atsushi Muraguchi and Hiroyuki Kishi
Department of Immunology, Graduate School of Medicine and Pharmaceutical Sciences (Medicine), University of Toyama, Toyama, Japan

Paola Vacca and Lorenzo Moretta
Department of Immunology, IRCCS Bambino Gesù Children's Hospital, Rome, Italy

Chiara Vitale
Department of Experimental Medicine (DIMES), University of Genoa, Genoa, Italy
UOC Immunology, IRCCS Ospedale Policlinico San Martino Genova, Genoa, Italy

Enrico Munari
Department of Pathology, Sacro Cuore Don Calabria Hospital, Negrar, Italy
Department of Pathology AOUI, University of Verona, Verona, Italy

Marco Antonio Cassatella
Department of Medicine, Section of General Pathology, University of Verona, Verona, Italy

Maria Cristina Mingari
Department of Experimental Medicine (DIMES), University of Genoa, Genoa, Italy
UOC Immunology, IRCCS Ospedale Policlinico San Martino Genova, Genoa, Italy
Center of Excellence for Biomedical Research (CEBR), University of Genoa, Genoa, Italy

Nishel M. Shah and Mark R. Johnson
Department of Surgery and Cancer, Imperial College London, Chelsea and Westminster Hospital, London, United Kingdom

Nesrina Imami
Department of Medicine, Imperial College London, Chelsea and Westminster Hospital, London, United Kingdom

Stefanie Ehrentraut, Karoline Sauss, Stefanie Langwisch, Ana Claudia Zenclussen and Anne Schumacher
Health Campus Immunology, Infectiology and Inflammation (GC-I3), Experimental Obstetrics and Gynecology, Medical Faculty, Otto-von-Guericke University, Magdeburg, Germany

Lydia Luley and Franziska Fettke
Health Campus Immunology, Infectiology and Inflammation (GC-I3), Experimental Obstetrics and Gynecology, Medical Faculty, Otto-von-Guericke University, Magdeburg, Germany
University Women's Clinic, Otto-von-Guericke University, Magdeburg, Germany

Romy Neumeister
Gynecologic Ambulance, Haldensleben, Germany

Anika Oettel and Serban-Dan Costa
University Women's Clinic, Otto-von-Guericke University, Magdeburg, Germany

Yi Xu, Gaurav Bhatti, Vanessa Topping, Haidy El-Azzamy, Christopher LaJeunesse and Zhong Dong
Perinatology Research Branch, Eunice Kennedy Shriver National Institute of Child Health and Human Development, National Institutes of Health, United States Department of Health and Human Services, Bethesda, MD, United States
Perinatology Research Branch, Eunice Kennedy Shriver National Institute of Child Health and Human Development, National Institutes of Health, United States Department of Health and Human Services, Detroit, MI, United States

Tinnakorn Chaiworapongsa
Perinatology Research Branch, Eunice Kennedy Shriver National Institute of Child Health and Human Development, National Institutes of Health, United States Department of Health and Human Services, Bethesda, MD, United States
Perinatology Research Branch, Eunice Kennedy Shriver National Institute of Child Health and Human Development, National Institutes of Health, United States Department of Health and Human Services, Detroit, MI, United States
Department of Obstetrics and Gynecology, Wayne State University School of Medicine, Detroit, MI, United States

Andrea Balogh and Gabor Szalai
Perinatology Research Branch, Eunice Kennedy Shriver National Institute of Child Health and Human Development, National Institutes of Health, United States Department of Health and Human Services, Bethesda, MD, United States
Perinatology Research Branch, Eunice Kennedy Shriver National Institute of Child Health and Human Development, National Institutes of Health, United States Department of Health and Human Services, Detroit, MI, United States
Systems Biology of Reproduction Lendulet Research Group, Institute of Enzymology, Research Centre for Natural Sciences, Hungarian Academy of Sciences, Budapest, Hungary

Nandor Gabor Than
Perinatology Research Branch, Eunice Kennedy Shriver National Institute of Child Health and Human Development, National Institutes of Health, United States Department of Health and Human Services, Bethesda, MD, United States
Perinatology Research Branch, Eunice Kennedy Shriver National Institute of Child Health and Human Development, National Institutes of Health, United States Department of Health and Human Services, Detroit, MI, United States
Department of Obstetrics and Gynecology, Wayne State University School of Medicine, Detroit, MI, United States
Systems Biology of Reproduction Lendulet Research Group, Institute of Enzymology, Research Centre for Natural Sciences, Hungarian Academy of Sciences, Budapest, Hungary
Maternity Private Department, Kutvolgyi Clinical Block, Semmelweis University, Budapest, Hungary
First Department of Pathology and Experimental Cancer Research, Semmelweis University, Budapest, Hungary

Kata Juhasz, Zsolt Gelencser, Janos Palhalmi, Amanda Demeter and Anett Szecsi
Systems Biology of Reproduction Lendulet Research Group, Institute of Enzymology, Research Centre for Natural Sciences, Hungarian Academy of Sciences, Budapest, Hungary

Zoltan Papp
Maternity Private Department, Kutvolgyi Clinical Block, Semmelweis University, Budapest, Hungary

Ilona Kovalszky
First Department of Pathology and Experimental Cancer Research, Semmelweis University, Budapest, Hungary

Roberto Romero
Perinatology Research Branch, Eunice Kennedy Shriver National Institute of Child Health and Human Development, National Institutes of Health, United States Department of Health and Human Services, Bethesda, MD, United States
Perinatology Research Branch, Eunice Kennedy Shriver National Institute of Child Health and Human Development, National Institutes of Health, United States Department of Health and Human Services, Detroit, MI, United States
Department of Obstetrics and Gynecology, University of Michigan, Ann Arbor, MI, United States
Department of Epidemiology and Biostatistics, Michigan State University, East Lansing, MI, United States
Center for Molecular Medicine and Genetics, Wayne State University, Detroit, MI, United States

Susan Land
Center for Molecular Medicine and Genetics, Wayne State University, Detroit, MI, United States

Adi Laurentiu Tarca
Perinatology Research Branch, Eunice Kennedy Shriver National Institute of Child Health and Human Development, National Institutes of Health, United States Department of Health and Human Services, Bethesda, MD, United States
Perinatology Research Branch, Eunice Kennedy Shriver National Institute of Child Health and Human Development, National Institutes of Health, United States Department of Health and Human Services, Detroit, MI, United States
Department of Obstetrics and Gynecology, Wayne State University School of Medicine, Detroit, MI, United States
Department of Computer Science, College of Engineering, Wayne State University, Detroit, MI, United States

Katalin Adrienna Kekesi, Balazs Andras Gyorffy, Attila Simor and Gabor Juhasz
Laboratory of Proteomics, Department of Physiology and Neurobiology, ELTE Eotvos Lorand University, Budapest, Hungary

Zhonghui Xu
Perinatology Research Branch, Eunice Kennedy Shriver National Institute of Child Health and Human Development, National Institutes of Health, United States Department of Health and Human Services, Bethesda, MD, United States
Perinatology Research Branch, Eunice Kennedy Shriver National Institute of Child Health and Human Development, National Institutes of Health, United States Department of Health and Human Services, Detroit, MI, United States
Channing Division of Network Medicine, Brigham and Women's Hospital, Harvard University, Boston, MA, United States

Ron Joshua Leavitt, Tzu Hung Chung and Manuel Krispin
Zymo Research Corporation, Irvine, CA, United States

Laszlo Orosz and Olga Torok
Department of Obstetrics and Gynaecology, University of Debrecen, Debrecen, Hungary

Eva Hunyadi-Gulyas and Zsuzsanna Darula
Institute of Biochemistry, Biological Research Centre, Hungarian Academy of Sciences, Szeged, Hungary

Katalin Eder and Andras Falus
Department of Genetics, Cell and Immunobiology, Semmelweis University, Budapest, Hungary

Szilvia Szabo
Systems Biology of Reproduction Lendulet Research Group, Institute of Enzymology, Research Centre for Natural Sciences, Hungarian Academy of Sciences, Budapest, Hungary
Department of Morphology and Physiology, Semmelweis University, Budapest, Hungary

Hamutal Meiri
TeleMarpe Ltd, Tel Aviv, Israel

Sorin Draghici
Center for Molecular Medicine and Genetics, Wayne State University, Detroit, MI, United States
Department of Clinical and Translational Science, Wayne State University, Detroit, MI, United States

Martin Knöfler
Department of Obstetrics and Gynecology, Medical University of Vienna, Vienna, Austria

Sonia S. Hassan
Perinatology Research Branch, Eunice Kennedy Shriver National Institute of Child Health and Human Development, National Institutes of Health, United States Department of Health and Human Services, Bethesda, MD, United States
Perinatology Research Branch, Eunice Kennedy Shriver National Institute of Child Health and Human Development, National Institutes of Health, United States Department of Health and Human Services, Detroit, MI, United States
Department of Obstetrics and Gynecology, Wayne State University School of Medicine, Detroit, MI, United States
Department of Physiology, Wayne State University School of Medicine, Detroit, MI, United States

Offer Erez
Perinatology Research Branch, Eunice Kennedy Shriver National Institute of Child Health and Human Development, National Institutes of Health, United States Department of Health and Human Services, Bethesda, MD, United States
Perinatology Research Branch, Eunice Kennedy Shriver National Institute of Child Health and Human Development, National Institutes of Health, United States Department of Health and Human Services, Detroit, MI, United States
Department of Obstetrics and Gynecology, Wayne State University School of Medicine, Detroit, MI, United States
Department of Obstetrics and Gynecology, Soroka University Medical Center School of Medicine, Faculty of Health Sciences, Ben-Gurion University of the Negev, Beer Sheva, Israel

Chong Jai Kim
Perinatology Research Branch, Eunice Kennedy Shriver National Institute of Child Health and Human Development, National Institutes of Health, United States Department of Health and Human Services, Bethesda, MD, United States
Perinatology Research Branch, Eunice Kennedy Shriver National Institute of Child Health and Human Development, National Institutes of Health, United States Department of Health and Human Services, Detroit, MI, United States
Department of Pathology, Wayne State University School of Medicine, Detroit, MI, United States
Department of Pathology, Asan Medical Center, University of Ulsan, Seoul, South Korea

Graham J. Burton
Centre for Trophoblast Research, Department of Physiology, Development and Neuroscience, University of Cambridge, Cambridge, United Kingdom

Ishan Paranjpe
Institute for Computational Health Sciences, University of California San Francisco, San Francisco, CA, United States

Index

www.ingramcontent.com/pod-product-compliance
Lightning Source LLC
LaVergne TN
LVHW082137200926
848484LV00008B/2066

* 9 7 9 8 8 8 7 4 0 3 7 9 3 *